# Assessing Older Persons

# ASSESSING OLDER PERSONS

## Measures, Meaning, and Practical Applications

*Edited by*

ROBERT L. KANE

ROSALIE A. KANE

*With the assistance of Marilyn Eells*

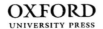

OXFORD
UNIVERSITY PRESS

# OXFORD
UNIVERSITY PRESS

Oxford   New York
Auckland   Bangkok   Buenos Aires   Cape Town   Chennai
Dar es Salaam   Delhi   Hong Kong   Istanbul   Karachi   Kolkata
Kuala Lumpur   Madrid   Melbourne   Mexico City   Mumbai   Nairobi
São Paulo   Shanghai   Taipei   Tokyo   Toronto

Copyright © 2000 by Oxford University Press, Inc.

First published in 2000 by Oxford University Press, Inc.
198 Madison Avenue, New York, New York, 10016
www.oup.com

First issued as an Oxford University Press paperback in 2004.
Oxford is a registered trademark of Oxford University Press.

Library of Congress Cataloging-in-Publication Data
Assessing older persons :
measures, meaning, and practical applications /
edited by Robert L. Kane, Rosalie A. Kane with the assistance of Marilyn Eells.
p. cm.
ISBN 978-0-19-517435-9 (pbk.)
1. Aged—United States—Social conditions.
2. Aged—Services for—United States.
I. Kane, Robert L., 1940–
II. Kane, Rosalie A.
HQ1061.A74 2000   305.26'0973—dc21   99-050148

3 5 7 9 8 6 4

Printed in the United States of America
on acid-free paper

# Preface

In 1981, we wrote a book called *Assessing the Elderly: A Practical Guide to Measurement.* Looking back at that book, we think it did three things. First, it compiled existing measures in a variety of areas: physical functioning, cognitive functioning, affective functioning, social functioning, and multidimensional measures. Second, it endorsed and gave supporting arguments for using systematic approaches and tools for assessing the well-being of older people. Third, it offered a cautionary tale, full of caveats, warnings, and recommendations about making assessments and interpreting the results. The 1981 book was in itself something of a by-product. At that time, we were designing a tool for a multidimensional assessment of resident outcomes of nursing home care and found that we needed to wade through voluminous but not easily accessible materials to examine what was out there. Having been forced to review the instruments and develop criteria against which to evaluate them, we had the rudiments of a book on hand.

The development of assessment tools and the growth of applications in the two decades since that book was written speaks volumes about how gerontology and geriatrics have matured. Given the enormous proliferation of measures in the last 20 years, the book long ago lost any claim to comprehensive inclusiveness, though many of the measures highlighted there are still in use, and the selection criteria, cautions, and caveats still apply.

This book is a sequel to rather than a new edition of our 1981 effort. It looks again at assessment in the content areas we dealt with two decades ago (function, health, emotion, cognition, and social well-being) and also treats entirely new content areas of assessment that were untouched in the previous book (such as family caregivers, physical environments, preferences, spirituality, and satisfaction). It also looks critically at various applications of assessment tools, singly or in comprehensive batteries, to guiding programs that serve older people.

Working on this volume as we approached the millennium, we had our own particular Y2K problem. The assessment terrain has expanded exponentially. Working by ourselves, it would not have been feasible for us to review the available materials. We lacked both the time and in some areas the specialized expertise. Instead, this book is a true team product that resulted from more than a year's work of a multidisciplinary seminar group at the University of Minnesota. Meeting weekly, this group functioned somewhat as an interdisciplinary assessment team is expected to function: We assessed the state of assessment tools and determined the content areas where summaries were needed; we developed criteria for examining each content area; and we reviewed one another's outlines and successive manuscript drafts. Each contributed chapter is the work of its author, but each is also part of what is intended to be a coherent approach to examining the assessment technology for older people. We hope we have avoided the curse of the edited book — lack of consistency and continuity. Decisions about which chapter should include particular content were sometimes arbitrary, but we have tried to provide ample cross-referencing.

The book is divided into two sections. The first addresses measures that comprise the set of tools needed to assess older persons. Most of these measures can be considered generic, but some are condition specific. The second section examines several of the applications for such measures.

Part I examines the major domains for assessing older people. We begin with physical function and physiological measures. The latter have been broadened to include a number of syndromes that commonly present problems for older persons. We then systematically move through cognition, affect, social functioning, quality of life, values and preferences, satisfaction, and spirituality. We have also included one chapter on assessment of family caregivers, many of whom are old themselves, and another on environment.

Part II looks at some of the common applications of assessment tools. These include comprehensive geriatric assessment, care coordination, and case management. We have also included a chapter on mandated assessment, focusing primarily on measures dealing with nursing homes, but also on those being advocated for other long-term care venues as well. Part II also contains a chapter on the special challenges of assessing persons who have substantial cognitive impairments. The concluding chapter outlines some of the challenges that still face those who seek to develop and implement better assessment.

A project of this magnitude leaves us in debt to those who helped us. Over the years, we have benefited from the generosity of gerontology scholars who have sent us their instruments for possible inclusion in any new work on assessment. We accelerated those efforts with general appeals in the last few years and are grateful for the response. We are extremely appreciative, too, of the patience and energy of the contributors to this volume, all of whom participated in the dialogue of the seminar and made the resulting book much richer than we could have done alone. Finally, executive secretary Marilyn Eells is the true heroine of this endeavor. She typed and retyped the manuscript with its many tables and references and even read and edited the content. Having spent so many hours on this project, she recently observed that there certainly are a lot of assessment tools out there, that it must be difficult for people to know about them, and even more difficult to decide which ones to use. If this book helps address her observation, we will have achieved our goal.

*Minneapolis, Minn.*　　　　　　　　　　　　　　　　　　　　　　　R. L. K.
　　　　　　　　　　　　　　　　　　　　　　　　　　　　　　　R. A. K.

# Contents

## PART II   APPLICATIONS OF ASSESSMENT

## PART III   CONCLUSION

# Contributors

LOIS J. CUTLER, PH.D., was a National Institute on Aging postdoctoral fellow and is now Research Associate at the University of Minnesota, where she works on determining the relationship between the physical environment and the quality of life of residents in assisted living facilities and nursing homes through the use of environmental assessment tools and post-occupancy evaluations.

MARILYN EELLS, C.P.S., is the Executive Secretary for Robert Kane in the Division of Health Services Research and Policy at the University of Minnesota School of Public Health. Her experience includes review and editing of numerous journal articles and book chapters in her work with Dr. Kane.

JENNIFER FRYTAK is a graduate student of Health Services Research and Policy. She is writing a dissertation on the relationship between health and aging in older persons.

PATRICIA FINCH-GUTHRIE, M.S., R.N., PH.D., practiced nursing for 21 years in acute care settings before becoming a doctoral candidate at the University of Minnesota School of Nursing. Her research interests focus on the prevention and management of care for hospitalized elderly patients who develop acute confusion. She is now a Professional Practice Specialist at North Memorial Health Center.

JOSEPH GAUGLER, PH.D., was National Institute on Aging Postdoctoral Fellow at the University of Minnesota, where he continued the work begun with his dissertation on elements of caregiving for older persons in need of long-term care. He is now an assistant professor at the University of Kentucky.

JEFFREY D. GRANN is a doctoral student in Educational Psychology at the University of Minnesota. His participation in the National Institute on Aging Pre-Doctoral Fellowship is contributing to his research into aspects of the aging process characterized by continued growth and resistance to decline.

GILLIAN HARPER, PH.D., was a postdoctoral student at the University of Minnesota where her work centered on physiological manifestations of stress in older people. She is now working on a project to test the use of physiological measures in assessing the quality of life for persons suffering from dementia. She is currently an assistant professor at the Ohio University College of Osteopathic Medicine.

ROBERT L. KANE, M.D., is a professor in the Division of Health Services Research and Policy at the University of Minnesota School of Public Health, where he holds an endowed chair in Long-term Care and Aging. He serves as the Director of the University's Center on Aging and the Clinical Outcomes Research Center. He is also the director of the University of Minnesota training program in aging, sponsored by the National Institute on Aging. His research includes work on various aspects of the health care of older people.

ROSALIE A. KANE, PH.D., is a professor in the Division of Health Services Research and Policy at the University of Minnesota School of Public Health, where she directs the National Long-term Care Resource Center. Her work has combined interests in long-term care and ethics. A pioneer in describing the emergence of assisted living as a major long-term care modality, she is now directing a major study to develop measures of quality of life for nursing home residents.

LINDA LANGLEY, PH.D., is a postdoctoral student at Duke University, where she is studying cognitive performance in older people.

JOAN LANGLOIS is working toward a Ph.D. in Social Administrative Pharmacy at the University of Minnesota.

CARRIE LEVIN is a graduate student in Health Services Research and Policy. She is working on a dissertation that examines the relationship between the preferences of older people and the preferences of other family members.

DOUGLAS OLSON is an assistant professor at the University of Wisconsin, Eau Claire. He is working toward a Ph.D. in Health Services Research and Policy at the University of Minnesota. His dissertation focuses on the relationship between leadership characteristics of long-term care institutions and quality of care.

VALINDA I. PEARSON, R.N., PH.D., was a doctoral candidate in the University of Minnesota School of Nursing, where she studied nursing interventions with older adults and their families, and stroke rehabilitation. She has worked extensively in the area of geriatric and adult rehabilitation and in acute, long-term care and community environments that provide rehabilitation and nursing services to older adults. She holds national certification as a Certified Rehabilitation Registered Nurse (CRRN). She is now an assistant professor at the College of St. Catherine.

MAUREEN A. SMITH, M.D., M.P.H., PH.D., studies the impact of managed care and other cost-containment measures on the quality of medical care and health outcomes for vulnerable populations. Dr. Smith received her M.D. and M.P.H. degrees from Yale University School of Medicine and her Ph.D. from the University of Minnesota in Health Services Research, Policy and Administration. She is an assistant professor at the University of Wisconsin. Specific interests include the relationship between health outcomes and other methods of quality measurement, the development of measurement tools to assess quality from the perspectives of the patient and provider, and the role of quality assessment in continuous quality improvement.

CRISTINA F. URDANGARIN, M.D., M.P.H., is a doctoral candidate in the Division of Epidemiology at the University of Minnesota and a National Institute on Aging trainee. She serves as a research assistant of the Minnesota GEM Study, a four-year randomized controlled trial of Outpatient Geriatric Evaluation and Management.

# 1

# Choosing and Using an Assessment Tool

ROBERT L. KANE

Assessment has become a central technology in the care of older persons. In the context of Rosemary Stevens' analysis of medical specialties, it is this technology that gives geriatrics a claim to specialty status (Stevens, 1971). At the same time, assessment is far from the exclusive purview of physicians or nurses who work with older persons. It is safe to argue that, at any age and in a variety of contexts (medical and social services), systematic assessment is preferred over haphazard practice. Despite the banality of such a simple statement, traditional care is not systematic. For many cases the lack of a systematic approach may not be critical (although few would rise to defend it), but in the care of and delivery of service to older persons, where presenting problems are often complex and multidimensional, systematic approaches are not merely preferable, they are necessary. For these reasons, systematic assessment has become an important part of geriatric and gerontological practice.

Assessment of older persons is more complicated than that of younger persons because there is often more to assess. Whereas the medical problems of younger persons are likely to be confined to a single organ system, older people typically have several simultaneous chronic problems. Moreover, these problems can be exacerbated by difficulties in other spheres, such as psychological and social.*

The growing body of knowledge demonstrates what should be intuitively clear, namely, the greater effectiveness of systematic assessments over routine care (see Chapter 13). The positive results of systematic assessment programs created a groundswell of enthusiasm for assessing older people in both the clinical and social service contexts. A major vehicle for such assessments has been case management. The underlying premise of case management is that persons with complex care needs will benefit from a systematic approach to identifying the various problems and their care implications and to continuing oversight to ensure that the problems are being systematically and adequately addressed. Unfortunately, case management has emerged as the modern cure-all for long-term care dilemmas. Assessment

*It would be incorrect to suggest that younger persons do not exhibit multisystem problems. For example, developmentally disabled children may present equally complex management challenges.

is seen as the basis for sorting out problems and assigning clients to their appropriate place. If only it were that easy. Assessment is a means of identifying client characteristics. Translating assessments into actions is still more an art than a science.

The demographic shift toward an aging population has also produced a tremendous spurt of research directed toward the delivery of services for older adults. Assessments are necessary at each phase of this research. They define baseline states. They measure outcomes of care, and they are used to adjust for differences to begin with, known as *case mix differences*. Good measures will improve such research. Knowing how to choose the right measures and how to use them wisely is the challenge addressed in this book.

Some measures have been developed for clinical use and others for research purposes. To some extent those developed for one purpose can be used for the other, but the user must act knowledgeably and cautiously. The burden of proof rests with the user. Choosing measures on the basis of attractive packaging or extravagant claims on the package is as hazardous in the world of assessment as it is in the rest of life. User training, competence, and insight are necessary. A few basic questions can help neophyte measurement consumers to think through what they are doing and what kinds of measures are best suited to their goals.

## WHY ASSESS?

Assessment is employed for different purposes. The criteria for the assessment vary with the purpose. Assessment can be used to decide on treatment, either a specific therapy or the best place to care for a client. It may serve as the basis for determining eligibility for care—either any care or various types and amounts of care. It may be the basis for an evaluation about the effectiveness of a program or a specific service.

In the clinical context, assessments are performed either to diagnose a case or to assess the effectiveness of care. Diagnosis is not an end in itself. The value of diagnosis lies in its ability to imply a course of treatment or (when there is no effective treatment) to offer a prognosis that will at least allow the patient to make appropriate plans to deal with what is expected. Screening is a variant of diagnosis. The goal of screening is not to definitively categorize, but to narrow down the field of potential people or issues to be more systematically evaluated. Most screening is performed on asymptomatic persons; hence, experts have suggested that one should not screen for problems that cannot be treated because one can raise anxiety levels. Screening can also, however, be used as part of the diagnostic evaluation process. When the definitive diagnostic test is expensive, screening can be used to winnow down the numbers of those who must undergo it, similar to the way one might use a low-power lens to define the field of vision before applying the high magnification lens.

Assessments are often used to determine eligibility for services. These assessments are usually set up to distinguish those on either side of an arbitrary threshold. As such, they are especially susceptible to bias. Those wishing to see people admitted to the program will tend to find enough points to push the applicant over the line, whereas those opposed to admission may find their applications clustered just below the threshold for eligibility. One way to avoid these artifacts is to move from a dichotomous situation to a more gradual one. If the amount of services moves from an all-or-none situation to one in which the amount of service is matched to the extent of need, a broader distribution of assessment results should follow. For example, eligibility for Medicaid is based on two fundamental criteria: poverty (a combination of income and assets) and disability. Once the latter has been established in terms of having reached a predetermined (but often arbitrarily defined) level, the individual (if he or she has achieved adequate levels of destitution) is eligible for a variety of services. Medicaid would work quite differently if it allowed a more flexible relationship between needs and eligibility, whereby clients could become more easily eligible for different amounts of care depending on their needs. Another strategy calls for separating the person performing the assessment from the act of determining eligibility, but it is naive to assume that the assessor can maintain a state of impartiality, knowing the consequences of such judgments.

Assessment is used in research to determine if the effect of an intervention is successful or to study the relationship of a phenomenon with other attributes. The better the measure, the greater the signal to noise ratio. In other words, good measures enhance researchers' abilities to detect differences as long as they are measuring the right things. The challenge lies in developing measures that can tap the phenomenon of specific interest without also bringing in extraneous information.

## WHAT TO ASSESS?

The targets of assessment boil down to risk factors and outcomes of various interventions. Risk factors can be positive or negative. Negative risk factors include all those elements that might be associated with an increased likelihood of developing an undesired condition. Positive risk factors, in contrast, constitute the array of characteristics that might have a protective effect. These are sometimes referred to as *strengths*. Given the large numbers of positive and negative potential risk factors, the question of what to assess is not simple.

The key to good assessment is using a strong conceptual model. This model should identify the specific attributes of interest. The model should include not only the attributes of the client but also related factors, such as the physical environment and informal support. Too often one encounters professionals who seem to begin with the measure and worked backward; because a measure seems to address a topic of interest, it is deemed appropriate for use. Choosing a measure, however, is no easier than making any other purchase when alternative products abound. One must have in mind the use of the measure and the likely circumstances of its use. A portable barbecue grill may be ideal for camping, but it would be a poor choice of appliance for daily cooking. Similarly, measures are best used to address specific spectrums of clients. Some are best suited to distinguish the sick from the well; others do better at discriminating among degrees of illness or disability.

One must examine the measurement product closely. Relying on a name or a reputation alone is dangerous. One would not bet on a horse simply because it is called "Speedy," but many people seem to accept a scale as measuring a concept simply because it has a name that evokes that concept. Most scales are, in fact, created after the fact. Responses to items are statistically manipulated to see how they aggregate. The aggregations are reviewed, and the extent to which they are judged to tap a given domain is determined. Finally, a name is applied to the dimension that is believed to have been addressed. It might be better to pass a rule forbidding the naming of scales and requiring that they be cited only by number. Life would be less colorful, but no one would inadvertently attribute meaning to these scales. Factor analysis and its variations are not inherently wrong—nor are their products invalid. The danger lies in believing too blindly that they measure the trait that their names suggest. In the end, they are simply the weighted responses to a series of questions. The investigator must examine the questions and decide if they tap the domain that is being explored.

The question of what to assess should be extended to include whom to assess. Here too the answer depends on the context and the purpose. The primary target for assessment should always be the client, but a comprehensive assessment of the client may not always be possible. In some cases the client may not be able to communicate effectively (see Chapter 17). Although some older people may be too confused to respond adequately, it is dangerous to decide too quickly that dementia prevents an older person from expressing valid feelings. This prematurely disenfranchises older people. In some cases the client's perceptions may be important but not altogether trustworthy. For example, older people may claim that they have more social support than is actually available. It may prove necessary to assess the availability of caregivers directly. It can also be pertinent for the assessment to probe why the older person claims more support than is available. Perhaps deep-seated preferences for a particular lifestyle combined with realistic and unrealistic fears about providers' suggestions are the reason for the exaggeration. Preferences and values, as Chapter 8 suggests, can also be the subject of assessment. Also, as this example shows, the validity of an assessment may be a function of the use the older person expects to be made of it. Older persons may deny problems or may have become inured to them. Direct observation and reports from other informed sources may be helpful in confirming older persons' self-reports.

## WHEN TO ASSESS?

Most assessments are performed in response to a precipitating event, as when an older person or an older person's family asks for care or help or applies for benefits. Some assessments, however, are done to uncover problems not yet perceived. These screenings are based on the belief that earlier detection can lead to more effective actions. Subsequent assessments can also be done to monitor the effects of treatment. Other triggers for assessment may be any change in status. For example, before people are sent to nursing homes it

might be helpful to assess their status to decide if that step is necessary or whether some other form of care might be feasible and preferred.

In a research context, assessments are often made at baseline (i.e., before an intervention) and at specific follow-up times after the intervention. Some analyses focus on the status at follow up, whereas others examine the change from baseline to follow up. The decision about when to collect follow-up information depends on the expected clinical course. The follow-up times should be designed to capture meaningful changes in status and should correspond to when most people can be expected to have reached that transition (i.e., when at least half should have shown the benefits of treatment). A common timing error is to compare treatments by timing the follow up from the end of the treatment (e.g., hospital discharge) instead of from its initiation. If part of the treatment difference is its duration, this effect will be obscured by such a strategy.

## WHO SHOULD ASSESS?

Many people conduct assessments. Some are highly trained professionals, and others are lay persons with little formal training. In general, the more structured the assessment, the less specialized the assessor needs to be. In some cases professional training is necessary to make informed inferences, but in many instances professional training can interfere with assessment accuracy. Professionals may be inclined to deviate from the protocol, preferring their insights to the strictures of the standardized approach.

It is important to match the measure and the measurer. Some assessments are designed to be applied by highly trained individuals who understand the limitations of the tools and the conditions under which they should be applied. Some assessments require generous application of expert judgment. Others are intended for use by a wide range of assessors. Still others are designed for self-administration. Older people themselves can use them, although some may need assistance with reading and interpretation.

Sometimes professionals from different disciplines want a role in the assessment process, but team assessments are very expensive. Often a better alternative is to achieve disciplinary representation through the creation of a questionnaire or protocol, but to use only one or two professionals who are trained specifically in the use and administration of the instruments to collect the information. Such an approach can ensure that the richness of each discipline's perspective is represented without the cost of each having to be present at every encounter.

For clinical purposes, the assessment can be organized as a preliminary screen, where trigger questions can identify the need for more detailed assessments. The latter assessments can be done by more specialized personnel, with the results brought back to interdisciplinary teams for incorporation in a plan of care.

## GENERIC AND CONDITION-SPECIFIC MEASURES

Outcome measures can be classified into two basic groups: generic and condition specific. Generic measures are designed to apply across populations, whereas condition-specific measures are used in a limited clinical context only. Each has its advantages and disadvantages, as summarized in Table 1.1. Generic measures address the bottom line effects of a treatment or the burden of an illness. They usually include such constructs as functioning, pain, psychological distress, and well-being. Often when they touch on multiple dimensions they are said to address quality of life. Generic measures provide both a measure of the ultimate effect and a basis for comparing across problems. In determining the cost effectiveness of alternative treatment strategies (i.e., whether to mount a campaign to address one problem or another), it is important to have a goal or outcome by which to measure the relative effectiveness of the different efforts.

The inclusive nature of generic measures also leads to their weakness. Because they are designed to cover a broad spectrum, they may not measure performance along all parts of that spectrum equally well. These limitations are referred to as *floor and ceiling effects*. For example, the SF-36 (Ware et al., 1993) may be useful in distinguishing sick from well persons, but it is less able to distinguish the sick from the very sick. Generic measures do not capture the upper or lower extremes of many problems well. They may address some domains better than others. They are less able to detect differences in specific areas than are measures designed for a specific problem.

Because they are designed to address a particular clinical problem, condition-specific measures are more apt to be able to detect clinically meaningful differences, but they are not useful to compare results across problems. Condition-specific mea-

**Table 1.1.** Relative Strengths and Limitations of Generic and Condition-Specific Measures

| Generic | Condition specific |
|---|---|
| Provides a Summary Measure (e.g., quality of life) | Usually based on Signs and Symptoms (but can address quality of life as well) |
| Enable comparisons across diagnoses | Address a specific diagnosis or a specific condition |
| Address bottom line effects of a problem | Highlight specific effects of a problem |
| Possess floor/ceiling limitations | Measure clinically meaningful changes |

sures are designed to detect the special effects of a given problem on the individual. For example, in the case of diabetes, the outcomes would address the specific complications of that disease (e.g., vascular problems, poor eyesight, and sores). Although one is accustomed to thinking of quality of life measures as generic, it is also feasible to create condition-specific quality of life measures that refer directly to the complications associated with a given condition (e.g., difficulties associated with managing a diabetic regimen).

At the same time, one might argue that condition-specific measures may be too sensitive. For example, finding a difference in the range of motion of a joint may be trivial if it is unrelated to any functional effect. Because generic and condition-specific measures complement each other, they are often best used in combination. Each can provide an aspect that the other does not address. The challenge lies in using them efficiently, avoiding duplication wherever possible.

## INFORMATION SOURCES

Measurements can be made in a variety of ways, relying on different types of information. The most widely used approach is probably the questionnaire (and interview schedule), where older people are asked about their situation. For many types of information, especially when the attitudes, feelings, or experiences of the older person are important, this may be the only way to obtain such information. Interviews and questionnaires, however, present problems. They have to be used in real time; that is, they must be part of the prospective design. (It is possible to ask clients about their past status or their use of services and exposure to potential threats, but such recollections may be biased by subsequent events and recall is subject to error. On the other hand, almost all clinical histories rely on just such recall.)

Because of cognitive limitations, some clients' responses are not trustworthy and other clients are unable to respond to questions. In these instances a proxy respondent may be used or another method of data collection employed. Although the issues surrounding the use of proxies and selection of appropriate proxies are discussed in greater detail in Chapter 17, a few comments are pertinent here. Proxies should be used only when there is convincing evidence that the respondent's reports are unreliable. Some people with cognitive deficits can still tell us a great deal about what they like and do not like, for example. The use of fixed strategies to determine when a person is too confused to be a reliable respondent has scientific appeal, but, because cognitive loss can be very spotty, it may be better to attempt to obtain a response from each respondent before or in addition to resorting to a proxy. When proxies are used, it is vital that they have had enough recent exposure to the client to be able to offer a meaningful report. It is also important to recognize that proxies may have a stake in the answers. If the information is going to be used to determine their success as caregivers, for example, their answers may be biased. It is thus critical to identify this potential source of bias and interpret the reports in that context.

Some information cannot be legitimately inferred from behaviors, and hence proxies cannot report it validly. Proxies derive their information from two sources: what they observe and what they hear. In most cases proxies rely on observations, but in some instances (e.g., when the primary respondent is not available) the proxy may be reporting on what they have heard previously from various sources (e.g., the older person, caregivers, or professionals). Some information is thus hard to derive from proxy reports. For example, although one may infer some extreme emotional states from behavior and facial expression, it would be unlikely that another person can really be sure someone is depressed or even in pain.

An alternative to using self-report or

proxies is reliance on observations. Observations can be obtained in several ways. At one extreme, observations become effectively proxy reports. Unstructured observations are translated into reports similar to the way in which the basis for a self-report is generated. Observations can be made more systematic by using a structured format for observing. This format dictates both how often to observe and what to observe. Structuring the observations in advance can make them more consistent, but the structure may limit the observations; the observer may force the observation to fit into the imposed structure.

The next level of structure is arranged or demonstrated performance, where the client is instructed in what to do. Usually these performances are done under structured conditions to improve comparability. In essence, these measures usually reflect the client's capability, whereas less structured observations or self-reports reflect actual performance. The differences in performances in structured and unstructured conditions may be due to the environment (e.g., the rules that govern activities or the incentives the staff or the client perceives). The simulated approach is designed to eliminate the effects of different environments. In so doing, however, it is limited to assessing only what a person can do under some arbitrary conditions; it says little about real-world functioning. In some settings, such as nursing homes, clients may not be allowed to do certain tasks themselves (e.g., bathing). Demonstrated performance is a standard tool of cognitive psychologists and others working in human behavior laboratories. When used for research purposes, these demonstrations have the advantage of standardization but the disadvantage of artificiality.

A common source of information in many studies and a basic component of clinical practice is the clinical record. As an information source, it is only as good as the structure and commitment to detail that went into it. Its greatest liability is the variation in recording from one person to another. Moreover, some recordings are difficult to interpret. For example, what does it mean when a clinician records "normal" or "unremarkable"? Without greater specifications about what precisely was examined and in what detail and about what constitutes the basis for calling something "normal," these conclusions are hard to compare from one client to another or one clinician to another.

## CHARACTERISTICS OF MEASURES

### Scales versus Judgments

Information about clients can be collected in different ways. Questions can be posed consistently and combined into scales. Clinical judgments can also be systematically collected. Some clinical judgments are more systematic than others. Diagnoses, for example, represent summary judgments presumably based on overt criteria; but the level of systematic assessment that goes into diagnoses varies greatly. At one extreme, psychiatry has attempted to compile a common explicit set of criteria for psychiatric diagnoses, the *Diagnostic and Statistical Manual*, a volume that lays out specific bases for each diagnosis. However, clinicians making a psychiatric diagnosis do not enter the specific elements into the clinical record. Rather, they enter the final conclusion.

Efforts to make medical records more systematic often result in a mixture of summarized clinical judgments and specific data elements. For example, one might ask about heart abnormalities (or even about cardiac rhythm) in an effort to collect more consistent information. Unless the questions are very specific (e.g., rate, regularity), however, much is still left to clinical judgment. There is an important role for systematic judgments, but they require (or assume) a high level of professional competence.

It may be informative to contrast the information obtained by asking older people about specific symptoms and asking clinicians about the presence of the conditions these symptoms represent. Such analyses can shed light on the thoroughness of clinicians and their ability to recognize pathology.

Another variant for structured clinical judgment is the rating score. Clinicians are asked to rate an aspect of a client on some numerical basis. In some cases, specific terms are applied to each level; in other instances the clinician is simply asked to use a Likert-like range (e.g., 1–5) to indicate severity. (For an example of such a scoring task, see the discussion of the Alzheimer's Disease Assessment Scale in Chapter 4.)

Clinicians may resist any systematic efforts to collect information, viewing them as an infringement on their professional prerogatives. They are likely to object more to detailed forms that resemble questionnaires in their specifics. Partly for this reason, clinicians often make poor interviewers. They feel obliged to go beyond the questions posed to add their own interpretations and insights, thus rendering the responses less reliable. In some instances, clinicians may adopt a protective role with the interviewee, wishing to spare him or her the anticipated embarrassment of some questions. In extreme cases they may simply assume what the responses would have been and complete the form without ever asking the questions. Such behavior is dangerous, but difficult to detect.

## Properties

A few basic concepts are usually employed to assess the usefulness of measures. These primarily address whether the measure is indeed measuring what it purports to measure (validity) and whether it yields consistent answers (reliability). Measures that are used to detect differences in the outcomes of a treatment may also be held to another standard: Are they *responsive* to meaningful changes in the intervention? Are they capable of detecting treatment effects when those effects are present?

### Reliability

Three broad types of reliability are typically examined. For scales composed of several discrete components, a basic concern is the extent to which the components converge on the general measure. This is usually referred to as *internal reliability* or *consistency*. In effect, the question is whether having a certain item as a part of the scale adds to the scale's overall coherence. This trait is usually measured by some type of item–scale correlation, often expressed in the form of a Chronbach's alpha statistic. The goal is to achieve a high level of internal reliability but not total convergence, which would mean that the item adds nothing to the scale or could simply be used in lieu of it.

Another type of reliability describes the extent to which the same measures perform as well in different hands (i.e., do different observers agree on what they are seeing?). This is called *inter-observer* (or *inter-rater*) reliability. The same question can be asked about the consistency of any given rater. The same observer can be asked to observe the same thing again (within a period when it should not have changed or on videotape).

Variation in response over time can result from several factors: *(1)* real change, *(2)* different reports from the client, or *(3)* intra-observer or inter-observer variation. A test that captures the latter two components involves test and retest. Here the same respondent is asked the same questions over a period of time designed to be long enough to forget the questions and short enough so that no significant change in status had occurred. Such a test combines the effects of client and observer variations. For example, a person may respond to a series of questions differently on two successive occasions. If no apparent reason for the change in the person's status can account for the discrepancy, one must assume that either the questions were asked differently (e.g., different phrasing, different emphasis, or different prompts) or the respondent was inconsistent in his or her answers. In either case, the questions are not reliable.

Much is made over the internal reliability of a measure, but it is important to appreciate that other forms of reliability are at least as important. For example, one might wax poetic over the reliability of a scalpel. It is made to perform within small tolerances and can cut sharply, but the ultimate reliability of its performance rests with the person using it. It will perform very differently in the hands of a skilled surgeon than in those of someone not trained to conduct surgery. One would hesitate to talk about the reliability of a hammer, knowing that carpentry skills are a major determinant of how well it is used. Likewise, while measures have a reliability of their own, they must be tested with those clinicians who will eventually use them. Reliability data from one experience has only limited transferability to another. In each case, it is necessary to establish the reliability of those who will use the measures in the given application. It is fairly safe to assume that a measure that was not previously reliable will not suddenly become reliable now, and likewise one cannot automatically assume that because the measure worked in one set of hands it will work in another.

## Validity

Validity refers to the capacity of a measure to accurately reflect the attribute it was intended to measure. Validity is an important concept but is often hard to prove. Although reliability is a prerequisite for validity, it is not sufficient. In the easiest case, one has the capacity to measure this attribute already albeit in a cumbersome fashion. The candidate measure is thus collected simultaneously with the standard, and the results are compared. The closer the relationship, the better the new measure. For many items, however, no such gold standard exists. Other stratagems must be used instead.

The most common test of validity is the so-called face validity. In essence, this means that the measures seem to be addressing the right items, and they make clinical or common sense "on the face of it." This test is usually necessary but rarely sufficient. A more subtle approach to establishing validity is assessing the measure's ability to discriminate between two groups identified on the basis of their a priori likelihood to have the characteristic or not, for example, sick versus well. The more subtle the distinction between the groups, the more sensitive the measure. Another way to approach discriminate validity is to test the measure's level of agreement with other measures that are believed to tap related domains and the measure's lack of concordance with those hypothesized to address different domains.

Still another test of a measure's validity lies in its ability to predict a client's subsequent status. Logically argued predictions that link current measurement of a domain with future changes in relevant other domains can establish that the first domain measure is indeed tapping a relevant area correctly.

## Responsiveness

A third basic criterion used to assess a measure is its responsiveness. In other words, can the measure detect real change when it occurs. In one sense, responsiveness is related to discriminate validity. The latter addresses the ability of a measure to discriminate between two groups that are believed to be different. The former addresses the ability to detect change over time. A measure may be able to discriminate but may not be useful for detecting change. For example, death is a good discriminator but may not be sensitive to real changes in conditions that are not fatal. Responsiveness (sometimes called *sensitivity*, although this term has another meaning in the context of screening, as discussed later) is difficult to establish. It requires a strong clinical model.

The only way to test a measure's responsiveness is to see if it detects changes when there is good reason to expect them. Therefore, it is usually assessed as part of a clinical trial, when there is every opportunity for endogenous reasoning. The failure to find responsiveness may lie in the impotence of the intervention. This attribute is closely linked to discriminant validity, but there are important differences. For example, death has strong discriminant features, but it may not be responsive to the effects of treating arthritis or even pneumonia.

*Sensitivity and Specificity*

Another set of criteria are used to evaluate screening measures. Here we seek sensitivity, specificity, and positive predictive accuracy. Sensitivity refers to a measure's ability to detect a problem when it is there. Specificity refers to the obverse, the ability to correctly state that a problem is absent. In the context of screening, these two attributes are assessed by comparing the screening or test results to a measure of truth, usually the result of a more comprehensive assessment or laboratory test. Table 1.2 illustrates the comparisons. Sensitivity is assessed as the proportion of true positives (a + b) the test correctly identifies, whereas specificity address the proportion of true negatives (c + d) identified. In general, sensitivity is obtained at the cost of specificity. Because these definitions can be manipulated by changing the level of measure that is said to represent a positive or negative state, moving the

threshold will increase one at the expense of the other. The pattern of this relationship in response to changes in threshold is displayed as a receiver–operator correspondence (ROC) curve, in which the sensitivity is graphed against (1 − specificity). The goal of such a measure is to maximize the area under the curve (Hanley & McNeil, 1982).

Sensitivity is emphasized when the consequences of missing a case are severe. For example, if a disease were highly contagious, it would be important to identify each case as quickly as possible. One would want to cast a wide net to identify possible cases and then rule out false positives. Likewise, if a serious disease with dire consequences was readily treatable if detected early, one would want a sensitive test. In contrast, if the cost of the subsequent evaluation were quite high and the condition less serious, one would aim for greater specificity and accept more false negatives.

*Positive Predictive Value*

An additional concept to sensitivity and specificity used in describing screening tools is the positive predictive value (PPV). In essence, this criterion asks how likely does a positive result from a screening test indicate the presence of real disease. Using the terminology from Table 1.2, PPV = a/(a + c). This information is very important in interpreting screening results and avoiding unnecessary alarm. The PPV is especially sensitive to the prevalence of the condition being screened for. The following example can illustrate the effect of prevalence.

Table 1.2.
Assessing Sensitivity and Specificity*

| True state | Test result | | Total |
| --- | --- | --- | --- |
| | Positive | Negative | |
| Positive | a | b | a + b |
| Negative | c | d | c + d |
| Total | a + c | b + d | |

*Sensitivity: a/(a + b); specificity: d/(c + d).

**Table 1.3.**
The Effects of Prevalence on Positive Predictive Value (PPV)

| | Test result | | |
|---|---|---|---|
| True State | Positive | Negative | Total |
| *Condition A (Prevalence 1/100)** | | | |
| Positive | 950 | 50 | 1000 |
| Negative | 4950 | 94,050 | 99,000 |
| Total | 5900 | 94,100 | 100,000 |
| *Condition B (Prevalence 1/1000)†* | | | |
| Positive | 95 | 5 | 100 |
| Negative | 4995 | 94,905 | 99,900 |
| Total | 5090 | 94,910 | 100,000 |

*PPV = 950/5900 = 16%.
†PPV = 95/5090 = 2%.

Let us assume that we have a test that is 95% sensitive and 95% specific. Table 1.3 shows the effects of two different prevalence rates. In both cases we will assume that we have screened 100,000 people. In condition A, the underlying prevalence is 1 in 100; in condition B, it is 1 in 1000. In both cases, despite what seem to be rather stringent criteria for sensitivity and specificity, the PPV is surprisingly low. A positive screening result under condition A is accurate only about 16% of the time and under condition B only about 2% of the time. The difference is attributable solely to the underlying prevalence of the problem. The greater the prevalence, the higher the PPV.

## GENERAL ISSUES IN THE ASSESSMENT OF OLDER PERSONS

### Establishing Communication

Common problems in interviewing older people involve difficulties with their hearing and vision. At the very least such problems may lead to poor performance. At worst they can lead to frustration for all parties, unnecessary use of proxies, and even misdiagnoses. A first rule of interviewing older people is to be sure that real communication has been established. Interviewers should ask questions even when they strongly believe they know the answers and wait for a response. They should speak slowly and enunciate carefully, facing the respondent. The older person needs to be wearing a hearing aid if one has been prescribed. Speaking loudly may help, and sometimes even using a portable amplifier is a possibility when hearing is a problem. If such a device is not available, a written form of the interview may be used. Similarly, to deal with vision problems, response cards or reading tests must be printed, and the interviewer must ensure that the older respondent is wearing reading glasses if they are needed (and they usually are).

### Time

In general, interviewing older subjects takes more time than usual. Not only is their response time longer, but some may have more difficulty focusing on the task. Lonely people may want to take advantage of the contact to talk about other things. Persons with minor cognitive deficits may need more prompts and reminders than unimpaired respondents. Interviewers need special training in learning how to accommodate some of this time delay but not get off track.

### Fatigue

Older respondents may tire easily. Fatigue will not only worsen their performance, it may place too great a strain on them. In some cases it can lead to an incomplete interview. Interviewers need to be trained to recognize indications of fatigue and to offer to stop for awhile or even to divide the session into multiple parts geared to the respondent's tolerance.

Clients with multiple medical problems will likely be at greater risk of fatigue. More attention should be paid to their condition as the interview continues. Some medications may affect the clients' level of consciousness or attention span.

### Embarrassment

Some older people may become upset when they cannot perform certain physical and cognitive tests. Interviewers need to be instructed in how to avoid and to cope with these reactions. It is not uncommon, for example, for older respondents to become upset when they cannot complete a simple cognitive test. Interviewers need to know how to provide reassurance that not everyone is expected to get each question correct or to complete all the tasks.

Likewise, some clients may not feel free to give honest answers. They may be embarrassed to admit certain problems and simply offer socially acceptable responses. They may be afraid that reporting certain things will have adverse consequences for them or others (e.g., in institutions). Some efforts may ameliorate these problems, such as assuring the clients of confidentiality (when such assurance is feasible) and emphasizing that many of the problems explored are common, but often the barriers will persist.

Oddly enough, however, interviewer embarrassment is an equally important factor. Even health professionals are uncomfortable asking people who resemble their parents or grandparents about continence or depression. When the interviewer is matter of fact and unruffled, the respondent is also more comfortable.

### Test Batteries

Often we use a battery of tests. In addition to considerations of fatigue and duplication, the order in which the tests are used

may be important. In general, it is better to begin with easier and less threatening material and allow the testing to proceed on the basis of adequate performance. This is easiest to accomplish within a given domain, such as cognition, but it also applies to the order of the domains tested. Areas, like cognition, where failure is more feasible should be presented as late as possible. Some people use cognitive batteries as screeners to determine if a person is competent to answer questions in other areas (or needs a proxy), but cognitive performance may be spotty. Not only does such screening potentially eliminate some people who might nonetheless be able to express meaningful opinions on various tokens, but the stress of the testing may also affect other areas. Likewise, a battery of questions about depression may cast a pall over the rest of the interview.

## STAKEHOLDERS AND CONTEXT

Assessments are used for various purposes. The nature of the stakeholders and the context in which questions are asked can dramatically influence the answers. Assessments can be used as both a means of entry and as a barrier. Assessments are also imprecise instruments capable of substantial manipulation. The same assessment can thus be employed by different stakeholders for opposite purposes. The aegis of the assessment can dramatically affect its conduct and its interpretation. Consider, for example, eligibility assessments. The predisposition of the assessor who is a stakeholder can play a great role in determining the outcome. If some arbitrary point score is needed to render a client eligible for services, an assessor who wishes to see the client receive the services can ask questions in a certain way or adjust judgments to achieve the target score. It is not surprising that wherever the level of eligibility is set, scores seem to cluster around that threshold.

Clients and their families are also major stakeholders. Their responses may be different depending on the context. They too may be sensitive to issues of eligibility and exaggerate difficulties to become eligible for desired services or minimize problems to avoid undesired treatments.

It is possible to obtain one set of responses when the family brings the client for treatment and another when a case manager asks the same questions as part of a formal eligibility evaluation. Clients may respond differently to a person they see as offering service and to one who is seen as an outside regulator. If the care provider also controls the older person's living environments, they may be reluctant to voice problems for fear of retaliation. Older people may also become accustomed to their situation and lose the basis for determining what represents difficulty or dissatisfaction.

## EFFICIENCY

It is also important to consider the costs of assessment. Assessments can be conducted in infinite detail, but the efficiency of such procedures must be judged in terms of the expected benefits. The measure of efficiency will depend on the context. In general, it is unwise to invest considerable energy uncovering more problems than can be addressed, either directly or indirectly. The latter refers to identifying external factors that may complicate care or that at least need to be addressed when the plan of care is developed. In some instances, however, extensive evaluations may be worth the expense. For example, if a treatment is expensive (or dangerous), one

wants to be sure that there is a sound basis for implementing it. Those who worry about the costs of long-term care may argue for more extensive evaluations first to identify potentially correctable problems whose repair may preclude the need for such extended care. Others may take a more programatically protective attitude by establishing admission barriers designed to allow entry to only the most severely disabled.

One's view of the role of evaluation and assessment depends in part on how one views the allocation of long-term care services. Those who see such care as composed of specific aliquots may be more inclined to emphasize assessment as a basis for strict care planning. They advocate closely matching treatments to cases. Extensive evaluation is needed to allow the proper titration of services. On the other hand, those who view long-term care services as more generic may be content with more limited assessments that allow an estimate of the total amount of care needed.

## REFERENCES

Hanley, J. A., & McNeil, B. J. (1982). The meaning and use of the area under a receiver operating characteristic (ROC) curve. *Radiology, 143*, 29–36.
——. Stevens, R. (1971). Trends in medical specialization in the United States. *Inquiry, 8*, 9–19.
——. Ware, J. E. Jr., Snow, K. K., Kosinski, M., & Gandek, B. (1993). *SF-36 health survey: Manual and interpretation guide.* Boston: The Health Institute, New England Medical Center.

# I

# Assessment Content

# 2

# Assessment of Function in Older Adults

VALINDA I. PEARSON

Over the years, physical functioning has come to mean a person's ability to perform those activities of daily living deemed necessary to survive adequately in modern society. Functional assessment includes three major domains: activities of daily living (ADLs) or self-care activities, instrumental activities of daily living (IADLs), and mobility (Spector, 1990). This chapter addresses the assessment of physical functioning in older adults.

Several aspects of assessing function in older adults need to be appreciated. First, assessment is not the exclusive domain of health professionals. Even before the health professional sees the patient, the patient has made his or her own assessment about what is normal and abnormal function for him or her. When the discrepancy between normal function and abnormal function becomes too large or unacceptable for the older adult, then the individual might think about seeking professional help. If the older person or the family believes that the discrepancy between normal and abnormal can be lessened or indicates possible future decline or pathology, then the older person may seek professional help.

Second, in the busy clinical practice setting, assessment of physical function is often based on verbal report of symptoms without observational data being systematically collected. This practice is understandable given the time constraints imposed on busy practitioners. Expectations of efficient use of time do not necessarily, however, make the practice of relying on verbal report either good medicine or efficient.

Third, the pathologic effects of disease are sometimes confused with the results of normal aging. When this happens, treatable consequences of disease are written off as the unavoidable and untreatable results of aging. Even within the normal decline of function associated with aging, it is often possible to either slow or modify the functional effects of aging by adapting the environment to the person or by helping the person adapt the task to his or her limitations. In some cases, functional decline can be slowed by altering lifestyle behaviors, for example exercise or dietary practices, of the older adult. In functional assessment, as in any other area of assessment of elderly persons, the tendency toward ageism and the resultant failure to consider the older person as an individual rather than a chronological age must be recognized and avoided.

The first part of this chapter covers functional assessment, the evolving conceptual models that have influenced the development of assessment instruments, and the strengths and weaknesses of various types of instruments. The second part reviews specific instruments that illustrate the variety of approaches to assessment, but the review does not claim to be an all-inclusive review of the more than 200 instruments that assess physical function.

## WHAT IS FUNCTIONAL ASSESSMENT?

In its simplest form, functional assessment is the evaluation of a person's ability to carry out the basic ADLs (Ikegami, 1995; Spector, 1990). Functional assessment includes both the physical capabilities demonstrated and the capabilities and the current deficiencies that the person reports. In other words, functional assessment is the systematic process of identifying or diagnosing the capabilities and deficiencies of

persons at risk from the consequences of aging and illness (Bernstein, 1992). At the individual level, this process focuses on how the older adult manages day-to-day activities and may lead to the development of individualized strategies to maintain quality of life. At the population level, aggregated functional assessments lead to development of programs designed to maintain the safety, security, and independence of elderly persons.

Evaluation is systematic and includes basic self-care activities such as bathing, dressing, eating, grooming, toileting, and continence (Boucher, 1989). In addition to the basic self-care activities or ADLs, functional assessment has expanded to include those activities necessary to survive as an individual in a community environment. These IADLs focus on three major areas: household chores including cooking, laundry, cleaning; mobility-related activities such as shopping and using transportation; and cognitive activities such as money management, using the telephone, and

**Table 2.1.**
Common Components of Functional Assessment

| Area* | Additional considerations for all performance components |
|---|---|
| ADLs | |
|   Dressing | |
|   Bathing | |
|   Eating | |
|   Grooming | |
|   Toileting | |
|   Continence | Amount of human assistance required |
|     Bladder |   Independent (no help) |
|     Bowel |   Supervision |
| IADLs |   Cuing/organization |
|   Cooking |   Hands-on help |
|   Cleaning |   Dependent (total help) |
|   Shopping | Speed of performance |
|   Money management | Degree of pain during performance; endurance |
|   Use of transportation | Quality of performance |
|   Use of telephone | Safety |
|   Medication administration | |
| Mobility | |
|   Walking (locomotion) | |
|   Stairs | |
|   Balance | |
|   Transferring† | |

*ADLs, activities of daily living; IADLs, instrumental activities of daily living.
†Often included in ADLs.

medication administration (Lawton & Brody, 1969). A third domain of functional assessment is mobility, also referred to as lower limb functioning. Within this area of assessment are evaluations of walking speed, balance, stair climbing ability, and transfer skills. Functional assessment can also include the evaluation of physical strength, endurance, and speed of performance (see Table 2.1).

Functional ability can be conceptualized as the dynamic interaction of an older adult's physiological status, the emotional or psychological environment, and the external or physical and social environment (Fig. 2.1). Each of the three components consists of numerous subcomponents. For example, physiological status includes disease conditions such as arthritis, congestive heart disease, or Alzheimer's disease and the limitations that disease and/or the process of aging place on functional ability. Psychological environment includes factors such as depression, hopefulness, mental status, problem-solving ability, expectations, values, safety concerns, and motivation. The ability to solve problems is a reflection of cognitive functioning, but it is also a factor of how the individual adapts the self, the task, or the physical environment to facilitate functioning. The external environment includes the physical setting and the social supports available to the individual. Thus, the lack of sufficient help (quantity or quality) is an environmental factor that influences functional status. How these three components and their subcomponents interact provides a picture of an older adult's functional ability at a given point in time. Other chapters in this book deal in depth with each of these components of functioning. This chapter deals with how to assess the functioning itself.

## RATIONALE FOR FUNCTIONAL ASSESSMENT

There are numerous reasons for the researcher or clinician to include an assessment of physical function in the battery of evaluations for the older adult. Function is the *lingua franca* of geriatrics (Applegate, Blass, & Williams, 1990). Regardless of where one practices within the realm of geriatrics and gerontology, concern with function and functional ability of older adults is the common pathway that all practitioners share. Functional assessment establishes the person's baseline abilities for purposes of future comparison and can be used to predict prognosis. From the perspectives of the researcher and the clinician, comparing results from baseline function to functional assessments done later in treatment objectively measures the results of treatment. This comparison forms a basis for continuation, modification, or termination of a treatment regime. Function is also assessed in order to determine which services or technological aids could compensate for functional deficits that cannot be altered by improvements in performance. Third, repeated measures of function permit one to determine changes that indicate deterioration of a disease state or recovery.

Functional assessment allows for the identification of physical strengths and abilities that can be positively emphasized and limitations that need to be considered as part of care planning. Practitioners such as occupational therapists, physical therapists, recreational therapists, physicians, and nurses use functional assessment to develop the initial plan of care and treatment goals and then to revise it. Functional assessment helps determine both the effectiveness of treatment and when

Functional ability = Physiological status + Psychological environment + Physical and social environment

**Figure 2.1.** An Equation of Functional Ability.

the patient is ready for discharge from treatment.

Functional ability constitutes the eligibility criteria for services provided by some organizations (Feinstein, Josephy, & Well, 1986). For the social worker or case manager, the results of functional assessment direct how resources and services are allocated. Patients and their families use the results of functional assessments to identify the progress made and the progress yet to be made. Changes in functional assessments provide objective information that helps patient and family plan for present and future needs. For the clinical researcher, changes in functional ability are frequently used as an outcome variable, a risk factor, or a case mix adjuster.

From the perspective of the practitioner or researcher interested in improving care, functional assessment provides a basis for evaluating and assuring quality of care. Comparisons of the results of repeated assessments of basic ADL functioning in groups of patients point to the effectiveness or ineffectiveness of treatment plans. When patients fail to maintain functional levels of performance without deterioration in physical or mental health, the possibility arises that the program of treatment is ineffective and needs to be revised.

For the program administrator, functional assessment increases the ability to predict future costs. There is a direct association between level of function and likelihood of dying, use of hospital days, and use of ancillary services (Spector, Katz, Murphy, & Fulton, 1987). More dysfunctional older adults use more services and die sooner than persons who are less dysfunctional in ADLs and IADLs.

Although the improvement of care is an important goal for the researcher, it is not the only reason for inclusion of functional assessment in research studies. For the researcher, four goals are met by functional assessment. Functional assessments serve as a baseline descriptor of research subjects. In addition, results of assessments also provide a mechanism for dividing groups of subjects according to preestablished levels of functioning (i.e., high functioning vs. low functioning). Level of functional ability may also determine whether an individual is appropriate for inclusion in a research study. A second goal is to test conceptual models of function in older adults. A frequently tested conceptual model has been the hierarchical model of ADL and IADL activities that posits that more complex activities such as shopping or cooking are lost sooner than more basic activities such as eating or bathing. A third goal is identifying the relationships between ability (can or could do an activity), performance (does do), and psychological variables such as cognitive ability, depression, optimism, helplessness, or hope. Finally, there is the goal of identifying relationships between function and other outcomes such as use of health services, number of hospital days, attendance at avocational activities, or general health status.

## THE INTENDED TARGET OF FUNCTIONAL ASSESSMENT

Functional assessment is not limited to older adults who are frail or living in institutional settings; it also useful with community dwelling older adults with chronic health problems (Zimmer, Rothenberg, & Andresen, 1997). If risk assessment and prevention are aims of gerontologists, then older well adults who are leading sedentary lifestyles and nondisabled older adults should also be assessed periodically for functional performance. Guralnik and associates (1995) found that older adults who did poorly on a battery of tests of lower limb functioning were at greater risk of decline after four years than other adults.

Older adults who are planning a move from one living environment to another would also benefit from functional ability screening. For many older adults, the decision to move from one's home of many years to another environment is triggered by the person's or family's recognition that the home environment is getting more difficult to maintain, that the older adult needs more help doing IADLs, or that he or she has given up doing activities. A functional assessment will point out areas where assistance in meeting ADLs and IADLs is needed and will also identify areas where environmental modifications are needed.

## CHALLENGES OF FUNCTIONAL ASSESSMENT WITH AN OLDER ADULT POPULATION

Carrying out a comprehensive, organized functional assessment of any person demands knowledge and skill. At a minimum, the assessor needs skill in administering the instrument and in communicating with older adults. The assessment tool has norms or standards for comparison that are appropriate to the age group being assessed. Not all of the functional assessment tools have norms that reflect the range of performance typical of older adults. Although most instruments have been used with persons over the age of 60 years, some instruments are more sensitive to early changes in function (IADL scales) while other instruments (ADL scales) have ceiling effects for community dwelling older adults.

Older adults in clinical settings often have multiple chronic health conditions that directly influence how the person functions. Chronic health conditions such as arthritis can influence the speed with which the older adult is able to complete tasks included in the assessment. Because speed of response can be a factor in some functional assessment measures such as the Physical Performance Test (Reuben & Siu, 1990) or the Timed Manual Performance Test (Williams, Gaylord, & Gerrity, 1994), taking a longer time to complete a task may be a predictor of performance problems. Given enough time, the older adult is able to carry out the task. Including speed as a performance criterion introduces the

question of when speed is relevant to performance. Slow performance may raise concerns about safety and also the practicality of doing an activity independently. Conversely, rapidity of performance can also lead to safety concerns, for example, when an individual transfers quickly from a wheelchair without locking the brakes.

In the research setting, chronic health conditions may contribute to the total amount of time required to complete a functional assessment even when speed is not a component of the assessment. The need to repeat directions or to provide directions one step at a time lengthens the time necessary to complete the assessment. When functional assessments are included as part of a battery of assessments, it may be necessary to schedule more time for the older individual to become familiar with the physical environment of the research setting so that the novel environment does not contribute to lower scores than would occur in a more familiar setting. The cognitive impairments associated with conditions such as multi-infarct dementia, Parkinson's disease or Alzheimer's disease may make functional assessment more challenging. Persons who are unable to understand directions or to retain directions long enough to complete the tasks involved in the assessment are likely to score more poorly than persons without cognitive impairments even though the person may be physically able to perform the task spontaneously as part of their daily activities. (For further discussion of assessment of cognitively impaired persons, see Chapter 4.)

Cognitive impairment in the older adult sometimes can make it necessary for proxy respondents to be used. The accuracy of proxy responses is influenced by the complexity of the activity; proxy reports of less physically demanding or complex ADLs are more accurate and less biased than are reports of IADLs (Dorevitch et al., 1992). (For a complete discussion of the role of proxy respondents, see Chapter 17.)

Some older adults are unfamiliar with

and suspicious of modern technology. Video cameras used to record performance and computer keyboards for inputting responses may be unfamiliar to some older adults, although the reported technophobia of older people may be exaggerated. For some older adults whose experiences with formal education were decades earlier, confronting an assessment situation in which they are told to "do their best" may be a stressful experience if they equate the assessment with a situation in which failure is possible. In addition, many older adults may not be motivated to perform at a level that represents their true ability to perform simply because they do not perceive the importance of the tests. For example, the inability to take a tub bath independently (an ADL) may not be important if the person has always "washed up at the sink." Inherent in the IADLs are traditional gender roles such as cooking and household maintenance that some older men have never performed and money management and transportation that may be unaccustomed tasks for older women.

A final challenge may be a difference in expectations between what the person doing the assessment hopes to accomplish and what the person being assessed expects. If the assessment is being done for research purposes and the assessor's goal is data collection, the older adult still may expect a service. That service might be information about current performance, suggestions for improving performance, or acknowledgment of the contribution made to humanity by participating in the study.

## DIMENSIONS OF FUNCTIONAL ASSESSMENT

No functional assessment tool is universally recognized as the "gold standard" in terms of range of activities included or performance indicators (Zimmer et al., 1997). Most tools, however, address some or most of the activities identified in Table

2.1. There are numerous functional assessment tools. Some of these tools are institution specific; some are disease specific. The types of instruments used in functional assessment vary from a single-item question that asks "Are you able to do the things that you want to do?" to domain-specific instruments that ask multiple questions about performance of a number of skills or tasks. The single-item question, often included as part of a larger questionnaire, acts as a screening device particularly for respondents who indicate that their performance is fair to poor. The response to the screening question triggers the completion of more a comprehensive and detailed assessment of physical function. Most multiple question instruments include either ADLs, IADLs, some combination of ADLs and IADLs, or mobility.

## USE OF A CONCEPTUAL FRAMEWORK TO UNDERSTAND AND MEASURE FUNCTION

A conceptual framework or model is a way of viewing the world. It provides the frame of reference for understanding the variables studied, for selecting the instruments used to collect information, and for interpreting results. It guides research and practice by identifying what is investigated or observed (the phenomena), what theories are tested, how phenomena and theories are investigated (methodology), and what data are collected. For example, one conceptual framework may state that the hierarchical nature of losing and recovering basic ADL functions is crucial to understanding function (Katz et al., 1963; Lawton & Brody, 1969), whereas a second conceptual framework may emphasize the person's ability to adapt to the environment.(Czaja, Weber, & Sankaran, 1993). A third conceptual framework may focus on the relationship between the person's desire to perform an activity versus actual ability to perform the activity (Glass, 1998).

## AN EVOLVING CONCEPTUAL FRAMEWORK OF FUNCTION AND FUNCTIONAL ASSESSMENT

Historically, the assessment of physical abilities and functioning has been closely tied to the assessment of functional disability. Although the first published use of the phrase "activities of daily living" was by Edith Buchwald in a 1949 issue of *Physical Therapy Review* (see Feinstein et al., 1986), the assessment of function became a major topic of interest during the mid-1960s. Two main areas of interest were Nagi's work on disability and function and the efforts of Katz, Barthel, and Lawton and their respective colleagues to identify the tasks that are now recognized as being components of physical functioning.

In 1965, Nagi presented one of the first conceptual frameworks for studying disability and function (Fig. 2.2). Nagi proposed a four-stage, sequential model as a basis for conceptualizing disability. The model begins with the underlying disease or pathology (stage 1) that may result in physiological impairment (stage 2). As a result of the physiological impairment, the person may develop physical and/or emotional constraints that limit performance (stage 3). These limitations in physical and emotional capacities may result in the inability of the person to carry out the tasks and role assignments that are associated with living independently and with work performance (stage 4).

In Nagi's model only one factor, disease, contributes to the development of physiological impairment and performance limitations that in turn lead to disability. As a single-factor model, it ignores other factors such as the environment, presence or

lack of social support, person's perception of health, or degree of motivation that may also contribute to the development of disability. A major assumption of the model is the unalterable sequential nature of progression from one stage to another. Although the time spent in each stage of the model may vary, the sequence remains unchanged unless death interrupts the progression through the model.

Although Nagi's work has been accepted as the traditional model of the disability process and has been the basis for more inclusive and descriptive models, many researchers and clinicians have criticized its failure to express the complex nature of disability and function. Perhaps the most widely known conceptual framework is the World Health Organization's (WHO) International Classification of Impairments, Disabilities, and Handicaps (ICIDH) (Kovar & Lawton, 1994; World Health Organization, 1976, 1980). The WHO model expanded on Nagi's model and the traditional medical model of etiology–pathology–manifestation by proposing a broader range of consequences of disease. According to the ICIDH, there are three possible outcomes of disease: impairment, disability, and handicap (Table 2.2).

As indicated in Table 2, *impairment* refers to the performance of an organ or body part and *disability* refers to the performance of an activity by a person. Not all impairments lead to disability. A person may have limited range of motion but still be able to carry out all normal activities independently.

The distinction between disability and handicap is a matter of severity and situation (Kovar & Lawton, 1994). A disability becomes a handicap when the person is no longer able to function in previously held

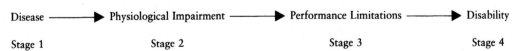

Disease ———▶ Physiological Impairment ———▶ Performance Limitations ———▶ Disability

Stage 1        Stage 2        Stage 3        Stage 4

**Figure 2.2.** Depiction of Nagi's conceptual model of the process of Disability (Nagi, 1965).

**Table 2.2.**
Definitions and Examples of Impairment, Disability, and Handicap

| Term | Definition | Example |
|---|---|---|
| Impairment | A loss or abnormality of physiological, psychological, or anatomical structure function | Loss of limbs<br>Limited range of motion<br>Mental impairment<br>Visual changes |
| Disability | A restriction or lack of ability, due to impairment, in performing an activity within the range considered normal for a person | Feeds self with adaptive equipment or is fed by another person<br>Drives using adapted brakes |
| Handicap | A disadvantage, due to an impairment or disability, that limits or prevents the fulfillment of a role that is normal for the person | Marital role dysfunction<br>Inability to function as grandparent |

Based on the World Health Organization's International Classification of Impairments, Disabilities, and Handicaps.

roles (Fig. 2.3). Within the framework provided by the WHO, it becomes important to assess how assistance, either human or equipment, can be utilized to prevent a disability from becoming a handicap.

Since the establishment of the WHO model, researchers and clinicians have provided additional dimensions to a conceptual framework of function and functional assessment. For example, Deniston and Jette (1980) have included the concepts of difficulty of performance and pain in performance. Czaja and associates (1993) have focused on the influence of the external environment on a person's functional ability. According to Czaja and associates, there is a three-way interaction between the capabilities of the person, the task or activity performed, and the structure and design of the environment. Modification of any one of the three components of this interaction will alter the degree of function that the person demonstrates in that environment. Fried and associates (1996) have operationalized the interaction between

functional ability and environment by assessing task and environmental modifications made by the older adult.

Glass (1998) has focused on the discrepancies between what the person reports being able to do, what the person can do in the laboratory or clinical setting, and what the person does in the home environment. Glass refers to this variation in performance as differences in the hypothetical tense (what the person reports being able to do), the experimental tense (the laboratory or clinical performance in the optimal environment), and the enacted tense (the in-home performance or what the person actually does). The distinction between can do (hypothetical tense) assessment and does in reality (enacted tense) lies at the root of differences in assessments based on self-report and direct observation. Many self-report instruments ask if the respondent can do an activity rather than when the person last did the activity or how the person does the activity. Direct observation or performance-based assessments

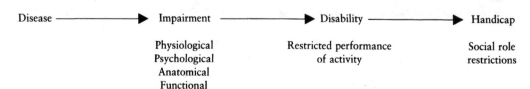

**Figure 2.3.** Outcomes of disease (based on the WHO's International Classification of Impairments, Disabilities, and Handicaps model).

make use of the enacted tense or the experimental tense to determine what the person can do. The difference between what a person can do and regularly does can be attributed to the effects of environment and motivation. Consideration of the need for assistance and the extent to which that need is met is a recent addition by Allen and Mor (1997) to the conceptual model of functional assessment.

## SPECIFIC TASKS TO BE ASSESSED

During the 1950s and 1960s, Katz and his colleagues at the Benjamin Rose Hospital in Cleveland began studying the functional abilities of a group of patients with hip fractures. Based on those observations, Katz developed the Index of Activities of Daily Living (ADL): feeding, continence, transferring, toileting, dressing, and bathing. According to Katz, these skills were learned in childhood in the order listed above and lost in the reverse order (the ontological assumption) as a result of neurologic damage or advancing age. Katz's studies led him and his associates to conclude that these six ADLs formed a hierarchy of performance. Since Katz' initial work, these six ADLs have come to be described as "early loss" and "late loss" ADLs (Morris & Morris, 1997). "Late loss" ADLs, eating and bed mobility, are the last functions lost by the person. "Early loss" ADLs are more complex ADLs such as bathing and dressing independently that originally were mastered by the person in late toddlerhood and are functions that are more susceptible to early cognitive decline.

Later work by Lawton and associates added the assessment of Instrumental Activities of Daily Living (IADLs)—use of a telephone, shopping, food preparation, housekeeping, laundry, use of transportation, medication administration, and money management—to the area of functional assessment (see Lawton & Brody, 1969). This inclusion was made to improve the usefulness of functional assessments of community dwelling elders. Although the basic ADLs were found to discriminate among levels of functioning in frail older adults or nursing home residents, ADLs were not useful in distinguishing levels of functioning in well older adults living in the community (Ward, Jagger, & Harper, 1998). The addition of IADLs helped identify those relatively well older adults at high risk for functional decline from other well older adults. Just as there is a hierarchical nature to ADLs, there is also a hierarchical relationship between the basic ADLs and the more complex IADLs and also within IADLs. Research studies have demonstrated this relationship by finding that persons who are dependent in ADLs are also dependent in IADLs, whereas persons who require assistance in performing IADLs will not necessarily need assistance with ADLs (Asberg & Sonn, 1988; Spector et al., 1987).

How much or how little assistance the person needs to perform ADLs is a factor in functional assessment. Consequently, most assessment tools, at a minimum, distinguish between being independent (requiring no assistance in performing an activity) and being dependent (requiring the help of another person or an object to perform the activity). Measurement metrics include consideration of the amount of help needed (or received). Some extend the measure by asking whether tasks that can be performed are difficult and what the amount of difficulty is associated with them. Some metrics allow the use of assistive devices; others do not.

## SELECTING A FUNCTIONAL ASSESSMENT MEASURE

Selecting the best functional assessment measure depends on what goal or purpose is to be achieved. The purpose of the measure and the population to be assessed have a direct impact on the instrument to be chosen. Whenever possible, instruments with good psychometrics are a better choice than instruments with poor or no reported psychometrics. The ease of administration and scoring, cost of administration, burden of performance, and demand placed on the subject are also factors to be considered.

## TYPES OF FUNCTIONAL ASSESSMENT INSTRUMENTS

Functional assessment instruments can be one of several types: single-item or two-item questions, self-report, proxy report, direct observation, and performance based. *Single-item* or *two-item questions* are used in multiple-item surveys in which functional performance is only one of several areas being assessed. The questions act as a screening device to determine the need for additional assessment. These tools are a relatively inexpensive way to screen out persons who do not need further assessment. A disadvantage of this method is that confusion may arise about what standard of comparison the respondent is using.

*Self-report questionnaires,* which draw on Glass's hypothetical tense (1998), that is, the respondents' reported performance rather than their actual performance, have the advantages of being easy to administer and low in cost; they can be done via the mail, over the telephone, or in face-to-face interviews. As the amount of personal contact increases, the cost of administration increases. Self-report measures, however, have several weaknesses. First, most lack sensitivity to change in function (Reuben, Siu, & Kimpau, 1992). Second, the cognitive status of the respondent has a direct impact on the ability to respond and on the quality of the response. Memory deficits influence the accuracy or completeness of responses. Discrepancies between self-report and actual ability to perform can be an issue with self-report measures. Discrepancies may represent overinflation of function when the respondent claims an ability to perform a task that is no longer done. Overinflation is frequently the result of a desire to maintain independence and

autonomy or to avoid placement in a group residential environment. On the other hand, underreporting of actual performance can also occur when the individual does the activity on some occasions but does not report the activity in order to appear more dependent or in need of assistance from family members or service providers. For example, if eligibility depends on being dependent, respondents may underreport their functioning. The mood state of the respondent can influence the accuracy of self-report measures, with depressed individuals tending to underreport abilities and euphoric individuals overstating abilities.

Any instrument that relies on self-report can also be used as a *proxy report measure* with minor changes in wording. Proxy reports are relatively inexpensive, easy to administer, and can be done in person, via telephone, or through the mail. The decision to use a proxy measure is often based on the assumption that the older subject of the report is too cognitively impaired to be a reliable respondent. Proxy measures assume that the person responding has had an adequate opportunity to observe the behavior being performed by the older adult and hence that the respondent knows enough about the older adult to be able to answer questions without guessing.

A disadvantage of proxy reports completed by family members is the discrepancy in ratings by the proxy when compared with the subject's reports. Proxy respondents who are family members tend to underrate functional performance and attribute poorer outcomes to the older adult than the adult would report (Dorevitch and coworkers, 1992; Magaziner, 1992; Magaziner et al., 1997). Proxies are subject to biased recall. Depending on the circumstances, they can exaggerate or minimize dependency. They may be influenced by a particularly dramatic episode. Responses from family members are usually based on unstructured or casual observations done in the natural setting or home environment. Proxy reports are sometimes completed by professional caregivers, and the same assumption about observing the activity applies in this situation. In many cases, the professional caregiver is also drawing on casual observations to complete the assessment and consequently may be no more reliable in observing than is a family member.

*Direct observation measures* require the subject to perform an activity at a time and place where the performance can be observed by a trained observer. Measures of direct observation tend to have structured criteria for observing and scoring the activity under consideration. This specificity contributes to the inter-rater reliability of such measures. Observers are trained to look for specific indicators, for example, speed, gait pattern, or sequencing, while assessing function. Among the advantages of these measures are their high degree of face validity and sensitivity to change over time. Direct observation measures are costly, however, in terms of performance time by the older adult and observation time of the observer. These measures tend to be more labor intensive than self-report and proxy measures. Observational measures require that the observer be able to present the directions one step at a time if the subject is unable to comprehend more complex directions. When the observation occurs in the clinic or laboratory setting, the environment is unfamiliar to the subject, which may influence the subject's performance. A major assumption of observation measures is that behavior seen in the clinic or laboratory setting is representative of behavior occurring in the subject's natural environment. For example, the older adult may demonstrate the ability to independently perform lower extremity dressing in the clinic setting with the observer present but may fail to carry out the same activity at home when the only observer is the spouse.

*Performance based measures* of physical function have been available for years. These tests usually focus on dimensions of physical functioning such as balance, strength, speed of performance, gait speed, or hand dexterity. The tasks assess both the physical and mental abilities of the subject because the subject must be able to understand the directions, recognize the props used, and demonstrate planning ability to carry out the physical task. The tasks included in these measures may be simulations rather than the actual activity being assessed. For example, the subject may be asked to transfer five beans, one at a time, with a spoon from a bowl to a plate (Physical Performance Test). This activity is used to simulate functional ability in eating. Performance-based measures are sensitive to change over time, can be used to assess function when recall is limited, and thus have better reliability for persons with mild to moderate cognitive impairment. They have excellent face validity for the tasks being performed (Zimmerman & Magaziner, 1994). A number of disadvantages can be attributed to these measures. Differences in subjects' motivation may create difficulties in assessing actual ability. When subjects do not complete a task, it is difficult to determine if the failure to complete the task is due to low level of motivation, inability to do the task, nonsupportive environment, or a combination of factors (Zimmer et al., 1997). As with direct observation measures, performance that occurs in the laboratory or clinic setting may not equal performance at home or in daily life. Because these measures are time and labor intensive for both the subject and the observer and require a trained observer, these are expensive measures to use.

## SCORING FUNCTIONAL ASSESSMENT MEASURES

Whether the clinician or researcher selects a self-report measure or an observational measure, scoring is an issue. Instruments that provide a summary score may be useful for describing overall function, but summaries can hide much information about the actual functioning of the individual (Morris & Morris, 1997). Changes in function of one or two items can cancel each other out without changing the summary score. Comparison of one subject's score of 43 to another subject's score of 43 tells little about the actual functioning of either subject.

Another approach to summary or aggregated scores is the hierarchical summary score that is produced when instruments, such as the Katz ADL Index, meet Guttman criteria. Theoretically, hierarchical summary scores should produce a score that more precisely describes functional performance of ADLs and IADLs than does a simple summary score (Kovar & Lawton, 1994). Implicit in hierarchical scales, however, are decisions about which tasks are more important. For example, is incontinence with good mobility worse than inability to feed and dress oneself? These decisions are value ladened and not universally accepted. Rather than being used to support decisions about hierarchical importance, most instruments are scored as summaries or profiles. The scoring is easy to construct but difficult to interpret.*

Profile scores consist of a series of separate scores, often called *axes* or *subscales,* that are not summarized into a single score. Profile scores present information about each task being rated and thus help clinicians identify areas of need and plan services to meet those needs.† Profiles are,

however, cumbersome to use in statistical analysis (Feinstein et al., 1986).

With few exceptions, ADL and IADL instruments treat all items equally for scoring purposes. Each item is assigned the same value or weight as every other item. The question arises, however, Should all tasks be weighted equally or should items be weighted unequally based on some predetermined factor? Many clinicians would agree that being dependent in eating is more limiting to the older person than being dependent in upper body dressing. An approach to scoring ADLs using magnitude estimation has been proposed (Finch, Kane, & Philp, 1995). When magnitude estimation is used as the scoring methodology, each item has its own weight that is determined based on its level of importance to the person doing the task. According to the authors, magnitude estimation provides a "more sensitive summation of the nature and extent of functional losses" (Finch et al., 1995, p. 883) than current scoring methods. The weights for the original scoring came from experts in the United States. Subsequent studies have examined patient weights (Kane et al., 1998b). In general, these two sources agree, but clients are more likely to give higher weights to IADL items (Kane et al., 1998a). No functional assessment instruments now in print use magnitude estimation as a basis for scoring.

Many instruments claim to be able to detect change in performance but use only a three-level interval scale such as "no help," "with help," and "unable." Such scales are too coarse to identify subtle changes in performance, especially in the "with help" level.

Another issue related to scoring is the use of assistance. Does the instrument discriminate between assistance provided by another person versus assistance provided by equipment? If the instrument does not make this differentiation, then care planning based on the results of the functional assessment becomes more difficult. Safety in performance is also a factor in assess-

*Reuben and colleagues have tried to extend the hierarchical nature of the ADL measure by creating a measure of Advanced ADLs. They used the answers to three questions to form a score: *(1)* Do you participate in any active sports such as swimming, jogging, tennis, bicycling, aerobics, exercise classes, or other activities that may cause you to work up a sweat or become winded? *(2)* How often do you walk a mile or more at a time, about eight blocks, without resting? *(3)* How often do you walk one quarter of a mile, about two or three blocks, without resting? (Reuben, Laliberte, Hiris, & Mor, 1990). Because this score emphasizes only physical activity, it is not really an extension of the usual ADLs, which generally do not include mobility.

†Think of the difference between a grade point average and grades in each course.

ment and is a factor that is rarely included in assessment instruments.

## SOME COMMONLY USED FUNCTIONAL ASSESSMENT MEASURES

The following discussion of functional assessment instruments examines ADL instruments, IADL instruments, combination instruments, and physical performance instruments. Comparisons of instruments in terms of content, administration, and psychometrics are presented in a series of tables. The instruments included meet the following criteria: reported psychometrics, use with older adults in clinical or research applications, applicable to community dwelling elders, and contribute to the development of a comprehensive assessment tool. Examples of self-report, proxy, direct observation, and performance measures are included among the instruments discussed. Taken as a whole, the group of instruments selected for review are representative of the range of instruments developed in the past 35 years. Instruments that are institution or disease specific are not included.

### Functional Assessment with Activities of Daily Living (ADL) Instruments

In this section, four ADL assessment tools— the Katz Index of Independence in Activities of Daily Living, the Barthel Index, the Rapid Disability Rating Scale-2, and the Functional Independence Measure—are presented. A summary of the administrative properties, contents, psychometrics, and uses of the instruments is presented in Table 2.3. A more detailed comparison of items assessed by each instrument is presented in Table 2.4.

### The Katz Index of Independence in Activities of Daily Living (Index of ADL)

The Katz Index observational tool is the foundation on which all other functional assessment instruments have been built. Originally developed to "study the results

of treatment and prognosis of the elderly and chronically ill" (Katz et al., 1963, p. 914), the tool has been widely used to evaluate the outcomes of treatment. The Katz Index is a measure of performance, what the person does rather than what the person is capable of doing. The trained observer assesses six activities: bathing, dressing, toileting, transferring, continence, and feeding. A three-category scoring model is used for each activity: independent, assistance limited in scope, and extensive assistance or does not do activity. The three categories can, however, be dichotomized into independent and dependent. Persons who are independent do the activity without human assistance but may rely on equipment. Dependence includes both supervision and hands-on help.

Central to the organization and scoring of the instrument is Katz' philosophical belief in the hierarchical nature of ADLs. Research by Katz and others has provided support for the existence of this hierarchical relationship in older adults (Katz et al., 1963; Katz et al., 1970; Siu, Reuben, & Hays, 1990). Given the hierarchical nature of the Katz Index it has been described by Katz as a Guttman Scale, that is, a cumulative scale that measures progressively higher levels of an attribute, in this case ADLs (DeVellis, 1991). For example, if an individual is dependent in feeding, he or she would be dependent in all other items included on the Index.

Spector and Takada (1991) claim, however, that the Index is not a true Guttman scale because the method of scoring described in Table 2.5 does not yield a hierarchical result. According to Siu and associates (1990), the hierarchical relationships found in the Index can be strengthened and the Guttman scalability of the Index improved when the item "continence" is removed. The rationale for the improvement lies in an understanding of the WHO definitions of impairment and disability. Continence is conceptualized as an impairment due to loss of physiological functioning, whereas the five other functions in the

**Table 2.3.**
Summary of the Properties of Four Activities of Daily Living (ADL) Assessment Instruments

| Name | Administration | Content | Reliability | Validity | Use |
|---|---|---|---|---|---|
| Katz ADL (Katz et al., 1963) | Self-report, trained observers | 3 point scale assesses ability to bathe, dress, toilet, transfer, feed self, and maintain bowel, and bladder continence; hierarchical scale | Scale reliability = 0.56 CR = 0.94–0.97* | Correlated with house confinement and mobility post-hospital | Community dwelling, outpatient, nursing home, and hospitalized elderly persons |
| Barthel Index (Roy et al., 1988) | Self-report, trained observers, proxy report, self-report take 2–3 min; in-home observation takes 10–15 min | 3 point scale assesses feeding, grooming, bowel and bladder continence, dressing, toileting, transfers, walking, stairs, and bathing | Inter-rater = 0.88–0.99 α = 0.95–0.96 | Low scores correlated with increased mortality (Beaton & Voge, 1998) | Inpatient and community dwelling older adults |
| Rapid Disability Rating Scale-2 (Linn, 1988) | Proxy report | 3 factors—ADLs, Disability, and Special Problems assessed on 3 point degree-of-severity scale | Inter-rater = 0.62–0.98 Test-retest at 3 days = 0.58–0.96 | Correlated with mortality in nursing home residents | Community dwelling and institutionalized older adults; used in studies of performance change over time |
| Functional Independence Measure (Smith et al., 1996) | Self-report, proxy, observation, telephone survey | 18 items include upper and lower body functioning, communication, and social cognition assessed on 7 point scale | α = 0.97 Subscales = 0.85–0.98 except for social cognition Kappa greater than 0.45 for all noncognitive items | Correlated with success in living in community post-rehabilitation | Inpatient and outpatient older adults with various neurologic and musculoskeletal deficits |

*CR = coefficient of reliability.

**Table 2.4.** Comparison of Content Items Included in Four Activities of Daily Living Assessment Instruments

| Area Assessed/Instrument | Katz | BI | FIM | RDRS-2 |
|---|---|---|---|---|
| Eating/feeding | x | x | x | x |
| Bathing | x | | x | x |
| Grooming/hygiene | | x | x | x |
| Dressing | x | x | x | x |
|   Upper body | | | x | |
|   Lower body | | | x | |
| Toileting | x | x | x | x |
| Transferring | x | x | x | |
|   Chair | x | x | x | |
|   Tub/shower | | | x | |
|   Toilet | | | x | |
| Locomotion | | | | |
|   Walking | | x | x | x |
|   Stairs | | x | x | |
|   Wheelchair | | x | | x |
| Bed mobility | | | | |
| Continence | | | | |
|   Bladder | x | x | x | x |
|   Bowel | x | x | x | x |
| Other | | | x | x |
| Response range | 3 | 2–4 | 7 | 4 |
| Number of items | 6 | 10 | 18 | 18 |
| Type of instrument | Self-report | Observation | Observation | Proxy |

Katz, Katz Index of Independence in Activities of Daily Living; BI, Barthel Index; FIM, Functional Independence Measure; RDRs-2, Rapid Disability Rating Scale-2.

Index—bathing, dressing, transferring, toileting, and feeding—are disabilities resulting from an impairment in physiological function or structure. Thus, continence is a more primitive or basic concept than are the other functions included in the Index. Based on the results of the assessment, persons are assigned a letter score from A to G, with A being the most independent in functioning and G being the most de pendent in functioning. Table 2.5 depicts the classification scheme proposed by Katz.

### The Barthel Index (BI)

The Barthel Index is another classic instrument in ADL assessment (Table 2.6). Originally developed in the 1950s by Mahoney and Barthel, the Barthel Index has been described by its developers as "a simple index of independence to score the ability of a patient with a neuromuscular or musculoskeletal disorder to care for himself, and by repeating the test periodically, to assess his improvement" (Mahoney & Barthel, 1965, p. 61). This 10 item, observational instrument rates the subject according to whether a task can be performed independently or with help. Scores range from 0 to 100, with higher scores indicating greater independence in functioning. It is one of the few functional assessment tools to use a variable weighting scale for scoring. Weights are based on observations of the "actual amount of time and physical assistance required when the individual is unable to perform the activity" (Mahoney & Barthel, 1965, p. 61), although many clinicians who use the Index rely heavily on patient or proxy reports.

The Barthel Index includes definitions for each task, which makes it relatively easy for the trained observer to score. For example, for a patient to receive a score of 10 in ascending and descending stairs, the patient "is able to go up and down a flight of stairs safely without help or supervision. He may and should use handrails,

**Table 2.5.** Katz Index of Independence in Activities of Daily Living Scoring Scheme

| Score | Level of performance of activity |
|---|---|
| A | Independent in feeding, continence, transferring, toileting, dressing, and bathing |
| B | Independent in all but one of the activities listed in A |
| C | Independent in all but bathing and one other activity listed in A |
| D | Independent in all but bathing, dressing, and one other activity listed in A |
| E | Independent in all but bathing, dressing, toileting, and one other activity listed in A |
| F | Independent in all but bathing, dressing, toileting, transferring, and one other activity listed in A |
| G | Dependent in all six activities |
| Other | Dependent in at least two activities, but not classifiable as C, D, E, or F |

canes, or crutches when needed. He must be able to carry canes or crutches as he ascends or descends stairs" (Mahoney & Barthel, 1965, p. 64). A score of 5 means that the patient requires help or supervision in accomplishing any part of the activity.

The Barthel Index is simple to administer, easy to score, and produces a summary score; however, it is not very sensitive to change in performance. Compared with the Katz Index, the Barthel Index provides a more comprehensive assessment of mobility. Its psychometric properties are good (see summary in Table 2.3). For care planning or treatment purposes, the individual task scores are more useful in identifying patient needs than is the total score. With the passage of time, the Barthel Index has

been replaced in many clinical practice settings by more sophisticated and detailed instruments. In the research setting, the Barthel Index remains one of the ADL instruments to which newer instruments are compared. Recent research activities have focused on modifying the Barthel Index for telephone interviews (Shinar et al., 1987) and as an outcome measure in a study of older women with hip fractures (Levi, 1997).

### Rapid Disability Rating Scale-2 (RDRS-2)

The Rapid Disability Rating Scale-2 (Linn & Linn, 1982; Linn, 1988) is a retooled, 18 item version of the original Rapid Disability Rating Scale, an ADL measure. Three factors are included in the instrument: Assistance with Activities of Daily

**Table 2.6.**
The Barthel Index

| Task observed | Scoring (points per item) | |
|---|---|---|
| | With help | Independent |
| Feeding (if food needs to be cut up, score as "with help") | 5 | 10 |
| Moving from wheelchair to bed and return (includes sitting up in bed) | 5–10 | 15 |
| Personal toilet (grooming: wash face, comb hair, shave, clean teeth, and so forth) | 0 | 5 |
| Getting on and off toilet (handling clothes, wipe, flush) | 5 | 10 |
| Bathing self | 0 | 5 |
| Walking on level surface (or, if unable to walk, propel wheelchair) | 10 | 15 |
| | 0* | 5* |
| Ascend and descend stairs | 5 | 10 |
| Dressing (includes tying shoes, fastening fasteners) | 5 | 10 |
| Controlling bowels | 5 | 10 |
| Controlling bladder | 5 | 10 |

*Score only if unable to walk.

Source: Mahoney & Barthel (1965).

Living, 8 items; Degree of Disability, 7 items; and Degree of Special Problems, 3 items (Table 2.7). Each item is rated on a four point scale. A number of changes in design and administration are included in the revised scale.

First, scoring has been expanded from a three point response option to a four point response, which allows for greater discrimination between levels of function. Second, revised instructions focus on current ability and performance, that is, on what the individual actually does rather than what the individual could do. Third, three new items — mobility, toileting, and adaptive tasks — have been added. The item "walking" is still included; however, mobility is a broader concept than walking and includes wheelchair performance. Toileting was added in addition to the original item of continence because the two activities measure different functions. The item "adaptive tasks" was added to measure an area of instrumental ADLs that was common to persons living in the community or in institutional settings.

The RDRS-2 is designed to be completed by a proxy/family member or professional caregiver who has observed the subject performing the tasks. The developers of the instrument recommend that observers complete a training session to increase reliability. Responses are based on observations of the current functioning of the subject. Items are scored from 1 = none (completely independent) to 4 = total (person cannot or will not or may not

due to medical condition perform a behavior). Summated scores range from 18 to 72. According to Linn and Linn (1982), community dwelling older adults with minimal disabilities have scores averaging 21 to 22, whereas the average score of hospitalized elderly adults is about 32 and the average score of nursing home residents is about 36.

## The Functional Independence Measure (FIM)

The Functional Independence Measure, an 18 item Likert-like summated rating scale of ADLs, is the result of a collaborative effort begun by members of the American Academy of Physical Medicine and Rehabilitation in 1984 and continued by staff at the State University of New York at Buffalo (Black, 1998). The FIM is unique among ADL instruments in both the method of is development and in the establishment of a network of users through the Uniform Data System (UDS) for Medical Rehabilitation. Membership in the UDS has allowed institutions using the FIM to compare the outcomes of patients treated in their programs with the outcomes of patients treated in other programs around the country and internationally. The FIM has undergone extensive testing with older adults who have been diagnosed with a multitude of neurologic and orthopedic conditions (Pollak, Rheault, & Stoecker, 1996; Stineman et al., 1996). Currently, there are three versions of the FIM: a telephone version (FONE

Table 2.7.
Factor Composition of Rapid Disability Rating Scale-2

| Factor 1: Activities of Daily Living | Factor 2: Disability | Factor 3: Special Problems |
|---|---|---|
| Eating | Communication | Mental confusion |
| Walking | Hearing | Uncooperativeness |
| Mobility | Sight | Depression |
| Bathing | Diet | |
| Dressing | In bed during day | |
| Toileting | Incontinence | |
| Grooming | Medication | |
| Adaptive tasks | | |

FIM) used for self-report or family proxy report, a mail survey, and an in-person assessment. The FIM was designed to assess the "burden of care" based on an individual's need for assistance, either human or equipment, in six areas: self-care, transfers, sphincter control, locomotion, communication, and social cognition (Hamilton et al., 1987). Each area is scored on a seven level scale, with a score of 1 indicating that the person requires total assistance and a score of 7 indicating that the person can accomplish the task independently in a safe and timely manner (Table 2.8). Scores can be reported as a total score, as a motor score (13 items) and a cognitive domain score (5 items), or as a profile of the separate items (Bonwich & Reid, 1991).

Compared with other ADL instruments, the FIM takes more time to complete and score, but it is more sensitive to change than are other ADL instruments (Kidd et al., 1995). The FIM suffers from floor and ceiling effects for some groups of elders and disabled persons. The social cognitive items have poorer psychometrics than other items. Observers require training and experience in using it before being considered competent in its use. Written directions and decision trees for scoring the FIM are included in the scoring booklet that is provided to users.

## Instrumental Activities of Daily Living Instruments

Although there are many IADL instruments available and the concept of IADL is generally understood as describing those activities necessary for independent living in the community, there is no universally accepted operational definition (Ward et al., 1998). Both cultural and gender biases may be present in some IADL measures

Table 2.8.
The Functional Independence Measure

| Domain | Item | Scoring | | |
|---|---|---|---|---|
| | | Level | Numeric value | Description |
| Motor | Self-care | Independence | 7 | Complete independence |
| | Feeding | | | Timely, safely |
| | Grooming | | | Uses device |
| | Bathing | Modified | 5 | Supervision |
| | Upper body dressing | dependence | 4 | Minimal assistance |
| | Lower body dressing | | | (subject does 75% + of effort) |
| | Toileting | | 3 | Moderate assistance |
| | Sphincter control | | | (subject does 50% + of effort) |
| | Bladder management | Complete | 2 | Maximal assistance |
| | Bowel management | dependence | | (subject does 25% + of effort) |
| | Mobility transfers | | 1 | Total assistance |
| | Bed, chair, wheelchair | | | (subject does 0% of effort) |
| | Toilet | | | |
| | Tub, shower | | | |
| | Locomotion | | | |
| | Walk/wheelchair | | | |
| | Stairs | | | |
| Cognitive | Communication | | | |
| | Comprehension | | | |
| | Expression | | | |
| | Social cognition | | | |
| | Social interaction | | | |
| | Problem solving | | | |
| | Memory | | | |

Source: Kidd et al. (1995).

(Fillenbaum, 1985). Most assessments include items on cooking, housework, and laundry, which are activities generally performed by women, particularly in older cohorts. There is an underlying emphasis on cognitive functioning, as reflected by the inclusion of items such as ability to use the telephone and manage finances and medications, that may be appropriate to assess some groups of older persons (e.g., stroke survivors) but less relevant for other groups. In addition, some of the IADLs assessed are done voluntarily as a couple activity by older adults. For example, a couple may shop together or may divide housework activities voluntarily whether or not assistance is actually required. Measures of IADLs should be able to distinguish between this type of voluntary dependence from involuntary dependence occurring because the individual is physically or cognitively unable to perform the task in question. Table 2.9 presents psychometric and administrative information about three selected IADL measures. A detailed comparison of content items of the three IADL instruments is presented in Table 2.10.

### Instrumental Activities of Daily Living Scale (IADL)

Developed by Lawton and Brody (1969) and their associates at the Philadelphia Geriatric Center during the 1960s, the IADL Scale was the first assessment tool to measure the more complex ADLs that demonstrate a person's ability to adapt to the environment. It was intended to be used as a guide to determine the most appropriate living arrangement for an elderly person (Lawton, 1970). The Lawton IADL Scale is a measure of performance rather than ability (although this rule is frequently violated) that includes eight items for women and five items for men (Table 2.11).

The eight items of the Lawton IADL Scale form a Guttman scale with Item A, ability to use the telephone, being the lowest level item and Item H, handling finances, being the highest level functional

activity (Spector, 1990). The instrument produces a summary score with a range of 0 (low function) to 8 (high function). A score of 1 in some items does not, however, mean that the highest performance criteria in that item has been met. For instance, in the item "ability to use the telephone" a score of 1 can be assigned for three of the four criteria. Only the criterion "does not use telephone at all" is rated as 0. Similarly, in the area of housekeeping, only the criteria "does not participate in any housekeeping tasks" is rated as zero, while the other four criteria are assigned a rating of 1. On the other hand, three items — shopping, food preparation, and medication administration — require complete independence in order to be scored as a 1. Finally, a gender bias is reflected in the scoring of "mode of transportation" because women can achieve a score of 1 and be more dependent in using transportation than men. This inconsistency in scoring can obscure the actual degree of functional limitation being demonstrated by the older person.

### The Older Americans Resources and Services Multidimensional Functional Assessment Questionnaire — IADL (OARS-IADL)

Developed and revised during the 1970s, the Older Americans Resources and Services Multidimensional Functional Assessment Questionnaire (OMFAQ), assesses five dimensions of personal functioning — social, economic, mental health, physical health, and self-care capacity — and service utilization (Fillenbaum & Smyer, 1981). The IADL component of the OARS has been developed as a separate, seven item, self-report assessment tool (Table 2.12) adapted from the Lawton IADL Scale (Fillenbaum, 1985). Unlike the Lawton IADL Scale, all items are asked of both men and women. Each item has three response options: without help, with help, or unable. The response of "with help" does not, however, distinguish between help provided by human assistance and help pro-

**Table 2.9.**

Summary of the Properties of Three IADL Assessments

| Name | Administration | Content | Reliability | Validity | Use |
|---|---|---|---|---|---|
| Lawton IADL (Spector, 1990) | Self-report measure of performance rather than ability | Items for Guttman Scale; use of telephone, housekeeping, food preparation, laundry, transportation, medications, money management; all items used for women; food preparation, laundry, housekeeping eliminated for men. | Inter-rater = 0.85 CR = 0.96 for men and 0.93 for women | Correlations with ADLs, mental status, physical health = 0.77, 0.74, and 0.50, respectively | Community dwelling older adults; may be used for hospital-based discharge planning; not useful for assessment of institutionalized elderly persons |
| OARS-IADL (Fillenbaum, 1985) | Self-report, trained observer | 5 item Guttman Scale (housework, travel, shop, meals, finances) and telephone use, medication administration | Test–retest = 0.71 at 5 weeks | Correlation with physical health = 0.54–0.55, mental health = 0.54–0.60 | Screening tool for determining need for services by community dwelling older adults |
| DAFA (Karagiozis et al., 1998) | Direct observation of performance; requires use of special equipment; time of assessment ranges from 45 min to 1.5 h | 7 areas—money management, shopping, hobbies, meal preparation, awareness, reading, and transportation | Test–retest = 0.95 ICC = 0.95 | Statistically significant difference in performance between cognitively intact and demented older persons | Cognitively impaired older persons in outpatient setting |

IADL, Instrumental Activities of Daily Living; OARS-IADL, Older Americans Resources and Services Instrumental Activities of Daily Living; DAFA, Direct Assessment of Functional Abilities; CR, coefficient of reliability; ICC, inter-class correlation.

**Table 2.10.**
Comparison of Content Items Included for Assessment in Three IADL Instruments

| Name/area | Lawton IADL scale | OARS-IADL scale | DAFA |
|---|---|---|---|
| Use of telephone | x | x | |
| Shopping | x | x | x |
| Meal preparation | x | x | x–2 items |
| Housekeeping | x | x | x |
| Laundry | x | | |
| Transportation | x | x | x |
| Self-medication | x | x | |
| Money management | x | x | x–2 items |
| Other | | | |
|   Hobbies | | | x |
|   Awareness | | | x–2 items |
|   Reading | | | x |
| Number of items | 8 | 7 | 10 |
| Response range | 5 | 3 | 4 |
| Type | Self-report, observation | Self-report | Direct observation |

IADL, Instrumental Activities of Daily Living; OARS-IADL, Older Americans' Resources and Services Instrumental Activities of Daily Living; DAFA, Direct Assessment of Functional Abilities.

vided via devices. The instrument, either self-administered or interviewer administered, has been used as a screening tool to determine the need for further assessment in older adults and for resource allocation (Reuben et al., 1995; Ottenbacher et al., 1994).

The scoring range is from 14 (independent functioning) to 0 (dependent functioning). Based on the results of factor analysis, five of the items (housework, travel, shopping, meal preparation, and finances) included on the scale form a Guttman scale.

### Direct Assessment of Functional Abilities (DAFA)

The Direct Assessment of Functional Abilities is a newly developed, 10 item, observational measure of IADLs designed for use with persons with dementia (Karagiozis et al., 1998). It is based on the Pfeiffer Functional Activities Questionnaire (PFAQ), an indirect, self-report assessment tool. Like the PFAQ, the DAFA consists of 10 items that represent seven domains of interest: money management, shopping, hobbies, meal preparation, awareness, reading, and transportation (Table 2.13). With the DAFA, individuals are asked to perform the task being assessed in the presence of the observer, whereas with the PFAQ, individuals are asked to report if they can do the task. The DAFA has been used with elderly persons with dementia and with control group of elderly persons.

Although the DAFA is a new instrument

**Table 2.11.**
Lawton Instrumental Activities of Daily Living

| Item | No. of criteria | Score |
|---|---|---|
| Ability to use telephone | 4 | 1–0 |
| Shopping | 3 | 1–0 |
| Food preparation* | 3 | 1–0 |
| Housekeeping* | 5 | 1–0 |
| Laundry* | 3 | 1–0 |
| Mode of transportation | 5 | 1–0 |
| Medication administration | 3 | 1–0 |
| Handling finances | 3 | 1–0 |

*Items not scored for men.

**Table 2.12.** Components of the Older Americans Resources and Services Instrumental Activities of Daily Living

| Question | Response option | | |
|---|---|---|---|
| | Without help (2) | With help (1) | Unable (0) |
| Can you use the telephone? | | | |
| Can you get to places out of walking distance? | | | |
| Can you go shopping (groceries/clothing)? | | | |
| Can you prepare your own meals? | | | |
| Can you do your own housework? | | | |
| Can you take your own medications? | | | |
| Can you handle your own money? | | | |

and has been used only in a limited number of settings, the initial psychometrics are encouraging. A disadvantage of the tool is the length of time required to complete the assessment, 45 minutes for control subjects and 1.5 hours for persons with dementia. The DAFA does, however, provide a better indication of actual functional ability of persons with dementia than does self-report (overestimation) or proxy report (underestimation) (Karagiozis et al., 1998).

**Combination ADL-IADL Instruments**

Combination instruments are becoming more frequently used in the assessment of

function. Because these instruments include both ADL and IADL components, they tend to require more time to complete. Tables 2.14 and 2.15 present psychometric and content information on selected combination instruments.

*Questionnaire on Clinical and Preclinical Disability (QCPD)*

A promising recent self-report measure that combines both ADLs and IADLs is the Questionnaire on Clinical and Preclinical Disability (Fried et al., 1996), a 27 item instrument (Table 2.16). The uniqueness of the instrument lies in its inclusion of an assessment of Task Difficulty and

**Table 2.13.**
Components and Scoring of the Direct Assessment of Functional Abilities Measure

| Domain | Item No. | Task |
|---|---|---|
| Money management | 1 | Write a check, record it in a ledger, and subtract for correct balance |
| | 2 | Complete an insurance form |
| Shopping | 3 | Shop alone for basic necessities using a list of 3 items |
| Hobbies | 4 | Play bingo or checkers |
| Meal preparation | 5 | Make coffee |
| | 6 | Make a sandwich |
| Awareness | 7 | Talk about current events in politics, sports, or entertainment |
| | 9 | Report birth date, next national holiday, number and schedule of medication |
| Reading | 8 | Summarize three main points of a passage from a story |
| Transportation | 10 | Locate the cafeteria using directions provided |

| Scoring | Value | Definition |
|---|---|---|
| | 0 | Performs without difficulty or help |
| | 1 | "Difficulty": does task without cues but states that it is difficult; or becomes agitated, frustrated, self-centered |
| | 2 | "Assistance": needs verbal, visual, or other cues, repeated directions, or physical aid; uses three or fewer cues to complete task |
| | 3 | "Dependent": incorrectly performs, unable to perform, refuses to complete, or requires more than three cues to perform task |

Source: Adapted from Karagiozis et al. (1998).

**Table 2.14.** Summary of the Properties of Four Selected Activities of Daily Living (ADL) and Instrumental Activities of Daily Living (IADL) Combination Instruments

| Name | Administration | Content | Reliability | Validity | Use |
|---|---|---|---|---|---|
| QCPD (Fried et al., 1996) | Self-report screening tool | Assesses 27 ADLs and IADLs for difficulty in performance, task modifications made, and frequency of performance | Test–retest = 0.74–0.86 | Construct and criterion validity assessed as acceptable | Identification of subtle indicators of early functional decline in community dwelling elderly persons |
| FSI (Jette, 1980) | Self-report, interview | Assesses 18 items in 4 domains for degree of assistance, pain, difficulty | Test–retest = 0.65–0.81 inter-rater = 0.65–0.91 | Not given | Used with community dwelling older adults with degenerative joint disease and other musculoskeletal conditions |
| DAFS (Lowenstein et al., 1989) | Direct observation | Assesses time orientation, communication skills, transportation, financial skills, shopping, eating, dressing/grooming | Test–retest = 0.71–0.91, depending on subscale for cognitively impaired and 0.91–0.97 for controls | Correlation with Blessed Scale = −0.58 to 0.65; convergent validity with medical records = 0.59–0.65 | Screening for declining function in cognitively impaired elders living in community |
| UNI (Allen & Mor, 1997) | Self-report, interview proxy | Assesses 11 items for difficulty, need for additional help, | a = 0.78 (ADLs) and 0.79 (IADLs) | Not presented | Screening devise with community dwelling elders; used to identify service needs |

QCPD, Questionnaire on Clinical and Preclinical Disability; FSI, Functional Status Index; DAFS, Direct Assessment of Functional Status; UNI, Unmet Needs Indices.

**Table 2.15.** Comparison of Content Items Included in Four Activities of Daily Living (ADL) and Instrumental Activities of Daily Living (IADL) Combination Instruments

| Name/area | QCPD | FSI | DAFS | UNI |
|---|---|---|---|---|
| | | ADLs | | |
| Eating | x | | x | x |
| Grooming | x | | x | |
| Bathing | x | | | x |
| Dressing | x | x (2 items) | x | x |
| Toileting | x | x | | x |
| Transfers | | | | |
|   Bed | x | x | | x |
|   Car | x | | | |
| Locomotion | | | | |
|   Walk | x | x (2 items) | | x |
|   Stairs | x | x | | |
| Continence | | | | |
| Other ADL | | | | |
| | | IADLs | | |
| Heavy housework | x | | | x |
| Light housework | x | x (3 items) | | x |
| Shopping | x | x | x | x |
| Manage money | x | | x | |
| Telephone | x | | x | |
| Self-medication | x | | | |
| Open jars | x | | | |
| Lift/carry 10 pounds | x | x | | |
| Meal preparation | x | x | | x |
| Other | Assesses difficulty, modifications | Assesses amount of assistance, pain, difficulty; 3 social activities | Includes transportation, letter preparation, time orientation, 4 items related to finance | Includes transportation, use of help |
| Number of items | 27 | 18 | 7 domains | 11 |
| Response range | 4 | 4–5 | 104 points possible | 3 |
| Type | Self-report | Self-report | Direct observation | Self-report, proxy |

QCPD, Questionnaire on Clinical and Preclinical Disability; FSI, Functional Status Index; DAFS, Direct Assessment of Functional Status; UNI, Unmet Needs Indices.

Task Modification as well as assessment of Task Function for each of the 27 items. Drawing on the WHO definition of disability, this questionnaire asks the respondent whether he or she has difficulty or dependency in doing a task. If the individual reports no difficulty in performing a task, the individual is then asked if he or she has modified the way in which the task is done. This modification includes a change in the frequency of doing the task or a change in the method of doing the task due to underlying health problems. Inclusion of the dimension of Task Modification is particularly relevant in the assessment of physical function in older adults because many adults make subtle changes in how they perform tasks or in the frequency with which they do tasks in order to maintain independence. According to Fried and associates, task modification is a compensatory strategy that allows the older adult to continue to age in place. The occurrence of task modification is considered to be a sign of early or preclinical disability. Thus, data collected with the instrument may help the clinician identify persons who are in the early stages of functional decline.

**Table 2.16.** Tasks Assessed by the Questionnaire on Clinical and Preclinical Disabilities and Types of Questions Asked About Each Task

| Task (self-report) | Basic Activities of Daily Living (ADLs) |
|---|---|
| Mobility tasks | Dress self |
| Walk one-half mile | Bathe or shower |
| Get out of car (transfer) | Feed self |
| Walk 150 feet | Cut toenails |
| Walk around home | |
| Get out of bed | |
| Walk up 10 steps | |
| Walk down 10 steps | |
| Stoop, crouch, kneel | |

| | Instrumental ADLs |
|---|---|
| Do heavy housework | Upper extremity strength |
| Do light housework | Lift/carry 10 pounds |
| Do own shopping | Reach out with arms |
| Prepare own meals | Get down 5 pounds |
| Manage own money | Grip with hands |
| Give self-medications | Open jars |
| Read | |
| Drive | |

**Questions asked:**
1. Do you have any difficulty with (task)?
    0 = No
    1 = Yes
    2 = No longer do the task due to difficulty
    3 = Could do it but do not for nonhealth reasons
2. Have you changed how frequently (how often) you do (task)?
    0 = No
    1 = Yes, do more frequently
    2 = Yes, do less frequently
    3 = Yes, do not do it any more
3. Have you changed (modified) the method that you use to do (task) compared with how you did it before?
    0 = No
    1 = Yes, changed the way I do it (then ask what are the changes)
4. What is the main symptom that caused you to modify, change the frequency, or have difficulty with this task?
5. What is the main health condition that caused you to modify, change the frequency, or have difficulty with this task?

Source: Adapted from Fried et al. (1996).

## Functional Status Index (FSI)

The Functional Status Index was initially developed as a performance assessment instrument for the Pilot Geriatric Arthritis Project of the Michigan Regional Medical Program (Deniston & Jette, 1980). The unique contribution of the FSI is its focus on three aspects of function: dependence (the degree of help or assistance the person needs to perform an activity), difficulty (how easy or hard it is to perform an activity), and pain (the degree of discomfort or pain experienced when the person performs the activity). Although the original instrument consisted of 45 ADLs and IADLs grouped into three broad categories of Mobility, Personal Care, and Work that required one to one and a half hours to complete, the instrument has been revised to an 18 item, self-report measure that requires less than 15 minutes to complete. Through the use of structural analysis techniques, the items of the assessment can be grouped into five indexes of function (Table 2.17). The items of the Hand Activities index have been deleted from the self-report measure.

The FSI draws on the older adult's memories of the previous 7 days to answer questions about the amount of assistance

**Table 2.17.**

Five Indexes and Component Activities of the Functional Status Index

| *Mobility* | *Personal care* | *Home chores* |
|---|---|---|
| Walking outside* | Washing all body parts | Doing laundry |
| Walking inside* | Putting on pants | Reaching into low cupboard* |
| Climbing stairs* | Putting on shirt | Doing yard work |
| Transfers*: | Buttoning shirt | Vacuuming a rug |
| Bed to chair | Putting on socks† | Preparing meals† |
| Tub | Getting on and off toilet† | Washing dishes† |
| | Putting on shoes† | Doing light housework† |

| *Hand activities* | *Interpersonal activities* |
|---|---|
| Opening containers | Driving a car |
| Writing | Visiting friends or relatives* |
| Dialing a phone | Attending appointments or meetings* |
| | Performing your job |
| | Shopping for groceries† |
| | Carrying a heavy bundle† |
| | Taking care of other people† |
| | Using public transportation† |

*Item included in both original assessment measure and in revised self-report measure.

†Item added to revised self-report measure but not included in original performance measure.

(human or equipment) needed to perform each activity, the amount of difficulty experienced, and the amount of pain experienced. Each of the three dimensions has a separate rating scale (Table 2.18).

Scoring of the FSI results in three summary functional scores—assistance, pain, difficulty—that can be divided by the number of items in each category to obtain an average score. Combining the three functional scores to achieve a total score results in a meaningless number that masks the influence of assistance, pain, and difficulty on functional ability. The FSI has been used to measure change in functional ability in community dwelling and hospitalized older adults with arthritis and other conditions affecting the joints (Jette, 1980).

### Direct Assessment of Functional Status (DAFS)

The Direct Assessment of Functional Status was developed specifically to assess functional ability in persons with dementia (Lowenstein et al., 1989). The instrument was designed to assess higher order functional abilities required to live in a non-institutionalized environment and not included in other observational tools such as Lawton's IADL Scale or Kuriansky and Gurland's Performance Activities of Daily Living (1976). The DAFS is a behaviorally based, direct observation tool in which the subject is tested in performing specific tasks grouped into seven scales: Time orientation, 16 points; communication skills, 17 points; transportation skills, 13 points;

**Table 2.18.**

Rating Scales of the Functional Status Index

| Assistance: | 1 = independent; 2 = uses devices; 3 = uses human assistance; 4 = uses devices and human assistance; 5 = unable or unsafe |
|---|---|
| Pain: | 1 = no pain; 2 = mild pain; 3 = moderate pain; 4 = severe pain |
| Difficulty: | 1 = no difficulty; 2 = mild difficulty; 3 = moderate difficulty; 4 = severe difficulty |

**Table 2.19.**
Examples of Scales of the Direct Assessment of Functional Status

|  | Correct (1 point) | Incorrect (0 points) |
|---|---|---|
| *Scale II. Communication skills* |  |  |
| Part B. Preparing a letter for mailing |  |  |
| Fold in half | ——— | ——— |
| Put in envelope | ——— | ——— |
| Seal envelope | ——— | ——— |
| Stamp envelope | ——— | ——— |
| Address (must be exact duplicate of examiner's copy) | ——— | ——— |
| Return address (must place correct address in upper left hand corner) | ——— | ——— |
| *Scale IV. Financial* |  |  |
| Part D. Balancing a checkbook |  |  |
| Amount A ($500 − $350) | ——— | ——— |
| Correct: $150 |  |  |
| Amount B ($323 − $23.50) | ——— | ——— |
| Correct: $299.50 |  |  |
| Amount C ($21.75 − $3.92) | ——— | ——— |
| Correct: $17.83 |  |  |

Source: Adapted from Lowenstein et al. (1989).

financial skills, 21 points; shopping skills, 16 points; grooming, 13 points; and eating, 10 points. Discrete steps that must be observed in performance are included in each subscale. Examples of components of scales are presented in Table 2.19.

The DAFS takes 30–35 minutes to administer and results in a summary score of functional performance. According to the developers, the transportation scale may be considered as an optional scale because many elderly persons have never driven. For comparison purposes, the maximum score is 93 points, which is indicative of normal functional ability. The DAFS has shown the ability to discriminate between normal elderly adults and elderly adults with dementia due to multiple infarcts or to Alzheimer's disease.

### The Unmet Needs Indices (UNI)

A recent addition to the ranks of ADL-IADL measures, the Unmet Needs Indices is a self-report or proxy report instrument that is based on the Katz Index of ADL and Lawton's IADL Scale (see Table 2.20 for contents of UNI). Its unique contribution to assessment is its focus on whether the need for help is met or not met. The UNI measures functional status of the respondent and the respondent's perception of the adequacy of the help received with activities that the respondent cannot do alone (Allen & Mor, 1997). Eleven func-

**Table 2.20.**
Components of the Unmet Needs Indices

| Domain | Task | Domain | Task |
|---|---|---|---|
| Activities of Daily Living | Bathing<br>Dressing<br>Eating<br>Transferring<br>Toileting<br>Moving around indoors | Instrumental Activities of Daily Living | Cooking<br>Light housekeeping<br>Heavy housekeeping<br>Shopping<br>Transportation |

tional activities are assessed. For each activity assessed, the UNI asks the following questions:

1. Do you do the activity alone, or does someone help you?
2. Do you use special equipment to assist you in doing the activity?
3. Is the activity difficult, somewhat difficult, or very difficult to do alone?
4. Have you needed (additional) help with the activity in the past month?
5. Have there been times in the past month when you have not done the activity because no one was available to help you?

In addition to these five questions, questions about the consequences or adverse effects of not having sufficient help are also asked.

At this time, the UNI has been used only for research purposes. Its clinical practice usefulness has not been tested. The potential strength of the UNI, however, is its application in care planning with community dwelling older adults.

### Physical Performance Measures

Physical performance measures provide an objective, standardized way of evaluating performance without having to rely on self-report or proxy reports of function. Criteria for evaluating function are predetermined and concrete. As a rule, physical performance measures use speed of functioning as an essential component. There

**Table 2.21.**
Summary of the Properties of Three Physical Performance Measures

| Name | Administration | Content | Reliability | Comments |
|---|---|---|---|---|
| TMP Test (Zimmer et al., 1997) | Administration time = 15–20 min; uses trained observer and props; automated version available | Assesses upper body function | "Moderate" internal consistency is reported | Timed for dominant and nondominant hand; strong predictor of LTC and dependent living; William et al. (1990) found significant differences in performance due to age, race, education and income |
| PPT (Reuben & Siu, 1990) | Administered by trained observer; requires 10–15 min to complete; either 7 or 9 item format; has established timed performance criteria | Upper body fine and coarse motor function, balance, mobility, coordination, endurance | $\alpha = 0.87$ (9 item) and 0.79 (7 item) <br><br> Inter-rater = 0.99 (9 item) and 0.93 (7 − item) <br><br> Correlation with Katz = 0.65 (9 item) and 0.50 (7 item) <br><br> Scale reliability = 0.77 | 7 Item test omits stair climbing activities |
| PADL (Kuriansky & Gurland, 1976) | Trained observer; uses props; 2 min is allowed for subject to complete each activity; short form available | Upper body (14 activities) and lower body (2 activities) functioning | High correlations with proxy reports, psychiatric diagnoses, and physical health <br><br> Inter-rater = 0.90 | High predictive validity for future hospitalizations and mortality |

TMP, Timed Manual Performance; PPT, Physical Performance Test; PALD, Performance Activities of Daily Living.

are several disadvantages to these measures. They are time consuming, require special equipment and trained observers, and can be potentially injurious to the person being evaluated (Guralnik et al., 1989). Table 2.21 presents information on psychometrics and contents for three physical performance measures.

## Physical Performance Test (PPT)

The Physical Performance Test is a timed, nine item or seven item, direct observation measure of upper body and lower body physical functioning that can be completed within 5 to 10 minutes and requires one observer and a limited number of props (Reuben & Siu, 1990; Reuben et al., 1995). The PPT assesses upper body fine motor and coarse motor functions, balance, mobility, coordination, and endurance. Simulated ADLs include eating, dressing, and transferring. The nine items can be arranged in a Guttman scale according to degree of difficulty, with writing a sentence being the least difficult and stair climbing being the most difficult activity assessed. Scoring of each item is based on a five point scale (0–4), with 4 being "less than 10 seconds" to 1 being "more than 20 seconds" to 0 being "unable to do." In this instrument, longer time of performance is equated with increased difficulty of performance. The PPT has been used to assess performance of community dwelling older adults.

## Timed Manual Performance Test (TMP)

The Timed Manual Performance is a brief, relatively inexpensive, two part screening instrument that measures speed and dexterity in the performance of selected activities that are representative of everyday tasks (Williams et al., 1994). The instrument assesses upper body functioning and can be administered by a person with minimal training. The first part consists of opening and closing nine different types of fasteners. The second part consists of five measures of hand skill: copying a short

sentence; simulated page turning (turning over 3 × 5 index cards); picking up two paper clips, pennies, and bottle caps and placing them in a container; stacking four checkers; and simulated eating (transferring kidney beans from one bowl to another). Each task is timed for the dominant and nondominant hand. The TMP takes approximately 15 minutes to perform and yields 27 distinct measurements. The TMP has been standardized with a sample of 1300 community dwelling older adults.

## The Performance Activities of Daily Living (PADL)

The Performance Activities of Daily Living is a timed test of performance of selected ADL and IADLs. It was originally developed by Kuriansky and Gurland (1976) as part of the Comprehensive Assessment and Referral Evaluation project for use in a study of mental illness in older people in New York and London. The original PADL includes 16 items, and a shorter form uses five items (Table 2.22); it requires a trained observer as the assessor and specific props. During the assessment process, the individual has 2 minutes to complete each task. If a task is not com-

Table 2.22. Components of the Performance Activities of Daily Living

| Upper body |
| --- |
| Drink from cup* |
| Wipe nose with tissue |
| Comb hair* |
| File nails |
| Shave |
| Lift food onto spoon and into mouth* |
| Turn faucet on and off |
| Turn light switch on and off |
| Put on and take off jacket* |
| Put on and remove slipper* |
| Brush teeth |
| Make phone call |
| Sign name |
| Turn key in lock |

| Lower body |
| --- |
| Stand up and walk a few steps and sit down |

*Item included in short form of the measure.

pleted in 2 minutes, the next task is introduced. Items are scored as "2" or independent if no cuing is required, as "1" if verbal cues are needed, and as "0" if the task is attempted but not completed.

## STATE OF THE ART IN FUNCTIONAL ASSESSMENT

A plethora of instruments are available to assess function. Many, especially those created to meet a specific institutional need, lack adequate psychometric testing and a sound rationale in developmental methodology. Although some instruments are designed for a specific chronic health condition, as a rule the severity of illness and the complexity of chronic health problems are not considered in either the performance or the scoring of instruments. There is a focus on disability and dependence without a consideration of strengths. The impact of the environment also is not considered.

The future of functional assessment might well be served by calling a moratorium on developing new instruments and by weeding out instruments that have poor psychometric characteristics.

## REFERENCES

Allen, S., & Mor, V. (1997). The prevalence and consequences of unmet need. *Medical Care, 35*(11), 1132–1148.

Applegate, W. B., Blass, J. P., & Williams, T. F. (1990). Instruments for the functional assessment of older patients. *New England Journal of Medicine, 322*(17), 1207–1214.

Asberg, K., & Sonn, U. (1988). The cumulative structure of personal and instrumental ADL. *Scandanavian Journal of Rehabilitation Medicine, 21,* 171–177.

Beaton, S., & Voge, S. (1998). *Measurements for long-term care.* Thousand Oaks, CA: Sage.

Bernstein, L. (1992). A public health approach to functional assessment. *Caring* (December), 32–38.

Black, T. (1998). FIM system adapts to rehabilitation's changing needs. *ARN Network, 14*(1), 1–2.

Bonwich, E., & Reid, J. (1991). Medical rehabilitation: Issues in assessment of functional change. *Evaluation Practice, 12*(3), 205–215.

Boucher, R. (1989). Nursing process. In S. Dittmar (Ed.), *Rehabilitation Nursing Process and Application* (pp. 45–62). St. Louis: C.V. Mosby.

Czaja, S., Weber, R., & Sankaran, N. (1993). A human factors analysis of ADL activities: A capability-demand approach. *The Journals of Gerontology, 48*(Special Issue), 44–48.

Deniston, O., & Jette, A. (1980). A functional status assessment instrument: Validation in an elderly population. *Health Services, 15*(1), 21–34.

DeVellis, R. F. (1991). *Scale Development: Theories and Applications.* Newbury Park, CA: Sage.

Dorevitch, M. I., Cossar, R. M., Bailey, F. J., Bisset, T., Lewis, S. J., Wise, L. A., & MacLennan, W. J. (1992). The accuracy of self and informant ratings of physical capacity in the elderly. *Journal of Clinical Epidemiology, 45*(7), 791–798.

Feinstein, A., Josephy, B., & Well, C. (1986). Scientific and clinical problems in indexes of functional disability. *Annals of Internal Medicine, 105*(3), 413–420.

Fillenbaum, G. G. (1985). Screening the elderly. A brief instrumental activities of daily living measure. *Journal of the American Geriatrics Society, 33*(10), 698–706.

Fillenbaum, G. C., & Smyer, M. (1981). The development, validity and reliability of the ORS multidimensional functional assessment questionnaire. *Journal of Gerontology, 36*(4), 428–434.

Finch, M., Kane, R. L., & Philp, I. (1995). Developing a new metric for ADLs. *Journal of the American Geriatrics Society, 43*(8), 877–884.

Fried, L., Bandeen-Roche, K., Williamson, J., Prasada-Rao, P., Chee, E., Tepper, S., & Rubin, G. (1996). Functional decline in older adults: Expanding methods of ascertainment. *Journal of Gerontology: Medical Sciences, 51A*(5), M206–M214.

Glass, T. A. (1998). Conjugating the "tenses" of function: Discordance among hypothetical, experimental, and enacted function in older adults. *Gerontologist, 38*(1), 101–112.

Guralnik, J., Branch, L., Cummings, S., & Curb, J. (1989). Physical performance measures in aging research. *Journal of Gerontology, 44*(5), M141–M146.

Guralnik, J., Ferrucci, L., Simonsick, E., Salive, M., & Wallace, R. (1995). Lower-extremity function in persons over the age of 70 years as a predictor of subsequent disability. *New England Journal of Medicine,* 332(8), 556–561.

Hamilton, B. B., Granger, C. V., Sherwin, F. S., Zielezny, M., & Tashman, J. S. (1987). A uniform national data system for medical rehabilitation. In M. J. Fuhrer (Ed.), *Rehabilitation Outcomes: Analysis and Measurement.* Baltimore: Brookes Publishing Co.

Ikegami, N. (1995). Functional assessment and its place in health care. *New England Journal of Medicine,* 332(9), 598–599.

Jette, A. (1980). Functional Status Index: Reliability of a chronic disease evaluation instrument. *Archives of Physical Medicine and Rehabilitation,* 61(9), 395–401.

Kane, R. L., Rockwood, T., Finch, M., & Philp, I. (1998a). Consumer and professional ratings of the importance of functional status components. *Health Care Financing Review,* 19(2), 11–22.

Kane, R. L., Rockwood, T., Philp, I., & Finch, M. (1998b). Differences in valuation of functional status components among consumers and professionals in Europe and the United States. *Journal of Clinical Epidemiology,* 51(8), 657–666.

Karagiozis, H., Gray, S., Sacco, J., Shapiro, M., & Kawas, C. (1998). The Direct Assessment of Functional Abilities (DAFA): A comparison to an indirect measure of instrumental activities of daily living. *Gerontologist,* 38(1), 113–121.

Katz, S., Down, T., Cash, H., & Grotz, R. (1970). Progressive development of the Index of ADL. *Gerontologist,* 10, 20–30.

Katz, S., Ford, A. B., Moskowitz, R. W., Jackson, B. A., & Jaffee, M. W. (1963). Studies of illness in the aged. The index of ADL: A standardized measure of biological and psychosocial function. *Journal of American Medical Association,* 185(12), 914–919.

Kidd, D., Stewart, G., Baldry, J., Johnson, J., Rossiter, D., Petruckevitch, A., & Thompson, A. (1995). The Functional Independence Measure: A comparative validity and reliability study. *Disability and Rehabilitation,* 17(1), 10–14.

Kovar, M., & Lawton, M. (1994). Functional disability: Activities and instrumental activities of daily living. In M. P. Lawton & J. A. Teresi (Eds.), *Annual Review of Gerontology and Geriatrics* (vol. 4). New York: Springer.

Kuriansky, J. B., & Gurland, B. (1976). Performance test of activities of daily living. *International Journal of Aging and Human Development,* 7, 343–352.

Lawton, M. (1970). Assessment, integration, and environments for older people. *Gerontologist,* 10, 38–46.

Lawton, M. P., & Brody, E. M. (1969). Assessment of older people: Self-maintaining and instrumental activities of daily living. *Gerontologist,* 9, 179–186.

Levi, S. (1997). Posthospital setting, resource utilization, and self-care outcome in older women with hip fracture. *Archives of Physical Medicine and Rehabilitation,* 78(9), 973–979.

Linn, M. (1988). Rapid disability Rating Scale-2 (RDRS-2). *Psychopharmacology Bulletin,* 24(4), 799–800.

Linn, M., & Linn, B. (1982). The Rapid Disability Rating Scale-2. *Journal of the American Geriatrics Society,* 30(6), 378–382.

Lowenstein, D., Amigo, E., Duara, R., Guterman, A., Hurwitz, D., Berkowitz, N., Wilkie, F., Weinberg, G., Black, B., Gittelman, B., & Eisdorfer, C. (1989). A new scale for the assessment of functional status in Alzheimer's disease and related disorders. *Journal of Gerontology: Psychological Sciences,* 44(4), 114–121.

Magaziner, J. (1992). The use of proxy respondents in health studies of the aged. In R. B. Wallase & R. F. Woolsen (Eds.), *The Epidemiologic Study of the Elderly* (pp. 190–129). New York: Oxford University Press.

Magaziner, J., Zimmerman, S. I., Gruber-Baldini, A. L., Hebel, J. R., & Fox, K. M. (1997). Proxy reporting in five areas of functional status: Comparison with self-reports and observations of performance. *American Journal of Epidemiology,* 146(5), 418–428.

Mahoney, F. I., & Barthel, D. W. (1965). Functional evaluation: The Barthel Index. *Maryland State Medical Journal,* 14, 61–65.

Morris, J., & Morris, S. (1997). ADL assessment measures for use with frail elders. *Journal of Mental Health and Aging,* 3(1), 19–45.

Nagi, S. (1965). Some conceptual issues in disability and rehabilitation. In M. Sussman (Ed.), *Sociology and Rehabilitation.* Washington, DC: American Sociological Association.

Ottenbacher, K., Mann, W., Granger, C., Tomita, M., Hurren, D., & Charvat, B. (1994). Inter-rater agreement and stability of functional assessment in the community-based elderly. *Archives of Physical Medicine and Rehabilitation,* 75(12), 1297–1302.

Pollak, N., Rheault, W., & Stoecker, J. (1996). Reliability and validity of the FIM for persons aged 80 years and above from a multilevel continuing care retirement community. *Archives of Physical Medicine and Rehabilitation, 77*(10), 1056–1061.

Reuben, D., Laliberte, L., Hiris, J., & Mor, V. (1990). A hierarchial exercise scale to measure function at the Advanced Activities of Daily Living (AADL) level. *Journal of the American Geriatrics Society, 38*(8), 855–861.

Reuben, D., & Siu, A. (1990). An objective measure of physical function of elderly outpatients. The Physical Performance Test. *Journal of the American Geriatrics Society, 38*(10), 1105–1112.

Reuben, D., Siu, A., & Kimpau, S. (1992). The predictive validity of self-report and performance-based measures of function and health. *Journal of Gerontology: Medical Sciences, 47*(4), M106–M110.

Reuben, D., Valle, L., Hays, R., & Siu, A. (1995). Measuring physical function in community-dwelling older persons: A comparison of self-administered, interviewer-administered, and performance-based measures. *Journal of the American Geriatrics Society, 43*(1), 17–23.

Roy, C., Togneri, J., Hay, E., & Pentland, B. (1988). An inter-rater reliability study of the Barthel Index. *International Journal of Rehabilitation Research, 11*(1), 67–70.

Shinar, D., Gross, C., Bronstein, K., Licata-Gehr, E., Eden, D., Cabrera, A., Fishman, I., Roth, A., Barwick, J., & Kunitz, S. (1987). Reliability of the Activities of Daily Living Scale and its use in telephone interview. *Archives of Physical Medicine and Rehabilitation, 68*(10), 723.

Siu, A. L., Reuben, D. B., & Hays, R. D. (1990). Hierarchical measures of physical function in ambulatory geriatrics. *Journal of the American Geriatrics Society, 38*(10), 1113–1119.

Smith, P., Illig, S., Fielder, R., Hamilton, B., & Ottenbacker, K. (1996). Intermodal agreement of follow-up telephone functional assessment using the Functional Independence Measure in patients with stroke. *Archives of Physical Medicine and Rehabilitation, 77*(5), 431–435.

Spector, W. D. (1990). Functional disability scales. In R. Spilker (Ed.), *Quality of Life Assessments in Clinical Trials.* New York: Raven Press.

Spector, W. D., Katz, S., Murphy, J. B., & Fulton, J. P. (1987). The hierarchical relationship between activities of daily living and instrumental activities of daily living. *Journal of Chronic Diseases, 40*(6), 481–489.

Spector, W. D., & Takada, H. A. (1991). Characteristics of nursing homes that affect resident outcomes. *Journal of Aging and Health, 3*(4), 427–454.

Stineman, M., Shea, J., Jette, A., Tassoni, C., Ottenbacher, K., Fiedler, R., & Granger, C. (1996). The Functional Independence Measure: Tests of scaling assumptions, structure, and reliability across 20 diverse impairment categories. *Archives of Physical Medicine and Rehabilitation, 77*(11), 1101–1108.

Ward, G., Jagger, C., & Harper, W. (1998). A review of instrumental ADL assessments for use with elderly people. *Reviews in Clinical Gerontology, 8,* 65–71.

William, M., Gaylor, S., & McGaghie, W. (1990). Timed manual performance in a community elderly population. *Journal of the American Geriatrics Society, 38*(10), 1120–1126.

Williams, M., Gaylord, S., & Gerrity, M. (1994). The Timed Manual Performance test as a predictor of hospitalization and death in a community-based elderly population. *Journal of the American Geriatrics Society, 42*(1), 21–27.

World Health Organization. (1976). *The International Classification of Impairments, Disabilities, and Handicaps.* Geneva: World Health Organization.

World Health Organization. (1980). *International Classification of Impairments, Disabilities, and Handicaps: A Manual of Classification Relating to the Consequences of Disease.* Geneva: World Health Organization.

Zimmer, J., Rothenberg, B., & Andresen, E. (1997). Functional assessment. In E. Andresen (Ed.), *Functional Assessment in Assessing the Health Status of Older Adults* (pp. 1–41). New York: Springer.

Zimmerman, S. I., & Magaziner, J. (1994). Methodological issues in measuring the functional status of cognitively impaired nursing home residents: The use of proxies and performance-based measures. *Alzheimer's Disease and Associated Disorders, 8*(1), 281–290.

# 3

# Physiological Well-being and Health

ROBERT L. KANE

## WHAT ARE HEALTH AND PHYSIOLOGICAL MEASURES?

Health and physiological measures are the basic components of all medical evaluations. For physicians, history taking, physical examination, and laboratory tests comprise the diagnostic evaluation of a patient. But such measures are also important to others like social workers, psychologists, and health care administrators involved in assessing older persons. It is beyond the scope of this volume to attempt to reproduce the contents of a textbook of physical diagnosis. Several good examples of both general texts and specific ones for geriatrics are available (Kane, Ouslander, & Abrass, 1999; Hazzard et al., 1999). The goal of this chapter is to address selected areas of particular relevance to assessments of older persons, even when those assessments are not performed by clinicians. Although these areas are almost always included in relevant condition-specific measures, they can also be addressed as generic measures in many instances.

Much that is discussed in this chapter should be considered commonplace in clinical training, but few clinicians systematically inquire into these areas. Indeed, the basic act of inquiry may be the most productive step. The extent and details of that investigation may be less important than the act of doing it. Few clinical evaluations use systematic procedures to evaluate and record findings in the areas addressed here.

The core clinical information that should be available to virtually anyone working with older clients includes diagnoses (at least as reported by the client but even better from a professional source) and a complete list of medications taken (both prescribed and over the counter). Because polypharmacy is a major geriatric problem, a standard component of every geriatric evaluation should be a comprehensive assessment of *all* the drugs a patient is taking. A common device to achieve this end is the "brown bag assay," wherein patients are asked to bring in all the medications (e.g., prescribed, over the counter, and home remedies) they are taking, and these are reviewed for possible duplications and drug interactions. This exercise may only identify potential drug interaction problems, but it is also an opportunity to test whether patients understand their medication regimens and whether they are following the prescribed regimen. If not, clinicians need to examine potential barriers to compliance. Of interest, however, is how to summarize this information into meaningful measures of polypharmacy for either research or clinical purposes.

Building on this base of simple but effective clinical core information, the measures to be addressed in this chapter include selected signs and symptoms and laboratory values; general health status; pain and discomfort; nutritional status; skin condition; and some special geriatric emphasis issues: incontinence, falls, and sleep. Other important factors not addressed specifically in this chapter are hearing and vision. Any comprehensive clinical examination should include at least basic inquiry about these areas, with the opportunity to address each area in greater detail if the screening warrants it. In addressing each of these varied topics, at least three general areas can be explored: what is the extent of the problem (i.e., present/absent, severe/mild), what is the impact of a problem on aspects of the patient's life, what are the risk factors for developing the problem. Clearly, all three would not be asked at the same time because they address different aspects of the condition. Poor performance in any of these dimensions can affect performance on other measures and erroneously suggest problems. It is therefore important to establish that effective communication is occurring before attempting to apply various assessments.

The sources of health and physiological information are comparable to those of all clinical data. Information can come from patient reports (usually termed *symptoms*) and from physical examination or special tests (usually termed *signs*).

### WHY ARE HEALTH AND PHYSIOLOGICAL MEASURES IMPORTANT?

Health and physiological measures are of primary clinical concern. There is an old

joke that the goal of academic geriatrics is that the patient die in metabolic balance. Less cynically, most clinicians attach great importance to such measures. They are familiar, being the measures most often used to track clinical progress. They are often those most observable either directly or through standard laboratory tests. Nonclinicians who ignore them risk losing clinical credibility. Moreover, these measures may have an effect on other domains such as quality of life and functioning. It virtually goes without saying that these domains are extremely sensitive to clinical status. Diagnostic and clinical information implies both risk factors and prognosis. They can thus serve as both indicators of the outcomes of care and as independent variables that predict general health status.

These elements may point to treatable problems that can directly influence the care provided by indicating areas in need of more attention (i.e., underdetected problems) or by indicating areas that may represent outcomes on their own.

In the context of research, health and physiological status are usually treated as variables used for purposes of adjustment to identify comparable subgroups with equivalent prognoses. This is frequently referred to as *case mix adjustment*. In some instances, the physiological state of an individual will affect responses to other interventions, and hence statistical interactions are possible.

### WHERE ARE THESE MEASURES CARRIED OUT?

Health and physiological measures are actively used in virtually every setting where a clinical assessment is performed. Indeed, useful data can be collected as part of interviews in a client's living room. Basic questions about a person's general health status and the need to see a clinician for a more detailed evaluation can be obtained anywhere.

The data are most commonly utilized by

**Table 3.1.**
General Health Measures

| Health status concept | Example |
| --- | --- |
| Perceived health | Rating of overall health (E, VG, G, F, P)* |
| Prior utilization | Physician visits, hospital days in past year |
| Disability days | Days in bed, days sick in past year |
| Symptom checklist | Which of the following symptoms have you experienced in past 2 weeks? |
| Diagnoses | Which of the following diagnoses has a doctor ever told you that you had? (Possibly divided into currently active and history of having had them.) |

*E, excellent; VG, very good; G, good; F, fair; P, poor.

physicians and nurses, but people in other disciplines also use all or part of various measures. Nonclinicians usually employ some general measures of health that summarize a client's health status. Table 3.1 summarizes the common measures used for this purpose. Many of these measures, which are derived from those used in the National Health Interview Survey, may also be used in certain clinical contexts. They should be used to some degree in all long-term care settings. The major distinction in their use is the degree of systematic application. Although health and physiological domains are routinely addressed in clinical practice, their treatment is often cursory and not systematic.

### WHO IS THE INTENDED TARGET?

All people receiving long-term or geriatric care should be assessed, but the level of detail will depend on the underlying clinical situation and care goals. Measures like those that ask persons to rate their overall health status have been shown to be extremely predictive of subsequent problems, far more than clinicians can readily explain (Idler & Kasl, 1991). In many instances systematic branching is useful. Under this process, basic questions are used to sort respondents (e.g., Have you had trouble sleeping? Have you had urinary accidents?). Those who reply affirmatively to some general stem question are then directed into a series of more detailed ques-

tions that examine that area to obtain more detail. Those who respond negatively to the stem questions can proceed rapidly. Some patients are at greater risk for certain conditions. For example, persons confined to bed are at risk for skin problems such as pressure sores, but it would not be necessary to inquire about this aspect of care for active or ambulatory individuals. On the other hand, even active older persons may be at risk for poor nutrition.

### HOW TO CHOOSE WHICH MEASURE (OR VERSION) TO USE?

As with other areas, the purpose and context of the measurement will affect decisions about what and how much to measure, but the distinctions may be even sharper in this instance. Questions can be asked to screen for persons who are at risk for untoward events (e.g., falling). Some measures may be general probes to identify areas where deeper probing is needed (e.g., nutrition). At the other extreme, those measures that tap specific elements may be used to assess clinical progress as part of a systematic follow-up of an already identified problem (e.g., incontinence).

Whereas some measures can be used generically by virtually anyone (e.g., rating one's overall health status), others require different levels of clinical skill (e.g., taking a clinical history or performing a physical examination), and still others require special facilities (e.g., laboratory tests).

## COMMONLY USED HEALTH AND PHYSIOLOGICAL MEASURES

### Overall Health Status

Perhaps the single most useful measure of health status is the basic question, "How would you rate your overall health?" The response is usually recorded on a five point scale (Excellent, Very Good, Good, Fair, Poor). In some instances a variant is used, "Compared with other people your age . . ." This deceptively simple question appears to have tremendous predictive power. Persons indicating fair or poor health have been shown much more likely to die in the next year than those rating their health as excellent or very good. This effect persists even after other, more clinical measures of health are applied (Idler & Kasl, 1991). It is not surprising, then, that this question has been incorporated into most general health measures, including the SF-36 (see Chapter 7), where it is paired with a similar question about changes in health status over the past year.

### Pain

Several different approaches to collecting information about pain have been developed. None is completely satisfactory. Pain is an elusive concept. It is basically subjective. Although some people have tried to assess the pain experienced by others who cannot communicate (e.g., dementia patients, terminally ill patients as they lapse into death), there is no objective measure. At best one relies on inferences from such signs as facial expressions and labored effort. Inferring pain can be difficult and imprecise (Simons & Malabar, 1995), although observers can be trained to be reliable (Miller et al., 1996). Given the difficulty of inferring pain, it is important to avoid prejudging patients' ability to report pain. This error is especially common in nursing homes, where efforts to question demented patients are easily reduced to relying on behavior, especially under the pressures of the Nursing Home Minimum Data Set (Hawes et al., 1997), which is

treated extensively in Chapter 16. Several studies have suggested that many demented persons can still report their pain if sufficient effort is made to interview them (Ferrell, Ferrell, & Rivera, 1995; Sengstaken & King, 1993).

Pain measures vary in their level of detail. Traditionally, pain is described clinically in terms of its character (e.g., sharp, dull), frequency, duration, location, radiation, and intensity. Other components may include precipitating events or associated symptoms (e.g., eating or nausea). Certain pain syndromes can be characterized by other phenomena, such as the amount of analgesia assumed to relieve the pain. Indeed, in judging pain it may be important to know whether the patient is currently taking analgesics and what kind and amount. In some cases one is assessing the effects of analgesic therapy; in others one is seeking some underlying level of pain. Most pain measures that refer to specific pain usually include at least the components of severity and frequency. The question is how to combine these dimensions. One could use some version of the product of the scores for the ordinal version of each component, or one could create a matrix from the two components and seek zones of equivalency, where the combination of frequency and intensity are considered to represent a common net level of pain. For example, frequent episodes of mild pain may be rated as less of a problem than rare episodes of intense pain. The challenge here is to decide on the criteria for ordering the zones. Table 3.2 illustrates one effort to create such combinations. In this instance, which was developed for a study of hip surgery, the severity of the pain is combined with the number of activities that bring on the pain. High severity occurs when any activity produces the highest pain level. The intermediate zone is made up of low levels of pain that are associated with two or more activities.

One can measure pain by addressing its dimensions and then presumably recombining these components into a summary

**Table 3.2.**
Sample Composite Pain Score

| Sum of pain while walking, climbing, sitting, lying down | Severity of pain | | | | | |
|---|---|---|---|---|---|---|
| | None 0 | 1 | 2 | 3 | 4 | Worst pain 5 |
| 0 | 0 | 0 | 0 | 0 | 0 | 0 |
| 1 | 0 | 1 | 1 | 1 | 3 | 3 |
| 2 | 0 | 2 | 2 | 2 | 3 | 3 |
| 3 | 0 | 2 | 2 | 2 | 3 | 3 |
| 4 | 0 | 2 | 2 | 2 | 3 | 3 |

0 = No pain; 1 = Low severity and less frequent; 2 = Low severity and more frequent; 3 = High severity and any frequency.

score or by simply asking patients to indicate the severity of the pain along a simple continuum. The latter approach is favored by many clinicians looking for a quick way to assess pain. They frequently employ one of a variety of summary devices such as visual analog scales, numerical overall scoring systems, and pain thermometers. Some debate the superiority of vertical versus horizontal visual analogs. A comparison of several measures indicated that elderly persons preferred the visual descriptor scale developed by Melzack and Torgerson (1971) over the various summary measures; the respondents also found it easiest to use (Herr & Mobily, 1993). An example of a visual analog scale is shown in Figure 3.1. The severity of the pain is assessed by the distance away from "no pain." (The same effect can be achieved by using a 0–10 scale.)

Assessing pain in older persons is not necessarily different from assessing pain in younger ones, but a few differences must be appreciated. Many older people suffer from some level of chronic pain. Hence, new pains or exacerbations may be harder to detect. Older patients have often developed effective coping strategies for their pain. These may blunt the effects of new treatments.

Perhaps the most exquisite systematic pain measure is the McGill Pain Questionnaire developed by Melzack. This measure, which has undergone several revisions, attempts to capture a wide variety of descriptors of pain, including its character, intensity, and frequency. (Respondents are asked to select words that typify the pain, including colors and temperatures.) It employs body maps to locate the pain and its radiations (Melzack & Torgerson, 1971; Gagliese & Melzack, 1997).

At the other end of the spectrum, a section of the SF-36 uses a few questions to address pain in general.

- How much bodily pain have you had during the past 4 weeks? (6 levels: none to very severe)
- During the past 4 weeks, how much did pain interfere with your normal work (including both work outside the house and housework)? (5 levels: not at all to extremely)

Pain per se may not be the most disabling or only significant symptom. Other forms of discomfort can be serious problems as well. Indeed, itching, for example, can be so annoying that many people try to substitute pain (i.e., by scratching). Other kinds of aches can also represent impor-

*Instructions: Put an "X" on the point along the line below that corresponds to your current level of pain.*

No
pain
───────────────────────────────────────────────

Worst pain
imaginable

**Figure 3.1.** Visual analog scale for pain.

**Table 3.3.**

Pain and Discomfort Scale

*The respondent is asked, "During the past month, have you experienced any of the following? If so, how often did it occur?"*

| | Frequency | | |
| --- | --- | --- | --- |
| Pain/discomfort | Every day | Less than daily | Not at all |
| Aches/pains in joints or muscles | | | |
| Chest pain | | | |
| Shortness of breath | | | |
| Dizziness | | | |
| Itching/burning | | | |
| Headaches | | | |

tant problems for some patients. A scale designed to tap a wider variety of discomforts is shown in Table 3.3. This scale was originally used with nursing home patients in a more simplified version (Kane et al., 1983).

Pain measures can also be directed at specific groups of people. An example of such a condition-specific measure is the pain component of the Arthritis Impact Measurement Scale, which was originally developed to assess the impact of rheumatoid arthritis (Meenan, Gertman, & Mason, 1980). The questions, listed in Table 3.4, address clinical aspects of arthritis pain with special sensitivity to the nature of the pain associated with rheumatoid arthritis. These questions would not be useful for addressing pain in general.

### Nutritional Status

Several efforts to collect systematic information on older persons' nutritional status have been designed. Some are intended as general screening tools, with more detailed anthropometric measures used when indi-

cated. Some clinicians would not even apply these screens unless they suspected a problem, relying instead on basic observations. The measures vary in their focus. Some address the manifestations of nutrition per se, such as height and weight (which can be combined into various body mass indexes), skinfold thickness, and evidence of obesity or undernutrition; whereas others ask about factors that might contribute to malnutrition, such as problems with eating, sore mouth, and even buying food. Laboratory data (e.g., serum albumin level and lymphocyte count) can also be used to indicate nutritional deficits.

The Mini Nutritional Assessment (MNA), sponsored by the Nestec Ltd. (Nestle Research Center/Clintec), is shown as Figure 3.2. The MNA combines anthropometric measures (e.g., height, weight), a dietetic assessment, and a subjective assessment with an overall clinical summary. There have been several efforts to test the validity of this tool. When its results were compared with clinical judgments in different settings, it discriminated between frail

**Table 3.4.**

Pain Subscale of the Arthritis Impact Measurement Scale

During the past month, how long has your morning stiffness usually lasted from the time you wake up?

During the past month, how often have you had pain in two or more joints at the same time?

During the past month, how often have you had severe pain from your arthritis?

During the past month, how would you describe the arthritis pain you usually have?

*I. Anthropometric Assessment*

   1. BMI (Body Mass Index) (weight / (height)$^2$ in kg/m$^2$)
     0 = BMI < 19
     1 = 19 ≤ BMI < 21
     2 = 21 ≤ BMI < 23
     3 = BMI ≥ 23
   2. Mid arm circumference (MAC in cm)
     0.0 = MAC < 21
     0.5 = 21 ≤ MAC ≤ 22
     1.0 – MAC > 22
   3. Calf circumference (CC in cm)
     0 = CC < 31   1 = CC ≥ 31
   4. Weight loss during last 3 months
     0 = weight loss > 3 kg
     1 = does not know
     2 = weight loss between 1 and 3 kg
     3 = no weight loss

*II. Global Evaluation*

   5. Does the patient live independently in contrast to a nursing home?
     0 = no  1 = yes
   6. Does the patient take more than 3 prescription drugs (per day)?
     0 = yes  1 = no
   7. In the past 3 months has the patient suffered psychological stress or acute disease?
     0 = yes  1 = no
   8. Mobility
     0 = bed of chair bound
     1 = able to get out of bed/chair but does not go out
     2 = goes out
   9. Neuropsychological problem
     0 = severe dementia or depression
     1 = mild dementia
     2 = no psychological problems
  10. Pressure sores or skin ulcers
     0 = yes  1 = no

*III. Dietetic Assessment*

  11. How many full meals does the patient eat daily?
     0 = 1 meal  1 = 2 meals  2 = 3 meals

*III. Dietetic Assessment — continued*

  12. Does he consume:
     - At least one serving of dairy products (milk, cheese, yogurt) per day?   (Y/N)
     - Two or more servings of beans or eggs per week?   (Y/N)
     - Meat, fish, or poultry every day?   (Y/N)
     0.0 = if 0 or 1 yes
     0.5 = if 2 yes
     1.0 = if 3 yes
  13. Does he consume two or more servings of fruits or vegetables per day?
     0 = no  1 = yes
  14. Has the patient food intake declined over the past three months due to loss of appetite, digestive problems, chewing, or swallowing difficulties?
     0 = severe loss of appetite
     1 = moderate loss of appetite
     2 = no loss of appetite
  15. How many cups/glasses of beverages (water, juice, coffee, tea, milk, wine, beer. . . . ) does the patient consumer per day?
     0.0 = less than 3 glasses
     0.5 = 3 to 5 glasses
     1.0 – more than 5 glasses
  16. Mode of feeding
     0 = fed requires assistance
     1 = does not know or moderate malnutrition
     2 = self-fed without any problem

*IV. Subjective Assessment*

  17. Does the patient consider himself to have any nutritional problems?
     0 = major malnutrition
     1 = does not know or moderate nutrition
     2 = no nutritional problem
  18. In comparison with other people of the same age, how would the patient consider his health status?
     0.0 = not as good
     0.5 = does not know
     1.0 = as good
     2.0 = better

*TOTAL (max 30 points):*

Score:
≥ 24 points: well-nourished
17 to 23.5 points: at risk of malnutrition
< 17 points: undernutrition

**Figure 3.2.**  Mini Nutritional Assessment. Source: Guigoz et al. (1994).

and healthy aged persons both when the biochemical data were included and not (Guigoz, Vellas, & Garry, 1994).

    A consortium composed of the American Academy of Family Physicians, the American Dietetic Association, and the national Council on Aging formed the Nutrition Screening Initiative (NSI), which in turn created the 10 item DETERMINE screening tool (Table 3.5). The name is ac-

**Table 3.5.**

The DETERMINE Checklist for Nutritional Risk

| | Risk points* |
|---|---|
| I have an illness or condition that made me change the kind and/or amount of food I eat | 2 |
| I eat fewer than two meals per day | 3 |
| I eat few fruits or vegetables or milk products | 2 |
| I have three or more drinks of beer, liquor, or wine almost every day | 2 |
| I have tooth or mouth problems that make it hard for me to eat | 2 |
| I don't always have enough money to buy the food I need | 4 |
| I eat alone most of the time | 1 |
| I take three or more different prescribed or over-the-counter drugs a day | 1 |
| Without wanting to, I have lost or gained ten pounds in the last six months | 2 |
| I am not always physically able to shop, cook, and/or feed myself | 2 |

*Checklist score = sum (0–21).

tually an acronym for the risk factors for poor nutritional status among older persons: *d*isease, *e*ating poorly, *t*ooth loss or mouth pain, *e*conomic hardship, *r*educed social contact, *m*ultiple medications, *i*nvoluntary weight loss or gain, *n*eed for assistance in self-care, and *e*lderly. Persons deemed to be at risk would then be assessed further in two stages: *(1)* additional measures (including anemia, skinfold thickness, and height and weight) and *(2)* more questions and measurements of hematological and anthropometric characteristics. When the predictive validity of this checklist was tested, older persons with a score of 4 or more were more likely to be in

**Table 3.6.**

Nutrition Risk Index

*Mechanics of Food Intake*

   1. Do you have trouble biting or chewing any kind of food?
   2. Do you wear dentures?

*Prescribed Dietary Restrictions*

   3. Are there any kinds of foods you can't eat because they disagree with you?
   4. Are you on any kind of special diet?

*Morbid Conditions Affecting Food Intake*

   5. Do you now have an illness or condition that interferes with your eating?
   6. Do you have an illness that has cut down on your appetite?
   7. Have you ever had an operation on your abdomen?
   8. Have you ever been told by a doctor that you were anemic (had iron poor blood)?
   9. Do you smoke cigarettes regularly now?
  10. In the past month, have you taken any medicines prescribed by a doctor?
  11. In the past month, have you taken any medicines that were not prescribed by a doctor?

*Discomfort with the Outcomes of Food Intake*

  12. Have you had any spells of pain or discomfort for 3 days in your abdomen or stomach in the past month?
  13. Did you have any trouble swallowing at least 3 days in the past month?
  14. Did you have any vomiting at least 3 days in the past month?
  15. Do you have any troubles with your bowels that make you constipated or give you any diarrhea?

*Significant Changes in Dietary Intake*

  16. Have you gained or lost any weight in the last 30 days?

poor health at baseline and to be functionally disabled or depressed a year later, but the scores did not predict mortality or the use of hospital services (Boult et al., 1999). These findings do little to establish the checklist's value as a screener for nutrition. The areas covered address risk factors more than direct manifestations. These risk factors are likely to be associated with other phenomena that indicate functional problems.

The Nutrition Risk Index was developed especially for use with older persons (Wolinsky et al., 1986, 1990; Pendergast et al., 1989). It was modified from questions used in the National Health and Nutrition Examination Survey (NHANES). As shown in Table 3.6, it consists of 16 questions organized around five themes. It represents a mixture of topics that reflect treatment, symptoms, and potential problem areas.

## Skin

Substantial attention has been directed to the condition of skin among long-term care clients. Sustained immobility, especially in the presence of loss of sensation and poor circulation, can lead to the development of pressure sores. Skin condition is usually graded on a 4 point scale, where 1 indicates some reddening, the harbinger of serious problems, and 4 represents deep ulceration to the bone. Once they develop, these ulcers can be slow to heal; they can become infected and eventually cause death. It thus behooves caregivers to pay close attention to skin condition and to institute preventive programs, especially turning patients to alter their body position to prevent sustained pressure on key points. Several risk scores have been developed to identify those at high risk for developing pressure sores.

An early effort to assess the risk of developing pressure sores was the Norton score, where patients with a score of 14 or less out of a possible 20 points were considered to be at risk and those with a score less than 12 were at high risk. The score used five components (physical condition, mental state, activity, mobility, and incontinence; each was rated from 4 (for normal) to 1 (for very severe). (Age has sometimes been added as another component.) As can be seen in Table 3.7, the items rely on a great deal of interpretation by the rater. There is also no reason to assume that these categories represent equal contributions to the risk of developing pressure sores. Using a cut score of 14 correctly identified 89% of persons who went on to develop a pressure sore but only 36% of those who did not (Goldstone, 1982).

The Norton Scale has generally been replaced by the Braden Scale, which uses a 23 point score covering six areas (shown in Table 3.8) to predict pressure sore risk (Braden & Bergstrom, 1987). (Five areas can receive up to 4 points each, and the sixth is rated on a three point scale.) Higher scores were associated with increased likelihood of developing pressure sores. A score of 16 was associated with complete detection of all patients who went on to develop pressure sores with 90% sensitivity and 64% specificity. Interrater reliability studies suggest high levels of reliability (agreement rates of 88%) when two nurse raters are compared but much poorer reliability when licensed practical nurses are compared with nurses

Table 3.7.
Norton Scale Components

| | |
|---|---|
| Physical condition | Good = 4, fair = 3, poor = 2, very bad = 1 |
| Mental condition | Alert = 4, apathetic = 3, confused = 2, stupor = 1 |
| Activity | Ambulant = 4, walk with help = 3, chairbound = 2, stupor = 1 |
| Mobility | Full = 4, slightly limited = 3, very limited = 2, immobile =1 |
| Incontinent | Not = 4, occasional = 3, usually of urine = 2, doubly = 1 |

Source: Norton et al. (1962).

**Table 3.8.**

Components of the Braden Scale for Predicting Pressure Sore Risk

| | |
|---|---|
| Sensory perception | |
| Activity | |
| Mobility ⎫ | Rated on a 4 point scale where 1 = least favorable and 4 = most favorable |
| Moisture ⎬ | |
| Nutrition ⎭ | |
| Friction/shear | Rated on a 3 point scale |

aids (Bergstrom et al., 1987). When the Braden Scale's contribution to predicting pressure sores was tested, the results were equivocal. In a model that included age, temperature, blood pressure protein, and iron, addition of the Braden Scale value did not increase the sensitivity (0.91), but it did improve the specificity a little (from 0.41 to 0.49) (Bergstrom et al., 1987).

## Falls

Falls represent a serious threat to older persons. Additionally, a history of falling is itself an indicator of frailty. Careful comprehensive evaluations of older persons with a history of falling can produce improvements in their functional status, even if there is no change in their subsequent rate of falling (Rubenstein et al., 1990). Evidence of successful interventions (i.e., exercise, improving drug regimens, training programs) to reduce the risk of falling is just beginning to emerge (Campbell et al., 1997; Wolf et al., 1996; Province et al., 1995; Tinetti et al., 1994). These findings suggest that it may be worthwhile to identify those at high risk of falling in order to intervene. Active work on systematically trying to understand risk factors for falling and identifying those at high risk has been going on for a little more than a decade. Much of that work is associated with Mary Tinetti, who has developed and tested fairly complex approaches to clinically assessing fall risk (Tinetti, Liu, & Claus, 1993; Gill, Williams, & Tinetti, 1995; Tinetti, McAvay, & Claus, 1996). A more widely used assessment tool, the Get Up and Go Test, was developed in the United Kingdom (Mathias, Nayak, & Isaacs, 1986) and subsequently modified

(Podsiadlo & Richardson, 1991). Many long-term care institutions have established elaborate fall prevention programs, and risk screening for falls is part of the routine admission process.

The Tinetti assessment involves detailed observations of balance and gait. The main elements of these assessments are summarized in Table 3.9. In the Get Up and Go Test, subjects sit in a straight-backed chair and are asked to rise, to stand still momentarily, to walk toward the wall, to turn without touching the wall, to walk back to the chair, and to turn around and sit down (Mathias et al., 1986). The performance is scored on a 1–5 scale, where 1 = normal, 2 = very slightly abnormal, 3 = mildly abnormal, 4 = moderately abnormal, and 5 = severely abnormal. "Normal" means no risk of falling at any time during the test; "severely abnormal" means appearing at risk of falling during the test. Inter-rater reliability across disciplines was a problem; senior physicians rated videotape performance significantly higher than did physiotherapists. Within-group agreement rates were better. Efforts to validate the scores against more standard physiological and mechanical measures of gait generally showed good agreement levels (Mathias et al., 1986).

A more recent variant of this test is the Timed Up and Go Test, in which a patient is timed rising from an arm chair, walking 3 meters, and returning to the chair to sit down. The time from standing to sitting is measured. Inter-rater and intra-rater agreement is very high (inter-class correlation 0.99). Correlations with balance and gait speed are respectable (0.72 and −0.55, respectively (Podsiadlo & Richardson, 1991).

**Table 3.9.**
Main Components of the Tinetti Fall Risk Scale

*Balance Assessment*

Sitting balance (in a hard, straight-backed chair)
Arising from chair
Immediate standing balance (first 3–5 sec)
Standing balance
Balance with eyes closed (with feet as close together as possible)
Turning balance (360°)
Nudge on sternum (patient standing with feet as close together as possible, examiner pushes with light even pressure over sternum three times; reflects ability to withstand displacement)
Neck turning (patient asked to turn head sideways and look up while standing with feet as close together as possible)
One leg standing balance
Back extension (ask patient to lean back as far as possible, without holding onto an object if possible)
Reaching up (have patient attempt to remove an object from a shelf high enough to require stretching or standing on toes)
Bending down (patient is asked to pick up small objects, such as a pen, from the floor)

*Gait Assessment*

*Patient stands with examiner at end of obstacle-free hallway. Patient uses usual walking aid. Examiner asks patient to walk down hallway at usual pace. Examiner observes one component of gait at a time. For some components the examiner walks behind the patient; for other components, the examiner walks next to the patient. May require several trips to complete*
Initiation of gait (patient is asked to begin walking down hallway)
Step height (begin observing after first few steps; observe one foot then the other; observe from side)
Step length (observe distance between toe of stance foot and heel of swing foot; observe from side; do not judge first few or last few steps; observe one side at a time)
Step symmetry (observe the middle part of the patch not the first or last steps; observe from side; observe distance between heel of each swing foot and toe of each stance)
Step continuity
Path deviation (observe from behind; observe one foot over several strides; observe in relation to line on floor (e.g., tiles) if possible; difficult to assess if patient uses walker)
Trunk stability (observe from behind; side to side motion of trunk may be a normal gait pattern, need to differentiate this from instability)
Walk stance (observe from behind)
Turning while walking

Source: Tinetti (1986).

## Incontinence

Urinary incontinence is a common problem among older persons and can lead to severe limitations in social function for those in the community and eventually may be a major cause of admission to a nursing home if it becomes severe. Despite its central role in affecting function, any inquiry about its occurrence is frequently omitted, probably because of embarrassment. Clinicians are loathe to discuss the subject and may fear embarrassing their patients. Quite the opposite is often the case; patients are concerned about the problem and its consequences but are re-luctant to express it. They welcome the opportunity to discuss it.

Recognizing the problem is the first step to fixing it. The initial inquiries are directed at determining the etiology. Traditional questions address the timing and circumstances of urinary accidents to distinguish different types of incontinence. Several mnemonics have been developed to remember the likely external causes of urinary incontinence. Two are shown as Table 3.10. The Agency for Health Care Policy and Research has developed a set of clinical guidelines for the evaluation of urinary incontinence (Fanti et al., 1996).

**Table 3.10.**
Potential Causes of Urinary Incontinence

| D | Delirium | | D | Delirium/confusional state |
|---|---|---|---|---|
| R | Restricted mobility, retention | | I | Infection, urinary (symptomatic) |
| I | Infection, inflammation, impaction | | A | Atrophic urethritis/vaginitis |
| P | Polyuria, pharmaceuticals | | P | Pharmaceuticals |
| | | | P | Psychological |
| | | | E | Excessive urine output |
| | | | R | Restricted mobility |
| | | | S | Stool impaction |

DRIP: Source: Kane et al. (1994). DIAPPERS: Source: Resnick (1995).

Fecal incontinence can also be a troublesome problem that can cause major restrictions in social activity. Although fecal incontinence is often found as a more advanced stage of urinary incontinence, it can also arise independently and should be asked about on its own.

Both types of incontinence can be troublesome components of care for demented persons. In this case, the etiology is likely less physiological than due to a loss of inhibition. Discussions with caregivers should address these events.

Both types of incontinence can be managed. In some cases correcting the underlying problem can eliminate the incontinence, but in almost all cases behavioral steps can be taken to make the problem more controllable.

### Sleep

Sleep is an important component of life. Inadequate amounts of sleep can lead to emotional and physical strain (Ouslander et al., 1998). Poor sleep patterns are associated with aging, but they can be greatly exacerbated by environmental factors, especially in situations like nursing homes. Many older persons use some type of sleeping medication. In some instances the medication may exacerbate the problem rather than alleviate it. The importance of a good night's sleep is just beginning to be appreciated. As a result, few clinicians systematically examine an older patient's sleep patterns. Just evaluating carefully an older person's sleep/wake cycle may provide valuable information and may suggest underlying problems such as delirium. One

measure to explore this area was developed as part of the RAND Córporation Medical Outcomes Study (MOS). This measure (shown in Table 3.11) consists of 12 items that have been transformed into two scales, one with six items and one with nine. These two scales are highly correlated (r = 0.97). The psychometric properties of these scales have been well studied. Efforts to establish their validity rest with correlations with other health measures. Internal reliability coefficients were 0.78 for the shorter measure and 0.86 for the longer one (Hays & Stewart, 1992).

The Philadelphia Sleep Quality Index (PSQI) was not developed specifically for older persons, but it was tested on a broad sample of ages (Buysse et al., 1989). It consists of 19 self-reported items and five

**Table 3.11.  RAND Medical Outcomes Study Sleep Items**

Trouble falling asleep* (1) (2) (R)
How long to fall asleep† (2)
Sleep was not quiet (restless)* (2) (R)
Awaken during sleep* (1) (2) (R)
Snore*
Awaken short of breath or with a headache* (1) (2) (R)
Feel rested in the morning* (1) (2)
Get amount of sleep needed* (1) (2)
Drowsy during the day* (2) (R)
Trouble staying awake* (1) (2) (R)
Take naps*
Hours sleep each night

*Coded on 1–6, where 1 = all the time and 6 = none of the time. (1) indicates use in 6 item scale; (2) indicates use in 9 item scale; (R) denotes reverse coding.

†Coded on time scale, where 1 = 0–15 min and 5 = more than 60 min.

**Table 3.12.** Major Components of the
Philadelphia Sleep Quality Index

Subjective sleep quality
Sleep latency
Sleep duration
Habitual sleep efficiency
Sleep disturbances
Use of sleeping medication
Daytime dysfunction

questions rated by a bed partner or room-mate. The results are converted by a trained scorer into seven component scores, each weighted on a 0–3 scale (Table 3.12). These component scores can be summed to create a single summary score. The overall Chronbach's alpha coefficient was 0.83, but the range among the component scores was from 0.76 (habitual sleep efficiency and subjective sleep quality) to 0.35 (sleep disturbances). Test–retest reliability was strong. Validity was assessed by comparing the results with those from established measures of sleep. Controls were significantly different from persons with high scores on the Disorders of Initiating and Maintaining Sleep and Disorders of Excessive Somnolence scales. In a study comparing the PSQI results from older and younger persons, the measures of older persons did not correlate as highly with other direct measures of sleep as did those of younger subjects (Buysse et al., 1991).

Another sleep-related measure is the Eppworth Sleepiness Scale, which was developed to assess daytime sleepiness. Again, this measure was not designed specifically for older persons (Johns, 1991). This measure consists of asking the respondent to rate his or her likelihood of dozing while performing eight different types of activity, from sitting and reading to stopped in traffic in a car. Chronbach's alpha was 0.88. Test–retest reliability was 0.82 (Johns, 1992).

**Alcohol Usage and Effects**

Alcohol use is often overlooked as a source of problems in older persons. It can explain cognitive and psychological symptoms as well as be the result of these. Alcohol is less well tolerated by older persons, and its addiction may be well hidden. On the other hand, because the subject is rarely broached, few clinicians are aware of their older patients' drinking problems (O'Connor & Schottenfeld, 1998). Because such behavior is more easily reversed for older than for younger persons, such an oversight is especially unfortunate.

Few instruments have been well tested for use with older persons. A widely used measure of alcohol problems, which seems to work well with older persons as well, is the CAGE questionnaire. The name is a mnemonic (cut down, annoyed by criticism, experiencing guilt, eye-opener drink in the morning). A positive response to one or more of these four statements has proven useful in identifying persons with drinking problem (Table 3.13). A higher number of positive responses has been shown to distinguish those with drinking problems from those who do not have such problems (Ewing, 1984). Although they were not developed specifically for older persons, they have been used with this group.

**Other Topics**

Several aspects of communication are important to both evaluating older people and affecting their function. Problems with

**Table 3.13.**
CAGE Items

Have you ever felt you ought to Cut down on your drinking?
Have people Annoyed you by criticizing your drinking?
Have you ever felt bad or Guilty about your drinking?
Have you ever had a drink first thing in the morning or to steady your nerves or to get rid of a hangover (Eye opener)?

vision and hearing are common but may be overlooked unless they are specifically addressed. Some losses in these areas can be readily corrected with appropriate prosthetic devices (e.g., better glasses or a hearing aid). Some problems are less amenable to correction but must be recognized so that a communication problem is not misinterpreted as cognitive decline. At a minimum, problems with an older person's vision and hearing can interfere with other testing. Poor performance may arise from a failure to properly understand the task or the question. It is important to ensure that adequate communication is occurring before any assessment proceeds and to take appropriate actions to compensate for problems uncovered (e.g., amplification, larger type, reading the questions). Simple testing procedures are possible. For example, one can whisper a phrase standing behind a subject to see if it is heard, but for purposes of assessing adequate communication for interviewing, even this level is not necessary. Simply establishing that the older respondent can repeat back a question posed is sufficient. Likewise, for vision, the ability to read written words can be readily assessed. Formal testing of both near and distance vision can be done with eye charts.

Another area that is commonly overlooked is the older person's dental condition. Tooth and mouth problems can contribute to problems with eating and hence are often addressed as risk factors for malnutrition. Several of the relevant questionnaires used to assess this area (noted earlier) inquire specifically about oral problems. Poor dental hygiene can lead to mouth sores and tooth loss that can create unnecessary pain and suffering. A tool for assessing geriatric oral health is available (Atchison, 1990).

## CONCLUSIONS

The measures described in this chapter are largely drawn from the clinical literature. Consistent with this origin, most have never been subjected to any type of psychometric analysis. When they have been studied, their ability to discriminate among clinically different groups or their predictive powers to identify those who will get into trouble have usually been addressed.

Although it is usually better to be thorough in investigating each area of function, the potential list can be exhaustive (and exhausting). The largest benefit comes from recognizing an area of potential problem. Once that recognition is achieved, more complete follow-up investigations are possible, either by the person doing the assessment or through a referral. Thus, it is better to ask a single question on a topic than to omit the topic for lack of a comprehensive assessment tool or the time to use it. In essence, coverage trumps measurement properties through multi-item scales.

## REFERENCES

Atchison, K. A. (1990). Development of the geriatric oral health assessment index. *Journal of Dental Education, 54*(11), 680–687.

Bergstrom, N., Braden, B. J., Laguzza, A., & Holman, V. (1987). The Braden Scale for Predicting Pressure Sore Risk. *Nursing Research, 36*(4), 205–210.

Boult, C., Krinke, U. B., Urdangarin, C. F., & Skarin, V. (1999). The validity of a nutritional screening tool in detecting poor health and in predicting future disability and depression among older adults. *Journal of the American Geriatrics Society, 47,* 995–999.

Braden, B., & Bergstrom, N. (1987). A conceptual schema for the study of the etiology of pressure sores. *Rehabilitation Nursing, 12*(1), 8–12.

Buysse, D. J., Reynolds, C. F. I., Monk, T. H., Berman, S. R., & Kupfer, D. J. (1989). The Pittsburgh Sleep Quality Index: A new instrument for psychiatric practice and research. *Psychiatry Research, 28,* 193–213.

Buysse, D. J., Reynolds, C. F. I., Monk, T. H., Hoch, C. C., Yaeger, A. L., & Kupfer, D. J. (1991). Quantification of subjective sleep quality in healthy elderly men and women using the Pittsburgh Sleep Quality Index (PSQI). *Sleep, 14*(4), 331–338.

Campbell, A., Robertson, M., Gardner, M., Norton, R., Tilyard, M., & Buchner, D. (1997). Randomised controlled trial of a general practice programme of home based exercise to prevent falls in elderly. *British Medical Journal, 315*(7115), 1065–1069.

Ewing, J. A. (1984). Detecting alcoholism: The CAGE Questionnaire. *JAMA, 252*(14), 1905–1907.

Fanti, J. A., Kaschak Newman, D., Colling, J., DeLancey, J. O. L., Keeys, C., Loughery, R., McDowell, B. J., Norton, P., Ouslander, J., Schnelle, J., Staskin, D., Tries, J., Urich, V., Vitousek, S. H., Weiss, B. D., & Whitmore, K. (1996). *Urinary Incontinence in Adults: Acute and Chronic Management* (Clinical Practice Guideline, Number 2, 1996 Update AHCPR Publication No. 96–0682). Rockville, MD: U.S. Department of Health and Human Services, Public Health Service, Agency for Health Care Policy and Research.

Ferrell, B. A., Ferrell, B. R., & Rivera, L. (1995). Pain in cognitively impaired nursing home patients. *Journal of Pain and Symptom Management, 10*(8), 591–598.

Gagliese, L., & Melzack, R. (1997). Chronic pain in elderly people. *Pain, 70*(1), 3–14.

Gill, T. M., Williams, C. S., & Tinetti, M. E. (1995). Assessing risk for the onset of functional dependence among older adults: The role of physical performance. *Journal of the American Geriatrics Society, 43*, 603–609.

Goldstone, L. A. (1982). The Norton score: An early warning of pressure sores? *Journal of Advanced Nursing, 7*, 419–426.

Guigoz, Y., Vellas, B., & Garry, P. J. (1994). Mini nutritional assessment: A practical assessment tool for grading the nutritional state of elderly patients. In B. J. Vellas, Y. Guigoz, P. J. Garry, & J. L. Albarede (Eds.), *Facts and Research in Gerontology 1994, Nutrition in the Elderly, The Mini Nutritional Assessment (MNA)* (Vol. Supplement No. 2, pp. 15–59). Paris: Serdi Publishing Company.

Hawes, C., Morris, J. N., Phillips, C. D., Fries, B. E., Murphy, K., & Mor, V. (1997). Development of the nursing home Resident Assessment Instrument in the USA. *Age and Ageing, 26*(Suppl 2), 19–25.

Hays, R. D., & Stewart, A. L. (1992). Sleep measures. In A. L. Stewart & J. E. Ware (Eds.), *Measuring Functioning and Well-Being: The Medical Outcomes Study Approach* (pp. 235–400). Durham, NC: Duke University Press.

Hazzard, W. R., Bierman, E. L., Blass, J. P., Ettinger, W. H. J., Halter, J. B., & Ouslander, J. G. (Eds.). (1999). *Principles of Geriatric Medicine and Gerontology (4th ed.).* New York: McGraw Hill.

Herr, K. A., & Mobily, P. R. (1993). Comparison of selected pain assessment tools for use with the elderly. *Applied Nursing Research, 6*(1), 39–46.

Idler, E. L., & Kasl, S. (1991). Health perceptions and survival: Do global evaluations of health status really predict mortality? *Journal of Gerontology, 46*(2), S55–S65.

Johns, M. W. (1991). A new method for measuring daytime sleepiness: The Epworth Sleepiness Scale. *Sleep, 14*(6), 540–545.

Johns, M. W. (1992). Reliability and factor analysis of the Epworth Sleepiness Scale. *Sleep, 15*(4), 376–381.

Kane, R. L., Bell, R., Riegler, S., Wilson, A., & Kane, R. A. (1983). Assessing the outcomes of nursing home patients. *Journal of Gerontology, 38*, 385–393.

Kane, R. L., Ouslander, J. C., & Abrass, I. B. (1999). *Essentials of Clinical Geriatrics* (4th ed.). New York: McGraw Hill.

Mathias, S., Nayak, U. S. L., & Isaacs, B. (1986). Balance in elderly patients: The "Get-Up and Go" test. *Archives of Physical Medicine and Rehabilitation, 67*, 387–389.

Meenan, R. F., Gertman, P. M., & Mason, J. H. (1980). Measuring health status in arthritis: The arthritis impact measurement scales. *Arthritis and Rheumatism, 23*(2), 146–152.

Melzack, R., & Torgerson, W. S. (1971). On the language of pain. *Anesthesiology, 34*(1), 50–59.

Miller, J., Neelon, V., Dalton, J., Ng'andu, N., Bailey, D. J., Layman, E., & Hosfeld, A. (1996). The assessment of discomfort in elderly confused patients: A preliminary study. *Journal of Neuroscience Nursing, 28*(3), 175–182.

Norton, D., McLaren, R., & Exton-Smith, A. N. (1962). *An Investigation of Geriatric Nursing Problems in the Hospital.* London: National Corporation for the Care of Old People.

O'Connor, P. G., & Schottenfeld, R. S. (1998). Patients with alcohol problems. *New England Journal of Medicine, 338*(9), 592–601.

Ouslander, J. G., Buxton, W. G., Al-Samarrai, N. R., Cruise, P. A., Alessi, C., & Schnelle, J. F. (1998). Nighttime urinary incontinence and sleep disruption among nursing home residents. *Journal of the American Geriatrics Society, 46*(4), 463–466.

Pendergast, J. M., Coe, R. M., Chavez, M. N., Romeis, J. C., Miller, D. K., & Wolinsky, F. D. (1989). Clinical validation of a nutritional risk index. *Journal of Community Health, 14*(3), 125–135.

Podsiadlo, D., & Richardson, S. (1991). The timed "Up & Go": A test of basic functional mobility for frail elderly persons. *Journal of the American Geriatrics Society, 39,* 142–148.

Province, M. A., Hadley, E. C., Hornbrook, M. C., Lipsitz, L. A., Miller, J. P., Mulrow, C. D., Ory, M. G., Sattin, R. W., Tinetti, M. E., & Wolf, S. L. (1995). The effects of exercise on falls in elderly patients: A preplanned meta-analysis of the FICSIT trials. *JAMA, 273*(17), 1341–1347.

Resnick, N. M. (1995). Urinary incontinence. *Lancet, 346,* 94–99.

Rubenstein, L. Z., Robbins, A. S., Josephson, K. R., Schulman, B. L., & Osterweil, D. (1990). The value of assessing falls in an elderly population. *Annals of Internal Medicine, 113,* 308–316.

Sengstaken, E. A., & King, S. A. (1993). The problems of pain and its detection among geriatric nursing home residents. *Journal of the American Geriatrics Society, 41*(5), 541–544.

Simons, W., & Malabar, R. (1995). Assessing pain in elderly patients who cannot respond verbally. *Journal of Advanced Nursing, 22,* 663–669.

Tinetti, M., Baker, D., McAvay, G., Claus, E., Garrett, P., Gottschalk, M., Koch, M., Trainor, K., & Hurwitz, R. (1994). A multifactorial intervention to reduce the risk of falling among elderly people living in the community. *New England Journal of Medicine, 331*(13), 821–827.

Tinetti, M. D., McAvay, G., & Claus, E. (1996). Does multiple risk factor reduction explain the reduction in fall rate in the Yale FICSIT trial? Frailty and injuries cooperative studies of intervention techniques. *American Journal of Epidemiology, 144*(4), 389–399.

Tinetti, M. E. (1986). Performance-oriented assessment of mobility problems in elderly patients. *Journal of the American Geriatrics Society, 34,* 119–126.

Tinetti, M. E., Liu, W.-L., & Claus, E. B. (1993). Predictors and prognosis of inability to get up after falls among elderly persons. *JAMA, 269*(1), 65–70.

Wolf, S. L., Barnhart, H. X., Kutner, N. G., McNeely, E., Coogler, C., Xu, T., & Atlanta FICSIT Group. (1996). Reducing frailty and falls in older persons: An investigation of Tai Chi and computerized balance training. *Journal of the American Geriatrics Society, 44*(5), 489–497.

Wolinsky, F. D., Coe, R. M., Chavez, M. N., Pendergast, J. M., & Miller, D. K. (1986). Further assessment of the reliability and validity of a nutritional risk index: Analysis of a three-wave panel study of elderly adults. *Health Services Research, 20*(6 Pt 2), 977–990.

Wolinsky, F. D., Coe, R. M., McIntosh, W. A., Kubena, K. S., Prendergast, J. M., Chavez, M. N., Miller, D. K., Romeis, J. C., & Landmann, W. A. (1990). Progress in the development of a nutritional risk index. *Journal of Nutrition, 120*(Suppl 11), 1549–1553.

# 4

# Cognitive Assessment of Older Adults

## LINDA K. LANGLEY

The cognitive abilities of older adults are assessed largely because of two age-related changes. First, normal aging is accompanied by subtle but detectable changes in cognitive functioning (see Craik & Salthouse, 1992 for a comprehensive treatment of cognitive aging). The nature of these changes is incompletely understood, and there is considerable variability in the amount of decline experienced by older adults, but in some individuals they are substantial enough to disrupt daily functioning. Second, the incidence and prevalence of dementing disorders increases in late life (Jorm, Korten, & Henderson, 1987). Dementing diseases, in contrast to normal age-related cognitive changes, lead to severe, irreversible, and global deterioration. Cognitive assessment is an integral part of detecting dementia. A comprehensive assessment includes physical and neurologic examination, medical history, functional status assessment, and cognitive testing. When interpreted in the context of these other tests, cognitive assessment contributes to informed diagnoses of abnormal functioning.

Beyond its involvement in detecting dementia, formal cognitive assessment contributes to the specification of dementia.

For treatment purposes it is important to distinguish as early as possible between reversible dementias (e.g., depression, delirium) and irreversible dementias (e.g., Alzheimer's disease, vascular dementia, subcortical dementia). This chapter outlines the issues relevant to assessing cognitive dysfunction in older adults. Although assessment of age-related changes is an important area of research development, this chapter focuses on assessing abnormal (dementia-related) changes.

## DOMAINS OF COGNITIVE FUNCTIONING

Cognitive assessment evaluates current levels of mental functioning within the context of past levels to predict future levels. Mental functioning is commonly broken down into domains that pinpoint specific areas of impairment.

Table 4.1 describes these domains in brief detail. In each domain, the changes that accompany normal aging and irreversible dementia are described. It is important to be aware of the domains included when choosing an assessment instrument. Certain domains are more sensitive than others to the effects of aging and demen-

**Table 4.1.**

Domains of Cognitive Functioning

| Domain | Description | Changes with age and dementia |
|---|---|---|
| Attention | (a) Arousal or consciousness, (b) alertness for expected events, (c) maintenance of alertness over time (i.e., vigilance), (d) spatial orienting, (e) selection of information in the presence of distraction, and (f) division of limited mental capacities for processing of simultaneous events | Arousal, concentration, alertness, vigilance, and spatial orienting do not change with age or until the later stages of irreversible dementia<br><br>Selection of information in the presence of distraction and the division of attention decline with age and to a greater degree with dementia |
| Memory | The collection, storage, and retrieval of information. Contrary to early views, memory is not a unitary phenomenon but instead is divisible into distinct systems | Aging and Alzheimer's disease differentially affect memory systems. See below |
| Orientation | Orientation is memory for contextual and autobiographical information, some of which must be continually updated (date, season, time, current location) and the rest of which is relatively permanent (name, address, birth date) | Orientation is rather insensitive to age-related changes but is extremely sensitive to early dementia-related changes |
| Calculation/working memory | Working memory is considered a type of memory that involves manipulation or transformation of memorized information into another form. For example, in a mental calculation problem, two or more numbers (e.g., 3 and 9) must be held in memory while at the same time added together | Working memory shows moderate age-related changes and prominent dementia-related changes |
| Episodic and semantic memory | Episodic memory and semantic memory both involve conscious memory of known facts<br><br>Episodic memories have temporal and spatial components (e.g., remembering *when* and *where* an event occurred). Episodic memories can be further divided into immediate (short-term), recent (long-term), and remote memories<br><br>Semantic memories are verbally mediated memories that lack a spatial or temporal context (i.e., factual knowledge about the world) | Episodic memory is the type of memory most affected by aging and dementia. As a consequence, most memory measures tap episodic memories. Aging causes mild changes in episodic memory, and dementia causes prominent changes. With age, recent memories are more affected than immediate or remote memories. With dementia, immediate memories and remote memories also become affected, but later than recent memories<br><br>Findings are mixed regarding semantic memory. Most studies find no change or only moderate age-related changes for factual knowledge. Dementia shows notable changes in semantic memory, particularly changes in access. These changes occur a little later than changes in episodic memory |
| Implicit and procedural memory | Implicit memory is memory that occurs without awareness of something being remembered<br><br>Procedural memory is improvement on a task without recalling the specific skills needed to complete the task (e.g., riding a bike) | Findings are mixed regarding age-related changes. Some studies find small changes, but most studies suggest there are no age-related changes in implicit and procedural memory. Only small changes in implicit and procedural memory are found with dementia until late in the disease. Because this is not an area of impairment, it is not as heavily assessed as other areas of memory |

*(continued)*

**Table 4.1.** — Continued

| Domain | Description | Changes with age and dementia |
|---|---|---|
| Language | Language involves both production and comprehension of verbal materials. Language production can be further divided into the ability to produce words versus the ability to use them meaningfully<br><br>Tests of language include verbal repetition, object naming, vocabulary, verbal fluency, writing, reading, and following commands | Although vocabulary, articulation, and reading at a lexical level are relatively intact, comprehension shows mild impairment with aging and marked impairment with dementia. Language skills that are particularly susceptible to age-related effects and more so by dementia-related effects are object naming and verbal fluency |
| Visuospatial abilities | Visuospatial abilities pertain to abilities to perceive objects and their spatial locations as well as to manipulate spatial and figural relations. Examples include locating an object in space, tracing a figure, learning a route, and putting together a puzzle | Visuospatial abilities are mildly impaired in older adults, although less so when familiar stimuli are used. Visuospatial abilities are significantly compromised with dementia. Deficits are found in mental rotation, picture arrangement, and block design, although simple orientation abilities are intact |
| Psychomotor speed | The rate at which cognitive processing occurs and the rate at which responses are made | Age-related slowing occurs within each of the cognitive domains — simple attention as well as complex problem solving. Alzheimer's disease and other dementias are accompanied by generalized psychomotor slowing, but at an accelerated rate compared with normal aging |
| Executive/problem solving | This domain, to a certain extent, is a "catch-all" domain of higher cognitive functions. Executive functions refer to cognitive skills involved in the initiation, planning, organization, and monitoring of goal-directed behavior. Tests of abstraction (proverb interpretation, similarities), set shifting (e.g., card sorting, maze learning), and set maintenance (list generation) are included in this domain | Most of the cognitive functions described in this domain show notable changes with aging and to a further extent with dementia |
| Intelligence | Tests of intelligence measure general or global levels of cognitive functioning. Intellectual abilities of older adults have been historically divided into crystallized and fluid abilities | |
| | Crystallized intelligence reflects the knowledge obtained through education and the social environment, for example, communication skills, social intelligence, and cultural knowledge | Crystallized intelligence shows little decline with normal aging, at least until the 70s. Crystallized abilities decline in dementia |
| | Fluid intelligence consists of the skills that make a person adaptable to the environment. It involves flexible and rapid processing of novel information | Fluid intelligence shows gradual age-related declines as early as age 20 or 30 years and continues monotonically into older adulthood. Decline is accelerated with the onset of dementia |

tia. Specific instruments are discussed later in this chapter, and each is described in terms of the domains addressed. Domains of importance may vary depending on whether the purpose of the assessment is to detect cognitive impairment, to diagnose dementia, to discriminate between irreversible and reversible forms of dementia, or to detect change in cognitive functioning.

## CHOOSING A MEASURE

Cognitive measures are not casually interchangeable. A measure that is highly effective in one situation may not be at all appropriate in another situation. The choice of a cognitive measure must be guided by the purpose of the assessment.

### Clinical Purposes

In a clinical context, the primary reasons for testing the cognitive capabilities of older adults are for screening; diagnosis; ranking the severity of impairments (i.e., staging); evaluating change; and making practical decisions regarding competency, management, and placement.

Clinical screening distinguishes normal cognitive changes from abnormal changes (e.g., dementia, delirium, or depression). Screening tests come in two forms: mental status tests, which consist of objective questions asked of the patient; and informant reports, which consist of questions asked of someone close to the patient.

Once screening instruments have identified individuals with possible cognitive deficits, diagnostic instruments confirm or disprove these abnormalities. The first step is determining whether impairments are reversible or irreversible. Perhaps the two most common types of reversible syndromes are depression and delirium. Depression affects cognitive functioning to varying degrees, but it can be so severe as to be confused with dementia symptoms (Folstein & McHugh, 1978). Inspection of performance helps distinguish depression from irreversible dementia (Blau & Ober, 1988; Hart et al., 1987; Johnson & Magaro, 1987; Weingartner, 1986). For example, depressed people complain of memory problems more so than demented people, but they do better on memory tasks (Niederehe, 1986). Verbal fluency and naming abilities show little change with depression but are impaired in Alzheimer's disease (La Rue, 1989). Depressed individuals typically score within the normal range on tests of intelligence (e.g., WAIS-R), whereas demented individuals show early floor effects on such measures (La Rue, E'Elia, Clark, Spar, & Jarvik, 1986). Depression must be assessed as part of any dementia work-up. (See Chapter 5 for a discussion of depression instruments used with older adults). In reality, depression and irreversible dementia often occur together. Approximately 20% of dementia patients are depressed (Reifler et al., 1986; Roth, 1978), and it is difficult with these individuals to distinguish what proportion of their cognitive difficulties are attributable to depression versus dementia. Treating the depressive symptoms may alleviate some of the cognitive impairment.

Delirium, a reversible but dramatic change in cognitive functioning, results from treatable physical conditions such as drug intoxication, metabolic imbalance, nutritional deficiency, infection, fever, and cardiovascular disorder. Although delirium's course is drastically different from that of an irreversible dementia (e.g., an abrupt vs. slow onset, extreme fluctuation vs. steady state of symptoms), delirium is often misdiagnosed as an irreversible dementia and consequently left untreated. Clinicians who are called on to assess cognitive functioning in the hospital see the patient at one point in time and therefore do not see the hallmark changes in symptoms. Several measures have been developed to screen for delirium (Albert et al., 1992; Inouye et al., 1990; Neelon et al., 1996). These measures assess the primary symptoms of delirium, including disturbed awareness, disorientation, memory impairment, hallucinations and delusions, incoherent speech, disorganized thinking, and increased or decreased psychomotor activity. The key feature of these instruments is that they focus on fluctuations in symptoms, either by wording the questions as such or by re-administering the instrument in short periods of time (e.g., within 48 hours). Once delirium is distinguished from dementia, the underlying pathology is treated.

If reversible dementias have been ruled

out as the source of cognitive abnormality, irreversible dementia must be considered. Table 4.2 lists the most common types of progressive dementias found in older adults. Table 4.3 describes the cognitive characteristics of three of the most predominant types of dementia, Alzheimer's disease, vascular dementia (i.e., multi-infarct dementia), and subcortical dementia (e.g., Parkinson's disease). Because cognitive profiles for dementias vary, assessments of specific domains contribute to a differential diagnosis of dementia.

Cognitive measures do more than determine whether deficits are present; they grade the severity of impairments. Ratings of severity inform decisions regarding future treatment and care (e.g., ability to drive, nursing home placement, and efficacy of interventions). Clinicians describe severity in terms of stages (e.g., very mild, mild, moderate, severe, and profound) using rating instruments. Certain mental status tests and shortened batteries have also proven useful in determining severity.

Practitioners are commonly called on to make decisions regarding individuals' abilities to function in the community. Competency assessments concern ability to drive, work, live independently, perform daily activities, take medications, and make medical, legal, and financial decisions. Institutional placement and formal care may require a formal determination of dependence. Cognitive assessments can inform decisions, although no measures have been proven to correlate highly with competency or performance of everyday tasks.

**Table 4.2.** Irreversible Dementias Most Commonly Found in Older Adults

| |
|---|
| Alzheimer's disease |
| Vascular dementia |
| Lewy body dementia |
| Frontal temporal dementia |
| Pick's disease |
| Parkinson's disease |
| Progressive supranuclear palsy |

## Research Purposes

Cognitive assessment occurs within research contexts. The specific research aims dictate the appropriate choice of cognitive measure. Categorical scores (e.g., impaired vs. unimpaired, mild vs. moderate dementia) are likely desired if cognitive ability is the independent/predictive variable. A continuous variable is more often sought when cognition is the dependent variable. Choice of a measure depends on whether the research seeks to measure evidence of cognitive impairment (impaired vs. unimpaired), diagnostic outcome (e.g., Alzheimer's disease vs. delirium), severity of dementia (mild vs. moderate vs. severe), amount of change in functioning over time, or level of functioning within a specific area.

Cognition-related research is largely categorized into clinical versus basic research. Clinical research is largely devoted to developing measures that can detect, diagnose, and stage dementia. An additional thrust is to examine the relationships between cognitive functioning and tasks of daily living, such as dressing (Heacock et al., 1997), medication compliance (Isaac & Tamblyn, 1993), driving ability (Hunt et al., 1997; Rizzo et al., 1997), and falls (Lord & Clark, 1996). A newer area of clinical research examines the manner in which patients' cognitive impairments affect the ability of clinicians to assess patient functioning in other areas, such as vision and hearing (Gates et al., 1995), cardiovascular functioning (Garrett, 1997), and pain (Parmelee, 1996). This line of research is important for determining whether an individual is capable of participating in noncognitive studies and reporting reliable information about themselves, such as their histories, habits, and so forth.

The primary purpose of basic research on cognitive aging is to characterize the phenomenon. Researchers seek to describe the domains and processes of cognition that are impaired and preserved by aging and the *progression* of normal age changes

**Table 4.3.**

Comparison of Three Common Types of Irreversible Dementia

| Characteristic | Alzheimer's disease (AD) | Vascular dementia | Subcortical dementia |
|---|---|---|---|
| Causes of dementia | Cause unknown. AD marked by neuritic plaques and neurofibrillary tangles in the brain | Multiple occlusions of cerebral arteries ("mini-strokes"), small vessel disease, and brain hemorrhage | Subcortical dementias include Parkinson's disease, Huntington's disease, and progressive supranuclear palsy. Causes unknown |
| Progression of cognitive symptoms | Gradual | Acute onset, stepwise progression | Gradual, modest, and variable decline |
| Physical symptoms that accompany the disease | No prominent physical symptoms | High blood pressure, gait problems | Movement disturbances, tremor, rigidity, postural changes |
| Attention/working memory | Attention is subtly impaired. Vigilance and concentration are relatively intact, but selective and divided attention are impaired<br><br>Working memory is impaired | Findings conflict. Little information is available | Vigilance and concentration are OK<br><br>Higher order attention skills are very impaired (set shifting, divided attention, selective attention)<br><br>Working memory is relatively intact but very slow' |
| Memory | Memory impairment is the most pronounced early symptom<br><br>Encoding impaired. Retention poor. Retrieval impaired<br><br>Recall and recognition both clearly impaired | Findings vary. Impaired memory not as prominent a symptom as in AD. Memory problems are equal to or less than those in AD<br><br>Encoding impaired. Retention OK. Retrieval impaired<br><br>Recall impaired, recognition normal | Memory problems occur but are not as prominent as in AD<br><br>Encoding preserved, retention good, retrieval impaired<br><br>Recall impaired, recognition normal or relatively preserved |
| Language | Naming and verbal fluency are impaired early in the disease<br><br>Normal articulation. Word reading ability intact<br><br>Decreased reading comprehension<br><br>Intact writing ability in the early stages | Poor naming ability (aphasia) and decreased fluency, but better than in AD<br><br>Normal articulation. Word reading ability intact<br><br>Mechanical problems (e.g., writing) are greater than in AD | No naming/word finding difficulties except when dementia is relatively advanced<br><br>Greatly reduced fluency<br><br>Poor speech. Poor articulation. Decreased volume in speech. Voice becomes increasingly monotonic<br><br>Mechanical problems are greater than in AD |

*(continued)*

**Table 4.3.** — Continued

| Characteristic | Alzheimer's disease (AD) | Vascular dementia | Subcortical dementia |
|---|---|---|---|
| Visuospatial skills | Basic visual abilities (sensation and perception) are intact<br><br>Visuospatial abilities are impaired in midstages of the disease. In occasional cases impairment occurs earlier<br><br>Poor drawing and copying ability. Poor facial discrimination, mental rotation, and complex construction | Similar to AD<br><br>May show more sensory and motor deficits than in AD (e.g., picture arrangement, object assembly, block design) | Pronounced difficulty in visual analysis, pattern completion, copying, and spatial orientation<br><br>Deficits occur at the same time or later than in AD<br><br>Output is slow on motor tasks (e.g., visual construction and copying designs). Impaired spatial orientation and spatial relations |
| Speed of cognitive processing | Slowing occurs, but less than in other dementias | Slowing is early and prominent | Slowing is early and prominent |
| Problem solving/executive functioning | Deficits occur early, but after memory changes. Deficits in problem solving, concept formation, and abstraction | Executive functioning deficits are prominent. Problem solving, concept formation, and abstraction are compromised | Executive deficits are one of the earliest symptoms, although deficits are not greater than in AD. Impairments in planning and sequencing, shifting mental set, and forming concepts |
| Mood | Mood changes are not prominent. Some depression, apathy, and diminished insight | Depression, indifference, and emotional liability | More likely to be depressed, apathetic, and anxious. Flat affect. May have psychotic symptoms (delusions and hallucinations) |

**Table 4.4.**
Types of Cognitive Tests Used for Different Assessment Purposes

| Reason for assessment | Mental status tests | Informant reports | Full test batteries | Domain tests | Shortened test batteries | Dementia rating scales | Global change measures |
|---|---|---|---|---|---|---|---|
| Screening | XX | XX | | | X | | |
| Diagnosis | X | X | XX | X | X | X | |
| Assess change | X | X | X | X | XX | X | XX |
| Staging | X | | X | | X | XX | |
| Management/placement decisions | X | X | X | X | X | X | |
| Research | XX | X | | X | XX | X | XX |

X, used; XX, most often used.

covering the spectrum from young–old to old–old ages. The checklist in Table 4.4 indicates the appropriate test categories for different assessment purposes.

## ASSESSMENT FORMATS AND TYPES OF RESPONSES

### Assessment Formats

Cognitive assessments vary in the manner in which information is gathered. Cognition can be either directly or indirectly assessed. With direct assessment, information is gathered by giving participants cognitive tasks to perform. With indirect assessment, information is gathered by asking participants or their informants questions about their cognitive functioning. Although direct assessment of cognitive functioning may be more reliable than indirect assessment (i.e., less influenced by reporting factors), indirect assessment may offer greater ecological validity (less influenced by the artificiality of laboratory-type cognitive items).

### *Objective Psychological Tests*

Of the four assessment formats primarily used in cognitive assessment, objective psychological testing is the only format to directly assess cognitive functioning. With objective testing, tasks are given to participants that are designed to tap specific cognitive processes (e.g., attention, memory, or language). Responses are scored objectively (e.g., correct–incorrect, number of items generated, or time to complete the task). The strength of objective measures lies in minimizing the subjective analysis of a participant's performance. No one, including the examiner, the participant, and the caregiver, is asked to interpret the cognitive performance of the participant. Rather, each item is scored according to previously defined criteria.

A weakness of objective measures is that they do not allow consideration of outside factors on performance. For example, an older adult with arthritis is more likely to perform timed written tasks more slowly than is an older adult without arthritis. Another weakness of objective measures is that they typically require the participant to correctly understand the instructions of the task and to produce verbal or written responses. Therefore, floor effects will occur for those more severely impaired.

### *Informant Reports*

In the indirect assessment format of informant reporting, someone other than the older adult being assessed supplies the responses, such as a spouse, a nurse, or a trained observer. This format is particularly useful for assessing someone who can no longer understand test instructions, who can no longer communicate effectively, or who is no longer cooperative. Moreover, a family caregiver may be able to report cognitive deficits of the individual in question that occur in a natural setting and that occur within the context of past performance (e.g., difficulty balancing the checkbook, poor driving skills, forgetting names). The person in question may not recognize these cognitive deficits himself or herself or may not be able to successfully report them. Furthermore, caregivers can describe decline or *change* in functioning because the informant is familiar with the subject's previous level of functioning. The caregiver is able to provide information regarding the mode of onset of cognitive dysfunction (abrupt vs. gradual), progression of symptoms (stepwise vs. continuous), and duration of symptoms.

A weakness of this assessment format is that, although items can be worded objectively, responses require interpretation of an individual's behavior by another person. Although subjective bias may taint scoring, research has shown that results from informant reports correlate significantly with findings from objective test measures (Paulman, Koss, & MacInnes, 1996). (See Chapter 17 for further discussion of strengths and weaknesses of informant reports.)

## Unstructured and Semistructured Interviews

Unstructured and semistructured interviews are indirect measures of cognitive functioning. Trained professionals (e.g., neurologists, geriatricians, psychiatrists, or psychologists) typically conduct such interviews in clinical contexts to determine whether cognitive deficits are present and, if so, the source of these deficits. The examiner may interview the older adult being assessed, a family member, or both sources. If both sources are interviewed, the interviewer may choose to conduct the interviews separately to promote openness from each party and to compare the information gathered. In an unstructured interview, the examiner selects questions relevant to her or his estimate of the likely diagnosis. These questions pertain to symptoms and behaviors that are either consistent or inconsistent with the diagnosis in question. As the interview progresses, the examiner may change his or her line of questioning based on information already gathered. Semistructured interviews include objective measures such as mental status tests or informant reports, prepared questions, and unstructured questions by the examiner.

The strength of the interview format is that abundant information can be gathered that is highly individualized for the circumstances of the older individual being assessed. The weakness of this format is that only professionals trained to use such a format can conduct the interviews. Such a format is highly subjective. The examiner may ask questions and interpret responses based on the diagnoses they think most likely and thus miss important information leading to an alternative diagnosis. Furthermore, because the findings are in a nonquantitative form, findings cannot be compared across patients.

## Self-Report

Older adults are occasionally asked to assess their own cognitive functioning. This indirect measure is the least used of the four formats. It is useful for gathering initial information (i.e., basic screening) or determining the impact of disease. Individuals describe the nature of their cognitive difficulties in terms of the context in which they occur, the frequency with which they occur, and the level of concern it causes them. These questions are presented in either a structured format (e.g., self-report questionnaire) or an unstructured format (e.g., general questions from the examiner). Self-reports are seldom used clinically because memory complaints correlate only weakly with actual cognitive performance (Hermann, 1982; Roth et al., 1986). Personality and social expectations may unduly influence reports of memory complaints and overshadow true memory deficits. Furthermore, individuals with dementia are typically less than fully aware of their deficits and, moreover, may be unable to express the self-knowledge they have (Paulman et al., 1996).

## Types of Responses

In addition to the format of administration, assessments vary according to the response format.

### Accuracy

One way in which objective psychological tests tabulate responses is in terms of accuracy. Either the number of items answered correctly or the number of items answered incorrectly (e.g., errors) is counted.

### Time Scores

Objective psychological tests may involve a time component as well as an accuracy component. Time scores take different forms; a test may measure either the amount of time to complete either a single item or a series of items or the number of items completed in a specific amount of time.

### Ratings

Ratings are responses commonly used on self-reports and informant reports. Ratings can be dichotomous (e.g., yes–no, agree–

disagree) or Likert scale (e.g., declined a great deal, declined slightly, improved slightly, improved a great deal; never, rarely, often, very often). To obtain scores from rating scales, ratings must be transformed into numerical responses and summed across items.

### Clinical Judgments

Clinical judgments are categorical decisions made by trained professionals (e.g., dementia or no dementia). These judgments, particularly those related to diagnosis, arise primarily from unstructured or semistructured interviews. They may also be based on findings from objective psychological tests, informant reports, medical history, physical examination, and laboratory results.

## INTERPRETING OLDER ADULTS' SCORES ON COGNITIVE TESTS: EFFECTS OF NONCOGNITIVE VARIABLES

Performance on cognitive tasks is not solely determined by cognitive abilities but also by noncognitive factors. To avoid misinterpretation of performance for ability, examiners must consider factors specific to the test situation or to the individual.

### Effect of Test-Situation Variables on Performance

Features inherent to a test or the test situation influence test performance. Time constraints, anxiety, and fatigue effects are three such test-situation factors.

Time constraints adversely affect the performance of older individuals. All cognitive processes slow with age (Birren, Woods, & Williams, 1980; Salthouse, 1985); and tasks in which time limits are enforced hamper the performance of older adults more so than that of younger adults. This lower level of production may be misinterpreted as a deficit in a particular cognitive domain. For slowing to be evidence of a domain-specific impairment, it must be greater than that predicted by generalized cognitive slowing (Nebes & Brady, 1992). Misinterpretation of slowing as specific cognitive impairment is avoided by comparing timed performance of older adults against age-specific norms or, in the case of a longitudinal design, by comparing performance against earlier (baseline) performance.

Subtractive methodology assesses domain-specific slowing. With this methodology, an individual's speed of performance in a condition that tests the domain of interest is compared with speed of performance in a control condition that is similar but does not test the domain of interest. If slowing as measured by this subtractive methodology is much greater for one individual compared with other individuals of the same age, this suggests a domain-specific impairment. Tests without time constraints that focus on accuracy rather than on reaction time offer information as to whether the task *can* be performed rather than the speed with which it is performed. This allows the focus to be on the quality of the performance. This is not to suggest that timed tests should be avoided with older adults. Speed of processing is an important factor in cognitive processing, and slowing is actually a strong indicator of early dementia (Nebes & Brady, 1992). Although speed of performance has diagnostic strengths, slowed processing must not be interpreted as impairment in a specific domain (e.g., language impairment) but rather as an influence on performance in several domains.

Excessive anxiety disrupts concentration necessary for optimal cognitive performance. To reduce anxiety, examiners should familiarize older adults with the purposes and procedures of testing. Task instructions should be presented in simple and clear language. Examiners should strive to establish rapport and a sense of trust with patients and to reassure them during testing, acknowledging that some tasks are difficult. Assessments that begin with easier items allow participants to experience success early.

Fatigue unduly influences cognitive performance when tests are excessive in length, are administered without breaks, or require large amounts of concentration. Therefore, lengthy tests should be shortened, divided into separate sessions, or given with breaks as needed. Additionally, efforts should be made to test older individuals when they are well rested and most alert, frequently in the morning or early afternoon hours.

### Effects of Other Variables on Performance

Sensory impairments hamper an older adult's ability to perform at an optimal level. Hearing difficulties are particularly troublesome in testing situations because the examiner asks the participant questions. Establishing adequate hearing can be as easy as having a brief conversation with the participant. Vision is also important, particularly for tasks that require reading, writing, or manipulation of objects. If in doubt, a visual acuity test will confirm or disconfirm suspicions of poor vision. There are several suggestions for enhancing an older adult's sensory experience. Give participants prior notice to bring all assistive devices (glasses, hearing aids) to the testing session, and ensure they are worn during testing. Choose a quiet testing environment without background noise. Test in a well-lit room with the participant's back to the window if there is one (to reduce glare and distraction). Enlarge print of materials with a photocopy machine if necessary. Of course, in many clinical situations the examiner does not have control of the testing environment, but all practical efforts should be made to maximize the sensory experience of older participants. When sensory limitations are evident, they must be taken into consideration when a performance is interpreted.

Two final noncognitive factors must be considered in test interpretation: education and premorbid intelligence. Individuals with high levels of education and/or high premorbid intelligence may perform well on cognitive tasks yet perform below their previous level of functioning (i.e., ceiling effects prevent detection of decline). On the other end, individuals with low levels of education and/or low premorbid intelligence may historically perform at a low level, so present poor performance does not necessarily indicate decline. To address educational differences, many assessment tools have been normed for different levels of education. These norms should be utilized when available. It is more difficult to correct for differences in premorbid functioning because often an individual's level of intelligence previous to the onset of cognitive difficulties is unknown to the clinician. Premorbid intelligence can be estimated from such things as years of education and occupation, which are known to correlate with intelligence, but these are imperfect estimates. Alternatively, tests have been devised to estimate premorbid intelligence. One such test is the National Adult Reading Test (NART) (Nelson, 1982; Nelson & O'Connell, 1978) in which participants pronounce words that are irregularly spelled. Vocabulary is relatively preserved in dementia, so the NART provides an estimate of level of vocabulary achieved before the onset of brain impairment. With this estimate of premorbid intelligence, a clinician can compare a person's test results with an estimate of their past test results and use this information to make a determination of decline or no decline. It must be kept in mind, however, that although vocabulary is *relatively* preserved in dementia, it is not *absolutely* preserved, and the applicability of the NART in estimating premorbid intelligence has its limitations (Storandt, Stone, & LaBarge, 1995).

Caution must be used when making allowances for low scores of poorly educated individuals. Low education is a risk factor for dementia. Lifestyle factors of those with low education (occupational hazards, poor health care) may put them at greater risk for dementia, whereas high education may provide a reserve capacity that buffers formation or emergence of cognitive impairment. Farmer and associates (1995) noted greater cognitive decline over a 1-year period for those with lower education than for those with higher education. Thus it is unclear whether poor education makes people *appear* more impaired or if poorly educated people actually *are* more impaired. Adjusting scores for lower levels of education may not be the appropriate solution. For individuals with high or low levels of education who are suspected of experiencing cognitive impairment, tests should be used that avoid ceiling and floor effects, and follow-up visits should be scheduled to determine whether decline occurs over time.

## MEASURES OF COGNITIVE FUNCTIONING IN OLDER ADULTS

Screening tests were not designed to be diagnostic but to be sensitive to cognitive abnormalities that require further assessment. Screening tests take the form of *(1)* objective psychological tests termed *mental status tests* and *(2)* informant reports. Both types of screening tests sample the domains of orientation, calculation/working memory, short- and long-term episodic memory, language, and visuospatial abilities. Orientation, episodic memory, and language are heavily sampled because these domains are most susceptible to early and significant impairment in dementia.

A continuing controversy concerns whether sensitivity or specificity is a more important property of screening measures. In some circumstances, the hazards of committing false-negative errors (not detecting reversible dementing syndromes) are greater than those of committing false-positive errors (unnecessary follow-up testing for individuals with no impairment). But there are trade-offs with increased sensitivity and decreased specificity. With increased sensitivity, people are more likely to go through extensive and expensive neuropsychological and laboratory testing

to determine they are not impaired. This wears emotionally on the family and the patient. False positives are particularly troublesome in the context of wide screening of older adults. In such a context, a false-positive rate is unmanageable in terms of time and dollars spent putting large numbers of people through complete diagnostic work-ups. On the other hand, a sensitive screen detects someone in the earliest stages of dementia, which is the time when drug treatments offer the greatest benefit. Furthermore, early detection gives families more time to prepare emotionally, financially, and practically for the changes that will inevitably occur. At the same time, because treatments are few, delayed detection has few deleterious consequences beyond those mentioned. As the dementia progresses over time, screening instruments will eventually detect it.

### Mental Status Tests

Mental status tests are direct, objective, and quantitative. They require verbal responses and may further require reading and writing responses. A wide range of mental status tests is now available. For a comprehensive review of cognitive screening instruments, see Karuza, Katz, & Henderson (1997), Mitrushina & Fuld (1996), and Ritchie (1988).

Strengths of mental status tests are brevity and portability; reduced susceptibility to practice effects; modest training required for administration; and quantified presentation of results that allows comparisons across time and clinicians (Mitrushina & Fuld, 1996). Limitations of mental status tests are high false-negative rates; global items that reduce detection of isolated deficits; occasional false-positive results related to advanced age, ethnic background, low IQ, and poor English skills; and poor distinction between types of cognitive impairments. Some of these limitations may seem unjustified for tests meant only to be screening tools, but these tools are often used (correctly or incorrectly) for purposes such as diagnosing, detecting change, and rating severity of dementia.

No single mental status test is superior to the others; in fact, most mental status tests are similar in reliability and validity. Discussed below are the mental status tests most widely used and validated.

## Mini-Mental State Examination (MMSE) (Folstein, Folstein, & McHugh, 1975)

The *Mini-Mental State Examination* remains the standard against which other mental status tests are measured. It is the most widely employed mental status test; more than 90% of physicians who screen for dementia use the MMSE (Somerfeld et al., 1991). It takes approximately 10 minutes to administer and includes both verbal and nonverbal items. Scoring is based on the number of correct items, with thirty points possible. Domains assessed are orientation, immediate and delayed episodic memory, calculation/working memory, visuospatial ability, and language. Most errors are made in orientation to date, delayed memory (recall of three words), calculation (serial seven subtractions), and visuospatial abilities (figure copying) (Fillenbaum et al., 1987; Galasko et al., 1990; Magaziner, Bassett, & Hebel, 1987). Factor analysis reveals a two-factor structure of memory/attention and verbal comprehension (Zillmer et al., 1990). Items from the MMSE are presented in Table 4.5.

Administration and scoring of the MMSE varies, as illustrated by scoring of the calculation section. To assess calculation, some clinicians use serial subtractions of seven starting with the number 100. Other clinicians use *WORLD* spelled backward. Still others use the higher score from the two items or use the *WORLD* item only for those with education levels below 10 years. This variation in scoring is problematic because research shows that the *WORLD* item leads to higher scores than the serial subtraction item (Ganguli et al., 1990). Correlation between *WORLD* and subtraction is low (r = 0.37) (Holzer et al.,

1984), suggesting that these two items do not measure the same construct. The variability in MMSE scoring techniques limits the universality of score interpretation.

The appropriate MMSE cut-off score has been widely debated. The traditional score of 23 was chosen because it optimized sensitivity and preserved moderate to high specificity (Anthony et al., 1982). Later research found that this score lead to unacceptably high false-negative rates (Roper, Bieliauskas, & Peterson, 1996). Comparing various cut-offs, the highest diagnostic accuracy was found with a cut-off of 26 (Roper et al., 1996). Strict cut-off values have utility for research but not for clinical purposes. Scores on the MMSE vary as a function of age, race, and education (Karuza et al., 1997). Other characteristics to consider when interpreting MMSE scores are physical disabilities, sensory impairments, and command of the English language. A strict cut-off does not allow for these considerations and may lead to erroneous conclusions of abilities. Corrected norms have been offered that take age and education into consideration (e.g., (Crum et al., 1993) and should be consulted when appropriate.

More than 25 studies have examined the sensitivity and specificity of the MMSE (Tombaugh & McIntyre, 1992). In approximately 75% of studies, a sensitivity of 85% or better was found with dementia patients (Karuza et al., 1997). The MMSE is less sensitive for those with lower levels of impairment (Anthony et al., 1982), and, unfortunately, those people are in the greatest need of detection. Sensitivity is lower in community samples than in clinic or hospital samples because the incidence of dementia is lower. As outlined later in Table 4.8, the MMSE has high test–retest and inter-rater reliability. It correlates well with other mental status tests (e.g., Blessed IMC, CCSE, and SPMSQ), with tests of functional ability (e.g., ADL, IADL), and with shortened test batteries (e.g., ADAS).

**Table 4.5.**
Mini-Mental State Examination

*Orientation (10 points possible)*

1. What is the month?
2. What is the date?
3. What is the year?
4. What season is it?
5. What day of the week is it?
6. What is the name of this hospital?
7. What floor are we on?
8. What city are we in?
9. What county are we in?
10. What state are we in?

*Immediate Memory (3 points possible)*

11. Tell patient you will say three words (1 second each). Tell patient to repeat all three objects after you have said them and to remember them for later recall. Score one point for each correct repetition on first trial. Repeat until patient learns all three.

*Attention and Calculation (5 points possible)*

12. Tell patient to begin with the number 100 and count backward by 7s. Stop after five answers. Count correct each answer that is correctly subtracted by 7 from the previous response.

   If patient refuses to do the task, have patient spell *world* backwards. Score one point for each letter in correct ordinal position. (Some clinicians count the higher score of the two items; other clinicians administer the *world* item only to persons with education levels of 9 years or less.)

*Delayed Memory (3 points possible)*

13. Have patient recall three words. Score one point for each correct answer.

*Language (9 points possible)*

14. Show a pencil and have patient name it.
15. Show a watch and have patient name it.
16. Have patient repeat the following phrase: "No ifs, ands, or buts." Allow only one trial.
17. Have patient complete the following three stage command: "Take a piece of paper in your right hand, fold it in half, and place it on the floor" (1 point for each part correctly executed, 3 points possible). Allow only one trial.
18. Have patient read the following sign and do what it says: "CLOSE YOUR EYES."
19. Ask the patient to write a sentence. The sentence must contain a subject and a verb and be sensible. Correct grammar and punctuation are not necessary.
20. Ask patient to copy a drawing of two intersecting pentagons. All 10 angles must be present and 2 must intersect to score 1 point.

Total: 30 points possible

*Blessed Orientation-Memory-Concentration Test (BOMC) (Katzman et al., 1983)*

The Blessed Dementia Scale (Blessed, Tomlinson, & Roth, 1968) consists of a functional assessment and a mental status test. The mental status test (the Blessed Information-Memory-Concentration [IMC] Test) assesses orientation, delayed recall of a phrase, and working memory/calculation (reciting the months backward and counting backward). Scores range from 0 (best) to 37 (worst) and are based on the number of errors. Katzman and colleagues (1983) developed a six item version of the Blessed mental status test called the *Blessed Orientation-Memory-Concentration*

**Table 4.6.**
Blessed Orientation-Memory-Concentration Test

| Item | Possible error points | Weight | Possible weighted score |
|---|---|---|---|
| 1. What year is it now? | 1 | 4 | 4 |
| 2. What month is it now? | 1 | 3 | 3 |
| 3. Repeat this phrase after me:<br>John Brown, 42 Market Street, Chicago | (see item 7) | | |
| 4. What time is it now (within 1h)? | 1 | 3 | 3 |
| 5. Count backward from 20 to 1. | 2 | 2 | 4 |
| 6. Say the months in reverse order. | 2 | 2 | 4 |
| 7. Repeat the memory phrase in item #3. | 5 | 2 | 10 |
| Total | | | 28 |

Score 1 for each incorrect response; maximum weighted score = 28.

For items 5 and 6, score 2 for uncorrected errors, 1 for self-corrected errors, and 0 for no errors.

For item 3, score 1 point for each underlined element not correctly recalled. No separate score is calculated; it is part of item 7.

*Test* (BOMC; Table 4.6). This test takes 3–6 minutes to administer, counts errors, and has 28 possible points. It consists of all verbal items and can be administered bedside. The dementia cut-off score is 10 errors, according to Katzman and coworkers (1983). Sensitivity is reasonable with this cut-off, and test–retest reliability and convergent validity with other mental status tests are good (Davis, Morris, & Grant, 1990; Davous et al., 1987; Fillenbaum et al., 1987; Parmelee, Katz, & Lawton, 1989).

### Short Portable Mental Status Questionnaire (SPMSQ) (Pfeiffer, 1975)

The SPMSQ (see Table 4.7) originated from the Mental Status Questionnaire (MSQ) (Kahn et al., 1960). Both the SPMSQ and the MSQ consist of 10 items that assess orientation and general/

**Table 4.7.**
Short Portable Mental Status Questionnaire

*Items*

1. What is the month, date, year?
2. What day of the week is it?
3. What is the name of this place?
4. What is your telephone number (if no telephone, what is street address)?
5. How old are you?
6. When were you born (month, date, year)?
7. Who is the current president of the United States?
8. Who was the president just before him?
9. What was your mother's maiden name?
10. Subtract 3 from 20 and keep subtracting each new number you get, all the way down.

| Scoring | Level of Impairment |
|---|---|
| 0–2 errors | Intact |
| 3–4 errors | Mild impairment |
| 5–7 errors | Moderate impairment |
| 8–10 errors | Severe impairment |

Allow one more error if education does not go beyond grade school.

Allow one fewer errors if education is beyond high school.

Table 4.8.
Mental Status Tests

| Name of test | Domains covered | Testing and scoring | Sensitivity and specificity | Reliability | Validity |
|---|---|---|---|---|---|
| Mini-Mental State Examination (MMSE) | Orientation, immediate and delayed episodic recall, working memory, language, and visuospatial abilities | 11 items<br><br>Maximum score is 30 based on sum of correct responses<br><br>Higher score indicates less impairment<br><br>Administration time is 10 min | Sensitivity = 0.80–0.90 with a cut-off of 24 (Anthony et al., 1982; Davous et al., 1987; Dick et al., 1984; Foreman, 1987; Tombaugh & McIntyre, 1992)<br><br>Sensitivity is as low as 0.21–0.54 with early cases of dementia (Tombaugh & McIntyre, 1992)<br><br>Specificity = 0.80–1.0 (Anthony et al., 1982; Davous et al., 1987; Foreman, 1987) | Test–retest reliability = 0.85–0.95, 1 day – 3 months (Anthony et al., 1982; Dick et al., 1984; Fillenbaum et al., 1987; Folstein et al., 1975)<br><br>Inter-rater reliability = 0.85–0.95 (Dick et al., 1984, review by Karuza et al., 1997)<br><br>Internal reliability = 0.96 (Foreman, 1987) | Correlates with other screening tests, r = 0.70–0.90 (Tombaugh & McIntyre, 1992)<br><br>Correlates with the WAIS, r = 0.78 (Folstein et al., 1975); the Mattis Dementia Rating Scale, r = 0.87 (Foreman, 1987); and the ADAS-Cognitive, r = −0.90 (Burch & Andrews, 1987) |
| Blessed Orientation-Memory-Concentration Test (BOMC) | Orientation, immediate and delayed episodic recall, and working memory | 6 items<br><br>Maximum score is 28 based on sum of errors<br><br>Higher score indicates greater impairment<br><br>Administration time is 3–6 min | Sensitivity = 0.87, specificity = 0.94 (Davous et al., 1987; Parmelee et al., 1989) | Test–retest reliability (1 month) = 0.77 (Fillenbaum et al., 1987) | Correlates with the MMSE, r = −0.83 (Fillenbaum et al., 1987)<br><br>Correlates with the Clinical Dementia Rating Scale, r = 0.79–0.81 (Davis et al., 1990)<br><br>Correlates with cortical plaque count, r = 0.73 (Katzman et al., 1983) |

| Instrument | Domains | Description | Sensitivity/Specificity | Reliability | Correlates |
|---|---|---|---|---|---|
| Short Portable Mental Status Questionnaire (SPMSQ) | Orientation and calculation/working memory | 10 items<br><br>Maximum score is 10 based on sum of errors<br><br>Higher score indicates greater impairment<br><br>Administration time is 5–10 min | Better specificity (0.72–0.98) than sensitivity (0.34–0.92) (Albert et al., 1991; Baker, 1989; Fillenbaum, 1980; Roccaforte et al., 1994a,b)<br><br>Better sensitivity in clinical samples (0.92) than in community samples (0.45) (Nelson et al., 1986) | Test–retest reliability above 0.80 (Pfeiffer, 1975)<br><br>Inter-rater reliability = 0.62–0.87 (Fillenbaum & Smyer, 1981)<br><br>Internal consistency = 0.90 (Foreman, 1987) | Correlates with the MMSE, r = −0.40 to −0.81 (Hooijer et al., 1992; Roccaforte et al., 1994a,b)<br><br>Correlates with the Abbreviated Mental Test, r = −0.49 (Hooijer et al., 1992)<br><br>Correlates with the Mattis Dementia Rating Scale, r = −0.71 (Foreman, 1987)<br><br>Correlates with the Clinical Dementia Rating Scale, r = 0.79 (Davis et al., 1990)<br><br>Correlates with dementia diagnosis, r = 0.63–0.71 (Foreman, 1987; Haglund & Schuckit, 1976) |
| Cognitive Capacity Screening Exam (CCSE) | Orientation, calculation/working memory, immediate and delayed episodic recall, and reasoning | 30 items<br><br>Maximum score is 30 based on sum of correct responses<br><br>Higher score indicates less impairment<br><br>Administration time is 10–15 min | Sensitivity = 0.43–1.0 (Baker, 1989; Foreman, 1987; Kaufman et al., 1979; Strain et al., 1988; Webster et al., 1984)<br><br>Specificity = 0.30–1.0 (Baker, 1989; Foreman, 1987; Kaufman et al., 1979; Strain et al., 1988; Webster et al., 1984) | Test–retest reliability = 0.84 (Villardita & Lomeo, 1992)<br><br>Inter-rater reliability = 1.0 (Jacobs et al., 1977)<br><br>Internal consistency = 0.97 (Foreman, 1987) | Correlates with the MMSE, r = 0.82–0.88 (Villardita & Lomeo, 1992; Foreman, 1987)<br><br>Correlates with the Blessed IMC, r = −0.73 to −0.81 (Villardita & Lomeo, 1992)<br><br>Correlates with the SPMSQ, r = −0.63 (Foreman, 1987)<br><br>Correlates with diagnosis, r = 0.87 (Foreman, 1987) |

(continued)

**Table 4.8.**
Mental Status Tests — Continued

| Name of test | Domains covered | Testing and scoring | Sensitivity and specificity | Reliability | Validity |
|---|---|---|---|---|---|
| Abbreviated Mental Test (AMT) | Orientation | 10 items<br><br>Maximum score is 10 based on sum of correct responses<br><br>Higher score indicates less impairment<br><br>Administration time is 3–5 min | In a geriatric assessment clinic, sensitivity = 0.91–0.94 and specificity = 0.82–0.87 (Flicker et al., 1997; Hooijer et al., 1992; Little et al., 1987)<br><br>In a community sample, sensitivity = 0.71–1.0 and specificity = 0.89–0.99 (Hooijer et al., 1992; Little et al., 1987; MacKenzie et al., 1996) | Test–retest reliability = 0.92 (Qureshi & Hodkinson, 1974) | Correlates with the MMSE, r = 0.51–0.87 (Flicker et al., 1997; Hooijer et al., 1992)<br><br>Correlates with the SPMSQ, r = −0.49 (Hooijer et al., 1992)<br><br>Correlates with the IQCODE, r = −0.67 (Flicker et al., 1997)<br><br>Correlates with CAMCOG scores, r = 0.72 (MacKenzie et al., 1996) |

personal information. Additionally, the SPMSQ assesses working memory. A score is determined by counting the number of errors, and the maximum score is 10. Similar to the BOMC, the SPMSQ consists of all verbal items and is brief (5–10 minutes) and portable. Scoring takes into account years of education. Originally intended to map four levels of cognitive functioning (intact, mild, moderate, and severe), in practice, the SPMSQ does not distinguish between those who are mildly impaired and those who are intact or moderately impaired (Smyer, Hofland, & Jonas, 1979).

## Cognitive Capacity Screening Examination (CCSE) (Jacobs et al., 1977)

The Cognitive Capacity Screening Examination was designed to detect diffuse brain pathology in medical inpatients. It is more comprehensive than many other mental status tests in the domains that it assesses: orientation (time and place), concentration (digit span forward and backward), working memory/calculation (serial seven subtractions), immediate and delayed memory for words, and reasoning (abstractions). All 30 items are verbal, making bedside administration easy. Scores are based on the number of correct responses; a cut-off score of 20 is used to define diminished cognitive capacity. Practice effects are minimal (Villardita & Lomeo, 1992). The CCSE has been effective in detecting cognitive impairment in inpatient populations, even in individuals with psychosis (Foreman, 1987; Jacobs et al., 1977; Haddad & Coffman, 1987). The CCSE is superior to the MMSE and to the SPMSQ in detecting cognitive impairment in inpatients (Foreman, 1987). The efficacy of this screen in community populations is unclear because testing has been limited to hospital settings. The CCSE is the longest of the mental status tests described in this chapter; the response burden may be too much for those with moderate to severe impairments.

## Abbreviated Mental Test (AMT) (Hodkinson, 1972)

The Abbreviated Mental Test is derived from the Roth-Hopkins Test (Roth & Hopkins, 1953). It is brief (3–5 minutes) and limited in breadth, covering only orientation. As noted in Table 4.8, the AMT correlates highly with other screening measures and informant reports (Flicker et al., 1997; Hooijer et al., 1992; MacKenzie et al., 1996). With a maximum of 10 points, the typical cut-off is either seven or eight points (Hooijer et al., 1992; MacKenzie et al., 1996). The AMT is more susceptible to false-positive results than the MMSE (MacKenzie et al., 1996), but it is not as affected by education and depression (MacKenzie et al., 1996).

Table 4.8 describes the psychometric properties of the mental status tests described.

## Informant Reports

In contrast to mental status tests, informant reports do not directly assess the patient. Rather, family and friends report on the patient's cognitive functioning as evidenced by everyday behavior and activities. The strength of this assessment approach is that decline or *change* in functioning can be assessed because the informant is familiar with the patient's previous level of functioning. Another strength is that informant reports are less influenced than are objective mental status tests by effects of premorbid IQ and education (e.g., Christensen & Jorm, 1992; Jorm et al., 1991; Morales et al., 1997). Even patients who have lost their verbal skills are assessable with informant reports. A weakness is that reports of relatives and friends may be influenced by the informants' motivation for providing information, which may be to have the patient appear either cognitively intact or cognitively impaired. More than one informant interviewed separately may reduce this bias. Questions about specific behaviors within specific time frames may also reduce the amount of subjective interpretation.

### Dementia Questionnaire (Silverman et al., 1986)

The Dementia Questionnaire is a brief semistructured informant interview. The questionnaire covers the following domains: memory, language, daily functioning, physical and psychological problems, past treatment of problem, and family history of dementia. Table 4.9 presents the items that pertain to cognitive functioning. Minimal experience is required to administer the questionnaire, but a trained clinician must interpret the provided responses because no formal scoring is used. Instead, clinicians make a diagnosis based on information from the questionnaire. Lack of a scoring system suggests a more strictly clinical use of this instrument. Research applications would be possible if a scoring system was created, cut-off scores for optimal sensitivity and specificity were determined, and reliability and validity were established. The Dementia Questionnaire has been found to be highly sensitive (100%) in detecting dementia cases but not very specific (i.e., it has a high false-positive rate) (Kawas et al., 1994). This low specificity may result because the caregiver completes the questionnaire, and, in a dementia clinic, the caregiver likely initiated the evaluation process because he or

**Table 4.9.**

Cognitive Items from the Dementia Questionnaire*

Patient Name: _____ Age: _____ Date: _____

Informant: _____ Relation to Patient: _____

*Instructions*: For each of the items below, answer *yes, no, don't know,* and *date*

*Memory*

Does _____ have any problem with
1. Memory?
2. Remembering people's names?
3. Recognizing familiar faces?
4. Finding way about indoors?
5. Finding way on familiar streets?
6. Remembering a short list of items?
7. Did trouble with memory begin suddenly?
8. Has the course of the memory problems been a steady downhill progression, or have there been abrupt declines?

*Expression*

Does _____
9. Ever have trouble finding the right word or expressing self?
10. Talk less than in the past?
11. Have a tendency to dwell in the past?

*Daily Functioning*

Does _____ have
12. Trouble with household tasks?
13. Trouble handling money?
14. Trouble grasping situations or explanations?
15. Difficulty at work (check if N/A)?
16. Trouble dressing or caring for self?
17. Trouble feeding self?
18. Trouble controlling bladder and bowels?
19. Agitation and nervousness?

*The Dementia Questionnaire also includes noncognitive items addressing physical problems, drug abuse, emotional state, medical contacts, and family history.

she believed that the patient was declining cognitively. This belief may bias the information provided on the questionnaire. Utilizing other sources of information to validate caregiver report may strengthen the clinical and research potential of the Dementia Questionnaire.

*Informant Questionnaire for Cognitive Decline in the Elderly (IQCODE) (Jorm, Scott, & Jacomb, 1989)*

The IQCODE (Table 4.10) is a self-administered instrument completed by an informant close to the patient. The infor-

---

**Table 4.10.**
Informant Questionnaire for Cognitive Decline in the Elderly

| Read to the informant: |
| --- |

Now we want you to remember what your friend or relative was like 10 years ago and compare it with what he/she is like now. 10 years ago was 19 –. Below are situations where this person has to use his/her memory or intelligence and we want you to indicate whether this has improved, stayed the same, or gotten worse in that situation over the past 10 years. Note the importance of comparing his/her present performance with 10 years ago. So, if 10 years ago this person always forgot where he/she had left things, and he/she still does, then this would be considered 'Hasn't changed much.' Please indicate the changes you have observed by marking the appropriate answer.

Compared with 10 years ago how is this person at:

Answer each item as *much better (1)*, *a bit better (2)*, *not much change (3)*, *a bit worse (4)*, or *much worse (5)*.
1. Recognizing the faces of family and friends?
2. Remembering the names of family and friends?
3. Remembering things about family and friends, e.g., occupations, birthdays, addresses?
4. Remembering things that have happened recently?
5. Recalling conversations a few days later?
6. Forgetting what he/she wanted to say in the middle of the conversation?
7. Remembering his/her address and telephone number?
8. Remembering what day and month it is?
9. Remembering where things are usually kept?
10. Remembering where to find things that have been put in a different place from usual?
11. Adjusting to any change in his/her day-to-day routine?
12. Knowing how to work familiar machines around the house?
13. Learning to use a new gadget or machine around the house?
14. Learning new things in general?
15. Remembering things that happened to him/her when he/she was young?
16. Remembering things he/she learned when he/she was young?
17. Understanding the meaning of unusual words?
18. Understanding magazine or newspaper articles?
19. Following a story in a book or on TV?
20. Composing a letter to friends or for business purposes?
21. Knowing about important historical events of the past?
22. Making decisions on everyday matters?
23. Handling money for shopping?
24. Handling financial matters, e.g., the pension, dealing with the bank?
25. Handling other everyday arithmetic problems, e.g., knowing how much food to buy, knowing how long between visits from family or friends?
26. Using his/her intelligence to understand what's going on and to reason things through?

*Scoring:* Add scores for each item
Range = 26–130. Higher scores indicate greater impairment.

mant rates the patient's cognitive function as better or worse than 10 years ago using a 5 point Likert scale. The long form is 26 items; the short form is 16. The two forms correlate highly and have similar validities (Jorm, 1994). The subscales of the IQCODE map directly onto memory distinctions (episodic, semantic, remote memory, and learning).

In samples from the general population, the IQCODE performs as well as the MMSE as a screening test for dementia (Jorm, 1994; Jorm et al., 1991; Jorm et al., 1996). In contrast to mental status tests, the IQCODE is not influenced by premorbid intelligence, education level, or occupational status (Christensen & Jorm, 1992; Jorm et al., 1991, 1996; Jorm & Jacomb, 1989; Morales et al., 1997), but it is influenced by age (Jorm et al., 1996). Furthermore, characteristics of both the informant and the patient can influence scores, particularly affective state (depression and anxiety) and personality (neuroticism and introversion) (Jorm et al., 1996). Moreover, the quality of the relationship between the informant and the patient (amount of caring, control, and bonding) impacts IQCODE scores (Christensen & Jorm, 1992).

Because of its simple administration demands, the IQCODE has potential utility as a screening measure for epidemiological research and particularly for research using telephone screens. The 10 year frame may pose difficulties. Not all primary caregivers have known for 10 years the patient on whom they are reporting. Additionally, caregivers may not accurately remember the cognitive status of patients over that time frame. Memory for past events is malleable and easily influenced by subsequent events. Finally, over a 10 year span, cognitive changes are expected due to aging itself and may be misinterpreted as early signs of dementia. Although purely conjecture at this point, a constrained time frame, perhaps 5 years rather than 10, may improve the validity and practical applicability of the IQCODE.

## Minimum Data Set (MDS) Cognition Scales (Morris et al., 1993)

The Minimum Data Set is a mandated assessment of nursing home care (see Chapter 16 for a critique of mandated assessments) that is required by federal law to be administered to all patients at admission into a nursing home and every 3 months thereafter. Nursing staff score the MDS based on their observations of patient behaviors and medical record data. Two scales constructed of items from the MDS to identify cognitive impairment are the Cognitive Performance Scale and the MDS-COG. The Cognitive Performance Scale consists of five items from the MDS: comatose status, short-term memory, decision-making ability, communication, and eating. The items are scored on a scale from 0 to 6, with higher scores indicating greater impairment. The Cognitive Performance Scale poorly distinguishes later stages of dementia as measured by the Global Deterioration Scale, so a new scale called the MDS-COGS was developed to address this limitation (Hartmaier et al., 1994). This scale incorporates items that assess long-term memory, orientation, and dressing ability (Table 4.11) to distinguish residents with moderate versus severe dementia.

Both scales have reasonable sensitivity and specificity, as well as acceptable reliability and validity. The Cognitive Performance Scale correlates well with known objective measures of cognition such as the MMSE, the Blessed Information-Memory-Concentration Test, the Mattis Dementia Rating Scale, and the Global Deterioration Scale (Table 4.12). Both scales must be interpreted within their limitations, though. Collected data are based on second-hand behavior ratings (e.g., the charge nurse gathers information from medical records that were completed by the nurses' aides), which calls its validity into question. Furthermore, raters are likely to vary from one recording period to the next, and rater training is not controlled, so test–retest and inter-rater reliability are reduced. De-

**Table 4.11.**

Cognition Scales of the Minimum Data Set (MDS-COG and CPS)

| MDS-COG | | CPS | |
|---|---|---|---|
| *Cognitive Patterns* | | *Cognitive Patterns* | |
| Short-term memory | | Short-term memory | |
| Memory OK | = 0 | Memory OK | = 0 |
| Memory problem | = 1 | Memory problem | = 1 |
| Long-term memory | | Decision making | |
| Memory OK | = 0 | Independent | = 0 |
| Memory problem | = 1 | Modified independent | = 1 |
| Location of own room | | Moderately impaired | = 2 |
| Does recall | = 0 | Severely impaired | = 3 |
| Doesn't recall | = 1 | Comatose status | |
| Knows he/she is in a nursing home | | Not comatose | = 0 |
| Does recall | = 0 | Comatose | = 1 |
| Doesn't recall | = 1 | | |
| Orientation | | | |
| At least 1 item recalled | = 0 | | |
| None recalled | = 1 | | |
| Decision making | | | |
| Independent | = 0 | | |
| Modified independent | = 1 | | |
| Moderately impaired | = 2 | | |
| Severely impaired | = 3 | | |
| *Communication Patterns* | | *Communication Patterns* | |
| Making self understood | | Making self understood | |
| Understood | = 0 | Understood | = 0 |
| Usually understood | = 0 | Usually understood | = 1 |
| Sometimes understood | = 0 | Sometimes understood | = 2 |
| Never/rarely understood | = 1 | Never/rarely understood | = 3 |
| *Physical Functioning* | | *Physical Functioning* | |
| Dressing self performance | | Eating performance | |
| Independent | = 0 | Independent | = 0 |
| Supervision | = 0 | Supervision | = 1 |
| Limited assistance | = 0 | Limited assistance | = 2 |
| Extensive assistance | = 0 | Extensive assistance | = 3 |
| Total dependence | = 1 | Total dependence | = 4 |
| Total | = 10 | Total | = 12 |

spite these limitations, the Cognitive Performance Scale and the MDS-COGS represent initiatives to assess cognitive functioning in institutional settings. Without these data, scarce information would be available on residents' cognitive status because widespread administration of objective tests is unfeasible.

Table 4.12 compares and contrasts the psychometric features of the informant reports described earlier.

**Full Neuropsychological Test Batteries**

Although screening tests identify possible cases of cognitive impairment, further assessment (physical and clinical examinations, laboratory tests, medical history, and neuropsychological tests) is necessary to diagnose the source of impairment. Neuropsychological test batteries aid in diagnosis, particularly in cases in which *(1)* the patient presents with a complicated

**Table 4.12. Informant Report Screening Tests**

| Name of test | Domains covered | Testing and scoring | Sensitivity and specificity | Reliability | Validity |
|---|---|---|---|---|---|
| Dementia Questionnaire (DQ) | Memory, language, visuospatial skills, daily functioning, and mood | Informant endorses patient's cognitive symptoms from those listed<br><br>No scoring format used<br><br>Administration time is 20 min | Sensitivity = 1.0 and specificity = 0.90 when diagnosis based on questionnaire is compared with clinical diagnosis (Kawas et al., 1994) | Inter-rater reliability = 0.83–0.94 (Kawas et al, 1994; Silverman et al., 1986)<br><br>Inter-informant reliability = 0.91 (Kawas et al., 1994) | No studies have compared the DQ with other cognitive measures |
| Informant Questionnaire on Cognitive Decline in the Elderly (IQCODE) | Episodic memory, semantic memory, procedural memory, working memory, language comprehension, language production, and executive function | 26 item or 16 item version available<br><br>Questionnaire filled out by an informant who has known the subject for 10 yr<br><br>Informant rates statements on a 5 point Likert scale in terms of change in functioning<br><br>Scores range from 26 to 130 points on the 26 item version and 16 to 80 points on the 16 item version, based on sum of individual items<br><br>An alternative scoring procedure is to average ratings across items for a total score between 1 and 5 points<br><br>Higher scores indicate greater impairment | Sensitivity = 0.69–0.91 (Flicker et al, 1997; Jorm, 1994; Jorm et al., 1991; Morales et al., 1997; Thomas et al., 1994)<br><br>Specificity = 0.63–0.90 (Flicker et al., 1997; Jorm, 1994; Jorm et al., 1991, 1996; Morales et al., 1997; Thomas et al., 1994) | Test–retest reliability = 0.96, 1–2 days (Jorm et al., 1991)<br><br>One year test–retest reliability = 0.75 (Jorm et al., 1989)<br><br>Internal consistency = 0.93–0.95 (Jorm et al., 1989, 1991) | Correlates with the MMSE, r = −0.37 to −0.78 (Bowers et al., 1990; Flicker et al., 1997; Jorm, 1994; Jorm & Jacomb, 1989; Jorm et al., 1996)<br><br>Correlates with the Abbreviated Mental Test, r = −0.58 to −0.62 (Flicker et al., 1997; Thomas et al, 1994)<br><br>Correlates with the Wechsler Memory Scale – Revised Logical Memory, r = −0.42, and the WAIS, r = −0.26 to −0.33 (Jorm et al., 1996)<br><br>Long version of the IQCODE correlates with the short version, r = 0.98 (Jorm, 1994) |
| Minimum Data Set, MDS-COG and Cognitive Performance Scale (CPS) | Consciousness, orientation, short-term memory, language, decision making, eating and dressing. | MDS-COG has 8 items. Maximum score is 10<br><br>CPS has 5 items. Maximum score is 12<br><br>For both measures, a higher score indicates greater impairment<br><br>Items completed by nursing home staff based on direct observation and medical record data<br><br>Administration time is 5 min | Using the MMSE as the standard, the sensitivity and specificity were both 0.94 (Hartmaier et al., 1995)<br><br>Sensitivity of CPS = 0.90–0.94 and specificity = 0.85–0.94 (Morris et al., 1994) | Inter-rater reliability = 0.80–0.85 (Casten et al., 1998; Morris et al., 1994) | Correlates with the MMSE, r = −0.86, and the Blessed Information-Memory-Concentration Scale, r = 0.66 (Hartmaier et al., 1995; Lawton et al., 1998)<br><br>Correlates with the Mattis DRS, r = −0.43 (Hartmaier et al., 1995)<br><br>Correlates with the Global Deterioration Scale, r = 0.59–0.80 (Hartmaier et al., 1994) |

medical and/or psychiatric history, (2) education and/or intelligence is very high or very low, or (3) performance on mental status examination does not match performance on tasks of daily living. Neuropsychological batteries consist of combinations of domain tests. These domain tests assess cognitive areas in relative isolation from one another; hence they can be used to develop a profile of spared and impaired functions. Examples of domain tests are shown in Table 4.13.

## Shortened Neuropsychological Test Batteries

For many purposes, a shortened neuropsychological test battery will suffice. Shortened test batteries retain features of a full battery (e.g., objective assessment of different domains, normed and reliable measures, and standardized and portable administration), but they take less time. As a result, shortened batteries serve purposes other than diagnosis, such as charting progression over time, determining efficacy of behavioral/pharmaceutical interventions, staging severity of dementia, and screening. Screening is appropriate for individuals who have demonstrated ceiling effects on mental status tests (particularly individuals with high education and/or intelligence) but who have declined in everyday functioning. Shortened test batteries typically take 15–30 minutes to administer and may require specialized training. Described below are the most widely used shortened batteries.

### Mattis Dementia Rating Scale (MDRS) (Coblentz et al., 1973; Mattis, 1976)

The Mattis Dementia Rating Scale was designed to assess adults with suspected dementia whose extremely low scores on traditional neuropsychological batteries such as the Wechsler Adult Intelligence Scale (WAIS) made it difficult to determine their degree of deficit. The Mattis assesses attention, memory, visuospatial construction, conceptualization, and initiation/preservation (Table 4.14). In contrast to other shortened batteries, the Mattis is organized so that the most difficult items in each domain are given first. The purpose of this administration scheme is to save time when testing less impaired patients. If the first item is answered correctly, the domain is considered "passed," and the remaining questions are given credit and omitted. Although often classified as a screening instrument, the Mattis is too detailed to be an efficient screen. High functioning older adults can complete the battery in less than 10 minutes, but other participants may take as long as 45 minutes.

The Mattis shows high sensitivity and specificity, even in the early stages of dementia (Green, Woodard, & Green, 1995; Monsch et al., 1995). Memory and Initiation/Preservation items appear most sensitive to early dementia (Monsch et al., 1995). The MDRS also has utility in later stages of the disease. It detects decline among patients with advanced Alzheimer's disease better than several screening measures (e.g., the Blessed IMC and the MMSE) (Salmon, Thal, Butters, & Heindel, 1990). Because the most difficult items in each domain are given first, however, this battery may be too fatiguing and anxiety-provoking for individuals in moderate to severe stages of dementia.

In addition to high sensitivity, the MDRS has proved useful in distinguishing patterns of cognitive deficits associated with a variety of illnesses (Appollonio et al., 1993; Kovner et al., 1992; Stoudemire et al., 1991). As found with several mental status tests, scores on the MDRS are influenced by age and education (Monsch et al., 1995; Smith et al., 1994; Vangel & Lichtenberg, 1995). Surprisingly, items from the Mattis domains do not correlate highly with items from the MMSE (Bobholz & Brandt, 1993; Friedl et al., 1996). In the early 1990s, the Mattis was adopted as the cognitive measure to be used in the National Institute on Aging's multisite cooperative study of Alzheimer's disease special care units in nursing homes.

**Table 4.13.**
Examples of Domain Tests

| Attention tests | Memory tests | Orientation | Psychomotor speed |
|---|---|---|---|
| Attention Index of the Wechsler Memory Scale-III (Digit Span, Mental Control, Visual Memory Span) | Auditory Verbal Learning Test (AVLT) | Abbreviated Mental Test | Bender Motor Gestalt Test |
| Brief Test of Attention | Benton Visual Retention Test | Blessed Orientation-Memory-Concentration (BOMC) Test — Orientation Items | Finger Tapping Grooved Pegboard Trail Making Test |
| Continuous Performance Test (The "A" Test) | Brief Visuospatial Memory Test — Revised (BVMT-R) | MMSE — Orientation Items | |
| Digit Cancellation | California Verbal Learning Test (CVLT) | Short Portable Mental Status Questionnaire (SPMSQ) — Orientation Items | |
| Digit Span (WAIS-III) | Continuous Recognition Test | | |
| Letter Cancellation | Continuous Visual Memory Test | | |
| Trail Making Test | Delayed Recognition Span Test | | |
| | Delayed Word Recall Test | | |
| | Fuld Object Memory | | |
| | Guild Memory Test | | |
| | Hopkins Verbal Learning Test — Revised (HVLT-R) | | |
| | Kendrick Battery | | |
| | Misplaced Objects Test | | |
| | Paired Associate Learning Test | | |
| | Recognition Memory Test | | |
| | Rey-Osterrieth Complex Figure Test — Recall Condition | | |
| | Rivermead Behavioral Memory Test | | |
| | Selective Reminding Test | | |
| | WMS-III: Associate Learning | | |
| | WMS-III: Logical Memory | | |
| | WMS-III: Visual Reproduction | | |

| Visuospatial tests | Language tests | Executive/problem solving | Intelligence tests |
|---|---|---|---|
| Benton Facial Recognition Test | Aphasia Screening Test | Category Test | National Adult Reading Test (NART) |
| Benton Line Orientation Test | Boston Diagnostic Aphasia Examination (BDAE) | Delayed Alternation & Object Alternation | Primary Mental Abilities |
| Benton Spatial Relations Visual Retention Test (Copy Administration) | Boston Naming Test (BNT) | Digit Symbol Test | Wechsler Adult Intelligence Test — III (WAIS-III) |
| Developmental Test of Visual–Motor Integration (VMI) | Controlled Oral Word Association Test (COWAT) | Everyday Problem Solving Inventory | |
| Hooper Test of Visual Organization | Multilingual Aphasia Examination (MAE) | Modified Card Sorting Test | |
| Mattis Dementia Rating Scale (DRS) — Figure Copying | National Adult Reading Test (NART) | Picture Absurdities of Stanford-Binet | |
| Parietal Lobe Battery | Token Test | Porteus Maze Test | |
| Rey-Osterrieth Complex Figure — Copy Administration | Verbal Fluency | Proverbs Test | |
| WAIS-III Block Design | WAIS-III Vocabulary | Raven's Progressive Matrices | |
| WAIS-III Object Assembly | | Stroop Color–Word Interference Test | |
| WAIS-III Picture Completion | | Tower of Hanoi | |
| Clock Test | | Trail Making Test | |
| Brief Visuospatial Memory Test — Revised (BVMT-R) | | Visual–Verbal Test | |
| | | WAIS-III Comprehension | |
| | | WAIS-III Similarities Subtest | |
| | | Wisconsin Card Sorting Test (WCST) | |

**Table 4.14.**

Mattis Dementia Rating Scale

| Domains and tests | Points possible | Sample items |
|---|---|---|
| *Attention* | (37) | |
| Digit span | 8 | Repeat random digit strings (e.g., 25, 4792) forward and backward |
| Respond to command | 10 | Stick out your tongue and raise your hand |
| Counting distraction | 11 | Count all "A"s in an array of letters |
| Read word list | 4 | Read a list of words correctly |
| Match designs | 4 | Point to a design that is the same as one pointed to by the examiner |
| *Initiation and perseveration* | (37) | |
| Verbal fluency | 30 | Name items at a supermarket. 1 minute time limit |
| Alternating movement | 3 | Start with one palm down, the other palm up. Simultaneously and continuously switch hand positions |
| Graphomotor functions | 4 | Copy designs (e.g., X, O, XOXOXO) |
| *Construction* | (6) | |
| Copy geometric figure | 6 | Copy a square with a diamond in it |
| *Conceptualization* | (39) | |
| Similarities — verbal | 8 | How are an apple and a banana alike? |
| Priming inductive reasoning | 3 | Name 3 things people eat — how are these items (named by patient) alike? |
| Similarities — multiple choice | 8 | Apple, banana. Are they both animals, both fruit, or both green? |
| Similarities — nonverbal | 8 | Point to two of three objects that are the most alike |
| Differences — verbal | 3 | Which doesn't belong with the others? Dog, cat, car |
| Differences — nonverbal | 8 | Point to one of three items that doesn't belong: circle, oval, and square |
| Create a sentence | 1 | Make up a sentence using the words "man" and "car" |
| *Memory* | (25) | |
| Sentence recall 1 | 4 | Recall a simple sentence |
| Sentence recall 2 | 3 | Recall a sentence created using the words "man" and "car" |
| Orientation | 9 | Time, place, president |
| Verbal recognition | 5 | Forced choice format: Select which word in a pair was read previously |
| Design recognition | 4 | Forced choice format: Select which design in a pair was seen previously |
| *Total* | 144 | |

## Alzheimer's Disease Assessment Scale (ADAS) (Rosen, Mohs, & Davis, 1984)

As suggested by its name, the Alzheimer's Disease Assessment Scale was one of the first instruments specifically tailored for Alzheimer's disease. It was geared toward applications in pharmacological research on ameliorating memory decline. The ADAS is composed of a Noncognitive Behaviors (mood and behavior) section and a Cognitive Behaviors section. The Cognitive Behaviors section (outlined in Table 4.15) is a mix of objective measures and subjective clinical ratings. The objective section assesses orientation, word recall, word list recognition, object and finger naming, verbal commands, figure copying, and completing an overlearned task (mailing a letter). The subjective section assesses spoken language ability, comprehension,

**Table 4.15.**
Alzheimer's Disease Assessment Scale: Cognitive Behavior Section

| | Error points possible | Description |
|---|---|---|
| | | Objective Test Items |
| Word Recall | 10 | Read a list of 10 words individually, then recall the words immediately. Three trials with the same words |
| Naming Objects and Fingers | 5 | Name 12 objects and 5 fingers |
| Commands | 5 | Execute five verbal commands of increasing complexity (e.g., make a fist, point to the ceiling and then to the floor; tap each shoulder twice with two fingers keeping both eyes shut) |
| Constructional Praxis | 5 | Copy four line drawings of increasing complexity (circle, overlapping rectangles, rhombus, and cube) |
| Ideational Praxis | 5 | Complete the steps involved in an overlearned task (mailing a letter) |
| Orientation | 8 | Answer eight items of orientation (e.g., name, date, time) |
| Word Recognition | 12 | Read aloud a 12 item list of words. These words are then presented with 12 distractors. Respond to each item as "old" or "new." Three trials with the same word list, new distractors on each trial |
| | | Subjective Test Items |
| Language | 5 | Examiner rates the participant's ability to speak understandably. 5 point Likert scale |
| Comprehension of Spoken Language | 5 | Examiner rates the participant's comprehension during testing. 5 point Likert scale |
| Word Finding Difficulty | 5 | Examiner rates the participant's frequency of word-finding difficulty. 5 point Likert scale |
| Remembering Test Instructions | 5 | Examiner rates the number of times the participant needs to be reminded of the instructions for the Word Recognition Task. 5 point Likert scale |
| Total | 70 | |

remembering test instructions, and word-finding difficulty in spontaneous speech. Memory and language items comprise approximately 75% of the test. The cognitive test is administered by a trained clinician or assistant and takes approximately 20–30 minutes to complete. The score is based on error points (70 possible), with higher scores indicating worse performance.

The ADAS effectively distinguishes between impaired and unimpaired individuals, even in the early stages of the disease. Zec and associates (1992) found that the ADAS correctly classified 91% of mild cases of Alzheimer's disease and 100% of moderate and severe cases when a cut-off score of two standard deviations above the control group mean was used. All cognitive subtest scores except naming were worse for adults with Alzheimer's disease

than for neurologically healthy older adults. Memory and spontaneous language showed relatively greater decline early in the course of the disease, whereas praxis, commands, and naming exhibited greater declines later.

Beyond detecting early dementia, the ADAS has utility in staging dementia (Weyer et al., 1997; Zec et al., 1992) and detecting change (Weyer et al., 1997). The ADAS has become one of the most widely used cognitive tools in antidementia trials because of its sensitivity to change. For example, it was one of the primary outcome measures in the multicenter trials of tacrine, the first drug approved by the Federal Drug Administration for the treatment of cognitive symptoms in Alzheimer's disease (Davis et al., 1992; Farlow et al., 1992; Knapp et al., 1994a, b). No studies have yet determined whether the ADAS is useful in distinguishing different types of dementia. The influence of age and education on scores is unclear. Although Zec and colleagues (1992) found that age and education had only minimal effects on ADAS scores, Doraiswamy and coworkers (1997b) found that scores varied by age, gender, and educational level. Practice effects on the ADAS are minimal (Rosen et al., 1984), which is an important feature of an instrument intended to detect change. Because of its sound psychometrics, practical applicability, and past successes in detecting treatment effects, the ADAS is sure to have continued research and clinical applications in Alzheimer's disease.

### Consortium to Establish a Registry for Alzheimer's Disease (CERAD) Neuropsychological Assessment Battery (Morris et al., 1988)

The CERAD battery was developed to standardize the assessment of Alzheimer's disease across clinics and facilitate multicenter studies of Alzheimer's disease. Over 950 patients with Alzheimer's disease were originally enrolled in a nationwide registry of 16 university medical centers and assessed with the CERAD battery. Tests were included to characterize changes in cognitive, physical, and emotional functioning. As a result, the battery contains physical and laboratory examinations, drug inventories, a depression scale, medical history

questionnaires, and semistructured interviews with both patients and informants. To address cognitive functioning, the CERAD contains both the Clinical Assessment Battery (composed of the Blessed Dementia Scale, the Short Blessed Test, and the Clinical Dementia Rating Scale) and the Neuropsychological Assessment Battery (Table 4.16). The Neuropsychological Assessment Battery is administered independently by trained technicians. It consists of existing domain tests that were chosen to measure the principal cognitive manifestations of Alzheimer's disease. The tests were thought to have a range of difficulty sufficient to examine deficits throughout the course of the disease. The domains (memory, orientation, working memory/calculation, language functions, and visuospatial functioning) load on three primary factors: memory, language, and praxis (Morris et al., 1989). The battery takes approximately 20–30 minutes to administer. Instruction manuals and videotapes demonstrate the standard method of administration.

The CERAD distinguishes diagnosed cases of Alzheimer's disease from normal controls (Morris et al., 1988). Moreover, it distinguishes mild cases of Alzheimer's disease from moderate cases (Morris et al., 1989). It is unclear at present whether the CERAD is able to distinguish very mild from mild dementia or moderate from severe dementia because few individuals in

**Table 4.16** Consortium to Establish a Registry for Alzheimer's Disease Neuropsychological Assessment Battery

| Test | Points possible | Description |
| --- | --- | --- |
| Verbal Fluency | Varies | Name as many animals as possible in 1 minute. Score equals total number of items generated |
| Modified Boston Naming Test | 15 | Name 15 line drawings of objects |
| Mini-Mental State Examination | 30 | |
| Word List Memory | 30 | Read a list of 10 words. Recall list immediately after presentation. Three trials of the same words |
| Constructional Praxis | 11 | Copy (draw) four figures of increasing complexity |
| Word List Recall | 10 | Recall 10 items from Word List Memory task after a delay |
| Word List Recognition | 10 | Read 10 items from Word List Memory and 10 distractor items. Indicate whether each word was presented earlier or not |

the very mild and severe stages have been included in the registry (Morris et al., 1989). The measure of delayed recall included in the battery has been particularly effective in detecting early cases of Alzheimer's disease (Welsch et al., 1991), although this test shows floor effects early and is not effective for staging Alzheimer's disease. Other tests of the neuropsychological battery, such as verbal fluency, recognition, and visuospatial functioning (figure copying) have proved to be valuable for staging purposes (Welsch et al., 1992). Although the CERAD neuropsychological battery shows sensitivity to changes in scores over time due to progression of the disease, reliability is acceptable for observation periods only longer than 1 year (Morris et al., 1993). Still unknown is the efficacy of this battery in community samples or in clinical treatment trials with less experienced clinicians.

## CAMCOG (Roth et al., 1986)

The CAMCOG is one portion of the Cambridge Mental Disorders of the Elderly Examination (CAMDEX) (Roth et al., 1986). The CAMDEX is a structured interview schedule that was designed in Britain as a comprehensive assessment for the early diagnosis and measurement of dementia. The CAMDEX includes a psychiatric history section, an informant interview, and an objective neuropsychological battery (the CAMCOG). The CAMCOG is comprised of items from the MMSE plus items to assess attention, orientation, memory, working memory, language, visuospatial functioning, and reasoning. Evidence suggests that the CAMCOG is more effective than the MMSE in detecting dementia (Lazaro et al., 1995), and, when compared with clinical diagnosis, it has high sensitivity and specificity (Lazaro et al., 1995; Roth et al., 1986). Although used primarily with patient populations, the CAMCOG has also identified cases of dementia in community samples (O'Connor et al., 1989). Used together with the CAMDEX interview, the CAMCOG successfully distinguishes different types of dementia (e.g.,

Alzheimer's disease, multi-infarct dementia, and delirium) (Hendrie et al., 1988; Lazaro et al., 1995; O'Connor et al., 1989). In the United States, the CAMCOG has been used less extensively than the ADAS or CERAD batteries, but initial research suggests that the effectiveness of the CAMCOG in U.S. samples is comparable with that in British samples (Hendrie et al., 1988). A strength of this shortened battery is that, in contrast to the other batteries described here, it was designed to detect all dementias and not just Alzheimer's disease.

## Stage-Specific Tests

Two desired features of shortened test batteries are *(1)* discrimination of individual differences in ability levels and *(2)* detection of change in performance. For patients with either very mild or very severe cognitive impairment, the simplicity or difficulty of a battery causes scores to cluster at either tail, rendering the measure insensitive to individual differences or changes in performance. Stage-specific tests avoid these floor and ceiling effects. No specialized shortened batteries have been created and validated for early dementia, although it could be argued that most neuropsychological tests are "early dementia tests." Four batteries have been created to assess severe stages of dementia; these batteries assess basic cognitive abilities and minimize the need for expressive language skills. Because severe impairment tests are recent additions to the arsenal of cognitive batteries (all were created within the last decade), information on their utility, reliability, and validity is presently relatively modest.

## The Severe Impairment Battery (SIB) (Saxton et al., 1990)

The Severe Impairment Battery was the first battery developed to assess dementia in the late stages. It is a 20 minute test that uses downward extensions of standard instruments. The domains assessed are attention, orientation, memory, language, visuospatial ability, construction, praxis, and

Table 4.17.
Severe Impairment Battery

| Domain | Points possible | Sample items from domain |
|---|---|---|
| Attention | 6 | Digit span (spans of one to five items tested), auditory span (count finger taps), and visual span (count the number of fingers held up by the examiner) |
| Memory | 14 | Immediate and delayed recall of the examiner's name. Recognition from among three items of the item shown earlier |
| Orientation | 6 | Provide name, month, and city |
| Orient to Name | 2 | Turn when name is called |
| Language | 46 | Write own name. Copy own name. Name objects. Repeat short phrases. Name colors. Identify shapes |
| Visuospatial Ability | 8 | Color matching and color discrimination. Shape matching and shape discrimination |
| Construction | 4 | Draw a circle and a square |
| Praxis | 8 | Demonstrate how to use a cup and a spoon |
| Social Interaction | 6 | Shake hand of examiner. Follow command to sit in a chair |
| Maximum score | 100 | |

estimation of social interaction skills (Table 4.17). All items except one (verbal fluency) are untimed. Administration requires several objects, including colored blocks, pictures of a cup and spoon, and an actual cup and spoon. Initial studies suggest that this test is sensitive to differences in scores between members of even the most impaired subgroups, and it detects change in functioning over time (Panisset et al., 1994; Schmitt et al., 1997). Although the SIB is sensitive to differences between very impaired individuals, evidence suggests that ceiling effects occur for the less impaired. Individuals who score between 0 and 5 on the MMSE are differentiated from those who score between 6 and 11, but individuals who score between 6 and 11 are not distinguished from those who score between 12 and 17 or from those who score greater than 17. Although the range of the SIB is somewhat limited, it can detect both decline and improvement in performance as indicated by longitudinal tracking (Panisset et al., 1994).

*The Test for Severe Impairment (TSI) (Albert & Cohen, 1992)*

The Test for Severe Impairment was developed shortly after the SIB. It is a relatively quick battery (24 items, taking approximately 10 minutes). It covers several domains but with only a few items in each domain (Table 4.18). The three primary areas are memory, verbal function, and manipulation and identification of body parts. The test is geared toward individuals with MMSE scores under 10; even individuals with an MMSE score of 0 earn points on the TSI (Albert & Cohen, 1992). The need for language production skills is minimized; emphasis is placed on pointing at or manipulating objects. Small and common objects that are easily obtainable in different testing situations are used as stimuli. The TSI has good test–retest and internal reliability (Albert & Cohen, 1992). No significant correlations have been found with age or education (Albert & Cohen, 1992). The limited number of items within each domain may hamper meaningful conclusions regarding functioning within a domain and may weaken functional comparisons between domains.

*The Severe Cognitive Impairment Profile (SCIP) (Peavy et al., 1996)*

The most recent late-stage dementia scale, the SCIP was developed because other instruments had a limited number of cognitive domains and a limited range of difficulty. Administration takes approximately 30 minutes, and scores range from 0 to 245 points. The SCIP is similar to the SIB

**Table 4.18.**
Test for Severe Impairment

| Domain | Points possible | Sample items from domain |
|---|---|---|
| Motor Performance | 4 | Show how to use a comb, write name, put top on a pen, shake hands |
| Memory—Immediate | 3 | Identify in which hand a paper clip is (hands open, hands closed, hands behind back) |
| Memory—Delayed | 1 | Identify thread as something not used during testing (from among three objects: thread, key, and paper clip) |
| General Knowledge | 4 | Identify number of weeks in a year. Sing "Happy Birthday." Identify number of ears on a person. Count 10 fingers |
| Language Production | 4 | Name nose. Name a key. Name color of pens (red and green) |
| Language Comprehension | 4 | Close eyes. Point to ear. Point to pen of a specified color (red, green) |
| Conceptualization | 4 | Identify pen as different from two paper clips. Identify which of two pens is the same color as a target pen. Predict next two steps when an object is alternated between hands (i.e., which hand will it be in next?) |
| Maximum score | 24 | |

in that they both require several specialized objects and stimuli for administration. Eight domains are assessed: attention, memory, language, arithmetic, visuospatial ability, conceptualization, motor functioning, and social interaction skills (see sample items from each domain in Table 4.19). In contrast to the SIB and the TSI, each domain of the SCIP is comprised of several items of varying difficulty so that meaningful conclusions can be made about functioning within a domain. Inter-rater and test–retest reliability for this instrument are high, and construct validity is good (Peavy et al., 1996). The most difficult domain to assess is social interaction because

**Table 4.19.**
Severe Cognitive Impairment Profile

| Domain | Points possible | Sample items from domain |
|---|---|---|
| Attention | 44 | Digit span, visual span, name identification, and visual cancellation |
| Motor Speed | 10 | Put 10 large disks on a peg—timed |
| Memory | 17 | Remote memory: sing well-known songs, recall personal information |
| | | Immediate and delayed memory: free recall and recognition of verbal and spatial information (1 and 3 min delays) |
| Arithmetic | 10 | Count blocks, identify values of coins, and use coins to make change |
| Language | 88 | Name objects, show how to use them, write name, read words, repeat words and phrases, name pictures and match to words, follow motor commands |
| Visuospatial Functioning | 16 | Copy block designs, put dot in middle of a circle, copy a square, trace a triangle |
| Conceptual Reasoning/Executive | 26 | Sort pictures of fruits and clothing into categories, match objects based on color |
| Comportment (Social Interaction) | 34 | Cooperate with the examiner, give a greeting response, state name, display appropriate mannerisms and affective responses, and respond to questions |
| Maximum score | 245 | |

these skills are difficult to operationalize for standardized scoring. The memory domain demonstrates the lowest test–retest reliability of all the domains. The SCIP differentiates groups of severely impaired patients at different severity levels (as determined by the MDRS), whereas the SIB does not differentiate less severely impaired groups (Peavy et al., 1996). The SCIP shows little vulnerability to floor effects; even when a subgroup of severely impaired individuals was retested 1 year later, they were still able to answer more than 58% of the items of the SCIP correctly. The same individuals answered only 30% of the items from the MDRS and 20% of the items from the MMSE 1 year later. The mean annual change was 45 points (18%). The MDRS and MMSE showed relatively smaller annual changes due to floor effects (14% and 4%, respectively). Among the late-stage batteries described, the SCIP appears most able to track changes due to disease progression or to therapeutic intervention (Peavy et al., 1996).

*The Modified Ordinal Scales of Psychological Development (MOSPD) (Auer et al., 1994)*

The MOSPD were adapted from a cognitive assessment tool developed for infants (Uzgiris & Hunt, 1975). The premise behind the scale is that cognitive skills that were achieved earliest in infancy should be those preserved the latest in dementia (e.g., visually tracking movement of people, making eye contact, reaching for objects). With this instrument, no language skills are nec-

essary; instead, five sensorimotor functions are assessed (Table 4.20). Because they are so elementary, these functions are not easily translated into the domains discussed throughout the rest of this chapter.

Testing on the MOSPD takes about 30 minutes. Individual items are scored as either achieved (1) or not achieved (0). The MOSPD is a hierarchical scale; the highest rated task the patient can perform within each function area comprises the raw score for an individual scale, and the sum of raw scores comprises the total score. Scores range from 0 to 55. Patients in moderately severe to severe stages of Alzheimer's disease who scored zero or within one standard deviation of zero on the MMSE could successfully perform tasks on the MOSPD (Auer et al., 1994). Very few patients scored zero on the MOSPD, only those who were classified immobile on a functional scale. The MOSPD scores differed significantly between patients placed in different functional groups. This instrument is probably most useful for populations who have very severe dementia and who have lost all verbal capacity. Those who show floor effects on other late-stage dementia batteries may still be testable on this battery (Auer et al., 1994). This battery shows great promise in nursing home settings. A difficulty of this instrument is its limited comparability with findings from other instruments or with other cognitive domains. Everyone but the most severely demented individuals will show ceiling effects on this instrument. Table 4.21 summarizes various aspects of shortened neuropsychological test batteries.

Table 4.20.
Modified Ordinal Scales of Psychological Development

| Subscale | Description |
| --- | --- |
| Object permanence | Ability to keep track of an object and form an inner picture of the object |
| Means–ends | Ability to cause events in the environment or to obtain objects that are desired (e.g., ability to reach for an object) |
| Causality | Ability to perform actions that "make something happen" |
| Spatial relations | Ability to understand the relations between objects or persons located in different spatial positions (e.g., glance between two presented objects) |
| Schemes | Ability to interact with peoples and objects in the environment (e.g., look at an object held in his or her hands). |

**Table 4.21.**
Shortened Neuropsychological Test Batteries

| Measure | Domains covered | Testing and scoring | Sensitivity and specificity | Reliability | Validity |
|---|---|---|---|---|---|
| Mattis Dementia Rating Scale (DRS) | Attention (digit span, letter cancellation, word reading), episodic memory (orientation, sentence recall, verbal and design recognition), initiation and perseveration (verbal fluency, alternating movements, repeating designs), visuospatial construction (figure copying), and conceptualization (similarities and differences, creating a sentence) | 38 items<br><br>Maximum score is 144 based on correct responses<br><br>Higher score indicates less impairment<br><br>Administration time is 10–45 min<br><br>The most difficult items in a domain serve as screens. If they are passed, the remaining items in that domain are skipped | Sensitivity = 0.85–0.98 and specificity = 0.89–0.97 with a cut-off of 125 (Monsch et al., 1995; Vangel & Lichtenberg, 1995)<br><br>Sensitivity = 0.95 and specificity = 1.0 with a cut-off of 133 (Green et al., 1995) | Test-retest reliability = 0.97 (Gardner et al., 1981; Vangel & Lichtenberg, 1995)<br><br>Split-half reliability = 0.90 (Gardner et al., 1981)<br><br>Internal consistency is high for attention, memory, construction, and conceptualization (>0.65) (Vitaliano et al., 1984a,b)<br><br>Internal consistency is low for initiation and perseveration (<0.5) (Vitaliano et al., 1984a,b)<br><br>Internal consistency for total score >0.7 (Vitaliano et al., 1984a,b) | Correlates with the MMSE, r = 0.78–0.82 (Bobholz & Brandt, 1993; Salmon et al., 1990)<br><br>Correlates with the MMSE more weakly in a community sample, r = 0.29 (Friedl et al., 1996)<br><br>Correlates with the Blessed Information-Memory-Concentration Test, r = 0.79 (Salmon et al., 1990)<br><br>Correlates with the WAIS, r = 0.75 (Gardner et al., 1981)<br><br>Correlates with the Wechsler Memory Scale, r = 0.70 (Vitaliano et al., 1984a,b)<br><br>Correlates with Activities of Daily Living, r = 0.76 (Vitaliano et al., 1984a,b) |

| Measure | Description | | Reliability | Validity |
|---|---|---|---|---|
| Alzheimer's Disease Assessment Scale (ADAS) Cognitive Behaviors Section | Orientation, episodic memory (word recall and word recognition), language (naming ability, clinician rating of comprehension, clinician rating of production, and clinician rating of word-finding ability), visuospatial functioning and praxis (manipulation of objects, figure copying, and following commands) | Objective items and subjective ratings<br><br>Maximum score is 70 points, based on number of errors<br><br>Higher score indicates greater impairment<br><br>Administration time is 20–30 min | Sensitivity = 0.97, specificity = 0.98 with a cut-off of 2 SDs above the control group mean (Zec et al., 1992)<br><br>Sensitivity = 0.91 for mild Alzheimer's disease, 1.0 for moderate Alzheimer's disease, and 1.0 for severe Alzheimer's disease (Zec et al., 1992) | Test–retest reliability = 0.90–0.93 (Kim et al., 1994; Rosen et al., 1984; Weyer et al., 1997)<br><br>Inter-rater reliability = 0.90–0.97 (Rosen et al., 1984; Standish et al., 1996)<br><br>Internal consistency >0.80 (Weyer et al., 1997) | Correlates with the MMSE, r = −0.66 to −0.76 (Doraiswamy et al., 1997a; Weyer et al., 1997; Zec et al., 1992)<br><br>Correlates with the Sandoz Clinical Assessment–Geriatric Instrument, r = 0.67 (Rosen et al., 1984)<br><br>Correlates with the Geriatric Evaluation by Relatives Rating Instrument (GERRI), r = 0.40 (Doraiswamy et al., 1997a)<br><br>Correlates with the Blessed Dementia Rating Scale, r = 0.48 (Rosen et al., 1984) |

(continued)

**Table 4.21.**
Shortened Neuropsychological Test Batteries — Continued

| Measure | Domains covered | Testing and scoring | Sensitivity and specificity | Reliability | Validity |
|---|---|---|---|---|---|
| Consortium to Establish a Registry for Alzheimer's Disease (CERAD) Neuropsychological Assessment Battery | Episodic memory (immediate and delayed recall, recognition), language (naming and verbal fluency), visuospatial functioning (line drawings), and global functioning (MMSE) | Objective items. Oral and written responses<br><br>Maximum score is variable. Score is based on correct responses<br><br>Higher score indicates less impairment<br><br>Administration time is 20–30 min | Composite score is not particularly effective for staging purposes (Welsch et al., 1991), but individual measures have some utility in staging<br><br>Correctly classified 86% of patients with mild Alzheimer's disease and 94% of unimpaired individuals using the delayed recall measure (Welsch et al., 1992)<br><br>Correctly classified 69% of mildly impaired Alzheimer's patients and 73% of moderately impaired patients using delayed recall and line drawing measures (Welsch et al., 1992)<br><br>Correctly classified 80% of moderately impaired Alzheimer's patients and 82% of severely impaired patients using verbal fluency, line drawing, and recognition measures (Welsch et al., 1992) | No overall score for the instrument. Test–retest reliabilities for the various domains range from 0.43 to 0.90 (Morris et al., 1989)<br><br>Inter-rater reliabilities for domain tests range from 0.92 to 1.0 (Morris et al., 1989) | High correlations among subtests—higher for tests within the same domain than for tests from different domains (Morris et al., 1989)<br><br>Correlations among memory tests = 0.32–0.90. Correlations among language tests = 0.53–0.64. Line drawing poorly correlates with other measures, $r = 0.16–0.51$ (Morris et al., 1989)<br><br>The MMSE correlates with CERAD verbal fluency, $r = 0.77$, and word recall, $r = 0.36$ (Morris et al., 1989)<br><br>The Blessed Dementia Scale correlates with CERAD recall, $r = 0.16$, and with CERAD line drawing, $r = 0.34$ (Morris et al., 1989) |

| Cambridge Mental Disorders of the Elderly Examination (CAMDEX) Cognitive Battery (CAMCOG) | Attention, orientation, working memory, language, episodic memory, visuospatial functioning, and reasoning<br><br>Items from the MMSE plus 43 other items<br><br>Maximum score is 106 based on number of items correct<br><br>Higher score indicates less impairment<br><br>Administration time is 15 min | Detected deterioration of cognitive abilities over a 1 year period (Morris et al., 1989, 1993)<br><br>Sensitivity = 0.92–1.0, specificity = 0.96–0.97 with a cut-off of 79 (Hendrie et al., 1988; Roth et al., 1986)<br><br>Sensitivity = 1.0 and specificity = 0.97, with a cut-off of 60 for geriatric medical inpatients with low education (Lazaro et al., 1995) | No information on test–retest reliability<br><br>Inter-rater reliability = 0.88–0.97 (Hendrie et al., 1988; Roth et al., 1986) | Performs better than the MMSE in distinguishing between demented and nondemented older adults (Hendrie et al., 1988)<br><br>Correlates with the Newcastle Dementia score, $r = -0.77$ (Hendrie et al., 1988)<br><br>Scores vary significantly between Alzheimer's disease severity groups (mild, moderate, and severe) as determined by the Clinical Dementia Rating Scale (Hendrie et al., 1988)<br><br>CAMCOG scores distinguish Alzheimer's disease from vascular dementia, depression, and neurologically intact adults (Hendrie et al., 1988) |
| --- | --- | --- | --- | --- |

(continued)

**Table 4.21.**
Shortened Neuropsychological Test Batteries—Continued

| Measure | Domains covered | Testing and scoring | Sensitivity and specificity | Reliability | Validity |
|---|---|---|---|---|---|
| Severe Impairment Battery (SIB) | Attention, orientation, episodic memory, language, visuospatial abilities, and social interaction | 40 items<br><br>Maximum score is 100 points<br><br>Most items use ratings 0–2 based on quality of performance. Total score is sum of item ratings<br><br>Higher score indicates less impairment<br><br>Tests consist of primarily untimed objective measures that require little verbal production<br><br>Administration time is 20 min | Distinguished between two severely demented groups who were categorized based on MMSE scores (0–5 and 6–11). Does not differentiate between less severely impaired groups (6–11 and 12–17) (Peavy et al., 1996)<br><br>Sensitive to change over a 12 month period for those with moderate to severe dementia (Panisset et al., 1994) | Test–retest reliability = 0.87–0.90 (Panisset et al., 1994; Schmitt et al., 1997)<br><br>Inter-rater reliability with simultaneous scoring = 1.0 (Panisset et al., 1994) | Correlates with the MMSE, r = 0.83–0.84 (Panisset et al., 1994; Peavy et al., 1996; Schmitt et al., 1997)<br><br>Correlates with the Mattis Dementia Rating Scale, r = 0.89 (Peavy et al., 1996)<br><br>Correlates with the Severe Cognitive Impairment Profile, r = 0.93 (Peavy et al., 1996)<br><br>Correlates with the Global Deterioration Scale, r = −0.65 (Schmitt et al., 1997)<br><br>Correlates with the Clinical Dementia Rating Scale, r = −0.75 (Schmitt et al., 1997) |
| Test for Severe Impairment (TSI) | Episodic memory (immediate and delayed), language (production and comprehension), general knowledge, conceptualization, and motor performance | 24 items<br><br>Few items per domain<br><br>Maximum score is 24 points based on correct responses<br><br>Higher score indicates less impairment<br><br>Administration time is 10 min | No information is available | 2 week test–retest reliability = 0.96 for overall test, 0.74–0.97 for subscales (Albert & Cohen, 1992)<br><br>Internal consistency = 0.91 (Albert & Cohen, 1992) | Correlates with the MMSE, r = 0.83 (Albert & Cohen, 1992) |

| Test | Domains | Scoring | Validity/Sensitivity | Reliability | Correlation |
|---|---|---|---|---|---|
| Severe Cognitive Impairment Profile (SCIP) | Attention, calculation, episodic memory (remote, immediate, and delayed), language, visuospatial functioning, psychomotor speed, executive functioning, and social interactions | Maximum score is 245 based on correct responses. Higher score indicates less impairment. Administration time is 30 min | The SCIP is able to distinguish between 4 groups of severely impaired individuals who were categorized on the Mattis Dementia Rating Scale (Peavy et al., 1996). More sensitive to change over a 1 year period than the MMSE because it avoids floor effects (Peavy et al., 1996) | Test–retest reliability = 0.96 for overall test, 0.56–0.96 for subscales (Peavy et al., 1996). Inter-rater reliability = 0.99 for overall test, 0.77–1.0 for subscales. Reliability was the lowest for the social interaction subscale (Peavy et al., 1996) | Correlates with the MMSE, r = 0.84 (Peavy et al., 1996). Correlates with the Mattis Dementia Rating Scale, r = 0.91 (Peavy et al., 1996) |
| Modified Ordinal Scales of Psychological Development (MOSPD) | Visual pursuit and object permanence, means–ends, causality, spatial relations, and schemes | Scores range from 0 to 55. Higher scores indicate less impairment. For each of the five domains, the highest rated task is the score for that domain. Total score equals sum of domain scores. Administration time is 30 min | The MOSPD was able to test individuals who were untestable on the MMSE or the Blessed Information-Memory-Concentration Test (Auer & Reisberg, 1996) | No test–retest information is available. Inter-rater reliability = 0.96–0.99 (Auer & Reisberg, 1996). Internal consistency = 0.95 for total scale. Intercorrelations between subtests ranged from 0.75 to 0.98 (Auer & Reisberg, 1996) | Correlates with the substages of the Functional Assessment Staging Test (FAST), r = 0.77 (Auer & Reisberg, 1996) |

## Dementia Rating Scales

Dementia rating scales assess severity of dementia (e.g., mildly impaired, moderately impaired, or severely impaired). Two of the most popular rating scales, the Global Deterioration Scale and the Clinical Dementia Rating Scale, rely on subjective decisions made by clinicians. In contrast, a recently developed scale, the Dementia Severity Rating Scale, relies on judgments made by caregivers. To determine severity, clinicians and caregivers consider not only cognitive functioning but also behavior, social interactions, and functional status. Ratings within each of these areas are guided by broad categorical criteria and then summarized for an overall rating of severity. Because rating scales were designed to rate severity of dementia rather than to detect cases of dementia, it logically follows that little information is available on the sensitivity and specificity of these instruments.

Objective psychological tests that were not originally designed for staging have also proved useful markers of dementia severity (e.g., the MMSE and the ADAS) (Doraiswamy et al., 1997a; Forsell, Fratiglioni, Grut, Viitanen, & Winblad, 1992; Juva et al., 1994; Zec et al., 1992). Shorter mental status tests (e.g., the SPMSQ) are not as useful for staging dementia.

### Global Deterioration Scale (GDS) (Reisberg et al., 1982)

To complete the GDS, experienced clinicians make global categorical judgments based on semistructured interviews with the patient and/or caregiver. Patients are assigned to one of seven stages ranging from no impairment (GDS = 0) to very severe impairment (GDS = 7). Each stage is described in terms of its clinical characteristics and psychometric concomitants. The stages are easily identifiable and serve to enhance universal communication of severity. On the other hand, individuals of widely different ability levels are classified together into single broad stages, and therefore the GDS may not capture significant but small changes in levels of functioning. Although the GDS has high face validity, the scoring rules for the GDS have not been defined in great detail, and its empirical validity has not been widely established. The seven stages of the GDS are listed in Table 4.22.

### Clinical Dementia Rating Scale (CDR) (Hughes et al., 1982; Berg, 1988)

The Clinical Dementia Rating Scale stages severity of impairment specific to Alzheimer's disease. The CDR improves on the GDS in that functioning within several different domains is scored systematically and independently. These domains are orientation, memory, judgment/problem solving, community affairs, home and hobbies, and personal care. The CDR is not entirely comprehensive in that it lacks measures of language and behavior. An overall score on the CDR is derived from scores in each domain (Table 4.23); this overall score ranks the individual as not impaired (CDR 0), very mildly impaired (CDR 0.5), mildly impaired (CDR 1), moderately impaired (CDR 2), or severely impaired (CDR 3). Like the GDS, an experienced clinician (e.g., geriatrician, neurologist, psychiatrist, psychologist, or clinical nurse) must complete the CDR. The clinician makes subjective ratings based on a structured interview with the patient and/or a caregiver. Length of administration depends on the length of the interview desired by the examiner. The CDR has proved to be useful for describing severity ratings in samples included in longitudinal studies of dementia (Dooneief et al., 1996) and in clinical trials of experimental therapies (Morris et al., 1997).

The CDR is widely accepted and employed by clinicians and researchers. Although its reliability and validity have been substantiated to a greater degree than those of the GDS, the psychometrics of the CDR have by no means been extensively established. Inter-rater reliability is high when raters are given uniform training on the instrument (Morris et al., 1997), but

**Table 4.22.**
Global Deterioration Scale

*Stage 1: No Cognitive Decline*

Patients appear normal clinically. There are no complaints of memory deficit, and a clinical interview does not elicit evidence of memory deficit

*Stage 2: Very Mild Cognitive Decline*

Phase of forgetfulness. Patients complain of a memory deficit. They forget where familiar objects have been placed, and they forget names. No objective evidence of memory deficit in clinical interview or in employment or social situations

*Stage 3: Mild Cognitive Decline*

Earliest clear-cut clinical deficits. Memory and concentration deficits may be noted on clinical testing. Decreased performance becomes noticeable in social and employment situations. Difficulty in finding words and names becomes evident to others. They may become lost in unfamiliar locations. Anxiety and denial may accompany cognitive symptoms

*Stage 4: Moderate Cognitive Decline*

Late confusional phase. Concentration is poor as evidenced by performance on serial subtractions. Decreased knowledge of recent events, memory of personal history. Impaired in traveling alone and handling personal finances. May still be well-oriented to time and person. Can still travel to familiar locations. Flattening of affect and withdrawal from previously challenging situations

*Stage 5: Moderately Severe Cognitive Decline*

Early dementia. Can no longer survive without some assistance. Unable to recall a major aspect of their current lives (e.g., address, phone number, or names of grandchildren). Difficulty counting backwards. Retains knowledge of major facts regarding themselves and others. No assistance with toileting or eating. May display some difficulty choosing proper clothes to wear

*Stage 6: Severe Cognitive Decline*

Middle phase of dementia. May occasionally forget the name of spouse. Unaware of all recent events and experiences in their lives. Sketchy knowledge of the past. Unaware of surroundings, the year, and the season. Requires substantial assistance with tasks of daily living. May experience sleep disturbances. Still recall their own name and can distinguish familiar from unfamiliar people in the environment. Personality and emotional changes occur. May experience delusional behavior, anxiety, and loss of motivation

*Stage 7: Very Severe Cognitive Decline*

Late dementia. Most verbal abilities are lost. Incontinent to urine, requires assistance in toileting. Psychomotor skills (e.g., walking) are lost

reliability is unclear among clinicians untrained on the instrument. Test–retest reliability has not been established. In terms of validity, the CDR correlates well with dementia staging criteria outlined by the *Diagnostic and Statistical Manual* (DSM) of the American Psychiatric Association (Forsell et al., 1992; Juva et al., 1994). Furthermore, the CDR correlates moderately with stages generated by a categorized MMSE (Forsell et al., 1992).

Heyman and associates (1987) extended the CDR to include profound (CDR = 4) and terminal (CDR = 5) stages of dementia and found that this modified rating scale correlated with measures of dementia severity, nursing home residence, and predicted shortened survival (Dooneief et al., 1996). Although the CDR correlates with other staging instruments, its agreement with neuropsychological measures is variable. Two strictly "cog-

Table 4.23.  Clinical Dementia Rating Scale (CDR)*

| | Healthy (CDR 0) | Very mild dementia (CDR 0.5) | Mild dementia (CDR 1) | Moderate dementia (CDR 2) | Severe dementia (CDR 3) |
|---|---|---|---|---|---|
| Memory | No memory loss or slight inconsistent forgetfulness | Mild consistent forgetfulness, partial recollection of events; "benign" forgetfulness | Moderate memory loss more marked for recent events, defect interferes with everyday activities | Severe memory loss; only highly learned material retained; new material rapidly lost | Severe memory loss; only fragments remain |
| Orientation | Fully oriented | Fully oriented | Some difficulty with time relationships; oriented to place and person at examination but may have geographic disorientation | Usually disoriented in time, often to place | Oriented to person only |
| Judgment, problem solving | Solves everyday problems well; judgment good in relation to past performance | Only doubtful impairment in solving problems, similarities, differences | Moderate difficulty in handling complex problems; social judgment usually maintained | Severe impairment in handling problems; similarities, differences; social judgment usually impaired | Unable to make judgments or solve problems |
| Community affairs | Independent function at usual level in job, shopping, business, financial affairs, volunteer and social groups | Only doubtful or mild impairment in these activities | Unable to function independently at these activities though may still be engaged in some; may still appear normal to casual inspection | No pretense of independent function outside home. Appears well enough to be taken to functions outside a family home | No pretense of independent function outside of home. Appears too ill to be taken to functions outside a family home |
| Home, hobbies | Life at home, hobbies, intellectual interests well maintained | Life at home, hobbies, intellectual interests slightly impaired | Mild but definite impairment of function at home; more difficult chores abandoned; more complicated hobbies and interests abandoned | Only simple chores preserved; very restricted interests, poorly sustained | No significant function in the home |
| Personal care | Fully capable of self-care | (No 0.5 impairment level.) | Needs prompting for self-care | Requires assistance in dressing, hygiene, keeping of personal effects | Requires much help with personal care; often incontinent |

*Score only as decline from previous level due to cognitive loss, not impairment due to other factors.

nitive" domains of the CDR are orientation and memory. Orientation correlates well with independent neuropsychological measure of orientation, but memory scores do not correlate highly with neuropsychological measures of memory (Fillenbaum, Peterson, & Morris, 1996).

## Dementia Severity Rating Scale (DSRS) (Clark & Ewbank, 1996)

The DSRS is a relatively new rating scale that takes a different approach to assessing severity. Caregivers rather than clinicians complete the scale using a structured multiple choice format. Information comes solely from the caregiver and not from a variety of sources as in other rating scales (e.g., patient, caregiver, and clinician). The caregiver rates the patient's ability to function in the home environment within eleven domains (Table 4.24). Six domains were chosen to mirror those of the CDR (orientation, memory, judgment, social interactions, home activities, and personal care), and the remaining domains were added to broaden the areas of functioning assessed (language, recognition, eating, incontinence, and mobility).

Within each domain, several levels of functioning are described. Each description is assigned a number. The informant chooses the description that most closely matches the patient's level of functioning, and scores for each domain are summed for a total score. With this scoring procedure, the DSRS offers a quantitative rather than a qualitative index of severity. Because the DSRS is continuous rather than categorical, there are no firm cutpoints for categorizing people into different severity levels as of yet, but Clark and Ewbank (1996) offer some preliminary groupings. They found that DSRS scores of 21 or less roughly equaled a CDR of 0.5 or 1 (mild dementia), scores of 22 to 39 equaled a CDR of 2 (moderate dementia), and scores of 40 or more equaled a CDR of 3 (severe dementia). In their sample, there was some overlap of DSRS scores for people with different CDR scores. The question of whether DSRS scores can distinguish between very mild dementia and mild dementia has not yet been addressed (Clark & Ewbank, 1996).

The DSRS is practical and easy to use. The 11 item scale takes only 5–10 minutes to complete and can be mailed to and completed by the caregiver at home. The questionnaire may be useful in multicenter clinical research studies. It correlates with other cognitive measures, including the MMSE, the CDR, and the CERAD (Clark & Ewbank, 1996). It has high test–retest reliability and high inter-rater reliability when clinician ratings are compared with caregiver ratings. This suggests that caregivers rate patients in much the same way as trained clinicians. This point will need to be further researched because findings from the Informant Questionnaire for Cognitive Decline in the Elderly (IQCODE) that was described earlier suggest that characteristics of the caregiver may bias reports of patients' cognitive functioning (Christensen & Jorm, 1992; Jorm et al., 1996).

Other rating instruments that have proved useful for dementia are the Mini-Mental State Examination (MMSE) and the Alzheimer's Disease Assessment Scale (ADAS) (Doraiswamy et al., 1997a, b); Forsell et al., 1992; Juva et al., 1994; Zec et al., 1992). Similar to the DSRS, the MMSE and ADAS produce scores along a continuum that can be grouped into discrete categories. Zec and coworkers (1992) divided patients with Alzheimer's disease into severity groups based on MMSE scores. Patients with scores above 24 were considered very mildly impaired, patients with scores between 20 and 23 were considered mildly impaired, those with scores between 10 and 19 were considered moderately impaired, and those with scores below 10 were considered severely impaired. Mean ADAS scores were significantly different for each of these groups except for very mild and mild groups. Doraiswamy and colleagues

**Table 4.24.**
Dementia Severity Rating Scale

Patient name: _____

Person completing form: _____

Relationship to patient: _____

In each section, circle the number that most closely applies to the patient. Please circle only one number per section.

*Memory*

0 Normal
1 Occasional "benign" forgetfulness of no consequence.
2 Mild consistent forgetfulness with partial recollection of events.
3 Moderate memory loss, more marked for recent events and severe enough to interfere with everyday activities.
4 Severe memory loss; only well-learned material retained with newly learned material rapidly lost.
5 Usually unable to remember basic facts such as the day of the week, month and/or year, when last meal was eaten, or the name of the next meal.
6 Unable to test due to speech and language difficulty and/or ability to follow instructions.
7 Makes no attempt to communicate and is no longer aware of surroundings.

*Orientation*

0 Normal
1 Some difficulty with time relationships, but not severe enough to interfere with everyday activities.
2 Frequently disoriented in time and sometimes disoriented to new places.
3 Almost always disoriented in time and usually disoriented to place.
4 Unable to answer questions related to time of day or name of present location.
5 Is unaware of questioner and makes no attempt to respond.

*Judgment*

0 Normal
1 Only doubtful impairment in problem-solving ability.
2 Moderate difficulty in handling complex problems, but social judgment usually maintained.
3 Severe impairment in handling problems, social judgment usually impaired.
4 Unable to exercise judgment in either problem solving or social situations.

*Social Interactions/Community Affairs*

0 No alteration in ability to participate in community affairs.
1 Only mild impairment, of no practical consequence, but clearly different from previous years. Still able to work (if applicable), but performance not up to previous standards.
2 Unable to function independently in community activities, although still able to participate to some extent and, to casual inspection, may appear normal. Unable to hold a job or, if still working, requires constant supervision.
3 No pretense of independent function outside of home. Unable to hold a job but still participates in home activities with friends. Casual acquaintances are aware of a problem.
4 No longer participates in any meaningful way in home-based social activities involving people other than the primary caregiver.

*Home Activities/Responsibilities*

0 Normal
1 Some impairment in activities such as money management and house maintenance, but no effect on the ability to shop, cook or clean. Still watches TV and reads newspaper with interest and understanding.
2 Unable to perform activities related to money management (bill paying, etc.) or complex household tasks (maintenance). Some difficulty with shopping, cooking, and/or cleaning. Losing interest in the newspaper and TV.
3 No longer able to shop, cook, or clean without considerable help and supervision. No longer able to read the newspaper or watch TV with understanding.
4 No longer engages in any home-based activities.

*(continued)*

**Table 4.24.**
Dementia Severity Rating Scale — Continued

*Personal Care*

0 Normal
1 Needs occasional prompting but washes and dresses independently.
2 Requires assistance with dressing, hygiene, and personal upkeep.
3 Totally dependent for help. Does not initiate personal care activities.

*Speech/Language*

0 Normal
1 Occasional difficulty with word finding, but able to carry on conversations.
2 Unable to thinks of some words. May occasionally make inappropriate word substitutions.
3 No longer spontaneously initiates conversation but can usually answer questions using sentences.
4 Answers questions, but responses are often unintelligible or inappropriate. Able to follow simple instructions.
5 Speech usually unintelligible or irrelevant. Unable to answer questions or follow verbal instructions.
6 No response, vegetative.

*Recognition*

0 Normal
1 Occasionally fails to recognize more distant acquaintances or casual friends.
2 Always recognizes family and close friends but usually not more distant acquaintances.
3 Alert, but occasionally fails to recognize family and/or close friends.
4 Only occasionally recognizes spouse or caregiver.
5 No recognition or awareness of the presence of others.

*Feeding*

0 Normal
1 May require help cutting food and/or have limitations as to the type of food able to eat independently.
2 Generally able to eat independently but may require some assistance.
3 Needs to be fed. May have difficulty swallowing or requires feeding tube.

*Incontinence*

0 Normal
2 Rare incontinence. Bladder incontinence (generally less than one accident per month).
3 Occasional bladder incontinence (an average of two or more times a month).
4 Frequent bladder incontinence despite assistance (more than once per week).
5 Total incontinence.

*Mobility/Walking*

0 Normal
1 May occasionally have some difficulty driving or taking public transportation, but fully independent for walking without supervision.
2 Able to walk outside without supervision for short distances, but unable to drive or take public transportation.
3 Able to walk within the home without supervision but cannot go outside unaccompanied.
4 Requires supervision within the home, but able to walk without assistance (may use cane or walker).
5 Generally confined to a bed or chair. May be able to walk a few steps with help.
6 Essentially bedridden. Unable to sit or stand.

(1997a) found similar results using two MMSE severity groupings (19–23 and 12–18). Juva and colleagues (1994) used slightly different cut-off scores: 24+ = intact, 18–23 = mildly impaired, 12–17 = moderately impaired, and 0–11 = severely impaired. This categorized MMSE correlated with stages of the DSM of the American Psychiatric Association, k = 0.44, and with stages of the CDR, k = 0.33. The MMSE tended to rate individuals as more impaired than did the

**Table 4.25.**
Dementia Rating Scales

| Measure | Domains covered | Testing and scoring | Sensitivity and specificity | Reliability | Validity |
|---|---|---|---|---|---|
| Global Deterioration Scale (GDS)* | Orientation, episodic memory, working memory, language comprehension, visuospatial abilities, executive functioning, functional status, emotional functioning, social interactions, and problem behaviors | A rating is given based on clinical judgment (1 = no cognitive decline, 7 = very severe cognitive decline)  Judgment based on information gathered from objective testing, informant interview, and patient interview  Administration time is dependent on interview length | No information available | No information available | Correlates with the MMSE, r = 0.92 (Reisberg et al., 1986)  Higher ratings (e.g., GDS level 4) show greater likelihood of institutionalization, death, and clinical deterioration than lower ratings (Reisberg et al., 1986) |

| Clinical Dementia Rating Scale (CDR) | Orientation, episodic memory, judgment and problem solving, community affairs, home and hobbies, and personal care | A rating on a 5 point scale is given for each domain (0 = normal, 0.5 = very mild dementia, 1 = mild dementia, 2 = moderate dementia, and 3 = severe dementia). These ratings are weighted and averaged for a total CDR score between 0 and 3<br><br>Ratings are based on clinical judgments<br><br>Judgments are based on information gathered during informant interview and patient interview<br><br>Administration time depends on interview length | Inter-rater reliability = 0.74–0.97 (Burke et al., 1988; Morris et al., 1997) | Sensitivity = 0.95, specificity = 0.94 with a cut-off of CDR 1 (Juva et al., 1995) | Correlates with the MMSE, r = 0.55–0.78 (Forsell et al., 1992; Juva et al., 1994)<br><br>Correlates with the Blessed Information-Memory-Concentration Test, r = 0.57 (Dooneief et al., 1996)<br><br>Agreement with DSM staging, r = 0.60–0.65 (Forsell et al., 1992; Juva et al., 1994)<br><br>Moderate agreement for mild stages, $\kappa = 0.47$ (Forsell et al., 1992)<br><br>Correlates with the Blessed Dementia Rating Scale, r = 0.67 (Dooneief et al., 1996)<br><br>Correlates with Activities of Daily Living scores, r = −0.64 (Dooneief et al., 1996)<br><br>Relates to Alzheimer's disease diagnosis at autopsy (Berg, 1988)<br><br>Predicts nursing home admission and death (Dooneief et al., 1996) |

(continued)

**Table 4.25.**
Dementia Rating Scales—Continued

| Measure | Domains covered | Testing and Scoring | Sensitivity and Specificity | Reliability | Validity |
|---|---|---|---|---|---|
| Dementia Severity Rating Scale (DSRS) | Orientation, episodic memory, language, judgment, social interaction, home activities, personal care, eating, incontinence, and mobility | 11 multiple choice items completed by the caregiver<br><br>Scores range from 0 to 51<br><br>Higher score indicates greater severity<br><br>Administration time is 5–10 min | No information available | Test–retest reliability (2 weeks) = 0.90 (Clark & Ewbank, 1996)<br><br>Inter-rater reliability = 0.87 when caregiver ratings were compared with clinician ratings (Clark & Ewbank, 1996)<br><br>Internal consistency = 0.92. Each item correlates with total score, r = 0.56–0.83 (Clark & Ewbank, 1996) | Correlates with the MMSE, r = −0.77 (Clark & Ewbank, 1996)<br><br>Correlates with the CERAD, r = −0.73. Correlates with CERAD subtests, r = −0.39 (delayed word recall) to −0.65 (verbal fluency) (Clark & Ewbank, 1996)<br><br>DSRS scores vary significantly between individuals with different Clinical Dementia Rating scores (Clark & Ewbank, 1996) |

CDR. Doraiswamy and associates (1997b) used ADAS scores to predict the GDR scores of patients. Nearly 85% of GDS 4 patients and 69% of GDS 5 patients were classified correctly. Of all domains, ADAS orientation items best discriminated GDS stages 4 and 5. Table 4.25 summarizes several facets of dementia rating scales.

## Global Change Measures

Measures of global change evaluate shifts in functioning due to treatment effects or progression of dementia. Completing a global change measure itself takes only a minute; it involves a single global judgment of change (e.g., improved, much improved, worse, much worse, or no change). Collecting the information on which this global judgment is based, however, takes more time. An experienced clinician gathers information by using interviews with patients and caregivers, scores on mental status tests, and functional assessments. The global judgment is completely subjective but is assumed to be based on extensive clinical experience and to capture a clinically significant event not revealed by quantitative measures. Because of its clinical sensitivity, the Federal Drug Administration requires that global assessments be included as primary outcome measures in all trials of antidementia drugs (Knopman, Knapp, Gracon, & Davis, 1994).

### The Clinician Interview-Based Impression of Change (CIBIC)

The CIBIC was one of two primary outcome measures (along with the ADAS Cognitive Behaviors Section) included in several clinical trials of antidementia drugs for Alzheimer's disease (Knapp et al., 1994a, b). In terms of CIBIC procedure, a skilled clinician makes a global rating based on an interview with the patient. The rating is intended to assess change from baseline. At baseline, special attention is given to cognitive performance and behavior of the patient. Target domains of focus include (but are not limited to) con-

centration, orientation, memory, language, behavior, initiative, and activities of daily living. At follow-up visits, at which ratings are made, the clinician is not allowed exposure to opinions from caregivers or clinic staff or to data from cognitive tests before making the rating. Instead, an interview with the patient alone is the basis of the rating, although the clinician may review the baseline composite file. If improvement or decline is noted, the clinician indicates which domains contributed to the impression: memory, language, concentration, orientation, reasoning, praxis, behavior, appearance, or other. Ratings are made on a 7 point Likert-type scale (1 = very much improved, 7 = very much worse), although the extremes of the scale are rarely used. No guidelines or descriptors are provided to further define individual ratings. Ratings are modestly reliable on test–retest at 2 weeks, but less reliable than objective measures (Knopman et al., 1994). The CIBIC ratings weakly but significantly correlate with quantitative measures. There is no correlation between CIBIC ratings and patient sex, education, or age (Knopman et al., 1994).

The CIBIC is less sensitive to change than is the MMSE or the ADAS. In tacrine drug trials, 38% of patients were rated as worse at week 30 with the CIBIC, but 59% were rated worse by the ADAS and 55% were rated worse by the MMSE. Fewer patients were rated as improved by the CIBIC (19%) compared with the ADAS (31%) or the MMSE (27%) (Knopman et al., 1994). This result may be interpreted to suggest that the CIBIC is less sensitive to change than are objective measures, but it could also be argued that these CIBIC results demonstrate that the drug led to clinically significant differences in cognitive functioning that were documented independent of sensitive cognitive measures. Correlations between change scores on the CIBIC and MMSE ($r = -0.39$) and the CIBIC and the ADAS ($r = 0.33$) were small but significant. Knopman and associates (1994) suggest that inclusion of caregiver input and improved definition of ratings on the global scale may strengthen the CIBIC. In a subsequent antidementia drug trial, the "CIBIC-Plus" used caregiver input for ratings. Inter-rater agreement improved, but it still varied widely from patient to patient. Variability was influenced by caregiver information (Boothby, Man, & Barker, 1995). An issue that needs to be addressed if ratings from the CIBIC are to be compared between clinical trials is the basis of ratings: interview alone, input from staff, input from caregivers, review of psychometric data, or some combination of these (Meya et al., 1994).

## CONCLUSIONS AND FUTURE DIRECTIONS

### Recommendations by Purpose and Situation

This chapter's goal was to emphasize the care with which cognitive measures should be chosen, by clinicians and researchers alike. Factors influencing choice include the purpose of testing (e.g., clinical vs. research), the context of testing (e.g., who will make assessments and who will provide responses), and characteristics of the person being tested (e.g., sensory or motor deficits, verbal abilities, behavior problems). Instruments under consideration should be evaluated in terms of sensitivity, specificity, reliability, and validity.

### Clinical Purposes

Geriatricians, neurologists, psychiatrists, psychologists, and even nurses employ cognitive tests in the course of their clinical work with older adults. Assessments assist in various aspects of clinical workups, including screening, diagnosis, staging, and documenting change.

Mental status tests and informant reports are the tools used to screen for cognitive impairment. These formats contrast in strengths and weaknesses. For example, informant reports offer greater ecological validity in terms of assessing cognitive

functioning as it presents itself in everyday contexts. They allow assessment of *change* in functioning rather than just deficit in functioning because caregivers compare present and past performances of the patient. At the same time, informant reports are prone to contamination by noncognitive characteristics such as affective state and personality of both the informant and the patient. Mental status tests assess cognitive performance on objective items under controlled circumstances, so they are less prone to biased interpretation, but at the same time they are more artificial and less sensitive to change because they assess cognition at one point in time. Estimates of cognitive functioning are more affected by the effects of age, education, race, and socioeconomic status on mental status tests than on informant reports. Because of contrasting strengths and weaknesses of mental status tests and informant reports, the optimal screening strategy is to utilize both screening formats to detect impairment, but of course in screening situations there is often time realistically for only one measure.

When choosing between mental status tests, it is important to note that most are similar in reliability, validity, sensitivity, and specificity. The MMSE and the Cognitive Capacity Screening Exam (CCSE) are the most global of the mental status tests in terms of domains covered; the Abbreviated Mental Test (AMT) is the least comprehensive (covering only orientation items). The Blessed Orientation-Memory-Concentration (BOMC) Test and the Short Portable Mental Status Questionnaire (SPMSQ) fall somewhere in between these two extremes, covering fewer domains and taking less time than the MMSE and the CCSE but covering more domains and taking more time than the AMT. The CCSE has proved effective with inpatients but has not been tested extensively with outpatient or community populations; the other tests have been used with a variety of populations. MacKenzie and colleagues (1996) recommend the MMSE over other mental status tests because it has a lower false-positive rate. It takes slightly longer to administer than other mental status tests, but in the long run it may save time and money because fewer people will be subjected to comprehensive testing. Additionally, information on cut-off scores for different sensitivities and specificities has been provided most comprehensively for the MMSE. The MMSE is the most universally well known to clinicians, so communication of functioning between clinicians is optimized.

On informant report questionnaires, caregivers report on specific behaviors related to cognitive functioning. Of the three informant report questionnaires reviewed, the Informant Questionnaire for Cognitive Decline in the Elderly (IQCODE) has the most extensive psychometric data and has proved to be a reliable and valid measure. The IQCODE is similar in length and content to the Dementia Questionnaire, but it gives a specific time frame in which to evaluate patients' behaviors (10 years). More importantly, it has a scoring format, whereas the Dementia Questionnaire has none. At present, the Dementia Questionnaire is limited to use in clinical settings by trained personnel who can interpret the significance of responses. It is useful as a guide in the context of a semistructured interview for the purpose of obtaining a cognitive history. The Minimum Data Set (MDS) cognition scales were designed for nursing home residents, and they may have limited reliability and validity in other settings. Nursing home staff rather than family members complete these scales. A strength of the MDS scales is that data collected for the purpose of assessing nursing home care can be used to answer questions of cognitive functioning. Otherwise, little information is available on cognitive status of nursing home residents. This is an important step in screening the cognitive status of nursing home residents, but these scales probably will not prove valuable for purposes other than screening because they assess only the most cursory

information regarding cognitive functioning. Among the three informant reports, the IQCODE is the only measure that could possibly be used across patient settings (e.g., community residence vs. nursing home residence), although nursing home staff may find its time requirements too demanding.

Clinicians form diagnoses of dementia based on various sources of information, including results of physical examinations and laboratory analyses, medical history, and functional status. According to diagnostic guidelines, suspected cases of dementia require documentation with cognitive testing. Neuropsychological assessment is the most rigorous method for detecting cognitive deficits, but a full battery is usually time-intensive and expensive. Shortened batteries retain many of the features of a full battery while enhancing practicality and economy. Whether a full battery or a shortened battery is enlisted, clinicians must consider the domains of cognition assessed by a particular battery. The domains most sensitive to dementia are orientation, episodic memory for recent events, confrontational naming, visuospatial construction, and psychomotor speed. For the most part, the shortened batteries discussed in this chapter cover these domains (except that the ADAS does not contain speeded items, the CERAD Neuropsychological Battery does not contain orientation items, and the Mattis Dementia Rating Scale [MDRS] does not contain naming items).

Because the ADAS and the CERAD were specifically designed to test people with Alzheimer's disease, these shortened batteries may be of limited utility for distinguishing different types of dementia. Neither of these measures includes items of attention or psychomotor speed. Deficits in these two domains occur in depression, delirium, and subcortical dementias, and therefore the lack of such measures in the ADAS and the CERAD makes these measures less sensitive to diagnostic distinctions. In contrast, the MDRS and the cognitive battery of the Cambridge Mental Disorders of the Elderly Examination (CAMCOG) assess attention, and both have proved useful in distinguishing between different types of cognitive impairments. Of these four batteries, the CAMCOG has proved most capable of distinguishing between different types of dementia common among older adults. As another approach, clinicians can supplement shortened batteries with domain tests to specifically address the question of impairment under investigation.

To aid in diagnosing and tracking progression of symptoms specific to Alzheimer's disease, the ADAS and CERAD are most highly recommended among the four shortened batteries, although the other measures have sound psychometric properties. The ADAS and CERAD take a similar amount of time to administer and are fairly consistent across patients in the amount of time to complete the battery. In contrast, the MDRS takes anywhere from 10 to 45 minutes to administer. The length of the battery and its administration format (i.e., most difficult items first) makes the MDRS potentially too frustrating for many of the more impaired patients. On the other hand, the MDRS has proved sensitive to later decline, as have the ADAS and CERAD. The ADAS offers an overall score, in contrast to the CERAD, which provides scores only for each subtest.

For purposes of staging severity of cognitive impairment, several instruments are available. Rating scales determine severity by taking into account daily functioning and social interactions as well as cognitive performance. The Global Deterioration Scale (GDS) and the Clinical Dementia Rating Scale (CDR) are two well-known rating scales. Clinicians complete these rating scales based on semistructured interviews with patients and caregivers. The CDR is recommended over the GDS because CDR ratings are based on ratings in several subareas, whereas GDS ratings are global, making them more prone to subjective bias. Furthermore, the validity of

the CDR has been more extensively established than that of the GDS. The Dementia Severity Rating Scale (DSRS) is a relatively new and appealing rating instrument. In contrast to the CDR and GDS, informants rather than clinicians complete the DSRS. The DSRS covers more domains than the CDR and gives a continuous rather than a categorical score. As another means of staging, objective measures such as the MMSE, the ADAS, and the CERAD have proved useful. Objective measures take longer to complete than rating scales and require determination of the appropriate cut-points, but they may be useful for rating severity based solely on cognitive performance without reference to social or functional limitations.

To be useful for charting the progression of cognitive impairments or determining the effectiveness of treatments, cognitive instruments must be sensitive to change. For global measures of change, the Clinician Interview-Based Impression of Change (CIBIC) has proved sensitive to clinically notable effects of antidementia drugs. On the CIBIC, clinicians document their overall impressions of improvement or decline using a single Likert scale rating. Although the CIBIC was developed for research purposes, there is no reason to believe that it cannot be used for charting change in clinical contexts. It is not as sensitive to change as are certain objective measures, but it may be a practical measure of observable change (in contrast to statistically significant change). Other global measures, such as dementia rating scales (the GDS, the CDR, and the DSRS), are not particularly useful as measures of change because they categorize functioning into broad categories (e.g., three or four stages of cognitive impairment).

Objective measures that have proved effective for detecting change are the MMSE, the ADAS, the MDRS, and the CERAD. With the MMSE, annual drops of one to three points can be seen among patients newly diagnosed with Alzheimer's disease. The rate of decline increases as the disease progresses, up to four or five points in later stages of the disease (Morris et al., 1993; Teri et al., 1995); (US Department of Health and Human Services, 1997). The MMSE has been criticized for poor discrimination of change in both the very early and very late stages of dementia (Albert & Cohen, 1992). Full or shortened neuropsychological batteries provide comprehensive appraisal of the baseline level of functioning and can be used for follow-up comparisons. Shortened batteries such as the ADAS and CERAD may be more sensitive to early- and late-stage changes in Alzheimer's disease than is the MMSE. The MDRS, for example, detects longitudinal decline better than mental status tests (Salmon et al., 1990). For moderate to severe dementia, most mental status tests and shortened batteries will show floor effects and therefore be less sensitive to change. Under these circumstances, late-stage batteries should be employed that contain downward extensions of standard batteries and that rely more heavily on nonverbal items.

There are four late-stage batteries. Although all four are sensitive to change in even the latest stages of dementia, the Severe Impairment Battery (SIB) and the Modified Ordinal Scales of Psychological Development (MOSPD) show unusually early ceiling effects for less severe impairments. The MOSPD was designed to test the most basic cognitive abilities and is probably useful for testing only individuals who are no longer testable with other late-stage batteries. The Severe Cognitive Impairment Profile (SCIP) shows the greatest range of sensitivity; it detects longitudinal changes in the very late stages of dementia but also in the moderate stages of the disease. In terms of administration, the SIB and the SCIP require several specialized objects and stimuli. The Test of Severe Impairment (TSI) is more portable because it does not require specialized stimuli. The TSI takes less time to administer (10 minutes vs. 20 minutes for the other instruments), but, at the same time, it has fewer

items per domain and therefore may not provide meaningful information regarding functioning within a domain.

*Research Purposes*

The same instruments developed for clinical purposes are typically useful for research purposes. The same considerations for choosing clinical instruments apply to choosing research instruments in terms of choosing the best fit for the purpose of the research, constraints of the testing situation, and characteristics of the person being tested. Further considerations for research purposes are the level of cognition being measured (global vs. local) and the level of response required (categorical vs. continuous).

Mental status tests, informant reports, rating scales, and shortened neuropsychological batteries provide global estimates of cognitive functioning. Domain tests and domain subscales of neuropsychological tests provide local estimates of function. Domain subtests of mental status tests should be used with caution because only a few items represent each domain. If categorical scores are desired (which is often the case when cognition serves as a predictor variable), rating scales (the GDS or the CDR) may be appropriate for assigning individuals to discrete severity stages (e.g., mildly, moderately, or severely impaired). Continuous measures can be used categorically. The MMSE and the ADAS have been used for categorizing individuals into stages, as have other mental status tests and shortened batteries. Data are available on the sensitivities and specificities of different cut-off scores with these measures. Mental status tests and informant reports categorize people as impaired or unimpaired. Except for the CIBIC and rating scales, almost all other measures described in this chapter are continuous measures and are potentially appropriate as outcome variables. Perhaps the cognitive measures that have been used most for research purposes are the MMSE, the ADAS, the MDRS, and the Wechsler Adult

Intelligence Scale. The Informant Questionnaire for Cognitive Decline in the Elderly and the Dementia Severity Rating Scale are relatively new measures that have strong research potential. They are brief measures that caregivers can complete via the mail, over the phone, or in person to provide information regarding change in cognitive functioning and/or severity of impairment.

Researchers must be cautious when using clinical measures for research purposes. For example, sensitivity and specificity of mental status tests as determined in patient populations (e.g., hospital or clinic settings) are not the same in community populations (i.e., diagnostic accuracy is usually lower in community populations). Instruments chosen based on clinical psychometric properties may ill-serve particular research purposes. Epidemiological research has used mental status tests to estimate the prevalence of dementia in the general population (Robins et al., 1981). Mental status tests may underrepresent the true number of cases of dementia for certain subgroups (e.g., high education and high intelligence) and overrepresent the true number of cases for other subgroups (e.g., low education and low socioeconomic status). This leads to biased estimates of dementia in the population, but, due to the time and cost constraints of epidemiological research, a biased estimate may be better than no estimate at all. Nevertheless, these limitations must be spelled out when findings are interpreted. All in all, researchers should determine the psychometric properties of instruments for the contexts in which they will be used.

## Current and Future Directions

### Telephone Assessments

There is an increasing reliance on telephone assessments to gather information about older adults' cognitive functioning. In a clinical context, patients who are reluctant or unable to return to the clinic are occasionally assessed over the telephone.

For research purposes, telephone assessments facilitate screening (e.g., researchers invite only people who pass the telephone screen to participate in in-person portions of the study). Large-scale epidemiological studies take advantage of telephone assessments to reduce the time and money that is dedicated to sending interviewers to targeted households. Several telephone assessments have been developed and validated. For example, there is a phone version of the MMSE (Roccaforte et al., 1994a & b). Of necessity, some items have been dropped, such as asking patients what floor of the building they are on or asking them to copy a picture of intersecting pentagons. Although sensitivity and specificity are similar for the telephone and in-person versions of the MMSE, people who report having hearing difficulties score lower on the telephone version (Roccaforte et al., 1994a, b).

Another telephone instrument is the Telephone Interview for Cognitive Status (TICS) (Brandt, Spencer, & Folstein, 1988). This instrument is similar in format to various mental status tests, it correlates highly with the MMSE, and its test–retest reliability is high (Brandt et al., 1988). Other instruments have potential for over-the-phone administration. For example, instruments that gather information from caregivers, such as the Informant Questionnaire for Cognitive Decline in the Elderly (IQCODE) and the Dementia Severity Rating Scale (DSRS), could be easily adapted for telephone administration.

Although telephone assessments are reliable and valid as well as practical, there are limitations. Examiners have little control over the testing environment when conducting assessments over the phone. In patients' homes, there is noise from radios and televisions, interruptions from family members or pets, and access to cognitive aids such as calendars and paper and pencils. Although examiners ask that these external distractions and aids be removed before testing, there is no way to ensure that this request is heeded. Examiners must also be extremely sensitive to the hearing difficulties of persons being tested.

## New Technologies

The wave of technological advances experienced during the last quarter century has advantaged the field of cognitive assessment. Although it is true that most cognitive assessments are paper and pencil based, computerized assessments have made their way into use. Computers present stimuli with great precision and provide systematic feedback to the person being tested. A computer can score and analyze results accurately and efficiently, leading to less "human error." Touch-screens, millisecond timing, and voice recognition make it possible for a range of different responses to be recorded. An additional advantage of computerized measures is that they tailor assessment to the individual. For example, examiners can program the computer to skip questions too easy or too difficult for the individual. Working on a computer may seem more "game-like" to participants and therefore less anxiety provoking. Drawbacks to computerized assessment are the rapid rate at which technology is outdated, the greater expense required for computer equipment than for paper-and-pencil measures, poor portability of computers, and greater potential for "breakdowns." For older adults not previously exposed to computer technology, working on a computer could be intimidating. Future advances in computer technology may make these drawbacks less formidable.

Other technological advances that have informed the field of cognitive aging are neuroimaging techniques that allow a once impossible view of the functioning brain. Atrophy, lesions, and reduced blood flow are detectable on neuroimaging scans. These scans help pinpoint or rule out certain causes of dementia (e.g., stroke). Researchers are now able to relate scores on traditional cognitive measures with brain structure and function.

Videotapes are increasingly used for purposes of training standardized administration (e.g., clinicians watch a videotaped testing session to view correct administration procedures, and trainers view videotapes of clinicians administering tests to ensure correct administration). Potentially, in a research context, videotapes could be used to tape patients' behaviors for staging purposes or for viewing performance of everyday cognitive functions.

## Relating Cognitive Measures to Everyday Functioning

As assessments become more specialized, they become more artificial and perhaps more difficult to relate to everyday functioning. If the purpose of assessment is to make management and treatment decisions, it is important to determine whether cognitive limitations impede tasks of daily living such as balancing a checkbook, driving safely, cooking, taking medications, and staying home alone. Research addressing the interpretation of cognitive performance on standardized tests into everyday functioning has been sparse and unsystematic, but this approach is receiving more and more attention (see Poon, Rubin, & Wilson, 1989). Studies have compared performance on mental status tests with functional ability, finding only modest relationships between the measures (Vitaliano et al., 1984a, b). Domains that have been found most useful for predicting functional competence (e.g., recreation, communication, and self-maintenance) are attention and memory (Vitaliano et al., 1984a, b). As an example of a systematic study, Henderson, Mack, and Williams (1989) tested adults with Alzheimer's disease and found that visuoconstructive deficits on objective cognitive tests combined with memory loss were significant predictors of everyday spatial disorientation as evidenced by wandering, getting lost, and failing to recognize familiar surroundings.

Miller and Morris (1993) suggest that greater reliance should be placed on criterion-referenced measurement to assess everyday cognitive functioning. This format assesses whether a person accomplishes a task up to minimum standards and, if not, to what level the task is accomplished. This information guides decisions regarding the manner in which tasks or the environment should be adapted in order to compensate for cognitive limitations. More measures of everyday cognitive abilities are being created (e.g., Willis, 1996). The downside to advocating for assessment of everyday abilities is the potential for creating tests that have high face validity for assessing these functions but in reality are no better in doing so than are traditional tests. For example, a simulated driving test may be designed to determine driving abilities, but this task may not capture actual driving performance, or it may not do so any better than traditional measures of attention, memory, visuospatial abilities, and executive functioning.

*Examining Cognitive Strengths of Older Adults*

An emerging trend in the field of cognitive aging has been to explore cognitive strengths as well as cognitive deficits of older adults, born out of the realization that not all aspects of cognition exhibit uniform decline with age, and not all older adults experience similar levels of decline. The areas of cognition that appear particularly resistant to the effects of aging are crystallized knowledge, wisdom, expertise, and creativity. With respect to wisdom, Baltes and colleagues found that, contrary to folk lore, younger adults as well as older adults display wisdom, and there are no age-related declines in wisdom performance (Baltes & Staudinger, 1993; Baltes, Staudinger, Maercker, & Smith, 1995). "Successful aging" is the term applied to the study of individuals resistant to typical aging effects (Baltes & Baltes, 1990; Rowe & Kahn, 1987). Findings from the Seattle Longitudinal Study, which is the longest running longitudinal study of cognitive aging, suggests that healthy cardiovascular functioning, high educational attainment, above-average occupational status, and attitudinal flexibility are factors that protect against age-related cognitive declines (Schaie, 1990). The assessment of cognitive strengths and successful aging has potential clinical applications. For example, preserved cognitive abilities of individuals could be enlisted to compensate for cognitive deficits when tailoring a treatment or management plan. Future research will need to explore the relationship between cognitive strengths and beneficial outcomes.

## REFERENCES

Albert, M., & Cohen, C. (1992). The test for severe impairment: An instrument for the assessment of patients with severe cognitive dysfunction. *Journal of the American Geriatrics Society, 40,* 449–453.

Albert, M., Levkoff, S., Reilly, C., Liptzin, B., Pilgrim, D., Cleary, P., Evans, D., & Rowe, J. (1992). The delirium symptom interview: An interview for the detection of delirium symptoms in hospitalized patients. *Journal of Geriatric Psychiatry and Neurology, 5,* 14–21.

Albert, M., Smith, L., Scherr, P., Taylor, J., Evans, D., & Funkenstein, H. (1991). Use of brief cognitive tests to identify individuals in the community with clinically diagnosed Alzheimer's disease. *International Journal of Neuroscience, 57,* 167–178.

Anthony, J., LeResche, L., Niaz, U., von Korff, M., & Folstein, M. (1982). Limits of the "Mini-Mental State" as a screening test for dementia and delirium among hospital patients. *Psychological Medicine, 12,* 397–408.

Appollonio, I., Grafman, J., Schwartzt, U., Massaqoi, S., & Itallet, M. (1993). Memory in patients with cerebellar degeneration. *Neurology, 43,* 1536–1544.

Auer, S., & Reisberg, B. (1996). Reliability of the Modified Ordinal Scales of Psychological Development: A cognitive assessment battery for severe dementia. *International Psychogeriatrics, 8,* 225–231.

Auer, S., Sclan, G., Yaffee, R., & Reisberg, B. (1994). The neglected half of Alzheimer's disease: Cognitive and functional concomitants of severe dementia. *Journal of the American Geriatrics Society, 42,* 1266–1272.

Baker, F. (1989). Screening tests for cognitive impairment. *Hospital and Community Psychiatry, 40,* 339–340.

Baltes, P., & Baltes, M. (Eds.). (1990). *Success-*

ful aging: Perspectives from the behavioral sciences. Cambridge, England: Cambridge University Press.

Baltes, P., & Staudinger, U. (1993). The search for psychology of wisdom. Current Directions in Psychological Science, 2, 75–80.

Baltes, P., Staudinger, U., Maercker, A., & Smith, J. (1995). People nominated as wise: A comparative study of wisdom-related knowledge. Psychology and Aging, 10, 155–166.

Berg, L. (1988). Clinical Dementia Rating (CDR). Psychopharmacology Bulletin, 24, 637–639.

Birren, J., Woods, A., & Williams, M. (1980). Behavioral slowing with age: Causes, organization, and consequences. In L. Poon (Ed.), Aging in the 1980s (pp. 293–308). Washington, DC: American Psychological Association.

Blau, E., & Ober, B. (1988). The effect of depression on verbal memory in older adults. Journal of Clinical and Experimental Neuropsychology, 10, 81.

Blessed, G., Tomlinson, B. E., & Roth, M. (1968). The association between quantitative measures of dementia and senile change in cerebral gray matter of elderly subjects. British Journal of Psychiatry, 114, 797–811.

Bobholz, J. H., & Brandt, J. (1993). Assessment of cognitive impairment: Relationship of the Dementia Rating Scale to the Mini-Mental State Examination. Journal of Geriatric Psychiatry and Neurology, 6, 210–213.

Boothby, H., Man, A. H., & Barker, A. (1995). Factors determining interrater agreement with rating global change in dementia: The CIBIC-plus. International Journal of Geriatric Psychiatry, 10, 1037–1045.

Bowers, J., Jorm, A. F., Henderson, S., & Harris, P. (1990). General practitioners' detection of depression and dementia in elderly patients. Medical Journal of Australia, 153, 192–196.

Brandt, J., Spencer, M., & Folstein, M. (1988). The telephone interview for cognitive status. Neuropsychiatry, Neuropsychology, and Behavioral Neurology, 1, 111–117.

Burch, E. A., & Andrews, S. R. (1987). Cognitive dysfunction in psychiatric consultation subgroups: Use of two screening tests. Southern Medical Journal, 80, 1079–1082.

Burke, W. J., Miller, J. P., Rubin, E., Morris, J. C., Coben, L. A., Duchek, J., Wittels, I. G., & Berg, L. (1988). Reliability of the Washington University Clinical Dementia Rating (CDR). Archives of Neurology, 45, 31–32.

Casten, R., Lawton, M. P., Parmelee, P. A., &

Kleban, M. H. (1998). Psychometric characteristics of the Minimum Data Set I: Confirmatory factor analysis. Journal of the American Geriatrics Society, 46, 726–735.

Christensen, K., & Jorm, A. F. (1992). The effect of pre-morbid intelligence on the Mini-Mental State and IQCODE. International Journal of Geriatric Psychiatry, 7, 159–160.

Clark, C. M., & Ewbank, D. C. (1996). Performance of the Dementia Severity Rating Scale: A caregiver questionnaire for rating severity in Alzheimer's disease. Alzheimer's disease and Associated Disorders, 10, 31–39.

Coblentz, J. M., Mattis, S., Zingesser, L. H., Kasoff, S. S., Wisniewski, H. M., & Katzman, R. (1973). Presenile dementia: Clinical evaluation of cerebrospinal fluid dynamics. Archives of Neurology, 29, 299–308.

Craik, F. I. M., & Salthouse, T. A. (1992). The handbook of aging and cognition. Hillsdale: Erlbaum.

Crum, R. M., Anthony, J. C., Bassett, S. S., & Folstein, M. F. (1993). Population-based norms for the Mini-Mental State Examination by age and educational level. Journal of the American Medical Association, 269(18), 2386–2391.

Davis, K. L., Thal, L. J., Gamzu, E. R., Davis, C. S., Woolson, R. F., & Group, T. C. (1992). A double-blind, placebo-controlled multicenter study of tacrine for Alzheimer's disease. New England Journal of Medicine, 327, 1253–1259.

Davis, P. B., Morris, J. C., & Grant, E. (1990). Brief screening tests versus clinical staging in senile dementia of the Alzheimer type. Journal of the American Geriatrics Society, 38, 129–135.

Davous, P., Lamour, Y., Debrand, E., & Rondot, P. (1987). A comparative evaluation of the short orientation memory concentration test of cognitive impairment. Journal of Neurology, Neurosurgery and Psychiatry, 50, 1312–1317.

Dick, J.P.R., Guiloff, R. J., Stewart, A., Blackstock, J., Bielawska, C., Paul, E. A., & Marsden, C. D. (1984). Mini-Mental State Examination in neurological patients. Journal of Neurology, Neurosurgery and Psychiatry, 47, 496–499.

Dooneief, G., Marder, K., Tang, M. X., & Stern, Y. (1996). The Clinical Dementia Rating scale: Community-based validation of "profound" and "terminal" stages. Neurology, 46, 1746–1749.

Doraiswamy, P. M., Bieber F., Kaiser, L., Connors, B. S., Krishnan, K. R., Reuning-Scherer, J., & Gulanski, B. (1997). Memory, language, and praxis in Alzheimer's disease: Norms for outpatient clinical trial populations. *Psychopharmacology Bulletin, 33*, 123–128.

Doraiswamy, P. M., Bieber, F., Kaiser, L., Krishnan, K. R., Reuning-Scherer, J., & Gulanski, B. (1997). The Alzheimer's disease assessment scale: Patterns and predictors of baseline cognitive performance in multicenter Alzheimer's disease trials. *Neurology, 48*, 1511–1517.

Farlow, M., Gracon, S. I., Hershey, L. A., Lewis, K. W., Sadowsky, C. H., Dolan-Ureno, J., for the Tacrine Group (1992). A controlled trial of tacrine in Alzheimer's disease. *Journal of the American Medical Association, 268*, 2523–2529.

Farmer, M. E., Kittner, S. J., Rae, D. S., Barko, J. J., & Regier, D. A. (1995). Education and change in cognitive function: The Epidemiological Catchment Area study. *Annals of Epidemiology, 5*, 1–7.

Fillenbaum, G. C. (1980). Comparison of two brief tests of organic brain impairment, the MSQ and the short portable MSQ. *Journal of the American Geriatrics Society, 28*, 381–384.

Fillenbaum, G. C., Heyman, A., Wilkinson, W. E., & Haynes, C. S. (1987). Comparison of two screening tests in Alzheimer's disease: The correlation and reliability of the Mini-Mental State Examination and the Modified Blessed Test. *Archives of Neurology, 44*, 924–927.

Fillenbaum, G. C., Peterson, B., & Morris, J. C. (1996). Estimating the validity of the Clinical Dementia Rating Scale: The CERAD experience. *Aging, 8*, 379–385.

Fillenbaum, G. C., & Smyer, M. (1981). The development, validity and reliability of the ORS multidimensional functional assessment questionnaire. *Journal of Gerontology, 36*(4), 428–434.

Flicker, L., Logiudice, D., Carlin, J. B., & Ames, D. (1997). The predictive value of dementia screening instruments in clinical populations. *International Journal of Geriatric Psychiatry, 12*, 203–209.

Folstein, M. F., Folstein, S., & McHugh, P. R. (1975). Mini-Mental State: A practical method for grading the cognitive state of patients for the clinician. *Journal of Psychiatric Research, 12*, 189–198.

Folstein, M. F., & McHugh, P. R. (1978). Dementia syndrome of depression. *Aging, 7*, 87–93.

Foreman, M. D. (1987). Reliability and validity of mental status questionnaires in elderly hospitalized patients. *Nursing Research, 36*, 216–220.

Forsell, Y., Fratiglioni, L., Grut, M., Viitanen, M., & Winblad, B. (1992). Clinical staging of dementia in a population survey: Comparison of DSM-III-R and the Washington University Clinical Dementia Rating Scale. *Acta Psychiatrica Scandinavica, 86*, 49–54.

Friedl, W., Schmidt, R., Stronegger, W. J., Fazekas, F., & Reinhart, B. (1996). Sociodemographic predictors and concurrent validity of the Mini-Mental State Examination and the Mattis Dementia Rating Scale. *European Archives of Psychiatry and Clinical Neuroscience, 246*, 317–319.

Galasko, D., Klauber, M. R., Hofstetter, C. R., Salmon, D. P., Lasker, B., & Thal, L. J. (1990). The Mini-Mental State Examination in the early diagnosis of Alzheimer's dementia. *Annals of Neurology, 47*, 49–52.

Ganguli, M., Ratcliff, G., Huff, F. J., Belle, S., Kancel, M. J., Fischer, L., & Kuller, L. H. (1990). Serial sevens versus world backwards: A comparison of the two measures of attention from the MMSE. *Journal of Geriatrics, Psychiatry, and Neurology, 3*, 246–252.

Gardner, R., Oliver-Munoz, S., Fisher, L., & Empting, L. (1981). Mattis Dementia Rating Scale: Internal reliability study using a diffusely impaired population. *Journal of Clinical Neuropsychology, 3*, 271–275.

Garrett, A. P. (1997). Assessing cardiovascular status in the older adult with cognitive impairments. *Journal of Cardiovascular Nursing, 11*, 1–11.

Gates, G. A., Karzon, R. K., Garcia, P., Peterein, J., Storandt, M., Morris, J. C., & Miller, J. P. (1995). Auditory dysfunction in aging and senile dementia of the Alzheimer's type. *Archives of Neurology, 52*, 626–634.

Green, R. C., Woodard, J. L., & Green, J. (1995). Validity of the Mattis Dementia Rating Scale for detection of cognitive impairment in the elderly. *Journal of Neuropsychiatry, 7*, 357–360.

Haddad, L. B., & Coffman, T. L. (1987). A brief neuropsychological screening exam for psychiatric-geriatric patients. *Clinical Gerontologists, 6*, 3–10.

Haglund, R. M. J., & Schuckit, M. A. (1976). A clinical comparison of tests of organicity in elderly patients. *Journal of Gerontology, 31*, 654–659.

Hart, R. P., Kwentus, J. A., Taylor, J. R., & Harkins, S. W. (1987). Rate of forgetting in dementia and depression. *Journal of Consulting and Clinical Psychology, 55*, 101–105.

Hartmaier, S. L., Sloane, P. D., Guess, H. A., & Koch, G. G. (1994). The MDS cognition scale: A valid instrument for identifying and staging nursing home residents with dementia using the Minimum Data Set. *Journal of the American Geriatrics Society, 42,* 1173–1179.

Hartmaier, S. L., Sloane, P. D., Guess, H. A., Koch, G. G., Mitchell, C. M., & Phillips, C. D. (1995). Validation of the Minimum Data Set cognitive performance scale: Agreement with the Mini-Mental State Examination. *Journal of Gerontology: Medical Sciences, 50A*(2), M128–M133.

Heacock, P. R., Beck, C. M., Souder, E., & Mercer, S. (1997). Assessing dressing ability in dementia. *Geriatric Nursing, 18,* 107–111.

Henderson, V. W., Mack, W., & Williams, B. W. (1989). Spatial disorientation in Alzheimer's disease. *Archives of Neurology, 46,* 391–394.

Hendrie, H. C., Hall, K. S., Brittain, H. M., Austrom, M. G., Farlow, M., Parker, J., & Kane, M. (1988). The CAMDEX: A standardized instrument for the diagnosis of mental disorders in the elderly: A replication with a US sample. *Journal of the American Geriatrics Society, 36,* 402–408.

Hermann, D. J. (1982). Know thy memory: The use of questionnaires to assess and study memory. *Psychological Bulletin, 92,* 434–452.

Heyman, A., Wilkinson, W., Hurwitz, B., Hurwitz, B. J., Helms, M. J., Haynes, C. S., Utley, C. M., & Gwyther, L. P. (1987). Early-onset Alzheimer's disease: Clinical predictors of institutionalization and death. *Neurology, 37,* 980–984.

Hodkinson, H. M. (1972). Evaluation of a mental test score for assessment of mental impairment in the elderly. *Age and Ageing, 1,* 233–238.

Holzer, C. E., Tischler, G. L., Leaf, P. J., & Myers, J. K. (1984). An epidemiological assessment of cognitive impairment in a community population. In J. R. Greenley (Ed.), *Research in community and mental health* (pp. 3–32). London: JAI.

Hooijer, C., Dinkgreve, M., Jonker, C., & Lindeboom, J. (1992). Short screening tests for dementia in the elderly population. I. A comparison between AMTS, MMSE, MSQ, and SPMSQ. *International Journal of Geriatric Psychiatry, 7,* 559–571.

Hughes, C. P., Berg, L., Danziger, W. L., Coben, L. A., & Martin, R. L. (1982). A new clinical scale for the staging of dementia. *British Journal of Psychiatry, 140,* 566–572.

Hunt, L. A., Murphy, C. F., Carr, D., Duchek, J. M., Buckles, V., & Morris, J. C. (1997). Reliability of the Washington University Road Test. A performance-based assessment for drivers with dementia of the Alzheimer type. *Archives of Neurology, 54,* 702–712.

Inouye, S. K., van Dyck, C. H., Alessi, C. A., Balkin, S., Siegal, A. P., & Horwitz, R. I. (1990). Clarifying confusion: The Confusion Assessment Method. *Annals of Internal Medicine, 113,* 941–948.

Isaac, L. M., & Tamblyn, R. M. (1993). Compliance and cognitive function: A methodological approach to measuring unintentional errors in medication compliance in the elderly. *Gerontologist, 33,* 772–781.

Jacobs, J. W., Berhard, M. R., Delgado, A., & Strain, J. J. (1977). Screening for organic mental syndromes in the medically ill. *Annals of Internal Medicine, 86,* 40–46.

Johnson, M. H., & Magaro, P. A. (1987). Effects of mood and severity on memory processes in depression and mania. *Psychological Bulletin, 101,* 28–40.

Jorm, A. F. (1994). A short form of the Informant Questionnaire on Cognitive Decline in the Elderly (IQCODE): Development and cross-validation. *Psychological Medicine, 24,* 145–153.

Jorm, A. F., Broe, G. A., Creasey, H., Sulway, M. R., Dent, O., Fairley, M. J., Kos, S. C., & Tennent, C. (1996). Further data on the validity of the Informant Questionnaire on Cognitive Decline in the Elderly (IQCODE). *International Journal of Geriatric Psychiatry, 11,* 131–139.

Jorm, A. F., & Jacomb, P. A. (1989). The Informant Questionnaire on Cognitive Decline in the Elderly (IQCODE): Sociodemographic correlates, reliability, validity and some norms. *Psychological Medicine, 19,* 1015–1022.

Jorm, A. F., Korten, A. E., & Henderson, A. S. (1987). The prevalence of dementia: A quantitative integration of the literature. *Acta Psychiatrica Scandinavica, 76,* 456–479.

Jorm, A. F., Scott, R., Cullen, J. S., & MacKinnon, A. J. (1991). Performance of the Informant Questionnaire on Cognitive Decline in the Elderly (IQCODE) as a screening test for dementia. *Psychological Medicine, 21,* 785–790.

Jorm, A. F., Scott, R., & Jacomb, P. A. (1989). Assessment of cognitive decline in dementia by informant questionnaire. *International Journal of Geriatric Psychiatry, 4,* 35–39.

Juva, K., Sulkava, R., Erkinjuntti, T., Ylikoski, R., Valvanne, J., & Tilvis, R. (1994). Staging the severity of dementia: Comparison of clinical (CDR, DSM-III-R), functional (ADL, IADL) and cognitive (MMSE) scales. *Acta Neurological Scandinavica, 90,* 293–298.

Juva, K., Sulkava, R., Erkinjuntti, T., Ylikoski, R., Valvanne, J., & Tilvis, R. (1995). Usefulness of the Clinical Dementia Rating Scale in screening for dementia. *International Psychogeriatrics, 7,* 17–24.

Kahn, R. L., Goldfarb, A. I., Pollack, M., & Peck, A. (1960). Brief objective measures for the determination of mental status in the aged. *American Journal of Psychiatry, 117,* 326–328.

Karuza, J., Katz, P. R., & Henderson, R. (1997). Cognitive screening. In E. Andresen, B. Rothenberg, & J. G. Zimmer (Eds.), *Assessing the health status of older adults.* New York: Springer.

Katzman, R., Brown, T., Fuld, P., Peck, A., Schechter, R., & Schimmel, H. (1983). Validation of a short Orientation-Memory-Concentration Test of cognitive impairment. *American Journal of Psychiatry, 140,* 734–739.

Kaufman, D. M., Weinberger, M., Strain, J. J., & Jacobs, J. W. (1979). Detection of cognitive deficits by a brief mental status examination: The Cognitive Capacity Screening Examination: A reappraisal and a review. *General Hospital Psychiatry, 1,* 247–255.

Kawas, C., Segal, J., Stewart, W. F., Corrada, M., & Thal, L. J. (1994). A validation study of the Dementia Questionnaire. *Archives of Neurology, 51,* 901–906.

Kim, Y. S., Nibbelink, D. W., & Overall, J. E. (1994). Factor structure and reliability of the ADAS in a multicenter trial with linopiridine. *Journal of Geriatric Psychiatry and Neurology, 7,* 74–83.

Knapp, M. J., Gracon, S. I., Davis, C. S., Solomon, P. R., Pendlebury, W. W., & Knopman, D. S. (1994a). Efficacy and safety of high-dose tacrine: A 30-week evaluation. *Alzheimer's Disease and Related Disorders, 8*(Suppl 2), S22–31.

Knapp, M. J., Knopman, D. S., Solomon, P. R., Pendlebury, W. W., Davis, C. S., & Gracon, S. I. (1994b). A 30-week trial of high-dose tacrine in patients with Alzheimer's disease. *Journal of the American Medical Association, 271,* 985–991.

Knopman, D. S., Knapp, M. J., Gracon, S. I., & Davis, C. S. (1994). The Clinician Interview-Based Impression (CIBI): A clinician's global change rating scale in Alzheimer's disease. *Neurology, 44,* 2315–2321.

Kovner, R., Lazar, J. W., Lesser, M., Perecman, E., Kaplan, M. H., Hainline, B., &

Napolitano, B. (1992). Use of the Dementia Rating Scale as a test for neuropsychological dysfunction in HIV-positive IV drug abusers. *Journal of Substance Abuse Treatment, 9,* 133–137.

La Rue, A. (1989). Patterns of performance on the Fuld Object Memory Evaluation in elderly inpatients. *Journal of Clinical and Experimental Neuropsychology, 11,* 409–422.

La Rue, A., E'Elia, L. F., Clark, E. O., Spar, J. E., & Jarvik, L. F. (1986). Clinical tests of memory in dementia, depression, and healthy aging. *Psychology and Aging, 1,* 69–77.

Lawton, M. P., Casten, R., Parmelee, P. A., Van Haitsma, K., Corn, J., & Kleban, M. H. (1998). Psychometric characteristics of the Minimum Data Set II: Validity. *Journal of the American Geriatrics Society, 46,* 736–744.

Lazaro, L., Marcos, T., Pujol, J., & Valdes, M. (1995). Cognitive assessment and diagnosis of dementia by CAMDEX in elderly general hospital inpatients. *International Journal of Geriatric Psychiatry, 10,* 603–609.

Little, A., Hemsley, E., Bergman, K., Volans, J., & Levy, R. (1987). Comparison of the sensitivity of three instruments for the detection of cognitive decline in the elderly living at home. *British Journal of Psychiatry, 150,* 808–814.

Lord, S. R., & Clark, R. D. (1996). Simple physiological and clinical tests for the accurate prediction of falling in older people. *Gerontology, 42,* 199–203.

MacKenzie, D. M., Copp, P., Shaw, R. J., & Goodwin, G. M. (1996). Brief cognitive screening of the elderly: A comparison of the Mini-Mental State Examination (MMSE), Abbreviated Mental Test (AMT) and Mental Status Questionnaire (MSQ). *Psychological Medicine, 26,* 427–430.

Magaziner, J., Bassett, S. S., & Hebel, J. R. (1987). Predicting performance on the Mini-Mental State Examination: Use of age- and education-specific equations. *Journal of the American Geriatrics Society, 35,* 996–1000.

Mattis, S. (1976). Mental status examination for organic mental syndrome in the elderly patient. In R. Bellack & B. Karasu (Eds.), *Geriatric psychiatry* (pp. 77–121). New York: Grune & Stratton.

Meya, U., Raschig, A., Siegfried, K., & Wannanmacker, W. (1994). Primary outcome measures in dementia drug trials: Modified Clinical Interview-Based Impression of Change (CIBIC-M). *International Journal* of Methods in Psychiatric Research, 4, 189–192.

Miller, E., & Morris, R. (1993). Assessment of dementia, The psychology of dementia (pp. 91–109). Chichester, England: John Wiley and Sons.

Mitrushina, M., & Fuld, P. A. (1996). Cognitive screening methods. In I. Grant & K. Adams (Eds.), Neuropsychological assessment of neuropsychiatric disorders (pp. 118–138). New York: Oxford University Press.

Monsch, A. U., Bondi, M. W., Salmon, D. P., Butters, N., Thal, L. J., Hansen, L. A., Wiederholt, W. C., Cahn, D. A., & Klauber, M. R. (1995). Clinical validity of the Mattis Dementia Rating Scale in detecting dementia of the Alzheimer type: A double cross-validation and application to a community-dwelling sample. Archives of Neurology, 52, 899–904.

Morales, J. M., Bermejo, F., Romero, M., & Del-Ser, T. (1997). Screening of dementia in community-dwelling elderly through informant report. International Journal of Geriatric Psychiatry, 12, 808–816.

Morris, J. C., Edland, S., Clark, C., Galaski, D., Koss, E., Mohs, R., van Belle, G., Fillenbaum, G., & Heyman, A. (1993). The Consortium to Establish a Registry for Alzheimer's Disease (CERAD). Part IV. Rates of cognitive change in the longitudinal assessment of probable Alzheimer's disease. Neurology, 43, 2457–2465.

Morris, J. C., Ernesto, C., Schafer, K., Coats, M., Leon, S., Sano, M., Thal, L. J., Woodbury, P., & the Alzheimer's Disease Cooperative Study (1997). Clinical Dementia Rating training and reliability in multicenter studies: The Alzheimer's Disease Cooperative Study experience. Neurology, 48, 1508–1510.

Morris, J. C., Heyman, A., Mohs, R. C., Hughes, J. P., van Belle, G., Fillenbaum, G., Mellitis, E. D., Clark, C., and the CERAD investigators (1989). The consortium to establish a registry for Alzheimer's disease (CERAD). Part I. Clinical and neuropsychological assessment of Alzheimer's disease. Neurology, 39, 1159–1165.

Morris, J. C., Mohs, R. C., Rogers, H., Fillenbaum, G., & Heyman, A. (1988). Consortium to establish a registry for Alzheimer's disease (CERAD) clinical and neuropsychological assessment of Alzheimer's disease. Psychopharmacology Bulletin, 24, 641–652.

Morris, J. N., Fries, B. E., Mehr, D. R., Hawes, C., Phillips, C., Mor, V., & Lipsitz, L. A. (1994). MDS cognitive performance scale. Journal of Gerontology Medical Sciences, 49(4), M174–M182.

Nebes, R. D., & Brady, C. B. (1992). Generalized cognitive slowing and severity of dementia in Alzheimer's disease: Implications for the interpretation of response-time data. Journal of Clinical and Experimental Neuropsychology, 14, 317–326.

Neelon, V. J., Champagne, M. T., Carlson, J. R., & Funks, S. G. (1996). The NEECHAM Confusion Scale: Construction, validation, and clinical testing. Nursing Research, 45, 324–330.

Nelson, A., Fogel, B. S., & Faust, D. (1986). Bedside cognitive screening instruments: A critical assessment. Journal of Nervous and Mental Disease, 174, 73–83.

Nelson, H. E. (1982). National Adult Reading Test (NART): Test manual. Windson, United Kingdom: NFER Nelson.

Nelson, H. E., & O'Connell, A. (1978). Dementia: The estimation of pre-morbid intelligence levels using the new adult reading test. Cortex, 14, 234–244.

Niederehe, G. (1986). Depression and memory impairment in the aged. In W. Poon (Ed.), Clinical Memory Assessment of Older Adults (pp. 226–237). Washington, DC: American Psychological Association.

O'Connor, D. W., Pollitt, P. A., Hyde, J. B., Fellows, J. L., Miller, N. D., Brook, P. B., Reiss, B. B., & Roth, M. (1989). The prevalence of dementia as measured by the Cambridge Mental Disorders of the Elderly Examination. Acta Psychiatrica Scandinavica, 79, 190–198.

Panisset, M., Roudier, M., Saxton, J. & Boller, F. (1994). Severe Impairment Battery: A neuropsychological test for severely demented patients. Archives of Neurology, 51, 41–45.

Parmelee, P. A. (1996). Pain in cognitively impaired older persons. Clinics in Geriatric Medicine, 12, 473–487.

Parmelee, P. A., Katz, I. R., & Lawton, M. P. (1989). Depression among institutionalized aged: Assessment and prevalence estimation. Journal of Gerontology Medical Sciences, 44(1), M22–29.

Paulman, R. G., Koss, E., & MacInnes, W. D. (1996). Neuropsychological evaluation of dementia. In M. F. Weiner (Ed.), The dementias: Diagnosis, management, and research (pp. 211–232). Washington, DC: American Psychiatric Press.

Peavy, G. M., Salmon, D. P., Rice, V. A., Galasko, D., Samuel, W., Taylor, K. I., Ernesto, C., Butters, N., & Thal, L. (1996). Neuropsychological assessment of severely demented elderly: The Severe Cognitive Impairment Profile. Archives of Neurology, 53, 367–372.

Pfeiffer, E. (1975). A short portable mental status questionnaire for the assessment of organic brain deficit in elderly patients. *Journal of the American Geriatrics Society, 23,* 433–441.

Poon, L. W., Rubin, D. C., & Wilson, B. A. (Eds.). (1989). *Everyday cognition in adulthood and late life.* Cambridge, England: Cambridge University Press.

Qureshi, K. N., & Hodkinson, H. M. (1974). Evaluation of a ten-question mental test in the institutionalized elderly. *Age and Ageing, 3,* 152–157.

Reifler, B. V., Larson, E., Tei, L., & Poulsen, M. (1986). Dementia of the Alzheimer's type and depression. *Journal of the American Geriatrics Society, 34,* 855–859.

Reisberg, B., Ferris, S. H., deLeon, M. J., & Crook, T. (1982). The Global Deterioration Scale for assessment of primary degenerative dementia. *American Journal of Psychiatry, 139,* 1136–1139.

Reisberg, B., Ferris, S. H., Shulman, E., Steinberg, G., Buttinger, C., Sinaiko, E., Borenstein, J., de Leon, M. J., & Cohen, J. (1986). Longitudinal course of normal aging and progressive dementia of the Alzheimer's type: A prospective study of 106 subjects over a 3.6 year mean interval. *Progress in Neuro-Psyopharmacological and Biological Psychiatry, 10,* 571–578.

Ritchie, K. (1988). The screening of cognitive impairment in the elderly: A critical review of current methods. *Journal of Clinical Epidemiology, 41,* 635–643.

Rizzo, M., Reinach, S., McGehee, D., & Dawson, J. (1997). Simulated car crashes and crash predictors in drivers with Alzheimer disease. *Archives of Neurology, 54,* 545–551.

Robins, L. N., Helzer, J. E., Croughan, J., & Ratcliff, K. S. (1981). The National Institute of Mental Health Diagnostic Interview Schedule: Its story, characteristics and validity. *Archives of General Psychiatry, 38,* 381–389.

Roccaforte, W. H., Burke, W. J., Bayer, B. L., & Wengel, S. P. (1994a). Reliability and validity of the Short Portable Mental Status Questionnaire administered by telephone. *Journal of Geriatric Psychiatry and Neurology, 7,* 33–38.

Roccaforte, W. H., Burke, W. J., Bayer, B. L., & Wengel, S. P. (1994b). Validation of a telephone version of the Mini-Mental State Examination. *Journal of the American Geriatrics Society, 40,* 697–702.

Roper, B. L., Bieliauskas, L. A., & Peterson, M. R. (1996). Validity of the Mini-Mental State Examination and the Neuro-behavioral Cognitive Status Examination in cognitive screening. *Neuropsychiatry, Neuropsychology, and Behavioral Neurology, 9,* 54–57.

Rosen, W. G., Mohs, R. C., & Davis, K. L. (1984). A new rating scale for Alzheimer's disease. *American Journal of Psychiatry, 141*(11), 1356–1364.

Roth, M. (1978). Diagnosis of senile and related forms of dementia. In R. Katzman, R. D. Terry, & K. L. Bick (Eds.), *Alzheimer's disease: Senile dementia and related disorders* (vol. 7). New York: Raven Press.

Roth, M., & Hopkins, B. (1953). Psychological test performance in patients over sixty. *Journal of Mental Science, 99,* 439–450.

Roth, M., Tym, E., Mountjoy, C. Q., Huppert, F. A., Hendrie, H., Verma, S., & Goddard, R. (1986). CAMDEX: A standardized instrument for the diagnosis of mental disorder in the elderly with special reference to the early detection of dementia. *British Journal of Psychiatry, 19,* 698–709.

Rowe, J. W., & Kahn, R. L. (1987). Human aging: Usual and successful. *Science, 237,* 143–149.

Salmon, D. P., Thal, L. J., Butters, N., & Heindel, W. C. (1990). Longitudinal evaluation of dementia of the Alzheimer type: A comparison of three standardized mental status examinations. *Neurology, 40,* 1225–1230.

Salthouse, T. A. (1985). Speed of behavior and its implications for cognition. In J. Birren & E. Schaie (Eds.), *Handbook of the psychology of aging* (2nd ed.). New York: Van Nostrand Reinhold.

Saxton, J., McGiongle-Gibson, K., Swihart, A., Miller, V., & Boller, F. (1990). Assessment of the severely impaired patient: Description and validation of a new neuropsychological test battery. *Psychological Assessment, 12,* 298–303.

Schaie, K. W. (1990). The optimization of cognitive functioning in old age: Predictions based on cohort-sequential and longitudinal data. In P. B. Baltes & M. M. Baltes (Eds.), *Successful aging: Perspectives from the behavioral sciences* (pp. 94–117). Cambridge, England: Cambridge University Press.

Schmitt, F. A., Ashford, W., Ernesto, C., Saxton, J., Schneider, L. S., Clark, C. M., Ferris, S. H., Mackell, J. A., Schafer, K., Thal, L. J., & the Alzheimer's Disease Cooperative Study (1997). The severe impairment battery: Concurrent validity and the assessment of longitudinal change in Alzheimer's disease. *Alzheimer's Disease and Associated Disorders, 11,* S51–S56.

Silverman, J. M., Breitner, J. C., Mohs, R. C.,

& Davis, K. L. (1986). Reliability of the family history method in genetic studies of Alzheimer's disease and related dementias. *American Journal of Psychiatry, 143,* 1279–1282.

Smith, G. E., Ivnik, R. J., Malec, J. F., & Kokmen, E. (1994). Psychometric properties of the Mattis Dementia Rating Scale. *Assessment, 1,* 123–131.

Smyer, M., Hofland, B., & Jonas, E. (1979). Validity study of the short portable mental status questionnaire for the elderly. *Journal of the American Geriatrics Society, 27,* 263–269.

Somerfeld, M. R., Weisman, C. S., Ury, W., Chase, G. A., & Folstein, M. F. (1991). Physician practices in the diagnosis of dementing disorders. *Journal of the American Geriatric Society, 39,* 172–175.

Standish, T. I. M., Malloy, D. W., Bedard, M., Layne, E. C., Murray, E. A., & Strang, D. (1996). Improved reliability of the Standardized Alzheimer's Disease Assessment Scale (SADAS) compared with the Alzheimer's Disease Assessment Scale (ADAS). *Journal of the American Geriatrics Society, 44,* 712–716.

Storandt, M., Stone, K., & LaBarge, E. (1995). Deficits in reading performance in very mild dementia of the Alzheimer type. *Neuropsychology, 9,* 174–176.

Stoudemire, A., Hill, C. D., Morris, R., Martino-Saltzman, D., Markwalter, H., & Lewison, B. (1991). Cognitive outcome following tricyclic and electroconvulsive treatment of major depression in the elderly. *American Journal of Psychiatry, 148,* 1336–1340.

Strain, J. J., Fulop, G., Lebovits, A., Ginsberg, B., Robinson, M., Stern, A., Charap, P., & Gany, F. (1988). Screening devices for diminished cognitive capacity. *General Hospital Psychiatry, 10,* 16–23.

Teri, L., McCurry, S. M., Edland, S. D., Kukall, W. A., & Larson, E. B. (1995). Cognitive decline in Alzheimer's disease: A longitudinal investigation of risk factors for accelerated decline. *Journal of Gerontology, 45,* 58–63.

Thomas, L. D., Gonzales, M. R., Chamberlain, A., Beyreuther, K., Masters, C. L., & Flicker, L. (1994). Comparison of clinical state, retrospective informant interview and the neuropathic diagnosis of Alzheimer's disease. *International Journal of Geriatric Psychiatry, 9,* 233–236.

Tombaugh, T. N., & McIntyre, N. J. (1992). The Mini-Mental State Examination: A comprehensive review. *Journal of the American Geriatrics Society, 40,* 922–935.

U.S. Department of Health and Human Services (1997). Quick reference guide for clinicians: Early identification of Alzheimer's disease and related dementias. *Journal of the American Academy of Nurse Practitioners, 9,* 85–97.

Uzgiris, I., & Hunt, J. M. (1975). *Assessment in infancy: Ordinal scales of psychological development.* Urbana, IL: University of Illinois.

Vangel, S. J., & Lichtenberg, P. A. (1995). Mattis Dementia Rating Scale: Clinical utility and relationship with demographic variables. *The Clinical Neuropsychologist, 9,* 209–213.

Villardita, C., & Lomeo, C. (1992). Alzheimer's disease: Correlational analysis of three screening tests and three behavioral scales. *Acta Neurologica Scandinavica, 86,* 603–608.

Vitaliano, P. P., Breen, A. R., Albert, M. S., Russo, J., & Prinz, P. N. (1984a). Memory, attention, and functional status in community-residing Alzheimer type dementia patients and optimally healthy aged individuals. *Journal of Gerontology, 39,* 58–64.

Vitaliano, P. P., Breen, A. R., Russo, J., Albert, M., Vitiello, M. V., & Prinz, P. N. (1984b). The clinical utility of the Dementia Rating Scale for assessing Alzheimer patients. *Journal of Chronic Disorders, 37,* 743–753.

Webster, J. S., Scott, R. R., Nunn, B., McNeer, M. F., & Varnell, N. (1984). A brief neuropsychological screening procedure that assesses left and right hemisphere function. *Journal of Clinical Psychology, 40,* 237–240.

Weingartner, H. (1986). Automatic and effort-demanding cognitive processes in depression. In L. W. Poon (Ed.), *Handbook for Clinical Memory Assessment of Older Adults* (pp. 218–225). Washington, DC: American Psychological Association.

Welsch, K. A., Butters, N., Hughes, J. P., Mohs, R. C., & Heyman, A. (1991). Detection of abnormal memory decline in mild cases of Alzheimer's disease using CERAD neuropsychological measures. *Archives of Neurology, 48,* 278–281.

Welsch, K. A., Butters, N., Hughes, J. P., Mohs, R. C., & Heyman, A. (1992). Detection and staging of dementia in Alzheimer's disease. *Archives of Neurology, 49,* 448–452.

Weyer, G., Erzigkeit, H., Kanowski, S., Ihl, R., & Hadler, D. (1997). Alzheimer's disease assessment scale: Reliability and validity in a multicenter clinical trial. *International Psychogeriatrics, 9,* 123–138.

Willis, S. L. (1996). Everyday cognitive competence in elderly persons: Conceptual issues and empirical findings. *Gerontologist, 36,* 595–601.

Zec, R. F., Landreth, E. S., Vicari, S. K., Belman, J., Feldman, E., Andrise, A., Robbs, R., Becker, R., & Jumar, V. (1992). Alzheimer Disease Assessment Scale: A subtest analysis. *Alzheimer Disease and Associated Disorders, 6,* 164–181.

Zillmer, E. A., Fowler, P. C., Cutnick, H. N., & Becker, E. (1990). Comparison of two cognitive bedside screening instruments in nursing home residents: A factor analytic study. *Journal of Gerontology, 45,* 69–74.

# 5

# Assessment of Emotions in Older Adults: Mood Disorders, Anxiety, Psychological Well-being, and Hope

JEFFREY D. GRANN

## DIAGNOSIS AND SCREENING

Mental illness is diagnosed according to criteria in the American Psychiatric Association's *Diagnostic and Statistical Manual of Mood Disorders*, 4th edition (DSM-IV; American Psychological Association 1994), using information obtained via a psychiatric interview. Two decades of revisions to the DSM have yielded reliable and objective criteria for diagnosing depression, manic episodes, and anxiety. The hallmarks of these criteria are somatic symptoms, the exclusion of medical disorders, minimum time duration, and the interference with usual routine. Instruments used to assess diagnosable disorders should agree closely with psychiatric evaluations.

Most psychological constructs, such as hope and psychological well-being, do not have DSM-IV criteria. Researchers define these constructs differently, placing various emphasis on their cognitive, social, biological, and emotional aspects. These constructs are assessed via instruments that both define and measure the construct under investigation. Good instruments yield scores that are internally consistent and have predictable correlations with other related constructs.

### Case Identification

A common purpose for assessing psychological characteristics is differentiating mental illnesses, such as depression and anxiety disorders, from normal levels of sadness and worry. With psychological assessments, the most important source of information is the client. Simply talking with older adults about their mental health can be informative. To overcome the limitations of this approach, modern assessment methods have been made more structured and systematic. For example, the diagnosis of DSM-IV disorders has been aided by self-report assessment tools, such as screening instruments or structured interviews, that sample aspects of the criteria under investigation. Multidimensional constructs, such as hope and psychological well-being, are also measured via self-report instruments with items sampling relevant domains. Currently, no tools are considered completely adequate for this purpose, and none can replace clinical decision making, which relies on multiple types and sources of information. Because variability increases with

129

age, psychological assessments should be systematic and should cover all relevant domains under investigation if they are to avoid missing treatable cases of mental illness.

### Treatment Selection

Once an appropriate diagnosis is made, beneficial treatments can be prescribed to reduce morbidity. Not all therapies are equally effective for all people or diagnoses. Many treatments for mood disorders, such as psychotherapy and drug interventions, are effective with older adults (Lebowitz et al., 1997). Certain psychotherapies require a minimum level of cognitive capacity or type of personality attributes to be effective. Optimally, the assessment should help a health care professional decide which treatment would be most effective for specific presentations of affective disorders. Measures of hope and psychological well-being have the potential to contribute to this clinical decision-making process.

### Measuring Change

Measuring treatment outcomes and monitoring side effects require instruments capable of detecting subtle distinctions in the affective state over time. Clinicians and therapists can use assessments to monitor treatment of affective disorders and potentially debilitating affective side effects of other treatments. A unique challenge of assessing affect in this way is practice effects. Exposure to the same items many times may invoke in older adults a pattern of responding called a *response set* that distorts the construct being measured. Some instruments have multiple forms to avoid this problem.

### Research

Many gerontologists are interested in using affective assessments in research programs. When affect is used as an independent variable, researchers group people according to scores on a reliable and valid measure. Often screening instruments are used for this purpose. The best instru-

ments have their highest level of precision at the decision point. When affect is used as a dependent variable, researchers need a reliable way of distinguishing subtle levels of change along a single continuum. This requires using lengthier instruments.

### States versus Traits

Most psychological measures used in health care settings attempt to measure the current emotional condition of the patient. State conditions may be more informative within the context of typical or usual conditions, which are referred to as *traits*. Simply put, the distinction between a trait and a state is one of duration and persistence. Making this distinction can be aided by a history with the patient. If possible, the best method for noting changes is to compare individuals to themselves across time. Establishing psychological baseline measures during regular health check-ups enables health professionals to track changes associated with advancing age.

### Timing

In psychology, timing is crucial. Negative emotions, such as sadness and despair, are healthy emotional reactions contingent on certain life events, and yet these emotions can also represent a mood disorder creating significant amounts of morbidity and health problems. Emotions change often, contingent on major and minor life events, internal reflections, and interactions of the two. When they change too frequently and independent of life events, health professionals should be concerned. The periodicity of affective experiences can be as informative as their duration (Lawton, Parmelee, 1996).

## CHALLENGES OF ASSESSING PSYCHOLOGICAL CONSTRUCTS IN OLDER ADULTS

Prospective studies with primary care physicians conducting health check-ups have demonstrated the benefits of paying close attention to patients' affect (Callahan et al., 1994a; German et al., 1987). However, Health care professionals may encounter various challenges when assessing affect in older adults.

## Comorbidity

Many symptoms and signs of mood disorders can be attributed to common health problems of older adults. Some physical declines in late adulthood may resemble affect symptoms. For example, poor sleeping habits can result from psychological problems or changes in health. Instruments used to assess affect in older adults can help to differentiate the etiology of these symptoms, but ultimately the health professional has to decide the course of action. The most useful measures for this have high discriminate validity with related, but different, constructs.

## Personality

Certain signs of an affective disorder may result from enduring personality traits. A personality trait can present as a state condition necessitating an intervention, but the presentation of a trait in the clinical context does not always require action. Here, a long-term relationship with a patient or a close proxy can provide valuable information, such as the severity of the state condition or the likelihood of it occurring. Personality traits summarize behavioral consistencies in affective reactions across various situations and time.

## Ageism

Gerontologists must combat the stereotypes of aging. One maxim of gerontology is that variation increases with age. For psychology, this means that knowing how old someone is does not inform one about how that person feels. Health care professionals' expectations of older adults greatly influence any assessment of affect. Negative stereotypes concerning the aging process can be dangerous. If health care professionals expect an increase in negative affective states with age, they will be less sensitive to treatable affective disorders.

## Cohort and Cultural Differences

Clinical detection of mental illness in older adults continues to be a problem (Garrad et al., 1998). Cultural and cohort differences may obscure the intent and meaning of discussions about affective states. Nonverbal communication problems present unique challenges to assessing affect in older adults. Nonverbal expressions of emotions may be masked by aging processes such as psychomotor slowing, wrinkles, and restrictions in movement. These age-related changes increase the difficulty of psychological assessments, especially with demented older adults.

## Social Desirability

Older adults may not respond honestly to questions concerning their affective states. Because affective disorders carry negative connotations in our society, health care professionals need to be sensitive to older adults' psychosomatic and cognitive symptoms. Older adults may be reluctant to admit a negative mood or loss of interest in pleasurable activities, but they may be willing to admit sleeping disorders or trouble remembering. This challenge can be overcome by using measures that systematically include items beyond the affective experience.

## The Problem of Range

Like most constructs, it is easy to judge affect at the extremes of the continuum and more difficult to distinguish within the middle. It is clear when a person is ecstatic or severely depressed. Clinical decisions are more difficult when judgments must be made concerning less extreme presentations. Overcoming this challenge requires instruments with well-balanced sensitivity and specificity.

## Dementia and Pseudodementia

The suspected presence of a dementia complicates psychological assessments. Many symptoms of depression, mania, and anxiety overlap with symptoms of dementia. These affective disorders can occur independently from, or jointly with, dementia, making assessment even more challenging. Much work has been done on *pseudodementia,* a term that denotes presentations of dementia that are actually depressive symptoms in older adults. Some have tried to establish criteria to distinguish dementia from primary depressive symptoms (Feinberg & Goodman, 1984). Basic emotional experiences, such as pleasant versus unpleasant, persist at very low cognitive levels and thus should not be discounted. Instruments designed to differentiate these disorders should be written simply. They may utilize visual analogs of emotional states and/or behavioral observations. New promising areas of research are addressing biological tests of affective states (see Chapter 17).

## MOOD DISORDERS

Mood disorders are defined according to DSM-IV criteria and consist of two main disorders: unipolar depression and bipolar manic depression. Research has focused on depression more than on any other psychological construct (for review, see Ossip-Klein, Rothenberg, & Andersen, 1997).

### Depression

Although it is an important public health concern and has received considerable attention in the research literature (for review, see Salzman, 1997), depression is significantly underdiagnosed and undertreated in older adults (NIH Consensus Development Panel on Depression in Late Life, 1992). The consequences of unrecognized and untreated depression in older adults include increased use of health care services, longer hospitalization stays, poor treatment compliance, and increased morbidity and mortality from medical illness and suicide (Schneider & Olin, 1995). Proper identification and treatment of depressed older adults may both alleviate disability and distress and reduce nonpsychiatric medical care costs (Henk, Katzelnick, Koback, Griest, & Jefferson, 1996).

Although depression is a multidimensional construct, the most salient features are persistent sadness and diminished interest in pleasurable activity. The DSM-IV (1994) criteria for diagnosing a major depressive episode specifies the behavioral symptoms and magnitude (Table 5.1). Depression represents a complex combination of high negative affect and low positive affect.

### Is Depression a Spectrum Disorder or a Categorical Disease?

Conceptualizing depression as a disease or an end point on a spectrum has led to different assessment procedures and research conclusions. The DSM-IV abides by the medical tradition of disease classification, but the many screening instruments conceptualize depression via the spectrum approach.

The clinical diagnostic measurement approach has its roots in psychiatry and emphasizes the importance of drawing a categorical distinction between depressive disorders and subclinical affective state as well as different classes of depressive disorders. With this approach, depression is either absent or present. Measures adopting this model use branching and probing questions designed to distinguish normal sadness from clinical depression. Distinctions are based on a series of symptom probes that assess the presence or absence of various components of a depressive symptom during a fixed period. This approach can underestimate the prevalence of depression in older adults due to elderly patient's presumed reluctance to discuss psychological issues upon investigation (Harper et al., 1990).

Depression can also be thought of as an end point on a continuum ranging from major depression to contentment. With this approach, many questions or observations are needed. Usually, psychiatric interviews or other measures based on the medical classification model are used as the criterion measure, which screening instruments attempt to emulate. To offset this

**Table 5.1.**

DSM-IV Criteria for a Major Depressive Episode

A. Five (or more) of the following symptoms have been present during the same 2 week period and represent a change from previous functions; at least one of the symptoms is either (1) depressed mood or (2) loss of interest or pleasure

Note: Do not include symptoms that are clearly due to a general medical condition or mood-incongruent delusions or hallucinations

   (1) Depressed mood most of the day, nearly every day, as indicated by either subjective report (e.g., feels sad or empty) or observation made by others (e.g., appears tearful) Note: In children and adolescents, can be irritable mood

   (2) Markedly diminished interest or pleasure in all, or almost all, activities most of the day, nearly every day (as indicated by either subjective account or observation made by others)

   (3) significant weight loss when not dieting or weight gain (e.g., a change of more than 5% body weight in a month) or decrease or increase in appetite nearly every day. Note: In children, consider failure to make expected weight gains

   (4) Insomnia or hypersomnia nearly every day

   (5) Psychomotor agitation or retardation nearly every day (observable by others, not merely subjective feelings of restlessness or being slowed down)

   (6) Fatigue or loss of energy nearly every day

   (7) Feelings of worthlessness or excessive or inappropriate guilt (which may be delusional) nearly every day (not merely self-reproach or guilt about being sick)

   (8) Diminished ability to think or concentrate, or indecisiveness, nearly every day (either by subjective account or as observed by others)

   (9) Recurrent thoughts of death (not just fear of dying), recurrent suicidal ideation without a specific plan, or a suicide attempt or a specific plan for committing suicide

B. The symptoms do not meet criteria for a Mixed Episode

C. The symptoms cause clinically significant distress or impairment in social, occupational, or other important areas of functioning

D. The symptoms are not due to the direct physiological effects of a substance (e.g., a drug of abuse, a medication) or a general medical condition (e.g., hypothyroidism)

E. The symptoms are not better accounted for by Bereavement, i.e., after the loss of a loved one, the symptoms persist for longer than 2 months or are characterized by marked functional impairments, morbid preoccupation with worthlessness, suicidal ideation, psychotic symptoms, or psychomotor retardation

conservative estimation of depression in older adults, cut scores with screening measures of depression are set to be highly sensitive.

Research currently shows that depression acts more like a spectrum disorder than a categorical disease (Lebowitz et al., 1997). Symptom ratings seem generally to yield higher estimates of depression than do clinical diagnoses (Parmelee, Katz, & Lawton, 1989). The prevalence of depression in older adults varies according to whether symptoms, diagnoses, or ratings are measured (Gurland, 1976; Newmann, 1989). Those studies measuring depressive symptoms via a screening scale found a U-shaped relationship between aging and depression, with the youngest and oldest adults showing the most depression. Those

studies that used a clinical diagnostic approach found the opposite, with the youngest and oldest adults showing the fewest symptoms of depression.

This method variance has contributed to conflicting research conclusions and considerable confusion. Epidemiologic studies have reported prevalence rates for depression ranging between 10% and 65% in hospitalized and community-based older adults (Epstein, 1976). The NIMH Epidemiologic Catchment Area Program found affective disorder rates to be significantly lower in the older adults (Regier et al., 1988). Although this study may be the most extensive study of mental health in the older population, it uses a disease classification model approach to diagnosing depression, thus leaving some questions unanswered.

*Measuring Depression with Frail Older Adults: Cognitive and Somatic Symptoms*

Determining the origin of cognitive and somatic symptoms is difficult with any age group but is uniquely challenging with older adults. The National Institute of Health Consensus Development Panel on Depression in Late Life (1992, 1997) warns of overlooking diagnosable depression because neither the victim nor the health care provider may recognize its symptoms in the context of the multiple physical problems of many elderly persons. Many geriatric patients in need of psychiatric care initially present to primary care physicians with physical rather than psychiatric complaints (Harper et al., 1990; Shurman, Kramer, & Mitchell, 1985; Gatz & Smyer, 1992).

Cognitive symptoms of depression include disorientation, memory loss, and distractibility. Somatic symptoms of depression include loss of appetite, chronic pain, weight loss, and sleeplessness. These symptoms can also be caused by physical illness or the aging process (Kessler et al., 1992). Differentiating these multiple potential sources of diseases in older adults is hard. One of the most common somatic symptom of depressed older adults is chronic pain. Although depression rating scales responded to standard DSM-III criteria for depression, they did not include a number of commonly reported symptoms of depression in the oldest people (Gottfries, 1997; Weiss, Nagel, & Aronson, 1986). This gap may explain the lower prevalence of major depression diagnoses under the medical model than symptoms of depression when measured using screening scales.

*Minor Depression*

Subsyndromal depression is more prevalent in the older adults (Harper et al., 1990; Lebowitz et al., 1997). Longitudinal data demonstrate that depressive symptoms in elderly primary care patients is associated with increased physician visits and outpatient charges (Callahan et al., 1994b). Failure to recognize and treat subsyndromal depression risks creating a subpopulation of older adults that chronically utilize nonpsychiatric health resources.

*State of the Art*

Depression has been well researched, but screening measures in this domain can be improved (Reiger et al., 1998). Elderly patients generally seek mental health care from their primary care physicians (Shurman et al., 1985), but depression is often overlooked. Only 9% of depressed patients admitted with physical illness were identified as depressed by hospital staff (Rapp et al., 1988). The use of screening measures has been shown to significantly increase primary physicians' detection of mental health problems of older adults (German et al., 1987; Callahan & Wallack, 1981). Several instruments are described in the sections that follow.

*Geriatric Depression Scale (Yesavage & Brink, 1983)*

The strength of the Geriatric Depression Scale (GDS) lies in its simplicity. The scale (shown in Table 5.2) was the first depression scale developed explicitly for older adults and has been extensively researched and used in clinical settings. During scale construction, items were empirically selected from a pool of 100 potential questions to correlate most highly with the total score. This method statistically removed somatic complaint questions (e.g., sleep disturbance, anorexia, weight loss, and cardiac or gastrointestinal symptoms) because they did not correlate highly with the total score. The method of administration of the GDS seems to be important, with rater-administered versions producing lower scores than the self-administered versions (O'Neil et al., 1992).

A number of studies have investigated the discriminate validity of the GDS by comparing scores from depressed and nondepressed older adults (for review, see Montorio & Izal, 1996). In relation to

**Table 5.2.**
The Geriatric Depression Scale (GDS)

*Choose the best answer for how you felt over the past week.*

1. Are you basically satisfied with your life?*
2. Have you dropped many of your activities and interests?*
3. Do you feel that your life is empty?*
4. Do you often get bored?*
5. Are you hopeful about the future?
6. Are you bothered by thoughts that you just cannot get out of your head?
7. Are you in good spirits most of the time?*
8. Are you afraid that something bad is going to happen to you?*
9. Do you feel happy most of the time?*
10. Do you often feel helpless?*
11. Do you often get restless and fidgety?
12. Do you prefer to stay at home at night, rather than going out and do new things?*
13. Do you frequently worry about the future?
14. Do you feel you have more problems with memory than most?*
15. Do you think it is wonderful to be alive now?*
16. Do you often feel downhearted and blue?
17. Do you feel pretty worthless the way you are now?*
18. Do you worry a lot about the past?
19. Do you find life very exciting?
20. Is it hard for you to get started on new projects?
21. Do you feel full of energy?*
22. Do you feel that your situation is hopeless?*
23. Do you think that most people are better off than you are?*
24. Do you frequently get upset over little things?
25. Do you frequently feel like crying?
26. Do you have trouble concentrating?
27. Do you enjoy getting up in the morning?
28. Do you prefer to avoid social gatherings?
29. Is it easy for you to make decisions?
30. Is your mind as clear as it used to be?

*Included in the 15 item form of the GDS.

other screening tools, sensitivity and specificity are quite good for this measure (McDowell & Newell, 1996).

The usefulness of the GDS with cognitively impaired older adults has been questioned. Some have concluded that the GDS is not an effective tool with seriously cognitively ill older adults (Montorio & Izal, 1996). A prospective study compared scores on the 30 item GDS to blinded geriatric psychiatrists' ratings and found no differences in the accuracy of the GDS for those older adults scoring below or above 24 on the Mini-Mental State Examination (Burke et al., 1988). With nursing home residents, a two step procedure of first screening for minimal levels of cognitive ability and then administering the GDS increased

the utility of the GDS in detecting depression (McGivney, Mulvihill, & Taylor, 1994).

Using the single question for screening depression in older adults "Do you often feel sad or depressed?" was as accurate as the GDS in screening for depression (Mahoney et al., 1994). Thus, primary health care practitioners should consider at least a simple screening question for depression in older adults rather than overlooking a potential source of distress.

GDS-15, a shortened form of the GDS consisting of only 15 items, has been tested (Sheikh & Yesavage, 1986). One study found it to have highly acceptable properties for use as a screening instrument for major depression in older primary care patients (Lyness et al., 1997).

The starred items in Table 5.2 comprise the short form. Each of the questions is answered yes or no.

### Center for Epidemiological Studies Depression Scale (CES-D) (Radloff, 1977)

Originally, the Center for Epidemiological Studies Depression Scale was developed to measure depressive symptoms in community samples for epidemiologic studies, but it has been used extensively in clinical settings and research studies with older adults (Lewinsohn et al., 1997). The scale consists of 20 items expressing depressed mood (Table 5.3). Patients use a four choice scale to rate how often they have felt certain ways during the past week. The four choices range from "Rarely or None of the Time (Less than 1 Day)" to "Most or All of the Time (5–7 Days)" (Radloff, 1977).

Four factors have been extracted from the CES-D in large community samples (Radloff, 1977) and frail older people (Davidson, Feldman, & Crawford, 1994). These are shown in Table 5.3.

Studies using this measure have obtained sensitivity scores for major depression between 60% and 99% and specificity scores between 73% and 94% on predicting diagnosis via the Diagnostic Interview Survey (Beekman et al., 1997). A recent study using this scale with older primary care patients recommended its use for screening purposes (Lyness et al., 1997).

### Beck Depression Inventory (BDI) (Beck et al., 1961)

The Beck Depression Inventory is a 21 item self-report measure of the intensity of symptoms and attitudes concurrent with depression. Items are based on recorded symptoms and attitudes of depressed patients recorded during psychoanalytic psychotherapy sessions (shown in Table 5.4). Much research has been done with this instrument (for review, see Beck, Steer, & Garbin, 1988b). Items were chosen based on their relationship to behavioral manifestations of depression, thus reducing the importance of psychological theory and etiologic concerns. The BDI does not survey vegetative symptoms of depression. With older adult psychiatric inpatients the BDI yielded a 93% sensitivity and 81% specificity (Gallagher et al., 1983). A 13 item shortened version of the scale was constructed for clinical use. Some have criticized the BDI because of its complex items, which may not be appropriate for cognitively impaired older adults and may be difficult for many older people with communication or hearing problems.

### The Zung Self-Rating Depression Scale (SDS) (Zung, 1965)

The Zung Self-Rating Depression Scale continues to be used in studies with

**Table 5.3.**  Center for Epidemiologic Studies Depression Scale

| During the Past Week: |
| --- |
| 1. I was bothered by things that usually don't bother me. (S) |
| 2. I did not feel like eating; my appetite was poor. (S) |
| 3. I felt that I could not shake off the blues even with help from my family and friends. (D) |
| 4. I felt that I was just as good as other people. (P) |
| 5. I had trouble keeping my mind on what I was doing. (S) |
| 6. I felt depressed. (D) |
| 7. I felt that everything I did was an effort. (S) |
| 8. I felt hopeful about the future. (P) |
| 9. I thought my life had been a failure. (D) |
| 10. I felt fearful. (D) |
| 11. My sleep was restless. (S) |
| 12. I was happy. (P) |
| 13. I talked less than usual. (S) |
| 14. I felt lonely. (D) |
| 15. People were unfriendly. (I) |
| 16. I enjoyed life. (P) |
| 17. I had crying spells. (D) |
| 18. I felt sad. (D) |
| 19. I felt that people disliked me. (I) |
| 20. I could not get "going." (S) |

| Key |
| --- |
| The letter in parentheses indicates the factor subscale for the item. |
| D = Depressed affect |
| P = Positive affect |
| S = Somatic/vegetative signs |
| I = Interpersonal distress |

Source: Radloff (1977).

**Table 5.4.**

Beck Depression Inventory

A (Mood)
0  I do not feel sad
1  I feel blue or sad
2a  I am blue or sad all the time and I can't snap out of it
2b  I am so sad or unhappy that it is very painful
3  I am so sad or unhappy that I can't stand it

B (Pessimism)
0  I am not particularly pessimistic or discouraged about the future
1  I feel discouraged about the future
2a  I feel that I have nothing to look forward to
2b  I feel that I won't ever get over my troubles
3  I feel that the future is hopeless and that things cannot improve

C (Sense of Failure)
0  I do not feel like a failure
1  I feel I have failed more than the average person
2a  I feel I have accomplished very little that is worthwhile or that means anything
2b  As I look back on my life all I can see is a lot of failures
3  I feel I am a complete failure as a person (parent, husband, wife)

D (Lack of Satisfaction)
0  I am not particularly dissatisfied
1a  I feel bored most of the time
1b  I don't enjoy things the way I used to
2  I don't get satisfaction out of anything any more
3  I am dissatisfied with everything

E (Guilty Feeling)
0  I don't feel particularly guilty
1  I feel bad or unworthy a good part of the time
2a  I feel quite guilty
2b  I feel bad or unworthy practically all the time now
3  I feel as though I am very bad or worthless

F (Sense of Punishment)
0  I don't feel I am being punished
1  I have a feeling that something bad may happen to me
2  I feel I am being punished or will be punished
3a  I feel I deserve to be punished
3b  I want to be punished

G (Self Hate)
0  I don't feel disappointed in myself
1a  I am disappointed in myself
1b  I don't like myself
2  I am disgusted with myself
3  I hate myself

H (Self Accusations)
0  I don't feel I am any worse than anybody else
1  I am very critical of myself for my weaknesses or mistakes
2a  I blame myself for everything that goes wrong
2b  I feel I have many bad faults.

I (Self-punitive Wishes)
0  I don't have any thoughts of harming myself
1  I have thoughts of harming myself but I would not carry them out
2a  I feel I would be better off dead
2b  I have a definite plans about committing suicide
2c  I feel my family would be better off if I were dead
3  I would kill myself if I could

J (Crying Spells)
0  I don't cry any more than usual
1  I cry more now than I used to
2  I cry all the time now. I can't stop it
3  I used to able to cry but now I can't cry at all even though I want to

K (Irritability)
0  I am no more irritated now than I ever am
1  I get annoyed or irritated more easily than I used to
2  I feel irritated all the time
3  I don't get irritated at all at the things that used to irritate me

L (Social Withdrawal)
0  I have not lost interest in other people
1  I am less interested in other people now than I used to be
2  I have lost most of my interest in other people and have little feeling for them
3  I have lost all my interest in other people and don't care about them at all

M (Indecisiveness)
0  I make decisions about as well as ever
1  I am less sure of myself now and try to put off making decisions
2  I can't make decisions any more without help
3  I can't make any decisions at all any more

N (Body Image)
0  I don't feel I look any worse than I used to
1  I am worried that I am looking old or unattractive
2  I feel that there are permanent changes in my appearance and they make me look unattractive
3  I feel that I am ugly or repulsive looking

O (Work Inhibition)
0  I can work about as well as before
1a  It takes extra effort to get started at doing something
1b  I don't work as well as I used to
2  I have to push myself very hard to do anything
3  I can't do any work at all

P (Sleep Disturbance)
0  I can sleep as well as usual
1  I wake up more tired in the morning than I used to
2  I wake up 1-2 hours earlier than usual and find it hard to get back to sleep
3  I wake up easily every day and can't get more than 5 hours sleep

Q (Fatigability)
0  I don't get any more tired than usual
1  I get tired more easily than I used to
2  I get tired from doing anything
3  I get too tired to do anything

R (Loss of Appetite)
0  My appetite is no worse than usual
1  My appetite is not as good as it used to be
2  My appetite is much worse now
3  I have no appetite at all any more

S (Weight Loss)
0  I haven't lost much weight, if any lately
1  I have lost more than 5 pounds
2  I have lost more than 10 pounds
3  I have lost more than 15 pounds

T (Somatic Preoccupation)
0  I am no more concerned about my health than usual
1  I am concerned about aches and pains or upset stomach or constipation or other unpleasant feelings in my body
2  I am so concerned with how I feel or what I feel that it's hard to think of much else
3  I am completely absorbed in what I feel

U (Loss of Libido)
0  I have not noticed any recent change in my interest in sex
1  I am less interested in sex than I used to be
2  I am much less interested in sex now
3  I have now lost interest in sex completely

Source Beck et al. (1961).

older adults (Zung, 1965). Half of the items are positively worded; the other half are negatively worded. Items were written based on clinical observations of depressed people. Respondents indicate the frequency with which each symptom occurs on a four point scale (Table 5.5). Depression scores are computed by adding the points in the given direction. Older adults score higher on this scale than people in other age groups (Zung, 1967). Studies have found different factor structures for the SDS depending on the age of the respondent, which may be due to its high inclusion of somatic items (Norris et al., 1987).

**Table 5.5.** The Zung Self-Rating Depression Scale

1. I feel down-hearted and blue. (−)
2. Morning is when I feel the best. (+)
3. I have crying spells or feel like it. (−)
4. I have trouble sleeping at night. (−)
5. I eat as much as I used to. (+)
6. I still enjoy sex. (+)
7. I notice that I am losing weight. (−)
8. I have trouble with constipation. (−)
9. My heart beats faster than usual. (−)
10. I get tired for no reason. (−)
11. My mind is as clear as it used to be. (+)
12. I find it easy to do the things I used to. (+)
13. I am restless and can't keep still. (−)
14. I feel hopeful about the future. (+)
15. I am more irritable than usual. (−)
16. I find it easy to make decisions. (+)
17. I feel that I am useful and needed. (+)
18. My life is pretty full. (+)
19. I feel that others would be better off if I were dead. (−)
20. I still enjoy the things I used to do. (+)

*Statements are answered "a little of the time," "some of the time," "a good part of the time," or "most of the time." The responses are given a score of 1 to 4, arranged so that the higher the score, the greater the depression; the statements designated with (+) are given "1" for response "most of the time," and those with (−) are given "4" for "most of the time."*

Source: Zung (1965).

## Summary

The measures presented here have been used extensively and are useful for different purposes. The GDS was developed especially for older adults. The CES-D and the SDS scales include somatic items. The BDI was developed during psychotherapy and allows for quantification of the severity of each symptom. For older adults, the SDS contains too many somatic items to be recommended over other suitable instruments. Tables 5.6 and 5.7 summarize various aspects of the depression measures that have been used with older persons.

## Bipolar Disorder

Bipolar disorder is characterized by extreme changes in mood, from depression to mania. DSM-IV defines an acute manic episode as a distinct period of abnormally and persistently elevated, expansive, or irritable mood lasting at least 1 week or necessitating hospitalization (American Psychiatric Association, 1994; Table 5.8 lists the specific criteria). Symptoms of bipolar disorder include hallucinations and delusions, destructive behavior, dysphoria, and cognitive slowing. Older adults suffering from mania are often excited and have racing thoughts, hallucinations and delusions, destructive behavior, and dysphoria.

Almost half of all manic episodes in older adults are preceded by a diagnosable case of depression (Yassa, Nair, & Iskandar, 1988; Stone, 1989). One year prevalence rates for bipolar disorder were 0.1% with older adults (Weissman, 1991). Between 4.6% and 18.5% of psychiatric hospitalizations of older adults are due to manic episodes (Moak & Fisher, 1990). Older adults with bipolar disorder typically have poor outcomes, significant morbidity, and mortality (Shulman et al., 1992; Katona, 1994).

Mania is typically considered a mental disease of younger adults. The onset of the manic episode is thought to play an important role in the severity of the disorder. Late onset mania has been characterized as having a more severe course versus early onset (Young, 1992; Young & Klerman, 1992).

Systematic assessments can help determine the scope and severity of the disorder. Reviews of the state of the art in geriatric mania have concluded that more needs to be done (Young, 1992; Young & Klerman, 1992). Few self-rating instruments have been constructed to measure mania, and none are specific to older adults.

## Young Mania Rating Scale (Young et al., 1978)

The Young Mania Rating Scale is a structured interview designed to measure the breadth and severity of mania (Table 5.9) (Young et al., 1978). Severity ratings are determined by combinations of subjects' reports on condition and behavioral observations during the interview with an emphasis on the latter. Items were chosen

**Table 5.6.**

Comparison of Common Depression Measures

| Specific scale | Type of instrument | No. of items | Administration | Time reference | Norming populations | Areas covered |
|---|---|---|---|---|---|---|
| Geriatric Depression Scale (GDS) (Yesavage & Brink, 1983) | Self-report: Yes/No<br><br>Range: 0–30<br><br>More depression with higher scores | 30 | 5–10 min | Past week | Older adults: community, psychiatric, and medical | Not somatic |
| Center for Epidemiological Studies Depression Scale (CES-D) (Radloff, 1977) | Self-report: Respond on frequency of symptoms: 4 point scale | 20 | 10–15 min | Past week | Community samples | Four factors: depressed mood; psychomotor retardation and somatic complaints; lack of well-being; interpersonal difficulties |
| Beck Depression Inventory (BDI) (Beck et al., 1961) | Self-report, multiple choice | 21 | 5–10 min | Past week, including today | Psychiatric patients; medical patients; normal persons | 21 categories of symptoms/attitudes of depression |
| Zung Self-Rating Depression Scale (Zung, 1965) | Self-report: frequency of agreement with statement | 20 items: 10 positive, 10 negative; range, 20–80 | 10–15 min | Not specified | Psychiatric and medical patients; normal older adults | Includes somatic |

based on published descriptions of the core symptoms of the manic phase of bipolar disorder and include abnormalities experienced across the entire range of the illness from mild to severe. Depressive symptoms were not included based on poor correlation with severity of mania.

*Summary*

Clearly, more scales are needed. Studies using the Young Mania Rating Scale have found adequate levels of reliability and validity. Table 5.10 describes attributes of the scale and Table 5.11 presents some of its psychometric properties.

# ANXIETY

With community-living older adults, generalized anxiety is the most frequently encountered disorder, even more prevalent than depression (for review, see Blazer, 1997). Anxiety is most closely synonymous with worry. Although the DSM-IV lists criteria for a number of anxiety-related disorders, the most common among older adults is generalized anxiety disorder (GAD; for specific criteria, see Table 5.12). Compared with the amount of research concerning depression and dementia, little research concerning anxiety in older adults has been done.

**Table 5.7.**
Psychometric Properties of Depression Measures

| Scale name | Original purpose | Reliability | Validity | Sensitivity and specificity |
|---|---|---|---|---|
| Geriatric Depression Scale (GDS) (Yesavage & Brink, 1983) | Assess extent of depression and changes in level of depression | Split-half = 0.94, Test-retest = 0.85 (1 week) (Yesavage & Brink, 1983) | Discriminates between normal persons and mildly and severely depressed. Concurrent validity: r w/BDI = 0.85. (Norris et al., 1987) | With cut score 11, 84% sensitivity and 95% specificity; with cut score, 14, 80% sensitivity and 100% specificity (Yesavage & Brink, 1983) |
| | | | | Poor sensitivity in older adults with MMSE score <15 |
| | | | | For elderly medical patients: w/cut = 11, 90% sensitivity and 74% specificity w/cut = 14; 73% sensitivity and 91% specificity (Magni et al. 1986) |
| | | | | With older outpatients w/cut = 10 89% sensitivity and 73% specificity w/cut = 14 78% sensitivity and 86% specificity (Norris et al., 1987) |
| Center for Epidemiological Studies Depression Scale (CES-D) (Radloff, 1977) | Designed to assess extent of depressive symptoms in general population | Original study: Alpha = 0.85–0.90, Split-half = 0.76–0.85, Spearman-Brown = 0.86–0.92 Test-retest = 0.53 for different samples | Discriminated between psychiatric inpatients and general population | Major depression past month: CES-D → 16% Sensitivity 100% Specificity 55.3% CES-D → 18 Sensitivity 93.5% Specificity 65.6% CES-D → 20 Sensitivity 93.5% Specificity 73.5% (Beekman et al. 1997): |

**Table 5.7.** — Continued

| Scale name | Original purpose | Reliability | Validity | Sensitivity and specificity |
|---|---|---|---|---|
| Beck Depression Inventory (BDI) (Beck et al., 1961) | Assess extent of depression and changes in level of depression | Spearman-Brown split-half = 0.93; Gallagher test–retest reliability, normal N = 82, depressed N = 77 (normal elderly = 0.86, depressed patients = 0.79; Spearman-Brown split-half, normal = 0.74, patient = 0.58; coefficient alpha, normal = 0.76, depressed = 0.73) (Gallagher et al., 1982) | Correlates with clinical ratings (Depth of Depression). Reflects clinical changes in Depth of Depression. Predicts RDC diagnosis in older adult psychiatric patients (Gallagher et al., 1983). Concurrent validity: r w/GDS = 0.85 (Norris et al., 1987) | With older outpatients; DIS-III interview: BDI = 10 Sensitivity 89% Specificity 82% BDI = 17 Sensitivity 50% Specificity 92% (Norris et al., 1987) |
| Zung Self-Rating Depression Scale (SDS) (Zung, 1965) | Screening; assess change | Internal consistency = 0.71–0.85; Test–retest 0.68–0.91 | | Psychiatric examination Sensitivity 77% Specificity 82% (Okiomoto et al., 1982) |

**Table 5.8.**
DSM-IV Criteria for a Manic Episode

A.  A distinct period of abnormally and persistently elevated, expansive, or irritable mood, lasting at least 1 week (or any duration if hospitalization is necessary)

B.  During the period of mood disturbance, three (or more) of the following symptoms have persisted (four if the mood is only irritable) and have been present to a significant degree:
  (1)  Inflated self-esteem or grandiosity
  (2)  Decreased need for sleep (e.g., feels rested after only 3 hours of sleep)
  (3)  More talkative than usual or pressure to keep talking
  (4)  Flight of ideas or subjective experience that thoughts are racing
  (5)  Distractibility (i.e., attention too easily drawn to unimportant or irrelevant external stimuli)
  (6)  Increase in goal-directed activity (either socially, at work or school, or sexually) or psychomotor agitation
  (7)  Excessive involvement in pleasurable activities that have a high potential for painful consequences (e.g., engaging in unrestrained buying sprees, sexual indiscretions, or foolish business investments)

C.  The symptoms do not meet criteria for a Mixed Episode

D.  The mood disturbance is sufficiently severe to cause marked impairment in occupational functioning or in usual social activities or relationships with others, or to necessitate hospitalization to prevent harm to self to others, or there are psychotic features

E.  The symptoms are not due to the direct physiological effects of a substance (e.g., a drug of abuse or other treatment) or a general medical condition (e.g., hyperthyroidism)

*Manic-like episodes that are clearly caused by somatic antidepressant treatment (e.g., medication, electroconvulsive therapy, light therapy) should not count toward a diagnosis of Bipolar Disorder I.*

Source: American Psychological Associaton (1994).

**Table 5.9.**
Young Mania Rating Scale

1. Elevated Mood
   Absent (0)
   Mildly or possibly increased on questioning (1)
   Definite subjective elevation; optimistic, self-confident; cheerful; appropriate to content (2)
   Elevated, inappropriate to content; humorous (3)
   Euphoric; inappropriate laughter; singing (4)
2. Increased Motor Activity-Energy
   Absent (0)
   Subjectively increased (1)
   Animated; gestures increased (2)
   Excessive energy; hyperactive at times; restless (can be calmed) (3)
   Motor excitement; continuous hyperactivity (cannot be calmed) (4)
3. Sexual Interest
   Normal; not increased (0)
   Mildly or possibly increased (1)
   Definite subjective increase on questioning (2)
   Spontaneous sexual content; elaborates on sexual matters; hypersexual by self-report (3)
   Overt sexual acts (toward patients, staff, or interviewer) (4)
4. Sleep
   Reports no decrease in sleep (0)
   Sleeping less than normal amount by up to one hour (1)
   Sleeping less than normal by more than one hour (2)
   Reports decreased need for sleep (3)
   Denies need for sleep (4)
5. Irritability
   Absent (0)
   Subjectively increased (2)
   Irritability at times during interview; recent episodes of anger or annoyance on ward (4)
   Frequently irritable during interview; short, curt throughout (6)
   Hostile, uncooperative; interview impossible (8)
6. Speech (Rate and Amount)
   No increase (0)
   Feels talkative (2)
   Increased rate or amount at times, verbose at times (4)
   Push; consistently increased rate and amount; difficult to interrupt (6)
   Pressured; uninterruptible, continuous speech (8)

7. Language-Thoughts Disorder
   Absent (0)
   Circumstantial; mild distractibility; quick thoughts (1)
   Distractible; loses goal of thought; changes topics frequently; racing thoughts (2)
   Flight of ideas; tangentially; difficult to follow; rhyming, echolalia (3)
   Incoherent; communication impossible (4)
8. Content
   Normal (0)
   Questionable plans, new interests (2)
   Special project(s); hyperreligious (4)
   Grandiose or paranoid ideas; ideas of reference (6)
   Delusions; hallucinations (8)
9. Disruptive-Aggressive Behavior
   Absent, co-operative (0)
   Sarcastic; loud at times, guarded (2)
   Demanding; threats on ward (4)
   Threatens interviewer; shouting; interview difficult (6)
   Assaultive; destructive; interview impossible (8)
10. Appearance
    Appropriate dress and grooming (0)
    Minimally unkempt (1)
    Poorly groomed; moderately dishevelled; overdressed (2)
    Dishevelled; partly clothed; garish make-up (3)
    Completely unkempt; decorated; bizarre garb (4)
11. Insight
    Present; admits illness; agrees with need for treatment (0)
    Possibly ill (1)
    Admits behavior change, but denies illness (2)
    Admits possible change in behavior, but denies illness (3)
    Denies any behavior change (4)

Source: Young et al. (1978).

**Table 5.10.**

Description of the Young Mania Rating Scale

| | |
|---|---|
| Type of instrument | Structured interview: Rate along severity dimension |
| No. of items | 11 |
| Administration | 15–30 min |
| Time reference | Last 48 h |
| Populations | Verbal |
| Areas covered | Mania, somatic, social, cognitive, not depression |

Many of the same issues encountered in the assessment of depression are present in the assessment of anxiety in older adults. For GAD to be diagnosed, the symptoms of anxiety cannot be due to a medical condition or medication. This is particularly challenging with older adults because it is difficult to determine if symptoms of anxiety stem from GAD. Symptoms of anxiety may be due to a number of factors, including various medical conditions, treatment side effects, and life events. Measures of anxiety cover a range of domains such as affective (anxious, fear), cognitive (nervousness, worry), and somatic (shortness of breath and rapid heartbeat) symptoms.

Anxiety and depressive symptoms coexist and overlap in elderly patients, making the symptoms difficult to distinguish (Blazer, 1997; Clayton et al., 1997). Anxiety and depression may be expressed as sleeplessness or fatigue. Many have attributed this difficulty to the nonspecific nature of anxiety disorders. Sometimes anxiety presents as a general feeling in which even the respondent might have trouble determining its source.

## Specific Instruments

### State-trait Anxiety Inventory (STAI) (Spielberger, Gorusch, & Lushene, 1970)

The State-Trait Anxiety Inventory is a self-rated scale that was developed to distinguish between state and trait anxiety levels. The scale consists of two 20 item scales: the STAI-A-State scale and the STAI-A-Trait scale. Respondents check the response that matches the intensity of their feelings for each item on a scale of 1 (not at all) to 4 (very much so). The instrument has been used extensively in clinical and research settings. With this instrument, studies have obtained reliable and valid scores of anxiety for community dwelling older adults and for elderly psychiatric inpatients and outpatients (Himmelfarb & Murrell, 1983; Patterson, O'Sullivan, & Spielberger, 1980; Stanley, Beck, & Zebb, 1996). With older adults, a measure of worry was found to correlate 0.41 with the state version and 0.57 with the trait version of the STAI (Stanley et al., 1996). Because the STAI was developed for younger people, its content validity for older

**Table 5.11.**

Psychometric Properties of the Young Mania Scale

| | |
|---|---|
| Original purpose | Not intended to be used as a diagnostic instrument |
| Reliability | Inter-rater reliability r = 0.93 |
| Validity | Concurrent validity: r = 0.88 global ratings; r = 0.71 Beigel; r = 0.89 Petterson |
| | Predictive validity: No. of days in hospital, r = 0.66 |
| Sensitivity and specificity | Differentiates severity of illness |

**Table 5.12.**

DSM-IV Criteria for Generalized Anxiety Disorder

A. Excessive anxiety and worry (apprehensive expectation), occurring more days than not for at least 6 months, about a number of events or activities (such as work or school performance)

B. The person finds it difficult to control the worry

C. The anxiety and worry are associated with three (or more) of the following six symptoms (with at least some symptoms present for more days than not for the past 6 months). *Note:* Only one item is required for children
   (1) Restlessness or feeling keyed up, on edge
   (2) Easily fatigued
   (3) Difficulty concentrating or mind going blank
   (4) Irritability
   (5) Muscle tension
   (6) Sleep disturbance (difficulty falling or staying asleep or restless, unsatisfying sleep)

D. The focus of the anxiety and worry is not confined to features of an Axis I disorder, e.g., the anxiety or worry is not about having a Panic Attack (as in Panic Disorder), being embarrassed in public (as in Social Phobia), being contaminated (as in Obsessive-Compulsive Disorder), begin away from home or close relatives (as in Separation Anxiety Disorder), gaining weight (as in Anorexia Nervosa), having multiple physical complaints (as in Somatization Disorder), or having a serious illness (as in Hypochondriasis), and the anxiety and worry do not occur exclusively during Posttraumatic Stress Disorder

E. The anxiety, worry, or physical symptoms cause clinically significant distress or impairment in social, occupational, or other important areas of functioning

F. The disturbance is not due to the direct physiological effects of a substance (e.g., a drug of abuse, a medication) or a general medical condition (e.g., hyperthyroidism) and does not occur exclusively during a Mood Disorder, a Psychotic Disorder, or a Pervasive Developmental Disorder

---

adults needs to be studied with regard to differences in age-related symptom experiences. The STAI's responsiveness to treatment effects with older adults has not been studied. The more recent version of this scale, the State–Trait Anxiety Inventory–Form Y (Spielberger, 1985), has been used with older adults (Kabacoff et al., 1997). The STAI is copyrighted and published by Psychological Assessment Resources.

*Beck Anxiety Inventory (BAI)*
*(Beck et al., 1961)*

The Beck Anxiety Inventory is a 21-item self-report questionnaire of common anxiety symptoms. Respondents rate the intensity of each symptom on a four point scale ranging from 0 (not at all) to 3 (severely, I could barely stand it). The BAI has been evaluated with outpatient older adults in a psychiatric clinic (Kabacoff et al., 1997). Wetherell and Arean's investigation (1997)

of the BAI with a sample of disadvantaged elderly medical outpatients found high internal consistency and adequate discriminant validity. This scale is shown in Table 5.13.

*Zung Self-Rating Anxiety Scale (SAS)*
*(Zung, 1971)*

The Zung Self-Rating Anxiety Scale measures symptoms of anxiety. Items were written to reflect 20 (5 affective and 15 somatic) diagnostic criteria, based on reviews of descriptions of anxiety (Table 5.14). Scores on the instrument are determined by assigning a value of 1, 2, 3, or 4 to a response (none or a little, some of the time, a good part of the time, most or all of the time) depending on whether the item is positively or negatively worded. These raw scores are summed and then divided by 80, the total possible, and multiplying by 100.

**Table 5.13.**

Beck Anxiety Inventory Items

| | |
|---|---|
| Numbness or tingling | Hands trembling |
| Feeling hot | Shaky |
| Wobbliness in legs | Fear of losing control |
| Unable to relax | Difficulty breathing |
| Fear of worst happening | Fear of dying |
| Dizzy or lightheaded | Scared |
| Heart pounding or racing | Indigestion or discomfort in abdomen |
| Unsteady | Faint |
| Terrified | Face flushed |
| Nervous | Sweating (not due to heat) |
| Feelings of choking | |

Source: Beck et al. (1988a).

## Summary

Compared with the work done with measures of depression, anxiety is understudied in older adults. The measures presented here have been studied with older adults. Table 5.15 offers a comparison of the anxiety measures that have been used with older persons. Table 5.16 displays the psychometric properties of these anxiety measures.

## PSYCHOLOGICAL WELL-BEING

Is well-being the absence of disorder? More positively oriented measures of affect such as psychological well-being are too often overlooked, probably because the dimensions of psychological well-being are not well distinguished conceptually or empirically (Andrews & Robinson, 1991; Frijda, 1993, as per Filipp, 1996). Yet these measures address an important dimension in the lives of older people. The successful aging movement will require instruments designed to measure growth in individuals. Measures of psychological well-being are often used to predict and measure treatment outcomes (Kercher, 1992). Research into this area can yield better diagnostic measures of mental illness and increase sensitivity to changes in depressive and anxious states. Two broad approaches to measuring psychological well-being are presented: the circumplex model and measures of life satisfaction.

**Table 5.14.**

Zung Self-Rating Anxiety Scale

| | |
|---|---|
| 1. I feel more nervous and anxious than usual | 11. I am bothered by dizzy spells |
| 2. feel afraid for no reason at all | 12. I have fainting spells or feel like it |
| 3. I get upset easily or feel panicky | 13. I can breathe in and out easily* |
| 4. I feel like I'm falling apart and going to pieces | 14. I get feelings of numbness and tingling in my fingers, toes |
| 5. I feel that everything is all right and nothing bad will happen* | 15. I am bothered by stomachaches or indigestion |
| 6. My arms and legs shake and tremble | 16. I have to empty my bladder often |
| 7. I am bothered by headaches and neck and back pains | 17. My hands are usually dry and warm* |
| 8. I feel weak and get tired easily | 18. My face gets hot and blushes |
| 9. I feel calm and can sit still easily* | 19. I fall asleep easily and get a good night's rest* |
| 10. I can feel my heart beat fast | 20. I have nightmares |

*Reversed scoring.

Table 5.15.
Comparison of Anxiety Measures

| Specific scale | Type of instrument | No. of items | Administration | Time reference | Studied populations | Areas covered (content validity and factor analysis studies) |
|---|---|---|---|---|---|---|
| State–Trait Anxiety Inventory (STAI) (Spielberger et al., 1970) | Self report: 4 point intensity scale | 40 items, respond on intensity dimension, first 20 items on current state and second 20 items on how generally feel | 10–20 min | STAI-A-State: current emotional state; STAI-A-Trait: relatively stable personality trait | Patient and nonpatient groups: elderly psychiatric inpatients and outpatients | Apprehension Tensions Nervousness Worry |
| State–Trait Anxiety Inventory, Form Y (STAI-Y) (Spielberger, 1985) | Self report: 4 point intensity scale | 40 items, respond on intensity dimension, first 20 items on current state and second 20 items on trait | 10–20 min | State Trait | Older adults | Factor I: items scored in negative direction <br> Factor II: items worded in a positive direction (Kabacoff et al., 1997) |
| Beck Anxiety Inventory (Beck et al., 1988a) | Self-report Likert scale, 0 (not at all) to 3 (severely, I could barely stand it); 13 physiological, 5 cognitive, and 3 somatic and cognitive items (Beck et al., 1988a) | 21 items, score range: 0–63 | | | Medical patient and community older adults | 2 factors: I, somatic aspect (1–3, 6–8, 11–13, 15, 18–21); II, subjective (4, 5, 9, 10, 14, 16, 17) (Kabacoff et al., 1997) |
| Zung Self-Rating Anxiety Scale (SAS) (Zung, 1971) | Self report: frequency of symptoms | 20 items, score range: 20–80 | 10–15 min | Past Week | Psychiatric and medical patients; normal older adults | 20 diagnostic criteria (5 affective and 15 somatic) |

**Table 5.16.**
Psychometric Properties of Selected Anxiety Scales

| Scale name | Original purpose | Reliability | Validity | Sensitivity and specificity |
|---|---|---|---|---|
| State–Trait Anxiety Inventory (STAI) (Spielberger et al., 1970) | Measure State and Trait Anxiety | Original study internal consistency above 0.80 for both state and trait. Older adults community and psychiatric: adequate internal consistency (Himmelfarb & Murrell, 1983; Patterson et al, 1980). Older adults with GAD State alpha = 0.94, trait alpha = 0.85, Control State alpha = 0.88; Control State alpha = 0.85, trait alpha = 0.79; State test–retest = 0.62; Trait test–retest = 0.84 (Stanley et al., 1996) | Concurrent validity: STAI-A State/Trait with STAI-C (Children) r = 0.82/0.83; construct validity: STAI State/Trait with MIBS (behavioral ratings) r = 0.36/0.44; discriminate validity: STAI did not correlate with 10 other MIBS scales (such as hostility, excitement, regression, withdrawal, paranoid thinking, or confused communication) (Patterson et al., 1980) | Not reported |
| State–Trait Anxiety Inventory, Form Y (STAI-Y) (Spielberger, 1985) | | With older adults: S-Anxiety alpha = 0.92; T-Anxiety alpha = 0.90 (Kabacoff et al., 1997) | Discriminant validity with older adults: T-Anxiety, significant distinction; S-Anxiety, no difference between disorder group and nonanxiety disorder group (Kabacoff et al., 1997) | |
| Beck Anxiety Inventory (BAI) (Beck et al., 1988a) | Distinguish symptoms of anxiety from depression; sensitive to treatment changes | Psychiatric outpatients alpha = 0.92 (Beck et al., 1988a); outpatient psychiatric older adults alpha = 0.90 (Kabacoff et al., 1997); low-income elderly medical alpha = 0.92 (Wetherell & Arean, 1997) | Concurrent validity: with SCL-90-R anxiety subscale r = 0.81 (Steer et al., 1993), Hamilton anxiety rating scale r = 0.56 (Beck & Steer, 1991). Discriminant validity: good with older adult outpatients (Kabacoff et al., 1997) | Not reported |
| Zung Self-Rating Anxiety Scale (SAS) (Zung, 1971) | Measure severity of anxiety; predict outcomes | Split-half r = 0.71 | Differentiated anxiety disorder diagnosis from schizophrenia, depressive disorder, personality disorder, transient situational disturbances, and controls. Concurrent validity: Taylor Manifest Anxiety Scale r = 0.30 | Not reported |

GAD = generalized anxiety disorder.

### Circumplex Model: Positive and Negative Affect

Subjective well-being can be represented by a balance or regulation of emotional reactions. The circumplex model assumes this emotional relationship can be best represented by a distinction between positive affect (PA) and negative affect (NA) (Lawton, Kleban, Dean, Rajagopal, & Parmelee, 1992a). The model was statistically derived from self-report responses to a number of different affective states. Factor analysis of these data yielded two independent dimensions labeled *positive affect* and *negative affect*. The dimensions of pleasantness–unpleasantness and high and low intensity can also be distinguished. The circumplex model, shown in Figure 5.1, illustrates this relationship.

A central feature of the circumplex model is the independence of PA and NA. Factors at 90 degree angles are independent of one another, and those across from each pole are negatively correlated with one another. This means that a person's status on the PA continuum does imply their position along the NA continuum. Therefore, measuring only one continuum of PA or NA could be misleading.

Health professionals have been primarily concerned with mental disorders, such as depression and anxiety. Instruments designed to measure these constructs have

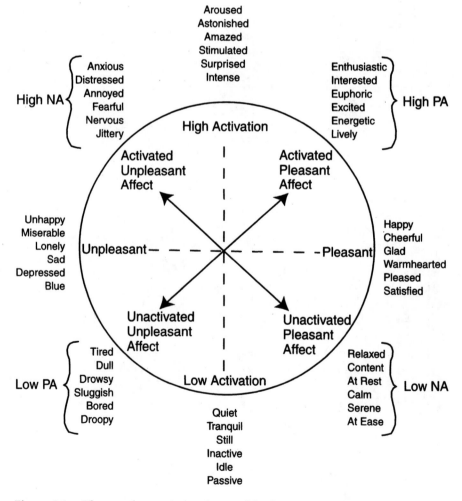

Figure 5.1.  The two-factor circumplex model of emotion. NA = negative affect; PA = positive affect. Source: Adapted from Larsen and Diener (1992).

tended to measure only the NA component of the disorder. According to the circumplex model, depression and anxiety are both characterized by high levels of NA, thus making them hard to distinguish. The PA component differentiates the two disorders. Tellegen (1985) attributes depression to low PA and high NA, with anxiety being a case of high NA independent of PA levels. Lawton, DeVoe, & Parmelee (1995) found PA to be related to external events and NA related to inner influences.

## Life Satisfaction

Subjective well-being can also be represented by more cognitive measures of life satisfaction. Life satisfaction measures ask respondents to reflect across multiple and broad domains and long time periods to arrive at judgments. Usually comparisons are elicited regarding expectations and perceptions of outcomes for salient components of life such as social situations, relationships, self-worth, and finances. Measures of life satisfaction are often used as dependent variables in outcome studies.

The distinction between life satisfaction and quality of life can be muddled, though quality of life measures usually are broad.

### Life Satisfaction Index A (LSI-A) (Neugarten, Havighurst, & Tobin, 1961)

The Life Satisfaction Index A is a widely used, 20 item, agree–disagree, self-report scale. The measure uses the respondent's own evaluations as the point of reference. The items of the LSI-A were selected to correlate most highly with an interview and expert rating assessment of life satisfaction. This measure taps trait characteristics, which are stable over time and not as responsive to treatment effects (Lawton, 1997). The limited response format (agree–disagree) reduces the complexity of the instrument for cognitively impaired older adults. Twelve items are positively worded, and eight are negatively worded. Scores are generated by adding together responses that match the keyed response. The full version of the LSI-A is shown in Table 5.17. The LSI-Z (Wood, Wylie, & Sheafor, 1969) is a 13 item shortened version of the LSI-A, which has

Table 5.17.
Life Satisfaction Index A

1. As I grow older, things seem better than I thought they would be (A)*
2. I have gotten more of the breaks in life than most of the people I know (A)*
3. This is the dreariest time of my life (D)*
4. I am just as happy as when I was younger (A)*
5. My life could be happier than it is now (D)
6. These are the best years of my life (A)*
7. Most of the things that I do are boring or monotonous (D)*
8. I expect some interesting and pleasant things to happen to me in the near future (A)
9. The things I do are as interesting to me now as they ever were (A)*
10. I feel old and somewhat tired (D)
11. I feel my age, but it does not bother me (A)
12. As I look back on my life, I am fairly well satisfied (A)*
13. I would not change my past life even if I could (A)
14. Compared to other people my age, I've made a lot of foolish decisions in my life (D)
15. Compared to other people my age, I make a good appearance (A)
16. I have made plans for things I'll be doing a month or a year from now (A)*
17. When I think back over my life, I didn't get most of the important things I wanted (D)*
18. Compared to other people, I get down in the dumps too often (D)*
19. I've gotten pretty much what I expected out of life (A)*
20. In spite of what people say, the lot of the average man is getting worse, not better (D)*

A, agree; D, disagree.

*Items in the Life Satisfaction Index Z (shortened) form.

Source: Neugarten et al. (1961).

**Table 5.18.**
Life Satisfaction in the Elderly

| Items* | | Responses | | | |
|---|---|---|---|---|---|
| | Anchor 1 | Anchor 2 | Anchor 3 | Anchor 4 | Anchor 5 |
| 1. My daily routine is: (1) | Very boring | Boring | Average | Satisfying | Very satisfying |
| 2. I am most satisfied with my life situation: (2) | Never | Almost never | Sometimes | Often | Always |
| 3. I think about what I would like to accomplish: (3) | Very often | Often | Sometimes | Seldom | Never |
| 4. I am ___ in a bad mood. (4) | Always | Often | Sometimes | Seldom | Never |
| 5. Physically I am: (6) | Unhealthy | Somewhat unhealthy | Average | Healthy | Very healthy |
| 6. I take medication: (6) | Very often | Often | Sometimes | Seldom | Never |
| 7. I have enough money to enjoy myself: (7) | Never | Rarely | Sometimes | Often | Always |
| 8. I try to spend time with people: (8) | Never | Rarely | Sometimes | Often | Always |
| 9. I have ___ friends. (8) | No | Few | Some | Many | A great many |
| 10. I generally plan ___ activities. (1) | No | Few | Some | Many | A great many |
| 11. In general I feel: (2) | Very satisfied | Unsatisfied | Average | Satisfied | Very satisfied |
| 12. I feel pain: (6) | Always | Often | Sometimes | Seldom | Never |
| 13. Compared to any other time in my life, I am now: (5) | Very unsatisfied | Unsatisfied | Average | Satisfied | Very satisfied |
| 14. In my life I have achieved: (3) | Nothing | Very little | Something | A lot | A great deal |
| 15. How important are you to others: (5) | Not at all important | Of little importance | Somewhat important | Important | Very important |
| 16. Being with other people is ___ pleasurable. (8) | Never | Rarely | Sometimes | Often | Always |
| 17. My current income is: (7) | Very inadequate | Inadequate | Fairly adequate | Adequate | Very adequate |
| 18. I find the company of others to be: (8) | Very uncomfortable | Usually uncomfortable | Somewhat comfortable | Usually comfortable | Very comfortable |
| 19. I worry about finances: (7) | Always | Often | Sometimes | Seldom | Never |
| 20. My financial situation is: (7) | Very bad | Bad | Fair | Good | Excellent |
| 21. In looking back, I feel that I have done ___ of the things that I've wanted to do. (3) | Very few | Few | Some | Almost all | All |

|  | | | | | |
|------|---|---|---|---|---|
| 22. My schedule of activities is: (1) | Very satisfying | Satisfying | Occasionally satisfying | Not really satisfying | Very unsatisfying |
| 23. As I look back on my life, I am: (3) | Very satisfied | Satisfied | Partially satisfied | Dissatisfied | Completely dissatisfied |
| 24. The things I do every day give me: (1) | A great deal of pleasure | A lot of pleasure | Some pleasure | Little pleasure | No pleasure |
| 25. My usual mood is: (4) | Always happy | Usually happy | Sometimes happy | Mild depression | Severe depression |
| 26. My intelligence is: (5) | Superior | Above average | Average | Below average | Far below average |
| 27. My physical appearance is: (5) | Very attractive | Somewhat attractive | Average | Somewhat unattractive | Very unattractive |
| 28. I am generally: (6) | Very healthy | Healthy | In average health | Ill | Quite ill |
| 29. The time I spend with friends is: (8) | Always satisfying | Usually satisfying | Sometimes satisfying | Usually unsatisfying | Completely unsatisfying |
| 30. People say that I am: (4) | Always in good spirits | Usually in good spirits | Sometimes moody | Often moody | Very moody |
| 31. My present situation is: (2) | Very pleasurable | Pleasurable | I get by | Difficult | Very difficult |
| 32. When it comes to taking care of myself, I: (5) | Am always independent | Am usually independent | Am sometimes independent | Often depend on others | Totally depend on others |
| 33. I regard my life as: (2) | Very meaningful | Meaningful | Having some meaning | Having little meaning | Without meaning |
| 34. People think that I am financially well off: (7) | Always | Often | Sometimes | Rarely | Never |
| 35. I visit my doctor: (6) | Almost never | Rarely | Sometimes | Regularly | Very often |
| 36. I am happy with the way things turn out: (3) | Very often | Often | Sometimes | Almost never | Never |
| 37. I consider myself to be: (4) | Always optimistic | Usually optimistic | Sometimes pessimistic | Usually pessimistic | Always pessimistic |
| 38. I am ___ with my outlook on life. (4) | Very satisfied | Satisfied | Somewhat dissatisfied | Dissatisfied | Very dissatisfied |
| 39. I am satisfied with the way things are: (2) | Very often | Often | Sometimes | Almost never | Never |
| 40. I am pleased with my daily activities: (1) | Always | Usually | Sometimes | Seldom | Never |

*Items marked with 1 = daily activity; 2 = meaning; 3 = goals; 4 = mood; 5 = self-concept; 6 = health; 7 = finances; 8 = social concept.

been found to correlate strongly (0.94) with the longer form (Lohmann, 1977b).

### Salamon-Conte Life Satisfaction in the Elderly Scale (LSES) (Salamon & Conte, 1984)

The Salamon-Conte Life Satisfaction in the Elderly Scale was designed especially for older adults. Five items were written for each of the following eight categories: daily activities, meaning, goals, mood, self-concept, health, finances, and social contacts. For each question, respondents select one out of five possible responses that best matches the way they feel. Subscale scores can be determined for each category by assigning the corresponding anchor weight to the marked item and adding across all items in that category. The total score is determined by adding all subscale totals together. The eight subscales are designed to aid in treatment selection and monitoring progress in older patients' well-being. Preliminary normative data are available for older adults (age range 55 to over 80 years). With older adults, the LSES correlated with self-report measures of health but found few significant relationships with implicit measures of motivation (Jacob & Guarnaccia, 1997). Table 5.18 shows the items in the scale and responses for each.

### Philadelphia Geriatric Center Morale Scale

The Philadelphia Geriatric Center Morale Scale—Revised was designed to measure psychological well-being in older adults in a simple two choice format (Lawton, 1975). The resulting 24 item scale measures three factors of psychological well-being: agitation, attitudes toward one's own aging, and loneliness—dissatisfaction (for scale, see Table 5.19). Scores are generated separately for each factor by adding together those responses matching the response in parentheses.

**Table 5.19.** Philadelphia Geriatric Center Morale Scale—Revised*

*Factor 1—Agitation*

1. Little things bother me more this year (No)*
2. I sometimes worry so much that I can't sleep (No)*
3. I have a lot to be sad about (No)
4. I am afraid of a lot of things (No)*
5. I get mad more than I used to (No)*
6. Life is hard for me most of the time (No)
7. I take things hard (No)*
8. I get upset easily (No)*

*Factor 2—Attitude Toward Own Aging*

1. Things keep getting worse as I get older (No)*
2. I have as much pep as I had last year (Yes)*
3. Little things bother me more this year (No)
4. As you get older you are less useful (No)*
5. As I get older, things are better/worse than I thought they would be (Better)*
6. I sometimes feel that life isn't worth living (No)
7. I am as happy now as when I was younger (Yes)*

*Factor 3—Lonely Dissatisfaction*

1. How much do you feel lonely? (Not much)*
2. I see enough of my friends and relatives (Yes)*
3. I sometimes feel that life isn't worth living (No)*
4. Life is hard for me much of the time (No)*
5. How satisfied are you with your life today? (Satisfied)*
6. I have a lot to be sad about (No)*
7. People had it better in the old days (No)
8. A person has to live for today and not worry about tomorrow (Yes)

*High morale response in parentheses. Items marked with an asterisk have the highest factor loadings and consist of revised PGMS.

Source: Lawton (1975).

### Bradburn Affect Balance Scale

The Bradburn Affect Balance Scale was one of the first instruments to distinguish between PA and NA and has been used extensively in geriatric settings (Bradburn, 1969). The scale consists of 5 PA questions and 5 NA questions. Respondents agree or disagree with each of these statements. Positive responses count toward the PA or NA score. An affect and balance score can be generated by subtracting the PA from the NA and adding 5. The scale correlates −0.63 with GDS and 0.57 with a self-esteem scale (Coleman, Philp, & Mulle,

**Table 5.20.**
Bradburn Affect Balance Scale*

*During the past few weeks, did you ever feel . . .*

1. Particularly excited or interested in something (P)
2. So restless that you couldn't sit long in a chair (N)
3. Proud because someone complimented you on something you had done (P)
4. Very lonely or remote from other people (N)
5. Pleased about having accomplished something (P)
6. Bored (N)
7. On top of the world (P)
8. Depressed or very unhappy (N)
9. That things were going your way (P)
10. Upset because someone criticized you (N)

*P, positive affect; N, negative affect.

Source: Bradburn (1969).

1995). The Affect Balance Scale (Table 5.20) has some undesirable psychometric characteristics with its response format (Watson, 1988) and high PA/NA correlations from using NA/PA mixed indicators (Kercher, 1992).

### Positive Affect and Negative Affect Schedule (PANAS) (Watson, Clark, & Tellegen, 1988)

The Positive Affect and Negative Affect Schedule is based on the circumplex model. Respondents rate the extent or intensity of emotions representing PA (10 items) and NA (10 items). Scores are calculated for the PA and NA separately by adding the responses for their respective items. State or trait measures of affect can be made using the seven different time periods (Table 5.21). No gender differences have been found. The PANAS relies on verbally understanding what the emotion words mean and may be difficult to use with cognitively impaired older adults. The PANAS has been recommended for use with older adults to assess psychological well-being (Kercher, 1992; Lawton, 1997). The scale yields reliable and valid scores with varying descriptors, time frames, and rating formats (Watson et al., 1988).

### Philadelphia Geriatric Center Positive and Negative Affect Scales

The Philadelphia Geriatric Center Positive and Negative Affect Scale (shown in Table 5.22) measures positive and negative emotions and is based on the circumplex model (Lawton et al., 1992b). The instrument was designed especially for use with older adults in clinical settings. This scale is very similar to the PANAS but samples

**Table 5.21.**
Positive Affect and Negative Affect Schedule*

*Indicate to what extent (very slightly or not at all, a little, moderately, quite a bit, or extremely) for each time period.*

| | | |
|---|---|---|
| Interested (+) | Hostile (−) | Nervous (−) |
| Distressed (−) | Enthusiastic (+) | Determined (+) |
| Excited (+) | Proud (+) | Attentive (+) |
| Upset (−) | Irritable (−) | Jittery (−) |
| Strong (+) | Alert (+) | Active (+) |
| Guilty (−) | Ashamed (−) | Afraid (−) |
| Scared (−) | Inspired (+) | |

Time instructions:
Moment (you feel this way right now, that is, at the present moment)
Today (you have felt this way today)
Past few days (you have felt this during the past few days)
Week (you have felt this during the past week)
Past few weeks (you have felt this during the past few weeks)
Year (you have felt this during the past year)
General (you generally feel this way, that is, how you feel on the average)

Source: Watson et al. (1988).

* + positive affect; − negative affect.

**Table 5.22.**

Philadelphia Geriatric Center Positive and Negative Affect Scales

*This scale is used in two different versions. In the trial version the question is posed as: "How often have you felt this way during this past year" and the response set is: Never, Rarely, Sometimes, Frequently, Very Frequently. In the state version the question is posed as: "How strongly have you felt that way during the past two hours" and the response set is: Not At All; Barely Noticeable; Present But Moderate; Fairly Strong; Very Strong.*

| Positive Affect—Pleasant | Negative Affect—Unpleasant |
|---|---|
| Energetic | Worried |
| Interested | Sad |
| Happy | Depressed |
| Warmhearted | Annoyed |
| Content | Irritated |

Source: Lawton et al. (1992b).

broader quadrants. Items were selected to represent two related domains: positive affect–pleasant and negative affect–unpleasant. These terms were thought to be more meaningful to older adults and useful in clinical settings than the purer orthogonal items of the PANAS. Scores for the PA and NA are generated by summing the 5 point ratings for the five affects in each index. High scores represent high PA and low NA, respectively.

## Summary

Measures of psychological well-being can be assessed using an emotional or cognitive approach. The instruments presented here use a variety of approaches. Table 5.23 presents the attributes of the psychological well-being scales discussed earlier. Table 5.24 summarizes the psychometric properties of these scales.

## HOPE AND HOPELESSNESS

### Hope

Although the prevalence of depression in older adults is lower than that that in any other age group (Regier et al., 1988), the highest suicide rate of any age group is among older adults, especially older Caucasian men who live alone (American Psychological Association, 1997). The loss of hope has been shown to predict suicidal ideation in depressed older adults after

controlling for depressive symptom levels are controlled for (Beck et al., 1993; Uncapher et al., 1998). Good measures of hope may predict suicide more efficiently than depressive symptoms. Most definitions of hope are enabling and beneficial, yet hope could be detrimental to one's health. Hope during grave situations may reduce one's effort to seek out cures. Denial could be ultimate hope or psychopathology.

Establishing content validity for any hope instrument is challenging because of hope's undetermined multidimensional nature. Many measures of hope emphasize its prospective or future-oriented nature. Stotland (1969) defined hope as an expectation greater than zero of success in attaining a goal. Similarly, Raleigh and Boehm (1994) claim that hope is a positive expectation; it is future oriented; it motivates the organism; and it is a means of coping with uncertainty.

Hope is a multidimensional construct (Herth, 1992). The multidimensional nature of hope has been operationalized into four central attributes: experiential, spiritual or transcendent, rational, and relational (Farren, Herth, & Popovich, 1995). Some instruments attempt to measure all of these domains, whereas others focus on one domain.

Typically, people do not have an opportunity to display hope. Hope is expressed only in the presence of a stressful event.

**Table 5.23.**
Comparison of Psychological Well-being Scales

| Specific scale | Type of instrument | No. of items | Administration | Time reference | Developing population | Areas covered |
|---|---|---|---|---|---|---|
| Life Satisfaction Index-A (LSI-A) (Neugarten et al., 1961) | Self-report; Range 0–20 | 20 | 10 min | Not specified; current | Adults aged 50+ years and sample of people from various social classes | 3 components: (1) Zest vs. apathy; (2) resolution and fortitude, congruence between desired and achieved goals, self-concept; (3) and mood tone |
| Salamon-Conte Life Satisfaction in the Elderly Scale (LSES) (Salamon & Conte, 1984) | Self-report: Varying 5 choice alternatives | 40 | 15 to 25 min | General; not specified | Older adults | 8 categories of items: Daily activities, Meaning, Goals, Mood, Self-concept, Health, Finances, Social contacts |
| Philadelphia Geriatric Center Morale Scale—Revised (Lawton, 1975) | Self-report: Agree or disagree format; Range 0–17 | 17 | Brief | Not specified | Older adults | 3 factors: Agitation, Attitude toward own aging, Lonely dissatisfaction |
| Bradburn Affect Balance Scale (Bradburn, 1969) | Self-report: Yes/no | 10 items: 5 PA, 5 NA | 5 min | Past few weeks | General population; suitable | Positive affect, Negative affect |
| Positive Affect and Negative Affect Scale (PANAS) (Watson et al., 1988) | Self-report: Rate on 5 point intensity of feelings or frequency | 20 items: 10 PA, 10 NA | Brief | Moment, Today, Past few days, Past few weeks, Year, General | College undergraduates | Positive affect, Negative affect |
| Philadelphia Geriatric Center Positive and Negative Affect Scales (Lawton et al., 1992a) | Self report: PA = 5 items; NA = 5 items; Score range = 5–25 | 10 items: 5 PA—pleasant, 5 NA—unpleasant | 2 or 3 min | State or Trait wording | State and Trait versions: Elderhostel older adults (60+ years), middle-aged (31–59), young adults (17–30); State only: Residential sample | Positive affect—pleasant, Negative affect—unpleasant |

NA, negative affect; PA, positive affect.

**Table 5.24.**

Psychometric Properties of Selected Psychological Well-being Scales

| Scale Name | Original purpose | Reliability | Validity |
|---|---|---|---|
| Life Satisfaction Index A (LSI-A) (Neugarten et al., 1961) | Measure life satisfaction using the individual's own evaluations as the point of reference independent of activity level or social participation | Internal not reported<br><br>Test–retest not reported | Convergent validity:<br>  Correlated 0.55<br>    with an interview<br>and expert assessment<br>  Correlated 0.39<br>    with clinical psychologists' ratings<br><br>Discriminant validity:<br>  Not reported |
| Salamon-Conte Life Satisfaction in the Elderly Scale (LSES) (Salamon & Conte, 1984) | Measure life satisfaction in older adults in a variety of settings and incorporate largest number of related domains | Community older adults alpha = 0.93; patient alpha = 0.92<br><br>Test–retest: Community dwelling older adults, 1 month r = 0.90; 6 month r = 0.67<br><br>Subscales alpha range = 0.60–0.79 | Convergent validity: not reported<br><br>Eight factors account for 60% of the total variance<br><br>Older adults:<br>  LSES r number of<br>    friends = 0.34<br>  LSES r Rand health<br>    survey = 0.45<br>  (Jacob & Guarnaccia,<br>    1997) |
| Philadelphia Geriatric Center Morale Scale — Revised (Lawton, 1975) | Measure three dimensions of psychological well-being: dissatisfaction–loneliness, agitation, attitude toward one's own aging | Agitation: alpha = 0.85<br><br>Attitude toward own aging: alpha = 0.81<br><br>Lonely dissatisfaction: alpha = 0.85 | Convergent validity: not reported (Lohmann, 1977a); average 0.73 correlation with 9 other well-being measures<br><br>Discriminant validity: not reported<br><br>Three factors can be combined into general subjective well-being (Liang & Bollen, 1985) |
| Bradburn Affect Balance Scale | A measure for general population | Test–retest: 0.80–0.97 | Discriminate elderly psychiatric patients and normals<br><br>Poor convergent correlations (Watson et al., 1988)<br><br>PA:<br>  Factor 1 = 0.50<br>  Factor 2 = −0.18<br>NA:<br>  Factor 1 = −0.21<br>  Factor 2 = −0.51 |

*(continued)*

Because ethical considerations prevent researchers from manipulating stressful conditions to elicit hope, studies of hope typically focus on a group believed to be experiencing a stressful event, such as cancer patients, nursing home residents, and prison inmates.

As a state condition expressed under stress, this measurement is simplified; self-report is a valid and useful measurement

**Table 5.24.**— Continued

| Scale Name | Original Purpose | Reliability | Validity |
|---|---|---|---|
| Positive Affect and Negative Affect Scale (PANAS) (Watson et al., 1988) | Measure positive and negative affect independently | Alpha across time ratings<br>PA: 0.86–0.90<br>NA: 0.84–0.87<br>Test–retest<br>Moment: PA = 0.54, NA = 0.45<br>General: PA = 0.68, NA = 0.71 | Discriminate validity:<br>PA/NA r = −0.12 to −0.23<br>Convergent and discriminant validity:<br>PA:<br>Factor 1 = 0.92<br>Factor 2 = −0.08<br>NA:<br>Factor 1 = −0.08<br>Factor 2 = 0.94<br>Concurrent validity:<br>HSCL past few weeks/NA r = 0.74; /PA r = −0.19<br>HSCL today/NA r = 0.65; /PA r = −0.29<br>BDI past few days/ NA r =0.56; /PA r = −0.35<br>BDI past few weeks/ NA r = 0.58; /PA r = −0.36<br>A-State past few weeks/NA r = .51; /PA r = −0.35 |
| Philadelphia Geriatric Center Positive and Negative Affect Scales (Lawton et al., 1992a) | Sample affects from 2 quadrants of the circumplex array, including affects used in longer lists. Short to use with broad range of competences and over multiple daily assessments | Alpha PA = 0.79; alpha NA = 0.81 | Discriminant validity:<br>PA/NA r = −0.23–0.48<br>Concurrent validity:<br>Bradburn + r w/PA = 0.41; NA = −0.26<br>Bradburn − r w/PA = −0.26; NA = 0.53 |

NA, negative affect; PA, positive affect; HSCL, Hopkins Symptom Checklist; BDI = Beck Depression Inventory.

approach. The state versus trait component of hope is manipulated via the time referent. Self-report state measures use an immediate (e.g., now, currently) time referent, and trait measures use a longer or open (e.g., usually, most of the time) time referent.

## Hopelessness

Many implicitly define hopelessness as the opposite, or a lack, of hope. Multiple definitions and scales of hope have been created, but few definitions of hopelessness exist. Given the variety, it may be difficult to validate one hope scale against another, despite recommendations to do so, and even less useful to validate hope against hopelessness (Stoner, 1991).

Validity studies usually require a number of measures to be taken on the same individual within a brief period. The assessment of hope is challenging because it appears to be sensitive to fatigue effects (Herth, 1992).

## Specific Instruments

### Herth Hope Scale (HHS) (Herth, 1991)

The Herth Hope Scale attempts to measure the multidimensional nature of hope. Items were generated to reflect three dimensions: (1) cognitive-temporal, the perception that a positive, desired outcome is realistically probable in the near or distant future; (2) affective-behavioral, a feeling of confidence, with initiation of plans to effect the desired outcome; and (3) affiliative-contextual, the recognition of interdependence and an interconnectedness between self and others and between self and spirit. With this framework, 40 dichotomously scored items were generated. These were reduced to 32 items, which were then pilot tested with 20 adults with cancer (mean age, 41 years; range, 24–69 years). Five items with low-item total correlations were replaced. Through further pilot testing with cancer patients, two items, which loaded on all three factors, were eliminated, and the scale was changed to a 4 point summated rating scale. The final HHS (Table 5.25) was administered to

well adults, older adults in the community, and a sample of elderly widow(er)s and found to obtain adequate levels of internal consistency and repeated measures reliability.

### Herth Hope Index (Herth, 1992)

The Herth Hope Index (see Table 5.26) is an abbreviated version of the HHS designed for clinical use. It assesses the current hope state of the respondent via 12 questions.

### Snyder Hope Scale (Snyder et al., 1991)

Snyder and associates define hope as a cognitive set containing two components of goal directed behavior: agency and pathways. The perception of successful agency, or goal-directed determination, is the will component of hope. The perception of successful pathways, or planning of ways to meet goals, is the pathway component of hope. Defining these constructs separately may foster more focused interventions. This scale has been used with older adults.

Scale construction attempted to measure both agency and pathways of hope. Forty-five items were written reflecting this construct of hope. These were worked down

Table 5.25.
Herth Hope Scale

*For each item, response set is Never Applies to Me, Seldom Applies to Me, Sometimes Applies to Me, or Often Applies to Me.*

| | |
|---|---|
| 1. I am looking forward to the future | 17. I am immobilized by fears and doubts |
| 2. I sense the presence of loved ones | 18. I know my life has meaning and purpose |
| 3. I have deep inner strength | 19. I see the positive in most situations |
| 4. I have plans for the future | 20. I have goals for the next 3 to 6 months |
| 5. I have inner positive energy | 21. I am committed to finding my ways |
| 6. I feel scared about the future | 22. I feel all alone |
| 7. I keep going even when I hurt | 23. I have coped well in the past |
| 8. I have faith that gives me comfort | 24. I feel loved and needed |
| 9. I believe that good is always possible | 25. I believe that each day has potential |
| 10. I feel at a loss, nowhere to turn | 26. I can't bring about positive change |
| 11. I feel time heals | 27. I can see a light even in a tunnel |
| 12. I have support from those close to me | 28. I have hope even when plans go astray |
| 13. I feel overwhelmed and trapped | 29. I believe my outlook affects my life |
| 14. I can recall happy times | 30. I have plans for today and next week |
| 15. I just know there is hope | |
| 16. I can seek and receive help | |

**Table 5.26.**
Herth Hope Index

*Response set is Strongly Agree, Disagree, Agree, or Strongly Disagree.*

| | |
|---|---|
| 1. I have a positive outlook toward life | 7. I can recall happy/joyful times |
| 2. I have short, intermediate, and/or long range goals | 8. I have deep inner strength |
| | 9. I am able to give and receive caring/ love |
| 3. I feel all alone | |
| 4. I can see a light in a tunnel | 10. I have a sense of direction |
| 5. I have faith that gives me comfort | 11. I believe that each day has potential |
| 6. I feel scared about my future | 12. I feel my life has value and worth |

Source: Herth (1992).

to 14 items with the highest item-remainder correlations (Harris, 1988). From this set, four items were selected to represent the agency component and four items for the pathway component of hope. The final scale consists of 8 hope items and 4 fillers (Table 5.27). Studies have found predictable relationships between the Hope Scale and other related scales (for review, see Snyder et al., 1991). Two factors, corresponding to agency and pathways, account for 52% to 63% of the variance in scores, validating a two factor solution.

*Nowotny Hope Scale (Nowotny, 1989)*

The Nowotny Hope Scale was designed to measure a multidimensional definition of hope after a stressful event. Hope is defined as a multidimensional dynamic attribute of the individual that includes the following six attributes: confidence in the outcome, relates to others, future is possible, spiritual beliefs, active involvement,

and comes from within. Respondents are asked to think of a stressful event, to imagine the event occurring right now, and indicate the response that best matches their feelings. The scale (shown in Table 5.28) has primarily been used with cancer patients (Rustoen & Moum, 1997). Psychometric properties of the scale have not been as thoroughly tested as some of the other scales.

*Beck Hopelessness Scale
(Beck et al., 1974)*

The Beck Hopelessness Scale was one of the first quantifications of hopelessness developed and continues to be used for clinical and research purposes. The 21 item scale (shown in Table 5.29) asks respondents to indicate if each statement is true or false for them. Scores are generated by adding together responses that match the response in parentheses. Higher scores indicate more hopelessness. This scale has

**Table 5.27.**
Snyder Hope Scale

*Response set is Definitely False, Mostly False, Mostly True, or Definitely True.*

| | |
|---|---|
| 1. I can think of many ways to get out of a jam (Pathways) | 7. I worry about my health (Filler) |
| 2. I energetically pursue my goals (Agency) | 8. Even when others get discouraged, I know I can find a way to solve the problem (Pathways) |
| 3. I feel tired most of the time (Filler) | |
| 4. There are lots of ways around any problem (Pathways) | 9. My past experiences have prepared me well for my future (Agency) |
| 5. I am easily downed in an argument (Filler) | 10. I've been pretty successful in life (Agency) |
| 6. I can think of many ways to get the things in life that are most important to me (Pathways) | 11. I usually find myself worrying about something (Filler) |
| | 12. I meet the goals that I set out for myself (Agency) |

Source: Snyder et al. (1991).

**Table 5.28.**
Nowotny Hope Scale

*Factor 1 — Confidence*

I can take whatever happens and make the best of it
I have a positive outlook
I know I can make changes in my life
I think I can learn (or I have learned) to adapt to whatever limitations I have (or might have)
I am ready to meet each new challenge
I feel the decisions I make get me what I expect
When faced with a challenge, I am ready to take action
I have confidence in my own ability

*Factor 2 — Relates to Others*

My family (or significant other) is always available to help me when I need them
I feel confident in those who want to help me
Sometimes I feel I am all alone
I share important decision making with my family (or significant other)
I know I can go to my family or friends for help

*Factor 3 — Future is Possible*

In the future I plan to accomplish many things
I feel confident about the outcome of this event/situation

*Factor 3–Continued*

I see a light at the end of the tunnel
I know I can accomplish this task
I look forward to the future

*Factor 4 — Spiritual Beliefs*

My religious beliefs help me most when I feel discouraged
I use prayer to give me strength
I use scripture to give me strength

*Factor 5 — Active Involvement*

I like to do things rather then sit and wait for things to happen
I lack confidence in my ability
I have important goals I want to achieve within the next 10–15 years
I like to sit and wait for things to happen
I have difficulty in setting goals

*Factor 6 — Comes from Within*

I like to make my own decisions
I want to maintain control over my life and my body
I expect to be successful in those tasks that concern me most

**Table 5.29.**
Beck Hopelessness Scale*

1. I look forward to the future with hope and enthusiasm (F)
2. I might as well give up because I can't make things better for myself (T)
3. When things are going badly, I am helped by knowing they can't stay that way forever (F)
4. I can't imagine what my life would be like in 10 years (T)
5. I have enough time to accomplish the things I most want to do (F)
6. In the future, I expect to succeed in what concerns me most (F)
7. My future seems dark to me (T)
8. I expect to get more of the good things in my life than the average person (F)
9. I just don't get the breaks, and there's no reason to believe I will in the future (T)
10. My past experiences have prepared me well for my future (F)
11. All I can see ahead of me is unpleasantness rather than pleasantness (T)
12. I don't expect to get what I really want (T)
13. When I look ahead to the future, I expect I will be happier than I am now (F)
14. Things just won't work out the way I want them to (T)
15. I have great faith in the future (F)
16. I never get what I want so it's foolish to want anything (T)
17. It is very unlikely that I will get any real satisfaction in the future (T)
18. The future seems vague and uncertain to me (T)
19. I can look forward to more good times than bad times (F)
20. There's no use in really trying to get something I want because I probably won't get it (T)

*T, true; F, false.

Source: Beck et al. (1974).

**Table 5.30.**

The Geriatric Hopelessness Scale

*Response set is True or False.*

1. If I allow myself to feel hopeful again, I'll probably be letting myself in for a lot more hurt in the future
2. I have faith that things will become better for me
3. I might as well give up because I can't make things better for myself or others
4. Although things are going badly, I know that they won't be bad all of the time
5. All I can see ahead of me is more grief and sadness
6. I believe that my days of grief and sadness are behind me
7. What's the point of trying; I don't think I can ever get back my energy and strength
8. These days there are many different foods and medicines to restore my energy
9. I will always be old and useless
10. Even as an elderly person, I can be useful and helpful to others
11. I don't think God will ever forgive me for my useless life on earth
12. I believe that God is kind and merciful toward older people
13. All I fear is God's punishment for my sins
14. I believe that God in His mercy will forgive me for all sins
15. There is no point in hoping that I will meet my loved ones after I die
16. I believe that after I die I will see my loved ones in God's care
17. The notion of ever being happy again is unclear and confusing to me
18. I believe that we all deserve the best of life, regardless of age
19. There is no point in hoping that any one here will remember me after I am gone
20. I believe that my family and friends will miss me after I'm gone
21. There is no use trying to get something I want because I'll be too tired and old to enjoy it if I get it
22. Although I'm getting older, I have enough time and energy to finish the things I really want to do
23. I've never had much luck in the past, and there's no reason to think I will now that I'm old and tired
24. I think I can make myself interesting and attractive to others
25. I cannot believe that anyone would take and interest in me now that I have little to say that is interesting to others
26. The future is full of peace and hope
27. The future seems very confusing to me
28. I will get more good things in life than most other persons my age
29. I see no reason why anybody would notice me
30. I believe my life has a definite purpose and that everyday I am getting closer to achieving it

Source: Fry (1984).

been used extensively as a criterion validity measure for new hope scales. The scale appears sensitive to change.

*Geriatric Hopelessness Scale( GHS) (Fry, 1984)*

The Geriatric Hopelessness Scale is a 30 item true–false self-report scale that attempts to measure general levels of hope. It is the only measure designed specifically for measuring hopelessness in older adults. The scale was constructed based on interviews with older adults concerning stressful episodes; 52 statements of hopelessness

were extracted. Those with high factor loadings were selected. The final version of the scale (shown in Table 5.30) contains 30 items, balanced for direction. The GHS effectively measures hopelessness in depressed and nondepressed older adults (Farren et al., 1995).

### Summary

The diversity of the measures of hope and hopelessness reflects the undefined nature of these emotions. Each measure is based on its own unique definition of hope. Thus, no one measure can be recom-

**Table 5.31.**
Comparisons of the Hope Scales

| Specific scale | Type of instrument* | No. of items/range of scores | Administration | Time reference | Populations studied | Areas covered |
|---|---|---|---|---|---|---|
| Herth Hope Scale (HHS) (Herth, 1991) | Self-report: 4 point summated rating | 30 items<br>Score range 0–90; higher scores denote greater hope | Brief | Past week or two | Cancer patients, acute and chronically ill adults, elderly widow(er)s, and well adults | Framework for generating items:<br>Cognitive–temporal<br>Affective–behavioral<br>Affiliative–contextual<br><br>3 subscales:<br>1. Temporality and future<br>2. Positive readiness and expectancy<br>3. Interconnectedness |
| Herth Hope Index (HHI) (Herth, 1992), | Self-report: Likert SA to SD | 12 items<br>Score range 12–48 | Few minutes | Right now | Acute, chronic, and terminally ill adults; family caregivers of terminally ill | 3 subscales:<br>1. Inner sense of temporality and future<br>2. Inner positive readiness and expectancy<br>3. Interconnectedness with self and others |
| Snyder Hope Scale (Snyder et al., 1991) | Self-report: Likert 4 point, DF, MF, MT, DT | 8 items with 4 filler items | Less than 10 minutes | Not specified | Undergraduates; one inpatient and one outpatient group, psychological treatment | 2 factors:<br>1. Agency (goal-directed determination)<br>2. Pathways (planning of ways to meet goals) |
| Nowotny Hope Scale (Nowotny, 1989) | Self-report: Likert 4 point, SA, A, D, SD | 29 items<br>Range of scores 29–116 | 15–20 min | Think of a previous stressful event | Well adults, cancer patients | Subscales 6:<br>1. Confidence in outcome<br>2. Relates to others<br>3. Future is possible<br>4. Spiritual beliefs<br>5. Active involvement<br>6. Inner readiness |

| Scale | Format/Scoring | Items | | Setting | Population | Dimensions/Factors |
|---|---|---|---|---|---|---|
| Beck Hopelessness Scale (Beck et al., 1974) | Self-report true/false scored 0 or 1 | 20 items Range of scores 0–20 | Brief | Not specified | Hospitalized patients recently attempting suicide; old, frail, multiply impaired nursing home residents (Abraham, 1991) | 3 dimensions of hopelessness: 1. Feelings about the future: Affective (lack of hope, enthusiasm, faith) items 1, 6, 13, 15, 19 2. Loss of motivation: Motivational (giving up, not trying) items 2, 3, 9, 11, 12, 16, 17, 20 3. Future expectations: Cognitive (lack of future expectations) items 4, 7, 8, 14, 18 |
| Geriatric Hopelessness Scale (Fry, 1984) | Self-report: True/false Range 0–30; higher the score, greater the hopelessness | 30; true = 15 items; false = 15 items | Brief | Reminisce about stressful episodes | Nonpsychiatric, nonpatient, and subclincally depressed older adults | 4 factors drawn from: 1. Recovering lost physical and cognitive abilities 2. Recovering lost personal and interpersonal worth and attractiveness 3. Regaining spiritual faith and grace 4. Receiving nurturance, respect, or remembrance |

*Responses abbreviated: SA, strongly agree; SD, strongly disagree; A, agree; D, disagree; DF, definately false; MF, mostly false; DT, definitely true; MT, mostly true.

**Table 5.32.**
Psychometric Properties of the Hope Scales

| Scale name | Original purpose | Reliability | Validity |
|---|---|---|---|
| Herth Hope Scale (HHS) (Herth, 1991) | Measure the multidimensional nature of hope | Alpha = 0.75–0.94 Test–retest (3 week) = 0.89–0.91 | Content: 2 expert panels, 4 judges with expertise in hope and 3 with expertise in measurement Divergent: r = −0.69 with hopelessness scale Construct: 3 factors (temporality and future, positive readiness and expectancy, and interconnectedness) explained 58% of variance |
| Herth Hope Index (HHI) (Herth, 1992) | Adaptation of HHS for clinical setting; Related to health changes | Alpha = 0.88 – 0.97 Test–retest = 0.87–0.91 | Criterion validity HHI/HHS r = 0.92 HHI/Existential Well-being Scale r = 0.84 HHI/Nowotny Hope Scale r = 0.81 Hopelessness scale r = −0.73 |
| Snyder Hope Scale (Snyder et al., 1991) | Develop a self-report scale of hope | Alpha = 0.74–0.84 Agency alpha = 0.71–0.76 Pathways alpha = 0.63–0.80 Test–retest, 3 week = 0.85 (Anderson, 1988) Test–retest, 8 week = 0.73 (Harney, 1989) Test–retest 10 week = 0.76 (Gibb, 1990); 0.82 (Yoshinobu, 1989) | Divergent validity (Gibb, 1990); r = −0.42 with Beck Depression Index; r = −0.51 hopelessness scale |
| Nowotny Hope Scale (Nowotny, 1989) | Measure the six dimensions of hope in response to stressful event | Cronbach alpha = 0.90 Test–retest = not tested | Concurrent validity: r = −0.47 with Beck Hopelessness Scale |
| Beck Hopelessness Scale (Beck et al., 1974) | Quantify hopelessness and represent respondent's negative expectancies | Alpha (KR-20) = 0.93 | Concurrent validity r = 0.74 clinical ratings |
| Geriatric Hopelessness Scale (Fry, 1984) | Assess hopelessness in non-psychiatric, nonpatient, and subclinically depressed older adults | Alpha = 0.69 Spearman-Brown = 0.73 | Concurrent validity r = 0.49 Geriatric Depression Scale; r = −0.55 self-concept scale Construct validity: 4 factors accounting for 67% of variance in scores |

mended over the others. Research should focus on finding a link between hope and outcome variables to help validate these measures. Table 5.31 summarizes aspects of the hope scales covered here. Table 5.32 contrasts the psychometric properties of these scales.

## CONCLUSIONS

Despite the large body of work on mood, much more needs to be done. In particular, the expression of anxiety by older adults needs more research. Research on the measurement of depression in older adults has yielded adequate instruments for clinical and research settings. These instruments make possible large-scale research studies into the psychological changes of, and life events specific to, older adults. The same can occur for the other measures surveyed in this chapter. Potentially useful research directions include exploring the relationship between depression and anxiety in frail adults to see if the distinction is maintained. The connection between cognitive declines and psychological constructs needs to be further explored (Lawton et al., 1992a). Positive measures of psychological adjustment, such as hope and psychological well-being, should more firmly establish their connections with other health outcome measures.

All health care professionals should be attentive to mental illness in older adults. The information presented in this chapter should be used as a guide in planning psychological assessments of older adults. Clearly, psychological instruments differ in their weighting of severity, duration, and spread of affect. Reflection on the purpose for the assessment can start this process and guide one to an appropriate instrument. Clear assessment questions and multiple assessment approaches are prerequisites to successful psychological assessments.

## REFERENCES

Abraham, I. L. (1991). The Geriatric Depression Scale and Hopelessness Index: Longi-tudinal psychometric data on frail nursing home residents. *Perceptual and Motor Skills, 72*(3), 875–880.

American Psychiatric Association (1994). *Diagnostic and statistical manual of mental disorders — revised (4th ed.).* Washington, DC: American Psychiatric Press.

American Psychological Association (1997). *What practitioners should know about working with older adults.* Washington, DC: American Psychological Association.

Anderson, J. R. (1988). *The role of hope in appraisal, goal-setting, expectancy, and coping.* Lawrence: University of Kansas.

Andrews, F. M., & Robinson, J. P. (1991). Measures of subjective well-being. In J. P. Robinson, P. R. Shaver, & L. S. Wrightsman (Eds.), *Measures of personality and social psychological attitudes* (pp. 61–114). San Diego, CA: Academic Press.

Beck, A. T., Epstein, N., Brown, G., & Steer, R. A. (1988a). An inventory for measuring clinical anxiety: Psychometric properties. *Journal of Consulting and Clinical Psychology, 56*, 893–897.

Beck, A. T., & Steer, R. A. (1991). Relationship between the Beck Anxiety Inventory and the Hamilton Anxiety Rating Scale with anxious outpatients. *Journal of Anxiety Disorders, 5*, 213–223.

Beck, A. T., Steer, R. A., Beck, J. S., & Newman, C. F. (1993). Hopelessness, depression, suicidal ideation, and clinical diagnosis of depression. *Suicide and Life-Threatening Behavior, 23*(2), 139–145.

Beck, A. T., Steer, R. A., & Garbin, M. G. (1988b). Psychometric Properties of the Beck Depression Inventory: Twenty-five years of evaluation. *Clinical Psychology Review, 8*, 77–100.

Beck, A. T., Ward, C. H., Mendelson, M., Mock, J., & Erbaugh, J. (1961). An inventory for measuring depression. *Archives of General Psychiatry, 4*, 561–571.

Beck, A. T., Weissman, A., Lester, D., & Trexler, L. (1974). The measurement of pessimism: The Hopelessness Scale. *Journal of Consulting and Clinical Psychology, 42*(6), 861–865.

Beekman, A. T. F., Deeg, D. J. H., Van Limbeek, J., Braam, A. W., De Vries, M. Z., & Van Tilburg, W. (1997). Criterion validity of the Center for Epidemiological Studies Depression Scale (CES-D): Results from a community-based sample of older subjects in the Netherlands. *Psychological Medicine, 27*, 231–235.

Blazer, D. G. (1997). Generalized anxiety disorder and panic disorder in the elderly: A review. *Harvard Review of Psychiatry, 5*(1), 18–27.

Bradburn, N. M. (1969). *The structure of psychological well-being.* Chicago, IL: Aldine.

Burke, W. J., Miller, J. P., Rubin, E., Morris, J. C., Coben, L. A., Duchek, J., Wittels, I. G., & Berg, L. (1988). Reliability of the Washington University Clinical Dementia Rating (CDR). *Archives of Neurology, 45,* 31–32.

Callahan, C. M., Handrie, H. C., Dittus, R. S., Brater, D. C., Hui, S. L., & Tierney, W. M. (1994a). Improving treatment of late life depression in primary care: A randomized clinical trial. *Journal of the American Geriatric Society, 42,* 839–846.

Callahan, C. M., Hui, S. L., Nienaber, N. A., Musick, B. S., & Tierney, W. M. (1994b). Longitudinal study of depression and health services among elderly primary care patients. *Journal of the American Geriatrics Society, 42*(8), 833–838.

Callahan, J., & Wallack, S. (Eds.). (1981). *Reforming the long-term care system.* Lexington, MA: Lexington Books.

Clayton, A. H., Holroyd, S., & Sheldon-Keller, A. (1997). Geriatric Depression Scale vs. Hamilton Rating Scale for Depression in a sample of anxiety patients. *Clinical Gerontologist, 17*(3), 3–13.

Coleman, P. G., Philp, I., & Mulle, M. A. (1995). Does the use of the geriatric depression scale make redundant the need for separate measures of well-being on geriatric wards? *Age and Ageing, 24,* 416–420.

Davidson, H., Feldman, P. H., & Crawford, S. (1994). Measuring depressive symptoms in the frail elderly. *Journal of Gerontology: Psychological Sciences, 49*(4), P159–P164.

Epstein, L. J. (1976). Depression in the elderly. *Journal of Gerontology, 31*(3), 278–282.

Farren, C. J., Herth, K. A., & Popovich, J. M. (1995). *Hope and hopelessness: Critical clinical constructs.* London, England: Sage.

Feinberg, T., & Goodman, B. (1984). Affective illness, dementia, and pseudodementia. *Journal of Clinical Psychiatry, 45*(3), 99–103.

Filipp, S. (1996). Motivation and emotion. In J. E. Birren & K. W. Schaie (Eds.), *Handbook of the psychology of aging* (4th ed., pp. 218–235). San Diego, CA: Academic Press.

Frijda, N. H. (1993). Moods, emotion episodes, and emotions. In M. Lewis & J. M. Hariland (Eds.), *Handbook of emotions* (pp. 381–403). New York: Guilford.

Fry, P. (1984). Development of a geriatric scale of hopelessness: Implications for counseling and intervention with the depressed elderly. *Journal of Counseling Psychology, 13*(3), 322–331.

Gallagher, D., Breckenridge, J., Steinmetz, J., &

Thompson, L. (1983). The Beck Depression Inventory and research diagnostic criteria: Congruence in an older adult population. *Journal of Consulting and Clinical Psychology, 51*(6), 945–946.

Gallagher, D., Nies, G., & Thompson, L. W. (1982). Reliability of the Beck Depression Inventory with older adults. *Journal of Consulting and Clinical Psychology, 50*(1), 152–153.

Garrad, J., Rolnick, S. J., Nitz, N. M., Luepke, L., Jackson, J., Fischer, L. R., Leibson, C., Bland, P. C., Heinrich, R., & Waller, L. A. (1998). Clinical detection of depression among community-based elderly people with self-reported symptoms of depression. *Journal of Gerontology Medical Sciences, 53A*(2), M92–M101.

Gatz, M., & Smyer, M. A. (1992). The mental health system and older adults in the 1990s. *American Psychologist, 47*(6), 741–751.

German, P. S., Shapiro, S., Skinner, E. A., Von Korff, M., Klein, L. E., Turner, R. W., Teitelbaum, M. L., Burke, J., & Burns, B. (1987). Detection and management of mental health problems of older people by primary care providers. *JAMA, 257,* 489–493.

Gibb, J. (1990). *The Hope Scale revisited: Further validation of a measure of individual differences in the hope motive.* Chicago: University of Chicago Press.

Gottfries, C. G. (1997). Recognition and management of depression in the elderly. *International Clinical Psychopharmacology, 12*(Suppl 7), S31–S36.

Gurland, B. J. (1976). The comparative frequency of depression in various adult age groups. *Journal of Gerontology, 31*(3), 283–292.

Harney, P. (1989). *The Hope Scale: Exploration of construct validity and its influence on health.* , Lawrence: University of Kansas.

Harper, R. G., Kotik-Harper, D., & Kirby, H. (1990). Psychometric assessment of depression in an elderly general medical population: Over- or underassessment? *Journal of Nervous and Mental Disease, 178*(2), 113–119.

Harris, C. B. (1988). *Hope: Construct definition and the development of an individual differences scale.* Lawrence: University of Kansas.

Henk, H. J., Katzelnick, D. J., Koback, K. A., Griest, J. H., & Jefferson, J. W. (1996). Medical costs attributed to depression among patients with a history of high medical expenses in a health maintenance organization. *Archives of General Psychiatry, 53,* 899–904.

Herth, K. (1991). Development and refinement of an instrument to measure hope. *Scholarly Inquiry for Nursing Practice An International Journal, 5*(1), 39–51.

Herth, K. (1992). Abbreviated instrument to measure hope: development and psychometric evaluation. *Journal of Advanced Nursing, 17*, 1251–1259.

Himmelfarb, S., & Murrell, S. A. (1983). Reliability and validity of five mental health scales in older persons. *Journal of Gerontology, 38*, 333–339.

Jacob, M., & Guarnaccia, V. (1997). Motivational and behavioral correlates of life satisfaction in an elderly sample. *Psychological Reports, 80*, 811–818.

Kabacoff, R. I., Segal, D. L., Hersen, M., & Van Hasselt, V. B. (1997). Psychometric properties and diagnostic utility of the Beck Anxiety Inventory and the State-Trait Inventory with older adult psychiatric outpatients. *Journal of Anxiety Disorders, 11*(1), 33–47.

Katona, C. L. (1994). Approaches to the management of depression in old age. *Gerontology, 40*(1), 5–9.

Kercher, K. (1992). Assessing subjective well-being in the old-old: The PANAS as a measure of orthogonal dimensions of positive and negative affect. *Research on Aging, 14*(2), 131–168.

Kessler, R. C., Foster, C., Webster, P. S., & House, J. S. (1992). The relationship between age and depressive symptoms in two national surveys. *Psychology and Aging, 7*, 119–126.

Larsen, R. J., & Diener, E. (1992). Promises and problems with the circumplex model of emotion. In M. S. Clark (Ed.), *Emotion: Review of personality and social psychology* (Vol. 13, pp. 24–59). Newbury Park, CA: Sage.

Lawton, M. P. (1975). The Philadelphia geriatric center morale scale: A revision. *Journal of Gerontology, 30*(1), 85–89.

Lawton, M. P. (1997). Measures of quality of life and subjective well-being. *Generations, 21*(1), 45–47.

Lawton, M. P., DeVoe, M. R., & Parmelee, P. (1995). Relationship of events and affect in the daily life of an elderly population. *Psychology & Aging, 10*(3), 469–477.

Lawton, M. P., Kleban, M. H., Dean, J., Rajagopal, D., & Parmelee, P. A. (1992a). The factorial generality of brief positive and negative affect measures. *Journal of Gerontology, 47*(4), 228–237.

Lawton, M. P., Kleban, M. H., Rajagopal, D., & Dean, J. (1992b). Dimensions of affective experience in three age stages. *Psychology and Aging, 7*(2), 171–184.

Lawton, M. P., Parmelee, P. A., Katz, I. R., & Nesselroade, J. (1996). Affective states in normal and depressed older people. *Journal of Gerontology Psychological Sciences, 51B*(6), P309–P316.

Lebowitz, B. D., Pearson, J. L., Schneider, L. S., Reynolds, C. F., Alexopoulos, G. S., Bruce, M. L., Conwell, Y., Katz, I. R., Meyers, B. S., Morrison, M. F., Mossey, J., Niederehe, G., & Parmelee, P. (1997). Diagnosis and treatment of depression in late life: Consensus statement update. *JAMA, 278*(14), 1186–1190.

Lewinsohn, P. M., Seeley, J. R., Roberts, R. E., & Allen, N. B. (1997). Center for Epidemiological Studies Depression Scale (CES-D) as a screening instrument for depression among community-residing older adults. *Psychology and Aging, 12*(2), 277–287.

Liang, J., & Bollen, K. A. (1985). Gender differences in the structure of the Philadelphia Geriatric Center Morale Scale. *Journal of Gerontology, 40*, 468–477.

Lohmann, N. (1977a). Correlations of life satisfaction, morale, and adjustment measures. *Journal of Gerontology, 32*, 73–75.

Lohmann, N. P. L. (1977b). *Comparison on life satisfaction morale, and adjustment scales on an elderly population.* Waltham, MA: Brandeis University.

Lyness, J. M., Noel, T. K., Cox, C., King, D., Conwell, Y., & Caine, E. D. (1997). Screening for depression in elderly primary care patients: A comparison of the Center for Epidemiologic Studies–Depression Scale and the Geriatric Depression Scale. *Archives of Internal Medicine, 157*(4), 449–454.

Magni, G., Schifano, F., & DeLeo, D. (1986). Assessment of depression in an elderly medical population. *Journal of Affective Disorders, 11*, 121–124.

Mahoney, J., Drinka, T. J. K., Alber, R., Gunter-Hunt, G., Matthews, C., Gravenstein, S., & Carnes, M. (1994). Screening for depression: Single question versus GDS. *Journal of the Geriatric Society, 42*, 1006–1008.

McDowell, I., & Newell, C. (1996). *Social Health. Measuring Health: A Guide to Rating Scales and Questionnaires* (2nd ed.). New York: Oxford University Press.

McGivney, S. A., Mulvihill, M., & Taylor, B. (1994). Validating the GDS depression screen in the nursing home. *Journal of the Geriatric Society, 42*, 490–492.

Moak, G. S., & Fisher, W. H. (1990). Alzheimer's disease and related disorders in state mental hospitals: Data from a nationwide survey. *Gerontologist, 30*(6), 798–802.

Montorio, I., & Izal, M. (1996). The Geriatric Depression Scale: A review of its development and utility. *International Psychogeriatrics, 8*(1), 103–112.

Neugarten, B. L., Havighurst, R. J., & Tobin, S. S. (1961). The measurement of life satisfaction. *Journal of Gerontology, 16,* 134–143.

Newmann, J. P. (1989). Aging and depression. *Psychology and Aging, 4*(2), 150–165.

NIH Consensus Development Panel on Depression in Late Life (1992). Diagnosis and treatment of depression in late life. *JAMA, 268*(8), 1018–1024.

Norris, J. T., Gallagher, D., Wilson, A., & Winogard, C. H. (1987). Assessment of depression in geriatric medical outpatients: The validity of two screening measures. *Journal of the American Geriatric Society, 35,* 989–995.

Nowotny, M. L. (1989). Assessment of hope in patients with cancer: Development of an instrument. *Oncology Nursing Forum, 16*(1), 57–61.

Okiomoto, J. T., Barnes, R. F., Veith, R. C., Raskind, M. A., Inui, T. S., & Carter, W. B. (1982). Screening for depression in geriatric medical patients. *American Journal of Psychiatry, 139*(6), 799–802.

O'Neil, D., Rick, I., Blake, P., Walsh, J. B., & Coakley, D. (1992). The Geriatric Depression Scale: Rater-administered or self-administered? *International Journal of Geriatric Psychiatry, 7,* 511–515.

Ossip-Klein, D., Rothenberg, D. M., & Andersen, E. M. (1997). Screening for depression. In E. Andersen, B. Rothenberg, & J. C. Zimmer (eds.), *Assessing the Health Status of Older Adults* (pp. 180–244). New York: Springer.

Parmelee, P. A., Katz, I. R., & Lawton, M. P. (1989). Depression among institutionalized aged: Assessment and prevalence estimation. *Journal of Gerontology Medical Sciences, 44*(1), M22–29.

Patterson, R. L., O'Sullivan, M. J., & Spielberger, C. D. (1980). Measurement of the state and trait anxiety in elderly mental health clients. *Journal of Behavioral Assessment, 2*(2), 89–97.

Radloff, L. S. (1977). The Center for Epidemiological Studies—Depression Scale: A self-report depression scale for research in the general population. *Applied Psychological Measurements, 3,* 385–401.

Raleigh, E. H., & Boehm, S. (1994). Development of the Multidimensional Hope Scale. *Journal of Nursing, 2*(2), 155–167.

Rapp, S. R., Parisi, S. A., Walsh, D. A., & Wallace, C. E. (1988). Detecting depression in elderly medical inpatients. *Journal of Consulting and Clinical Psychology, 56*(4), 509–513.

Regier, D. A., Boyd, J. H., Burke, J. D., Rae, D. S., Myers, J. K., Kramer, M., Robins, L. N., George, L. K., Karno, M., & Locke, B. Z. (1988). One-month prevalence of mental disorders in the United States: Based on five Epidemiologic Catchment Area Sites. *Archives of General Psychiatry, 45,* 977–986.

Reiger, M. S., Reiger, D. A., Kaelber, C. T., Rae, D. S., Farmer, M. E., Knauper, B., Kessler, R. C., & Norquist, G. S. (1998). Limitations of diagnostic criteria and assessment instruments for mental disorders: Implications for research and policy. *Archives of General Psychiatry, 55,* 109–115.

Rustoen, T., & Moum, T. (1997). Reliability and validity of the Norwegian version of The Nowotny Hope Scale: A nursing tool for measuring hope in cancer patients. *Scandinavian Journal Caring Science, 11,* 33–41.

Salamon, M. J., & Conte, V. A. (1984). *Salamon-Conte Life Satisfaction in the Elderly Scale (LSES).* Odessa, FL: Psychological Assessment Resources.

Salzman, C. (1997). Depressive disorders and other emotional issues in the elderly: Current issues. *International Clinical Psychopharmacology, 12*(Suppl 7), S37–S42.

Schneider, L. S., & Olin, J. T. (1995). Efficacy of acute treatment for geriatric depression. *International Psychogeriatrics, 7*(Suppl), 7–25.

Sheikh, J. I., & Yesavage, J. A. (1986). Geriatric Depression Scale (GDS) recent evidence and development of a shorter version. In T. L. Brink (ed.), *Clinical gerontology: A guide to assessment and intervention* (pp. 165–173). New York: Haworth Press.

Shulman, K. I., Tohen, M., Satlin, A., Mallya, G., & Kalunian, D. (1992). Mania compared with unipolar depression in old age. *American Journal of Psychiatry, 149*(3), 341–345.

Shurman, R. A., Kramer, P. D., & Mitchell, J. B. (1985). The hidden mental health network. *Archives of General Psychiatry, 42,* 89–94.

Snyder, C. R., Harris, C., Anderson, J. R., Holeran, S. A., Irving, L. M., Sigmon, S. T., Yoshinobu, L., Gibb, J., Langelle, C., & Harney, P. (1991). The will and the ways: Development and validation of an individual-differences measure of hope. *Journal of Personality and Social Psychology, 60*(4), 570–585.

Spielberger, C. D. (1985). Assessment of state and trait anxiety: Conceptual and methodological issues. *Southern Psychologist, 2,* 6–16.

Spielberger, C. D., Gorusch, R. L., & Lushene, R. E. (1970). *Manual for the State–Trait Anxiety Inventory.* Palo Alto, CA: Consulting Psychological Press.

Stanley, M. A., Beck, J. G., & Zebb, B. J. (1996). Psychometric properties of four anxiety measures in older adults. *Behavioral Research Therapy, 34*(10), 827–838.

Steer, R. A., Ranieri, W. F., Beck, A. T., & Clark, D. A. (1993). Further evidence for the validity of the Beck Anxiety Inventory with psychiatric outpatients. *Journal of Anxiety Disorders, 7*(3), 195–205.

Stone, K. (1989). Mania in the elderly. *British Journal of Psychiatry, 155,* 220–224.

Stoner, M. H. (1991). Response to "Development and refinement of an instrument to measure hope." *Scholarly Inquiry for Nursing Practice: An International Journal, 5*(1), 53–55.

Stotland, E. (1969). *The Psychology of Hope.* San Francisco: Jossey-Bass.

Tellegen, A. (1985). Structures of mood and personality and their relevance to assessing anxiety, with an emphasis on self-report. In A. H. Tuma & J. D. Maser (eds.), *Anxiety and the Anxiety Disorders* (pp. 681–706). Hillside, NJ: Erlbaum.

Uncapher, H., Gallagher-Thompson, D., Osgood, N. J., & Bonger, B. (1998). Hopelessness and suicidal ideation in older adults. *Gerontologist, 38*(1), 62–70.

Watson, D. (1988). The vicissitudes of mood measurement: Effects of varying descriptors, time frames, and response formats on measures of positive and negative affect. *Journal of Personality and Social Psychology, 55*(1), 128–141.

Watson, D., Clark, L. A., & Tellegen, A. (1988). Development and validation of brief measures of positive and negative affect: The PANAS Scales. *Journal of Personality of Social Psychology, 54*(6), 1063–1070.

Weiss, I. K., Nagel, C. L., & Aronson, M. K. (1986). Applicability of depression scales to the old old person. *Journal of the American Geriatric Society, 34,* 215–218.

Weissman, M. M. (1991). The affective disorders: Bipolar disorder and major depression. In A. Kerr & H. McClelland (eds.), *Concepts of Mental Disorder: A Continuing Debate* (pp. 103–111). London: Gaskell.

Wetherell, J. L., & Arean, P. A. (1997). Psychometric evaluation of the Beck Anxiety Inventory with older medical patients. *Psychological Assessment, 9*(2), 136–144.

Wood, V., Wylie, M. L., & Sheafor, B. (1969). An analysis of a short self-report measure of life satisfaction: Correlation with rater judgments. *Journal of Gerontology, 24,* 465–469.

Yassa, R., Nair, N. P. V., & Iskandar, H. (1988). Late-onset bipolar disorder. *Psychiatric Clinics of North America, 11,* 117–131.

Yesavage, J. A., & Brink, T. L. (1983). Development and validation of a geriatric depression screening scale: A preliminary report. *Journal of Psychiatric Research, 17*(1), 37–49.

Yoshinobu, L. R. (1989). *Construct Validation of the Hope Scale: Agency and Pathways Components.* Lawrence: University of Kansas.

Young, R. C. (1992). Geriatric mania. *Clinics in Geriatric Medicine, 8*(2), 387–399.

Young, R. C., Biggs, T., Ziegler, V. E., & Meyer, D. A. (1978). A rating scale for mania: Reliability, validity and sensitivity. *British Journal of Psychiatry, 133,* 429–435.

Young, R. C., & Klerman, G. L. (1992). Mania in late life: Focus on age at onset. *American Journal of Psychiatry, 149*(7), 867–876.

Zung, W. K. (1967). Depression in the normal aged. *Psychosomatics, 8,* 287–292.

Zung, W. K. (1971). A rating instrument for anxiety disorders. *Psychosomatics, 12,* 371–379.

Zung, W. W. K. (1965). A self-rating depression scale. *Archives of General Psychiatry, 12,* 63–70.

# 6

# Social Functioning

## CARRIE LEVIN

### WHAT IS SOCIAL FUNCTIONING?

Although there are well-established assessment tools within certain domains of assessment such as physical functioning, there is no gold standard for assessing social functioning. Progress toward using a common approach to measure social functioning began with the OARS Social Resources Scale, part of the Older Americans Resources and Services (OARS) Multidimensional Functional Assessment Questionnaire (Pfeiffer, 1975) a formal tool to assess older adults' social resources by measuring their contact with friends and family. Clinicians and researchers often, however, use much simpler methods, such as asking their patients questions regarding the amount of social activity in which they engage and the number of social contacts they have. This chapter explores the use of both formal assessment tools and less formal measures of social functioning.

Social functioning is the dimension of health and well-being that reflects how individuals get along with others, how others react to them, how well they perform socially expected roles, and how they interact with social institutions (McDowell & Newell, 1996; Froland et al., 1979).

There are both subjective and objective measures of social functioning. Clinicians and researchers may want to quantify different aspects of social functioning such as how many activities in which an older adult engages, how many hours of care he or she receives from family members, or how many friends are in his or her social network. This is the objective side of measuring social functioning. The subjective side relates to older adults' perceptions of their social functioning. This includes how satisfied they are with the activities and roles in which they participate, whether they feel they have adequate social support, and whether their social functioning provides pleasure and meaning in their lives.

There is no simple conceptual model of social functioning because it embraces all of social life. Social support, social networks, social resources, social roles and role functioning, and social activities are overlapping domains of social functioning that are discussed in detail in this chapter. Different aspects are salient in the lives of older adults depending on the context and the therapeutic goal. This chapter first explores reasons to assess social functioning in older adults, the goals of such measurement, and the issues that are associated with assessment of social functioning. Then the various domains of social functioning are examined, and tools used for assessment in each domain are discussed.

## REASONS TO ASSESS SOCIAL FUNCTIONING IN OLDER ADULTS

Social functioning affects health directly and indirectly. Persons who have diversified social networks have better scores on measures of activities of daily living, instrumental activities of daily living, vision, and perceived health (Litwin, 1998). The reciprocal is also true: Health affects social functioning (House, Landis, & Umberson, 1988; Kane & Kane, 1981). Persons who become bedbound will no longer be able to engage in activities that involve leaving their homes.

Clinicians and researchers investigate social functioning to determine how it may contribute to illnesses or disease, treatment, and rehabilitation (predictor variable) as well as to see how individuals with illnesses or disabilities function socially (outcome variable) (Kane, Kane, & Arnold, 1985). Thus, social functioning can be viewed as either an outcome (dependent) variable or a predictor (independent) variable.

As a predictor variable, social functioning affects outcomes such as health, physical functioning, and everyday activity. First, examining social functioning as a predictor variable can help determine if an older adult has become socially isolated or lacks the necessary social support to maintain health (Kane, 1995). For example, an extremely frail, community dwelling older adult loses his wife, who has been his primary caregiver. This man will need additional support in order to remain in his home. Second, social functioning as a predictor variable is examined to determine whether it will enhance an individual's satisfaction and well-being or hinder recovery (Kane & Kane, 1981). An individual who is overburdened by caregiving roles may

not recover from an acute episode as fast as someone who has no caregiving responsibilities. Assessing social functioning as a predictor variable can assist providers in understanding the values and preferences an older adult has regarding his or her social situation. Finally, social functioning as part of a clinical assessment is used to identify the individual's social resources, including finances, in order to determine if he or she can live independently in the community (Kane, 1995). Often, social functioning is examined as a risk factor for nursing home placement.

Because older adults often have chronic conditions that are not curable, clinicians are interested in providing interventions that can assist in functional improvement. To do this, social functioning is measured as a treatment outcome. This is done to evaluate the effect an individual's treatment plan has on his or her social well-being. This assessment is done so that alterations in care plans can be made in order to achieve "optimal" social functioning (Kane, 1995). In addition, social functioning can be used as an outcome to determine what the risk factors are for poor functioning. Clinicians may ask older adults about changes in their activity levels because, if a person is no longer getting out and being active, it may be a sign of depression or a mobility problem. Assessment of social functioning is important because it may be used in a descriptive sense to assess the social "state" in which a person is to determine what services that person requires or just to describe where that person is.

Providers assess baseline levels of social functioning to monitor changes over time as an outcome of treatment or intervention or to prescribe an intervention such as adult day care. For the latter purpose, the provider is setting a goal to expand an older adult's social functioning by sending him or her into a social situation where he or she may be able to establish relationships. There is some danger that assessment of social function for this purpose may lend itself to social judgments about what appropriate levels of social functioning are. We should not force individuals who are not interested in being social to do so.

## THE GOALS OF MEASURING SOCIAL FUNCTIONING

A primary goal of assessing social functioning is to determine how older adults function after an acute episode or how they cope with chronic illnesses or disability. Assessment of an older adult's social functioning is done to determine whether or not he or she has adequate social support to recover from an acute episode or maintain a chronic condition. Clinicians can obtain information regarding the amount of social resources, including information about finances and social support, to assess whether the older adult will be able to handle his or her condition. In addition, clinicians may need to establish baseline measurements. It is crucial to make baseline measurements of social function so that subsequent measurements can be compared with it in order to determine if an older adult is getting back to where he or she was before the acute episode.

A goal of a successful aging movement in terms of desired social functioning is to see what older adults want and need socially in their lives and whether they have it. There is a certain amount of social engagement (people, activities, stimulation) that is necessary in order to live. Therefore, it is important to assess whether older adults are functioning adequately. In addition, older adults have societal expectations to fulfill certain roles such as grandparenting and caregiving for a spouse. Assessing social functioning helps to monitor whether older adults' expectations are being met, and, if not, interventions can be prescribed to better fulfill them.

Identifying how socially active the older adult is and has been throughout his or her lifetime is important. Total isolation is bad, yet individuals will vary in the amount of social interaction that they need. If an older adult has never been gregarious, we should not intervene, but intervention is necessary for a vivacious person who is no longer socially active. Clinicians must, however, be aware that individuals can change their minds regarding the amount of social activity in which they want to participate, but there may be people who have been depressed for their entire lives and have always required intervention but never received it. It is important that clinicians not withhold an intervention that may have always been needed.

An additional goal of social functioning assessment is to determine if an older adult has the social resources, including social support and social networks, to remain living independently in the community. It has become increasingly important to assess social functioning for this purpose because care received in acute care institutions and residential long-term care facilities is expensive (McDowell & Newell, 1996; Gallo, Reichel, & Andersen, 1995). Case managers and discharge planners want to know what resources are available and provided, so they can plan for provision of additional services as needed.

Another goal of measuring social functioning is to identify individuals in both the community and long-term care facilities who are isolated and vulnerable. As a result, their quality of life may be low. Over a 9 year follow-up period, Berkman and Syme (1979) found that individuals who are socially isolated are more than twice as likely to die than are individuals who have limited social contacts. Increased social functioning leads to improved health, so it is important to identify individuals who are isolated and vulnerable.

## ISSUES, PROBLEMS, AND CONCERNS WITH SOCIAL FUNCTIONING ASSESSMENT

Because social functioning is a multidimensional concept, assessment can be difficult. A major problem with measuring social functioning in older adults is selecting an appropriate standard to determine whether an individual is adjusted or functioning adequately. For older adults this can be problematic because of the increase in variation among individuals as they age. Norms and expectations vary among individuals based on differences in educational level, physical health status, age, sex, and ethnicity (McDowell & Newell, 1996). These factors make it very difficult to judge whether an individual is socially adjusting.

One of the greatest challenges encountered when measuring social functioning is that social functioning has both an objective and subjective component and determining which type of measurement is most relevant in a particular context. The objective component quantifies a particular amount of a predictor variable included in social functioning such as how many people are in the individual's social network, how often the individual socializes with others, the number of hours that the individual receives care from others, and the amount of social activity in which the individual engages. The subjective component of social functioning is the individual's evaluation of whether his or her social situation is satisfying (Kane, 1987, 1995; Kane & Kane, 1981). Table 6.1 identifies the objective and subjective components included in each domain of social functioning that are discussed in this chapter.

Aggregating and weighting measures into scores that have meaning can be a challenge in both clinical and research assessments (Kane & Kane, 1981). If an overall score is achieved by summing individual scores, there is an underlying assumption that all questions are weighted equally. This can potentially bias results. What does it mean for a particular individual to have a particular score on an instrument? Can we base scores on societal norms? Each score depends on the individual, his or her expectations, and baseline social functioning level. Researchers and clinicians often look at change scores, so baseline scores must be established in order to do comparisons. It may be difficult to identify what the changes really mean, and this, too, can potentially bias results if causal inferences are made.

Threshold values and cut-off points can be an additional concern. An acceptable level of social functioning for one individual may not be adequate for someone else. The same holds true for levels of support. All measures of social functioning are unique to the individual who is being assessed, so investigators and clinicians must be aware that scores have little meaning if taken out of context of each individual's particular case.

Assessing social functioning in individuals with cognitive impairments can also be a challenge. This is especially true for subjective measures dealing with satisfac-

**Table 6.1.**
Assessment of the Social Functioning Domains

| Domain | Subjective component | Objective component |
| --- | --- | --- |
| Social Support | Amount of support available, provided, and received | Perceptions, satisfaction, and adequacy of support |
| Social Networks | Number of systems and people in network | Perceptions, satisfaction, and adequacy of network |
| Social Resources | Amount of resources available | Perceived availability of resources and adequacy of those resources |
| Social Roles and Role Functioning | Number and type of roles | Perception and satisfaction with roles |
| Activities | Number of activities, group memberships, and organizations in which individual is involved | Perception, satisfaction, and adequacy of activities |

tion, adequacy, and quality of social functioning. It is not, however, difficult to measure objective components of social functioning. This can be done by simply asking proxies to answer questions or to make direct observations of the cognitively impaired individual (Newsom, Bookwala, & Schulz, 1997).

Measuring social functioning can be challenging because there are a variety of different informants to provide information. The interactive nature of social functioning makes information-gathering burdensome. For a clinician or researcher with limited time and resources, it is often necessary, but not feasible, to consult the older adult, other family members, or close friends in order to make necessary assessments. To extend the group further is too time consuming and costly. Another difficulty with having more than one possible informant is to determine whose perspective should be used in the assessment when differences exist between the two (Kane, 1995; Kane & Kane, 1981).

Factors that make up social functioning, such as social roles and social support, are vague and abstract, which make them difficult to measure. Many measures purport to measure a single construct such as social support yet really assess more than one construct such as social support and social networks, and, therefore, results differ. The reverse is also true. Some measures appear to assess dissimilar aspects of social functioning but really measure the same things; for example, social network scales and social support scales often measure the same thing (Kane, 1987; Kane & Kane, 1981).

There are a number of practical problems associated with assessing social functioning in older adults. Kane & Kane (1981) describe these problems as falling into the following categories: limits of self-report; choice of time window; dealing with the hypothetical; and degree of specificity. Limits of self-report refer to the fact that there are socially desirable responses to assessment questions. An older adult may exaggerate quality or quantity of support or amount of social resources available to him or her. In addition, there may be problems with older adults' abilities to remember particular information. Choice of a recent time window increases the likelihood of accuracy in the individual's reply. There are, however, problems with establishing a short time window when dealing with older adults because special events, outings, or activities may happen more infrequently, particularly if the individual is institutionalized. Thus, if the time window includes only the past 24 hours or even the past week, valuable information may be missed.

In dealing with the hypothetical, measurements of social functioning have subjects pretend that they are in a particular situation that forces the respondent to make a guess as to what his or her behavior would be in the given situation. These types of questions can evoke socially desirable responses that may not be reliable because what an individual might do in a hypothetical situation often differs from what he or she will do in a real situation. Finally, degree of specificity is important because it can be difficult to quantify responses. For example, if an individual has one primary person who provides support, a spouse perhaps, and that individual provides support 24 hours a day, how does this compare with an individual whose social network consists of 10 friends who visit and provide support on a less frequent basis? This is a difficulty in determining what to measure: is quality or quantity more important? It is argued that a small number of individuals who provide intensive support are more important than a large number of individuals who provide only minimal support (Gallo et al., 1995). Henderson and Brown (1988) have shown that quality rather than quantity of social support is the best mediator of physiological distress.

## THE DOMAINS OF SOCIAL FUNCTIONING AND THE PURPOSES AND IMPLICATIONS OF ASSESSING THEM

The domains of social functioning include social support, social networks, social re-

**Table 6.2.**
Assessment of the Social Functioning Domains

| Domain | What is assessed |
| --- | --- |
| Social Support | Forms of support, including esteem, information, companionship, instrumental, and global |
| Social Networks | Formal and informal system(s) that provide support; reciprocity of relationships |
| Social Resources | Contact with others, employment, income, assets, spending, and insurance |
| Social Roles and Role Functioning | Different roles: mentor, grandparent, retiree, widow, dependent, care provider, spouse, parent, member of a particular group |
| Activities | Present or former occupation, leisure activities, religiosity, participation in volunteer work or social clubs, entertainment |

sources, social roles and role functioning, and activities. Table 6.2 identifies what is assessed in each of the five social functioning domains. Within each of the domains, both subjective and objective assessments can be made (see Table 6.1).

Tables 6.3 and 6.4 summarize the assessments described in this section. Table 6.3 summarizes the assessment tools by domain, and Table 6.4 is a quick review of the properties of each scale discussed.

## Social Support

Social support has been defined as the assistance that is provided through older adults' social networks (actual support) and the subjective interpretation of contributions made by others (perceived support) (Antonucci, Sherman, & Vandewater, 1997; Kane, 1995). Social support appears to be a buffer for stress in addition to being a moderator of both physical and psychological well-being (Heitzmann & Kaplan, 1988; Berkman & Syme, 1979). Social environmental stressors affect the neuroendocrine balance, which leads to increased susceptibility to disease. Therefore, people who lack meaningful social contact do not get necessary information and feedback, whereas people who have adequate social support are able to cope with changes in their lives and with crises (Cassel, 1976). Social support can be divided into the categories of emotional support, information and advice, tangible help, and

social stimulation (Antonucci et al., 1997; Kane, 1987, 1995.

There is little agreement in the definition of social support (O'Reilly, 1988). In addition, the concept is either not defined or ill-defined in the literature, and there is often definitional confusion between social network and social support both in conceptual models and in instruments. Some instruments that purport to be assessing social networks are really measuring social support, whereas other may attempt to measure both domains while really only tapping one. However, O'Reilly (1988) found that many definitions included part or all of five categories identified by Cohen and Wills (1985), including esteem, information, companionship, instrumental, and global/undifferentiated social support (Table 6.5).

These five categories of social support fall into two broad classifications of support: everyday support and support provided in times of crises. Both types of support are difficult to measure. Everyday support is often overlooked until it is no longer available. Support in times of crisis is difficult to measure because it does not exist until the crisis occurs, so it must be measured retrospectively (O'Reilly, 1988).

There are problems with measures of social support that simply identify a number of social contacts rather than specifying the intensity, quality, and quantity of that contact. An older adult who has a strong

**Table 6.3.**
Summary of Social Functioning Assessment Tools

| Domain | Tool | What is assessed | For use in |
|---|---|---|---|
| General Social Functioning | PAIS | Social and psychological adjustment to illness including attitude toward illness, affect on vocational environment, sexual relations, family relations, social environment, and psychological distress | Clinical setting |
| Social Networks | LSNS | Number and frequency of contact with friends and family, living arrangements | Clinical setting |
| Social Support | ISSB | Social factors, instrumental support, informational support, companionship | Clinical setting, research |
| Social Support | ISSI | Availability and perceived adequacy of social relations: esteem, instrumental, and companionship support; quality and quantity of support | Clinical setting, research |
| Social Support | PSS-Fa, PSS-Fr | Individual's perception of support from family and friends | Research |
| Social Support | MSPSS | Support from family, friends, and significant others: subjective assessment of social support adequacy | Research |
| Social Support | SSQ | Availability and satisfaction with social support: esteem, global, informational, structural, and provisional support | Research |
| Social Support | NSSQ | Social, global, esteem, companionships, instrumental, perceived, orientation, and structure of social support | Research |
| Social Support | SDRS | Negative aspects of an individual's adjustment: meaningfulness in life, goals, satisfaction | Research |
| General Social Functioning | OARS | Social resources and economic resources, including contact with others, employment, income, assets, spending, and insurance | Clinical setting, research |
| Social Roles and Role Functioning | RCI | Determine an individual's roles by counting the number of his or her relationships | Research |
| Activities | Activity and membership | Club membership and attendance, TV viewing, reading, listening to radio, telephone use, visits in the building, visits in the city, attendance at religious activities | Research |

PAIS, Psychosocial Adjustment to Illness Scale; LSNS, Lubben's Social Network Scale; ISSB, Inventory for Socially Supportive Behaviors; ISSI, Interview Schedule for Social Interaction; PSS-Fa, Perceived Social Support—Family Scale; PSS-Fr, Perceived Social Support—Friends Scale; MSPSS-Multidimensional Scale of Perceived Social Support; SSQ, Social Support Questionnaire; NSSQ, the Norbeck Social Support Questionnaire; SDRS, Social Dysfunction Rating Scale; OARS, Older Americans Resources and Services; RCI, Role Count Index.

relationship with a spouse and few other social contacts may be functioning at a higher level than an older adult who has a number of friends with whom to socialize occasionally, yet no companion with whom to spend time on a more regular basis (Barrera, Sandler, & Ramsay, 1981). Barrera and colleagues hypothesized that the actual number of individuals who are available to provide support for someone is not as important to an older adult's well-being as whether the receiver of the support is satisfied with the support pro-

vided (Barrera et al., 1981). Quantity does not necessarily imply quality (Heitzmann & Kaplan, 1988).

There is negative as well as positive social support. Elder abuse is a growing problem in the United States. Overburdened caregivers may provide negative support through either abuse or neglect. Also, many older adults may suffer financial losses from providers who take advantage of them. There is a negative aspect of support that deals with the reciprocal nature of relationships. Perhaps one spouse is

**Table 6.4.**
Properties of Social Functioning Assessment Tools

| Tool | Self-administered or interview | Reliability | Subjective or objective | No. of items |
|---|---|---|---|---|
| PAIS | Interview<br>Self-administered | IC = 0.12–0.93<br>IRR = 0.33–0.86 | Objective | 45 |
| LSNS | Self-administered | A = 0.70 | Subjective and objective | 10 |
| ISSB | Self-administered | TR = 0.44–0.91<br>IC = 0.93–0.94 | Subjective and objective | 40 |
| ISSI | Interview | TR = 0.75–0.79<br>IC = 0.67–0.81 | Subjective and objective | 52 |
| PSS-Fa, PSS-Fr | Self-administered | TR = 0.83<br>IC = 0.88 for PSS-Fr and 0.90 for PSS-Fa | Subjective | 40 |
| MSPSS | Self-administered | TR = 0.85<br>A = 0.87, family<br>A = 0.85, friends<br>A = 0.91, significant others | Subjective | 12 |
| SSQ | Self-administered | TR = 0.90 (N)<br>TR = 0.83 (S)<br>A = 0.97 (N)<br>A = 0.94 (S) | Subjective and objective | 27 |
| NSSQ | Self-administered | TR = 0.85–0.92<br>IC = 0.69–0.98 | Subjective and objective | 9 for each relation |
| SDRS | Interview | IRR = 0.54–0.86 | Subjective | 21 |
| OARS | Interview | TR = 0.91<br>IRR = 0.67–0.87 | Subjective and objective | 13, Social resources<br>20, Economic resources<br>24, Services received |
| RCI | Interview | N/A | Objective | 8 |

TR, test–retest; A, alpha; IC, internal consistency; IRR, inter-rater reliability; N/A, not applicable; N, number score; S, satisfaction score. PAIS, Psychosocial Adjustment to Illness Scale; LSNS, Lubben's Social Network Scale; ISSB, Inventory for Socially Supportive Behaviors; ISSI, Interview Schedule for Social Interaction; PSS-Fa, Perceived Social Support—Family Scale; PSS-Fr, Perceived Social Support—Friends Scale; MSPSS, Multidimensional Scale of Perceived Social Support; SSQ, Social Support Questionnaire; NSSQ, the Norbeck Social Support Questionnaire; SDRS, Social Dysfunction Rating Scale; OARS, Older Americans Resources and Services; RCI, Role Count Index.

no longer able to care for himself or herself. The nonimpaired spouse then becomes the sole caregiver of that person, and this may lead to extreme feelings of guilt on behalf of the spouse receiving the care because he or she can no longer provide as much physical support in return. Negative social support refers to support that results in unwanted or ineffective intervention (Kane, 1995). Often negative interaction comes from people with whom individuals have close relationships. Nega-

tive as well as positive aspects of support should be included in assessments of social support (Antonucci et al., 1997).

Social support may influence health outcomes. If an individual has an active social support network that assists in treatment adherence, then the older adult is more apt to manage his or her chronic illness or disability successfully (Heitzmann & Kaplan, 1988). Emotional support has been seen to influence recovery of functional capacity (Glass & Maddox, 1992). Simply having

**Table 6.5.**

Type of Social Support

| Type | Description |
|------|-------------|
| Esteem (emotional) | The support an older adult receives from being esteemed, respected, and accepted by others — approval, encouragement, sympathy, and affection are often included (Winemiller et al., 1993) |
| Informational (intangible) | Involves advice, referral, guidance, encouragement, and education of the older adult receiving support (Heitzmann & Kaplan, 1988; Cohen & Wills, 1985) |
| Companionship | Refers to spending time with others in both recreational and leisure activities (Winemiller et al., 1993) |
| Instrumental (tangible) | Includes physical support, financial support, and transportation (Heitzmann & Kaplan, 1988) |
| Global (undifferentiated) | Used for measures of support that are broad and cover one or more of the types of support previously described (Winemiller et al., 1993) |

someone around to remind an older adult to take his or her medication will aid in compliance.

Traditionally, measures of social support encompass two types of questions because measures of objective and subjective support differ. The first type of question regards the amount of support an individual receives, such as the number of caregivers and the frequency of care provided (see Zimet et al., 1988); (Procidano & Heller, 1983; Sarason, et al., 1983; Barrera et al., 1981; Norbeck, Lindsey, & Carrieri, 1981; Henderson, et al., 1980; Linn, et al., 1969). The second type of question includes assessments of how satisfied the individual is with the amount, frequency, and adequacy of social support that he or she receives (Kane, 1995; Sarason et al., 1983; Barrera et al., 1981; Norbeck et al., 1981; Henderson et al., 1980). Therefore, it is important to establish the context and purpose for assessing social support. The purpose could be to assess the frequency and sources of support that an individual receives from others or to determine if there are individuals who are available to perform specific tasks. There can be limitations to measuring social support in institutional settings because older adults who reside in institutions tend to be more physically and cognitively impaired than individuals living in the community. Being in-

stitutionalized means that there is greater availability of formal support (Newsom et al., 1997).

Social support can be assessed with the Inventory for Socially Supportive Behaviors (Barrera et al., 1981), Interview Schedule for Social Interaction (Henderson et al., 1980), Perceived Social Support–Family and Friends Scale (Procidano & Heller, 1983), Multidimensional Scale of Perceived Social Support (Zimet et al., 1988), Social Support Questionnaire (Sarason et al., 1983), Norbeck's Social Support Questionnaire (Norbeck et al., 1981), or the Social Dysfunction Rating Scale (Linn et al., 1969).

### Inventory for Socially Supportive Behaviors (ISSB) (Barrera et al., 1981)

The ISSB was developed as a general measure of social support and includes social factors, instrumental support, informational support, and companionship (Table 6.6). It uses a self-report format and consists of 40 items. The respondent is asked to report on a five point scale the frequency with which other people provided support for him or her or engaged in activities with him or her during the previous month. The ISSB has been used on a variety of populations, including older adults (Barrera et al., 1981).

The psychometric properties of the ISSB

**Table 6.6.**

The Inventory of Socially Supportive Behaviors

Indicate how often these activities happened to you during the past 4 weeks:

   A. Not at all
   B. Once or twice
   C. About once a week
   D. Several times a week
   E. About every day

During the past 4 weeks, how often did other people do these activities for you, to you, or with you:

1. Looked after a family member when you were away
2. Was right there with you (physically) in a stressful situation
3. Provided you with a place where you could get away for awhile
4. Watched after your possessions when you were away (pets, plants, home, apartment, etc.)
5. Told you what she or he did in a situation that was similar to yours
6. Did some activity with you to help you get your mind off of things
7. Talked with you about some interests of yours
8. Let you know that you did something well
9. Went with you to someone who could take action
10. Told you that you are OK just the way you are
11. Told you that she or he would keep things that you talk about private—just between the two of you
12. Assisted you in setting a goal for yourself
13. Made it clear what was expected of you
14. Expressed esteem or respect for a competency or personal quality of yours
15. Gave you some information on how to do something
16. Suggested some action that you should take
17. Gave you over $25
18. Comforted you by showing you some physical affection
19. Gave you some information to help you understand a situation you were in
20. Provided you with some transportation
21. Checked back with you to see if you followed the advice you were given
22. Gave you under $25
23. Helped you understand why you didn't do something well
24. Listened to you talk about your private feelings
25. Loaned or gave you something (a physical object other than money) that you needed
26. Agreed that what you wanted to do was right
27. Said things that make your situation clearer and easier to understand
28. Told you how he or she felt in a situation that was similar to yours
29. Let you know that he or she will always be around if you need assistance
30. Expressed interest and concern in your well-being
31. Told you that she or he feels very close to you
32. Told you who you should see for assistance
33. Told you what to expect in a situation that was about to happen
34. Loaned you over $25
35. Taught you how to do something
36. Gave you feedback on how you were doing without saying it was good or bad
37. Joked and kidded to try to cheer you up
38. Provided you with a place to stay
39. Pitched in to help you do something that needed to get done
40. Loaned you under $25

include test–retest reliability on a sample of 71 undergraduates of 0.88 after 2 days. Correlation coefficients ranged from 0.44 to 0.91, and alphas ranged from 0.93 to 0.94. Validity has been established through a correlation between the ISSB and Moos' Cohesion subscale of the Family Environment Questionnaire and network size of 0.36. There was also a 0.42 correlation between the ISSB and the Arizona Social Support Interview Schedule (Barrera et al., 1981).

One important feature of the ISSB is that it examines both the subjective and objective components of social support. It is a relatively short instrument that respondents can answer without the assistance of an interviewer or provider. This makes it a tool that can be used in both clinical and research settings.

### Interview Schedule for Social Interaction (ISSI) (Henderson et al., 1980)

The ISSI was developed as a research instrument to measure the availability and perceived adequacy of social relationships (Table 6.7). This scale is based on the concept that attachment is provided by close relationships and gives individuals a sense of security. It includes four dimensions of social support: esteem; instrumental; companionship; and global dimensions of social support that measure both quantity and quality. In addition, it measures perceived, provisional, and structural support (Henderson et al., 1980). The ISSI is an interview with closed-ended questions to which the respondent answers "yes" or "no." It takes about 45 minutes to complete (Heitzmann & Kaplan, 1988).

The ISSI assesses the close intimate relationships that individuals have with their families, parents, and close friends as well as relationships with others such as neighbors, coworkers, and acquaintances. In addition to assessing the number of relationships that the individual has, satisfaction with these relationships is also assessed. The interviewer suggests a specific type of social relationship and asks the respondent

if he or she has had such a relationship. Then the interviewer asks if the intensity of the relationship is adequate. In addition, the interviewer asks the respondent to name the person who is the main provider of the particular type of relationship. The information is then summarized in a table that records the degree of closeness of the respondent to each of the individuals to whom he or she mentioned having ties. The table is then used to indicate the accessibility of support resources available to the respondent as well as indicating the extent to which support is concentrated on many or few individuals in the respondent's social network (Henderson et al., 1980).

Each question is answered dichotomously (yes or no), and the questions allotted to each dimension are added up, with each item being given equal weighting (Henderson et al., 1980). The psychometric properties include internal consistency ranging from 0.67 to 0.79. Test–retest correlations after 18 days range from 0.71 to 0.76 (Henderson et al., 1980). Validity was established by showing significant differences between groups. The scales were able to discriminate between individuals who were new to a city compared with individuals who were permanent residents. A separate study showed that the ISSI was able to differentiate between married individuals and individuals who were separated or divorced (Henderson, 1981; Henderson et al., 1980). Validity has been extensively investigated and has shown that the schedule is likely to be measuring those constructs that it purports to examine. Correlations between the scale scores and the Eysenck Personality Inventory ranged from 0.18 to 0.31, and correlation between the respondent's scores and an informant's score reflecting his or her perception of the respondent's social behavior ranged from 0.26 to 0.59 (Henderson et al., 1980).

The ISSI attempts to identify the frequency of contacts with intimate relatives and friends as well as acquaintances. It

**Table 6.7.** Selected Questions from the Interview Schedule for Social Interaction*

Now let's consider people you exchange a word or two with: that is, someone serving you in a shop or in an office, but whom you normally don't see apart from at their work.

1. Most days, how many people like this do you see?
2. Would you like more or less of this, or is it about right?
3. On most days, how many people do you see whom you know just a little, to smile or wave to, or to say good morning to? People you do not know well—you may not know their names—but you greet each other when you pass by.
4. Is this about right for you, or do you wish you saw more or fewer such people?
5. These days, how many people with similar interests to you do you have contact with?
6. Would you like more or less of this, or is it about right? (persons, duration, or frequency)
7. In an ordinary week, how many people whom you know would you say you have contact with?
8. Would you like more or less of this, or is it about right for you? (persons, duration, or frequency)
9. At present, do you wish there were more or less or are there about the right number of people in your day-to-day life?
10. I have been talking about people you may know a little but not call them all close friends. At this time last year, would you have said there were more such people in your life than now, fewer than now, or about the same number as now?
11. How many friends do you have who could come to your home at any time and take things as they find them—they wouldn't be embarrassed if the house were untidy or you were in the middle of a meal?
12. Would you prefer more or less of this, or is it about right for you?
13. How many friends do you have whom you could visit at any time without waiting for an invitation. You could arrive without being expected and still be sure you would be welcome.
14. Would you like to have more or fewer friends like this, or is it about right for you?
15. Overall, would you say you belong to a close circle of friends—a group of people who all keep in close touch with each other—or not?
16. Would you like more or less of this, or is this about right for you? (persons, duration, or frequency)
17. People differ in how much they need friendship. Would you say you are the sort of person who can manage without friends or not? If the answer is cannot manage without friends: A) Do you prefer to do without friends or would you prefer to have them?
18. Among your family and friends, how many people are there who are immediately available to whom you can talk with frankly, without having to watch what you say? If the answer is not none: A) Would you like to have more or less people like this, or is it about right for you? B) With the one (those) you have, would you like to feel more free to be frank or is it about right? C) Who is this mainly (fill in one only on the Attachment Table) If no one: D) Do you wish there were someone or not?
19. Would you say you have a single, lasting relationship, someone you intend to go on sharing your life with or not? If yes: A) Who is this (fill in only one on the Attachment Table)? B) Do you wish you felt more certain of this or not? If no one: C) Do you wish there were someone, or do you prefer to be unattached right now?
20. May I ask if anyone close to you has died in the last few years? If yes: A) Who was it (fill in on Attachment Table)? B) When was that? C) Would you say you still think about this person?

*Scoring of ISSI is done on the basis of dividing the questions into four dimensions: AVAT, the Availability of Attachment; ADAT, the perceived Adequacy of Attachment; AVSI, the Availability of Social Integration; ADSO, the Adequacy of Social Integration.

also addresses the number of unpleasant interactions that individuals have with others as well as the number of relationships that have been lost and the reasons for these losses (Kane et al., 1985). Intended uses of the ISSI include continuing to study the relationship between social relationships and morbidity (Henderson et al., 1980; Berkman & Syme, 1979), assessing the adequacy of an individual's social network, and assessing the social resources of individuals such as older adults who are already at increased risk of morbidity (Henderson et al., 1980).

### Perceived Social Support–Family and Friends Scale (PSS-Fa; PSS-Fr) (Procidano & Heller, 1983)

The combined PSS scales were developed to measure an individual's perception of support (Table 6.8). The scale consists of two parts, one part to assess the support that an individual perceives to receive from family and a second part to assess perceived support received from friends. In addition, there are some items that measure the reciprocity of support that the respondent provides to individuals in his or her network (Lindsey, 1997). Each part is a 20 item self-report scale that assesses whether the individual perceives that his or her needs for support, information, and feedback are being met by his or her family and friends. In addition, the scale measures perception, provision, and orientation of social support (Procidano & Heller, 1983).

The psychometric properties of the scale include a test–retest reliability over a 1 month period of 0.83. The Cronbach's alpha for the PSS-Fr was 0.88, and for the PSS-Fa it was 0.90. Reliability was established based on a sample of 222 students. Construct validity was shown by both subscales, proving to be a better predictor of psychiatric symptomatology than life events or structural characteristics of support networks (Procidano & Heller, 1983).

This tool measures the reciprocity of social support by asking the respondent questions about both the support that they receive and the support they provide to others. These scales are also unique in that they separate the support received from family members from the support that they receive from friends. The premise of this separation is that the sources of these two categories of support represent different aspects of an individual's social relations (Lindsey, 1997).

### Multidimensional Scale of Perceived Social Support (MSPSS) (Zimet et al., 1988)

The MSPSS is a 12 item battery that assesses the adequacy of an individual's perceived social support from family, friends, and significant others (Table 6.9). Respondents use a Likert-type scale to rate each item from Very Strongly Agree to Very Strongly Disagree.

Psychometric properties have been tested and are sound for use in nonpsychiatric samples (Dahlem, Zimet, & Walker, 1991; Zimet et al., 1988). Internal consistency has been established with undergraduates, adolescents, and pediatric residents. Chronbach's alphas have been obtained for the scale as a whole (0.88) and for each subscale: significant other (0.91), family (0.87), and friends (0.85; Zimet et al., 1988). Test–retest after 2 to 3 months was 0.85 for the entire scale and 0.72 for the significant other subscale, 0.85 for the family subscale, and 0.75 for the friends subscale (Zimet et al., 1988). Construct validity has also been established when social support measured in the MSPSS has been shown to correlate negatively with both depression and anxiety. In addition, the MSPSS correlates only minimally with other measures of social desirability, showing that it has convergent validity (Zimet et al., 1988; Cecil, et al., 1995). Cecil and colleagues have shown that the psychometric properties hold for psychiatric patients as well as the general public.

Because it is short, reliable, and valid, the MSPSS is useful as a research tool, and it can be used in research and clinical prac-

**Table 6.8.** The Perceived Social Support—Friends (top) and Family (bottom) Scales

---

*Directions: The statements that follow refer to feelings and experiences that occur to most people at one time or another in their relationships with friends. For each statement there are three possible answers: Yes, No, Don't Know. Please circle the answer you choose for each item.*

1. My friends give me the moral support I need
2. Most other people are closer to their friends than I am
3. My friends enjoy hearing about what I think
4. Certain friends come to me when the have problems or need advice
5. I rely on my friends for emotional support
6. If I felt that one or more of my friends were upset with me, I'd just keep it to myself
7. I feel that I'm on the fringe in my circle of friends
8. There is a friend I could go to if I were just feeling down, without feeling funny about it later
9. My friends and I are very open about what we think about things
10. My friends are sensitive to my personal needs
11. My friends come to me for emotional support
12. My friends are good at helping me solve problems
13. I have a deep sharing relationship with a number of friends
14. My friends get good ideas about how to do things or make things from me
15. When I confide in friends, it makes me feel uncomfortable
16. My friends seek me out for companionship
17. I think that my friends feel that I'm good at helping them solve problems
18. I don't have a relationship with a friend that is as intimate as other people's relationships with friends
19. I recently got a good idea about how to do something from a friend
20. I wish my friends were much different

*Directions: The statements that follow refer to feelings and experiences that occur to most people at one time or another in their relationships with their families. For each statement there are three possible answers: Yes, No, Don't Know. Please circle the answer you choose for each item.*

1. My family gives me the moral support I need
2. I get good ideas about how to do things or make things from my family
3. Most other people are closer to their family than I am
4. When I confide in the members of my family who are closest to me, I get the idea that it makes them uncomfortable
5. My family enjoys hearing about what I think.
6. Members of my family share many of my interests
7. Certain members of my family come to me when they have problems or need advice
8. I rely on my family for emotional support
9. There is a member of my family I could go to if I were just feeling down, without feeling funny about it later
10. My family and I are very open about what we think about things
11. My family is sensitive to my personal needs
12. Members of my family come to me for emotional support
13. Members of my family are good at helping me solve problems
14. I have a deep sharing relationship with a number of members of my family
15. Members of my family get good ideas about how to do things or make things from me
16. When I confide in members of my family, it makes me uncomfortable
17. Members of my family seek me out for companionship
18. I think that my family feels that I'm good at helping them solve problems
19. I don't have a relationship with a member of my family that is as close as other people's relationships with family members
20. I wish my family were much different

**Table 6.9.** Multidemensional Scale of Perceived Social Support

1. There is a special person who is around when I am in need
2. There is a special person with whom I can share my joys and sorrows
3. My family really tries to help me
4. I get the emotional help and support I need from my family
5. I have a special person who is a real source of comfort to me
6. My friends really try to help me
7. I can count on my friends when things go wrong
8. I can talk about my problems with my family
9. I have friends with whom I can share my joys and sorrows
10. There is a special person in my life who cares about my feelings
11. My family is willing to help me make decisions
12. I can talk about my problems with my friends

Source: Dahlem et al. (1991).

tice as a way to assess social support. Eker and Arkar (1995) found that that factor structure of the MSPSS was stable in a cross-cultural study in Turkey. The measure had good internal consistency as well as construct validity.

*Social Support Questionnaire (SSQ)*
*(Sarason et al., 1983)*

SSQ is a measure of both the availability of social support and the respondent's satisfaction with the support that he or she receives (Table 6.10). The questionnaire was designed to study the association between social support and health because

**Table 6.10.** Items from the Social Support Questionnaire

1. Whom can you really count on to listen to you when you need to talk?
2. Whom could you really count on to help you out in a crisis situation, even though they would have to go out of their way to do so?
3. Whom can you really count on to be dependable when you need help?
4. With whom can you totally be yourself?
5. Who do you feel really appreciates you as a person?
6. Whom can you count on to console you when you are very upset?

Source: Sarason et al. (1983).

Sarason and colleagues (1983) postulate that social support leads to personal development and positive adjustment and serves as a buffer against life stress. The questionnaire was designed as a self-administered, 27 item research instrument to measure esteem and global, informational, perceived, structural, and provisional social support. Each item has two responses: *(1)* list the individuals who provide support under specific circumstance and *(2)* rate the level of satisfaction with the support that is available. The scale yields two scores, a number (N) score and a satisfaction (S) score. The number score is the sum of the numbers of persons who provide support in each of the six items divided by six. The satisfaction score is obtained by rating each item from a 1, Very Dissatisfied, to a 6, Very Satisfied. The average of the six items is then the satisfaction score (Sarason et al., 1983).

The psychometric properties of the SSQ include a test–retest reliability of 0.90 overall and 0.83 for the satisfaction score based on 105 students after a 4 week period. Interitem correlations for the number scores had a mean of 0.54 (range 0.35–0.71). The alpha coefficient for internal reliability was 0.97. For satisfaction scores, the interitem correlations ranged from 0.21 to 0.72, and the alpha coefficient was 0.94. Validity was established by comparing the SSQ with the Multiple Affect Adjective Check List (MAACL) and the Lack of Protection Scale (LP). Negative correlations between the SSQ-S and the SSQ-N and items in the MAACL that measured emotional discomfort were found to be significant. Additionally, there were also negative correlations between items measuring recollections of separation anxiety in childhood on the LP and items on the SSQ. Further validation comes from a comparison of the Extroversion and Neuroticism scales of the Eysenck Personality Inventory that resulted in negative correlations with the SSQ-S but were only significant for women (McDowell & Newell, 1996; Sarason et al., 1983).

This scale counts the number of individuals who are available to the respondent to provide support as well as asks the respondent how satisfied he or she is with the support. It is important to assess both the subjective and objective components, and this scale does both. In addition, it is a short, self-administered format, which makes it easy to use in research.

*Norbeck Social Support Questionnaire (NSSQ) (Norbeck et al., 1981; Norbeck, Lindsey, & Carrieri, 1983)*

The NSSQ was designed to measure the multiple dimensions of social support, including the social, esteem, global, companionship, and instrumental aspects of social support, as well as the perception, orientation, and structure of the support (Table 6.11). This questionnaire is a self-report measure that takes about 10 minutes to complete. The questionnaire first asks the respondent to think about and identify all of the people who provide personal support or who are important to them and about the relationship of those people to the respondent. After listing up to 20 network members, respondents are asked to rate each of their network members on nine questions about the functional properties of social support (affect, affirmation, and aid), the duration of their relationship, the frequency of contact, and recent losses in social support. Responses are on a Likert scale from Not at All to A Great Deal. Scoring is done by transferring responses from the questionnaire onto a one page scoring sheet. For the first eight questions, the respondent's ratings for each network member are summed to determine the score for that item. If the number in the network reported by the respondent is eight, then the score for that item is eight. Question nine regarding recent losses of important relations is a dichotomous yes/no answer; the number of losses is determined by summing the number of categories that the respondent checks, and the quality of the losses is scored by transferring the respondent's rating on the 5 point scale provided (Norbeck et al., 1981).

Psychometric properties of this scale have been well tested (Norbeck et al., 1981, 1983) and include test–retest reliabilities ranging from 0.85 to 0.98. Internal consistency coefficients ranged from 0.69 to 0.98. Concurrent validity for the NSSQ was established based on a modest ($-0.03$ to 0.56) positive correlation with Shaefer, Coyne, and Lazarus' Social Sup-

**Table 6.11.** Questions for Rating Network Members on the Norbeck Social Support Questionnaire

1. How much does this person make you feel liked or loved? (Affect)
2. How much does this person make you feel respected or admired? (Affect)
3. How much can you confide in this person? (Affirmation)
4. How much does this person agree with or support your actions or thoughts? (Affirmation)
5. If you needed to borrow $10, a ride to the doctor, or some other immediate help, how much could this person usually help? (Aid—short term)
6. If you were confined to bed for several weeks, how much could this person help you? (Aid—long term)
7. How long have you know this person? (Duration of the relationship)
8. How frequently do you usually have contact with this person? (Phone calls, visits, or letters) (Frequency of contact)
9. During the past year, have you lost any important relationship due to moving, a job change, divorce or separation, death, or some other reason? (Recent loss)
   a. If Yes, check the category(s) of persons who are no longer available to you. (9 categories listed)
   b. How much support did this person (or persons) provide for you during the past 6 months?

Source: Norbeck et al. (1981).

port Questionnaire. In addition, discriminate validity was established by the lack of correlation between the NSSQ and relevant segments of the Profile of Mood States that deal with psychiatric symptomatology and negative mood. The authors also found no correlation between the NSSQ and the Marlowe-Crowne Social Desirability Scale, which shows that there is no response bias in the measure (Norbeck et al., 1981).

The NSSQ is a short, self-report measure that taps many important aspects of social support. For this reason it is a good tool to use if one is interested in assessing loss, network, and functional aspects of support (Lindsey, 1997). The NSSQ is one of the few measures of social support that has been used successfully with residents

in nursing homes (Newsom et al., 1997). This makes this questionnaire a desirable tool for researchers interested in examining social support within an institutional setting.

### Social Dysfunction Rating Scale (SDRS) (Linn et al., 1969; Linn, 1988)

The SDRS was developed as an interview tool to assess the negative aspects of an individual's social adjustment, and it takes 30 minutes to administer (Table 6.12). It was designed as a research tool for use with elderly individuals to assess the meaningfulness in their lives, their goals, and their satisfaction. This assessment contains 21 items that deal with the respondent's self-image, interpersonal relationships, and lack of success and dissat-

**Table 6.12.**
Social Dysfunction Rating Scale

*Directions: Score each of the items as follows: 1, Not Present; 2, Very Mild; 3, Mild; 4, Moderate; 5, Severe; 6, Very Severe.*

| Self System |
|---|
| 1. Low self-concept (feelings of inadequacy, not measuring up to self ideal) |
| 2. Goallessness (lack of inner motivation and sense of future orientation) |
| 3. Lack of a satisfying philosophy or meaning of life (a framework for integrating past and present experiences) |
| 4. Self-health concern (preoccupation with physical health, somatic concerns) |

| Interpersonal System |
|---|
| 1. Emotional withdrawal (degree of deficiency in relating to others) |
| 2. Hostility (degree of aggression toward others) |
| 3. Manipulation (exploiting of environment, controlling at others' expense) |
| 4. Overdependency (degree of parasitic attachment to others) |
| 5. Anxiety (degree of feeling of uneasiness, impending doom) |
| 6. Suspiciousness (degree of distrust or paranoid ideation) |
| 7. Lack of satisfying relationships with significant persons (spouse, children, kin, significant persons serving in family role) |

| Performance System |
|---|
| 1. Lack of friends, social contacts |
| 2. Expressed need for more friends, social contacts |
| 3. Lack of work (remunerative or nonremunerative, productive work activities that normally give a sense of usefulness, status, confidence) |
| 4. Lack of satisfaction from work |
| 5. Lack of leisure time activities |
| 6. Expressed need for more leisure, self-enhancing, and satisfying activities |
| 7. Lack of participation in community activities |
| 8. Lack of interest in community affairs and activities that influence others |
| 9. Financial insecurity |
| 10. Adaptive rigidity (lack of complex coping patterns to stress) |

Source: Linn et al. (1969) and Linn (1988).

isfaction in social situations. The scale uses a combination of the interviewer's evaluations with the respondent's own evaluation. For example, the interviewer will first rate the availability of social contacts and then ask the respondent if he or she feels that he or she needs more friends (Linn et al., 1969). Scoring of the SDRS is based on the subjective answers to questions on a scale from 1, Not Present, to 6, Very Severe (Gallo et al., 1995).

The psychometric properties of the SDRS include inter-rater reliability that ranged from 0.54 to 0.86. Validity was demonstrated by distinguishing between psychiatric and nonpsychiatric subjects with a 93% success rate. Significant correlations (0.89) between the total score on the scale and global judgments of adjustment made by social workers have been demonstrated (Linn et al., 1969).

The scale is useful in a research context when it is necessary to assess the changes that occur due to treatment, and it can also be used as an independent measure of social dysfunction (Linn et al., 1969). This scale is broad in nature and will be similar to measures designed to measure satisfaction and quality of life (McDowell & Newell, 1996).

## Social Networks

Social networks are the web of individuals and services, both formal and informal, in which older adults interact (O'Reilly, 1988). Social networks are necessary but not sufficient for social support. A social network can be in place without providing adequate social support for an older adult.

Interactive relationships that individuals have can be formal, informal, and semiformal. Informal support networks are made up of individuals the older adult selects or who select the older adult and are often based on long-term relationships with friends and family members. Formal support includes adults in social welfare programs, such as Medicare, Medicaid, and Social Security, that provide support to older people (Gallo et al., 1995). Formal

support also includes professionals such as social workers, physicians, and other health care professionals. Finally, semiformal support is provided by community organizations such as religious organizations and senior citizen centers (Gallo et al., 1995).

Social networks fulfill both social and emotional needs. Social networks function in many ways to provide informational support, affective support, social support and stimulation, and tangible help (Kane, 1995). Social networks are often family based across the entire lifespan. There is a notion of filial obligation in which families have a duty to care for their members. Children are supported by their parents, and older adults are supported by their children. As individuals age, their nonfamily interactions decrease so that the family becomes the most important source of social support (Lindsey & Hughes, 1981). When examining social networks, it is important to look at the weight of reciprocity and beneficence in an older adult's life (Antonucci, 1990). Individuals both receive and provide support for one another, and the amount of care received and supplied differs for each individual. There are cultural variables that need to be considered when assessing older adults' social networks. Some ethnic and cultural groups have a great sense of filial obligation, while others do not. This can lead to a greater feeling of obligation to provide care, and, therefore, larger social networks and more available support for some people. In addition, certain ethnic and cultural groups have more of a tradition of respect for elders, which can translate into larger social networks and more support.

Social networks are extremely important for chronically ill and disabled older people who live independently in the community. These networks may help individuals cope with their illnesses, prevent isolation, and provide resources (emotional, physical, and financial) that enable community dwelling older people to remain in their own homes (Lindsey & Hughes, 1981).

Threats to social networks include retirement, bereavement, decreased financial resources, relocation, and declining health. All of these events may reduce social contact and create voids in an individual's social network (Kane & Kane, 1981).

Generally, assessments of social networks cover two types of information: *(1)* quantitative information regarding social networks such as their size, frequency of contact with others, number of activities an individual engages in, and how often the individual participates in those activities, as well as loneliness and social isolation (Kane, 1995); and *(2)* information regarding the older adult's satisfaction with contacts, activities, and interactions, as well as the satisfaction with the frequency with which they occur. Social networks

can be assessed with *Lubben's Social Network Scale* (LSNS; Lubben, 1988).

The LSNS was created as a modified version of the Berkman-Syme Social Network Index (BSNI) for use as a composite measure of social networks among elderly populations (Table 6.13). The BSNI consists of four components: *(1)* marital status, *(2)* nature of relationships with relatives and friends, *(3)* church membership, and *(4)* membership in other organizations and clubs. Lubben dropped the marital status variables and membership in organizations that are part of the BSNI because there is limited variation between these two variables for older adults.

A total score for the LSNS is derived by adding up the total of the individual items for each of the 10 questions, with a sum

Table 6.13.
Lubben's Social Network Scale

1.  How many relatives (including in-laws) do you see or hear from at least once a month? 0 = zero; 1 = 1; 2 = 2; 3 = 3–4; 4 = 5–8; and 5 = 9+

2.  Tell me about the relative with whom you have the most contact? How often do you see or hear from that person? 0 = <monthly; 1 = monthly; 2 = a few times a month; 3 = weekly; 4 = a few times a week; 5 = daily

3.  How many relatives do you feel close to? That is, how many of them do you feel at ease with, can talk to about private matters, or can call on for help? 0 = zero; 1 = 1; 2 = 2; 3 = 3–4; 4 = 5–8; and 5 = 9+

4.  Do you have any close friends? That is, do you have any friends with whom you feel at ease, can talk to about private matters, or can call on for help? 0 = zero; 1 = 1; 2 = 2; 3 = 3–4; 4 = 5–8; and 5 = 9+

5.  How many of these friends do you see or hear from at least once a month? 0 = zero; 1 = 1; 2 = 2; 3 = 3–4; 4 = 5–8; and 5 = 9+

6.  Tell me about the friend with whom you have the most contact. How often do you see or hear from that person? 0 = <monthly; 1 = monthly; 2 = a few times a month; 3 = weekly; 4 = a few times a week; 5 = daily

7.  When you have an important decision to make, do you have someone you can talk to about it? 5 = always; 4 = very often; 3 = often; 2 = sometimes; 1 = seldom; 0 = never

8.  When other people you know have an important decision to make, do they talk to you about it? 5 = always; 4 = very often; 3 = often; 2 = sometimes; 1 = seldom; 0 = never

9a. Does anybody rely on you to do something for them each day? For example, shopping, cooking dinner, doing repairs, cleaning house, providing child care. If yes, score 5 points and go on to Q10. If no, go on to Q9b

9b. Do you help anybody with things like shopping, filling out forms, doing repair, providing child care, etc.? 5 = always; 4 = very often; 3 = often; 2 = sometimes; 1 = seldom; 0 = never

10. Do you live alone or with other people? 5 = lives with spouse; 4 = lives with other relatives or friends; 1 = lives with other unrelated individuals; 0 = lives alone

Source: Lubben (1988).

between 0 and 50. This tool can be used as a screening tool for examining whether an older adult is at risk of isolation. A score under 30 indicates that the older adult may be socially isolated (Lubben, 1988). All 10 items in the scale are highly correlated, which means that they represent a common construct — social networks — with a Chronbach's alpha of 0.70. Validity was established by comparing the relationship between the LSNS and three other indicators of health, including the dichotomous variable of whether a respondent had been hospitalized during 6 or more days during the year after the survey; the LSI-A, which is a measure of mental health; and the Belloc-Breslow checklist of seven health practices. The correlations between the LSNS and the three other health measures were significant (Lubben, 1988).

This scale is a short measure of social networks that was specifically designed for use in research on older adults. Because the tool has only 10 questions and is easy to administer and score, it can be easily adapted for use in clinical settings as well (Lubben, 1988).

## Social Resources

Social resources are the tangible resources available to older adults. They include financial, housing, neighborhood, and community resources (Kane, 1995). Most geriatric assessment tools do not include measures of social resources (Kane, 1995). Inclusion of social resources in general measures of social functioning is necessary because, without adequate social resources, an individual is not able to function. In addition, assessment of social resources may trigger inclusion in publicly funded programs for services such as Social Security Income (SSI) and Medicaid if an older adult meets eligibility requirements. Older adults may not know that they are eligible for such programs and thus these tools can be used as screening instruments. It is important to collect information about social resources when assessing social functioning because it helps

determine the options available for the older adult (Kane, 1987). Like social support, social resources appear to provide a buffer against the stressors in individuals' lives as well as acting as moderators of physical and psychological health and well-being (Heitzmann & Kaplan, 1988). Gathering this information can assist in determining whether the older adult is able to function independently and what sort of interventions and services may be needed but not provided.

Instead of using a particular scale for assessment of social resources, clinicians and researchers often ask questions about the information in which they are interested, such as the older person's income, assets, housing, and community (Kane, 1995). Additionally, questions about the composition of the household, available resources for support, adequacy of housing, and availability of transportation should be asked. Subscales of the Older Americans Resources and Services Multidimensional Functional Assessment Questionnaire (Pfeiffer, 1975) can be used to assess social resources. The OARS questionnaire is discussed later.

## Social Roles and Role Functioning

Atchley (1997) defines roles as behaviors that are associated with positions within the organization of a group. Some activities do not involve interaction with other individuals such as being a painter or writer, but ordinarily roles come from a particular relationship between individuals. Adults have marital, parental, familial, occupational, and community roles (Weissman, 1975).

Assessing social roles and role functioning is difficult because both are complex. Over the lifespan, people occupy many roles that continually change with circumstance. Individuals have involuntary roles such as those brought by age, gender, and ethnicity and by their specific position within the family (e.g., sibling, grandparent) as well as achieved roles such as spouse, caregiver, volunteer, parent, and vocation (Kane, 1995). Because individuals occupy many roles simultaneously and relationships between roles are complex, it is difficult to include every aspect of an individual's position when making assessments regarding social roles and role functioning.

Social role theory states that a person is adjusted socially if he or she can perform adequately compared with standard social expectations (Barrabee, Barrabee, & Finesinger, 1995). This makes assessment of social roles and role functioning difficult because determining what is adequate for an individual, as well as determining what standard social expectations are, is complex. For an individual recovering from an acute episode, standard social expectations relate to fulfilling the roles that the individual had before the acute episode. One way to define social expectations is to compare an individual's roles and functioning with that of other individuals with the same chronic illness or disability. If a person cannot meet social expectations, he or she is said to be socially disabled (McDowell & Newell, 1996).

There are two hypotheses regarding how social roles affect health. One hypothesis states that having many roles strains and overloads an individual, which may result in poorer physical and mental health. The opposing hypothesis states that multiple roles provide individuals with purpose and meaning, which may result in positive physical and mental health outcomes. Empirical evidence supports the second hypothesis (Rushing, Ritter, & Burton, 1992).

Lindsey & Hughes (1981) found that as individuals age, there is a decrease in the number of roles that they may have. This in turn decreases the number of networks to which individuals can relate, as well as the amount of interaction and variety of social contacts. Retirement is an example of an event that leads to a decrease in the number of roles an older adult has as well as potentially decreasing an older adult's social network.

Assessment of social roles and role functioning is done to evaluate the number of different types of roles older adults have, such as mentor, grandparent, retiree, widow, dependent, mediator, resident of a long-term care facility, peer counselor, financial manager, friend, pet owner, member of a particular cultural group, leader in the community, parent, and spouse. It is also important to assess whether older adults are able to function in their social roles or whether some physical or mental health problem inhibits their ability to function. In addition, the older adult's satisfaction with his or her social roles and role functioning should be assessed. One conceptual issue that needs to be dealt with concerning assessment of social roles and role functioning is how to evaluate an individual's functioning. Should expectations and ability be compared with the individual's aspirations or with society's expectations (McDowell & Newell, 1996)? This is especially compelling when dealing with older adults because of the extreme variations in health, wealth, interests, and abilities among individuals in this cohort. We cannot assume that the number of roles an individual has represents functioning. Therefore, it is vital to assess both subjectively and objectively in order to ensure that the older adult has roles, is functioning in his or her roles, and is satisfied with the roles he or she has. Rather than using a formal assessment instrument, clinicians often simply ask their patients what their roles are and whether or not their illnesses or disabilities interfere with their regular role functioning. Roles can be assessed using the *Role Count Index* (RCI).

The RCI (Cumming & Henry, 1961) was created to determine the number of roles that an older adult has as part of an extensive interview for the Kansas City Study of Adult Life, which was used to study older adults' engagement. The index is sensitive to age differences as well as age-specific patterns of relationships (Cumming & Henry, 1961). To determine a score for the RCI, a short questionnaire about social interactions, the *Lifespace Measure*, needs to be administered (Table 6.14). Following the administration of the Lifespace Measure, the interviewer can determine the score for the Role Count Index (Table 6.15).

Because the RCI is short, user friendly, and easy to score, it is a useful tool for assessing older adults' social roles. The main drawback to this index is that its validity and reliability have not been formally tested.

## Activities

There are two general reasons that an older person's social activities are assessed. Clinicians and researchers may be interested in an older adult's preferences, expectations, and level of activity before they make suggestions for treatment or evaluate how effective a particular treatment has been. Social activity is also assessed because it allows clinicians and researchers to estimate the needs of older adults and determine whether they have an adequate level of social stimulation and involvement or whether there are limitations (physical, mental, social) that keep them from enjoying valued activities (Kane, 1987). These assessments can be used to determine what adaptations should be made in order for the older adults to overcome their limitations.

In assessing an older adult's activities, it is necessary to obtain specific information regarding the individual's present or former occupation, his or her leisure-time pleasures, how often the individual leaves home, whether the individual still drives, religiosity, participation in volunteer work or social clubs, and what types of entertainment the individual enjoys (Kane, 1987). This establishes whether the older adult is doing what he or she likes and being active or if he or she is inactive and, therefore bored and/or lonely. In addition, information regarding the older adult's expectations for participation in activities such as sports, reading, game playing, watching television, shopping, and working as well as his or her level of satisfac-

---

**Table 6.14.**

Lifespace Measure

1. When you were last interviewed, there were ___ (No. in household) living here. Are the same number of persons living here now?
2. Last time, you mentioned _____ (whoever mentioned in Interview 2) as the relatives you feel closest to. Is that right?
3. How often do you get together with these relatives?
4. How many people whom you know do you consider close friends — that is, people you can confide in and talk over personal matters with? (Get respondent to give you a specific number if possible.)
5. Now, about the friends you're closest to — about how often do you get together with any of them?
6. Now, about people you see for certain specific purposes-like storekeepers, bus drivers, waiters, salespeople, and so on — about how many of these people do you see fairly regularly? Would you say _____?
7. Last time, you mentioned _____ (whoever was mentioned in Interview 1) as the neighbors you know best. Is that right?
8. How often do you get together with these neighbors?
9. In the course of a day's work, about how many people do you see and talk to?
10. How often do you attend church?
11. Do you belong to any committees, auxiliaries, or anything like that? (If yes, get a list of all activities.)
12. Now, I'd like you to think over very carefully and tell me if you belong to any groups, clubs, or associations, or anything like that. Do you belong to any such groups? If yes, what are the groups and how often do you attend each? What do you do at each of the groups?

**Table 6.15.**

Scoring of the Role Count Index

1. Number in household: If only one person other than the respondent who lives in the household, count 1. For two or more people, count 2
2. Relatives: For each category of relatives mentioned in Interview 1, count 1. If none, count 0
3. Friends: Count 1 if any friends are mentioned, 0 if none are mentioned
4. Neighbors: Score as for friends
5. Fellow workers: Score 1 if employed, 0 if unemployed
6. Specific people: Score 1 if any mentioned, 0 if none are mentioned
7. Church: Score 1 for membership, 0 if not a member
8. Organizations: Score 1 for each attended, 0 if none

tion with his or her participation should be collected. As is done when assessing social resources and social roles, clinicians may simply ask their patients about their activities and their evaluations of whether or not they are satisfied with them.

Graney and Graney (1974) developed an instrument to measure activity and membership. This instrument was developed for research purposes based on the theory that communicative activity will be substituted for age-related decreases in physical activity, financial losses, and social losses. Graney and Graney (1974) hypothesized that conversing with family and friends, reading newspapers, magazines, and books, listening to the radio and watching television, and belonging to voluntary or religious groups increase as individuals experience decreases in physical activities and losses in other social and financial activities (Kane & Kane, 1981). A longitudinal study was initiated using a 9 item questionnaire (Table 6.16). The measurements were quantitative and divided into a trichotomous measure of low, moderate, and high of the frequency in which individuals engaged in all of the activities (Graney, 1975).

**Table 6.16.**

Activity and Membership Questions

1. About how many hours would you say you watched TV on a day like yesterday? ( ) hours
2. About how many hours would you say you listened to the radio yesterday? ( ) hours
3. About how many hours would you say you read yesterday? ( ) hours
4. Do you visit with your neighbors in the building often? More often than once a day ( ), daily ( ), less than daily ( ), never ( )
5. All in all, how often do you see any of your friends and relatives in the Twin Cities—I mean, people you know pretty well? Several times a week ( ), about once a week ( ), several times a month ( ), less often than once a month ( ), never ( )
6. Do you recall about how many phone calls you made or received yesterday? ( ) calls in and out
7. Do you go to church (or temple)? If yes, about how often? More often than weekly ( ), weekly ( ), monthly ( ), less often than monthly ( ), never ( )
8. Do you attend meetings of any clubs, civic groups, other organizations? If yes, which ones? If yes, do you attend these kinds of meetings often? Weekly ( ), monthly ( ), less often than monthly ( )
9. Do you maintain any organizational memberships? ( ) number of organizational memberships*

*Question addressed, but not directly stated (Graney, 1975; Graney & Graney, 1974).

## General Social Functioning

There have also been some tools developed to assess social functioning in general. Two of these measures are the Psychosocial Adjustment to Illness Scale (Morrow, Chiarello, & Derogatis, 1978) and the OARS questionnaire (Pfeiffer, 1975).

### Psychosocial Adjustment to Illness Scale (PAIS; Morrow et al., 1978)

The PAIS was developed as a multidimensional, semistructured clinical interview to assess the social and psychological adjustment of patients and their families to the patients' illnesses. There are 46 items covering seven domains addressed in the PAIS (Table 6.17).

The PAIS was designed as a semistructured clinical interview because the authors thought this format would increase the flexibility and depth of the assessment of the patient's adjustment. There is also a self-report version of the instrument called the PAIS-SR (Table 6.18) (Derogatis, 1986). Both forms of the PAIS instrument are scored on a four-point scale. For example,

in the extended family relationships domain, patients are asked, "Do you depend on those members of your family for any help or assistance, particularly since your illness?" The possible response set ranges from "totally independent of extended family" to "marked dependency, beyond degree of family commitment." There are independent scores for each domain as well as an overall adjustment score (Morrow et al., 1978).

Psychometric properties of the PAIS include internal consistency of each of the subscales with coefficients ranging from 0.12 to 0.93 (Derogatis, 1986). Inter-rater reliability falls in the "acceptable" range between 0.52 to 0.86 (Derogatis, 1986; Morrow et al., 1978). Validity was established through testing the correlation between the domains and the total score. The coefficients showed a consistent pattern of low intercorrelations among domain scores with high correlations with the total score (Derogatis, 1986). Convergent validity was established through the correlation with external criteria. The PAIS was tested against the Global Adjust-

**Table 6.17.** The Seven Domains Included in the Psychosocial Adjustment to Illness Scale

| Domain | What is assessed |
| --- | --- |
| Health care orientation | The nature of the patient's attitude toward his or her state of health |
| | Whether patient's attitude will promote a positive or negative adjustment to the patient's illness |
| | The patient's overall perception of health care |
| Vocational environment | How the illness will affect the patient's vocational environment, which can include traditional work, school, or home environment |
| Domestic environment | The impact of the illness on the domestic environment is assessed and is oriented toward difficulties that may arise at home or within the family due to illness-related issues |
| Sexual relationships | How the illness will affect the quality of sexual functioning or relationships |
| Extended family relationships | Disruptions of family interactions caused by the illness |
| | Whether the illness has a negative impact on the interactions and relationships within the family |
| Social environment | The adjustment that the patient's illness requires on current social and leisure activities |
| Psychological distress | The negative thoughts and feelings that the patient has that are associated with illness |

**Table 6.18.** Items from the Psychosocial Adjustment to Illness Scale — Self-Report

*Domestic environment (8 items)*

Example: To what degree has your illness interfered with your duties and tasks around the house?

0 = No interference
1 = Slight interference, easily overcome
2 = Substantial impairment in some domestic tasks
3 = Marked impairment, affecting all or nearly all tasks

*Extended family relationships (5 items)*

Example: Do you normally depend on members of your extended family for physical or financial assistance? Has this changed at all since your illness?

0 = No physical or financial dependency on extended family
1 = Some physical or financial dependency on extended family; however, consistent with degree of family commitment
2 = Some physical or financial dependency on extended family, beyond the level of family commitment
3 = Marked physical or financial dependency on extended family, clearly beyond the degree of family commitment

*Social environment (6 items)*

Example: Have you maintained your interests in social activities since your illness (e.g., social clubs, church groups, going to the movies)?

0 = Same level of interest as previously
1 = Slightly less interest than before
2 = Significantly less interest than before
3 = Little or no interest remaining

---

ment to Illness Scale, with a resulting correlation of 0.81 (Derogatis, 1986). It has been shown to be reliable using a diverse group of interviewers (Morrow et al., 1978).

The PAIS is a tool that is good for clinicians and discharge planners who want to know if an individual is able to adjust to his or her illness. This scale is useful to clinicians to compare different patient's adjustment to illness as well as measuring the effectiveness of psychotherapeutic interventions (De-Nour, 1982).

*Older Americans Resources and Services (OARS) Multidimensional Functional Assessment Questionnaire (Pfeiffer, 1975)*

The OARS is often used to assess social functioning in older adults. The OARS Social Resources Scale and Economic Re-sources Scale are two parts of the OARS assessment developed at Duke University. The OARS is probably the most widely used and studied assessment tool for measuring social functioning in older adults. The instrument includes sections to assess economic resources, mental health, activities of daily living, and instrumental activities of daily living. The questionnaire is divided into two parts, the Multidimensional Functional Assessment Questionnaire (MFAQ) and the Services Assessment Questionnaire (SAQ) (Fillenbaum, 1975). Social functioning and social resources are both part of the MFAQ, which consists of 70 questions. The social resources section measures the frequency and depth of social interactions, including satisfaction with social contacts, loneliness, availability of a confidant, and availability of help in case of illness. All of the answers to the social interactions questions are summarized into an overall rating on social resources in a 6 point scale. This score is a weighted combination of objective and subjective information collected by the interviewer. The resulting score rates the individual as having excellent social resources, good social resources, mildly socially impaired, severely socially impaired, or total social impairment (Pfeiffer, 1975).

The economic resources section focuses on evaluating the respondent's employment status, earnings, sources and amount of total income, and home ownership, as well as the respondent's subjective assessment of his or her financial situation. All of the information is compiled into an economic functioning rating on a 6 point scale ranging from Excellent to Satisfactory, Mildly Impaired, Moderately Impaired, Severely Impaired, or Completely Impaired (Pfeiffer, 1975).

The second element in the OARS questionnaire is the SAQ, which measures the amount of services that an individual receives as well as who provides the service, the frequency of the service, and the respondent's perceived need for service (whether he or she is receiving what he or she needs). Some of the generically defined services include transport, social/recreation, employment, health care, homemaker, financial, shopping, housing, and coordination and information services (Fillenbaum, 1975).

The psychometrics of the OARS questionnaire have been extensively tested, and the result is sound reliability and validity. The test–retest reliability after a 5 week interval was 0.91. Inter-rater correlations have been 0.80 or higher, and consistency has also been shown. Validity has been shown by comparison of interviewer summary ratings with external measures and ratings of professionals. Sensitivity has been shown, for the MFAQ has demonstrated discriminatory ability to differentiate between community dwelling older adults and institutional residents (Fillenbaum, 1975).

The OARS instrument is a well-designed, psychometrically proven tool. Because it was designed to measure functioning in older adults, it is an excellent tool for assessing social functioning. This instrument has been psychometrically tested over time, on numerous samples of older adults, and has proved to be a useful tool in both clinical and research settings. The drawback to using the OARS methodology is that it has to be administered by trained interviewers, and, when done in its entirety, it is rather lengthy. An alternate version of the OARS is available for use with individuals who are in institutions. This version adds questions about whether or not a spouse also resides in the institution, how often they leave the facility, how much social interaction they have with others, and whether they have someone outside the institution who could provide assistance if needed (Kane & Kane, 1981; Pfeiffer, 1975).

## CONCLUSION

There are a number of different tools available for researchers and clinicians who want to examine social functioning, but there is no gold standard. No one instrument has been created that taps overall social functioning and includes all of the domains of interest: social support and social networks (number of members, frequency, and adequacy of relationships); activities (frequency and satisfaction); social resources (quantity as well as adequacy); and roles and goals (what they are and whether they are fulfilling and adequate). Is this a problem, or is it satisfactory that there remains to be established a measure of social functioning? In research contexts this can be problematic because researchers want a reliable and valid scale that can be used to measure underlying concepts such as social functioning. Presently, researchers have to include measures from each domain in which they are interested rather than having an aggregate measure of social functioning. In a clinical setting this is much less worrisome. This is because clinicians are often more concerned with specific aspects of social functioning: whether there is support available to assist an older adult or whether an individual has become less active, indicating a physical or psychological illness that is causing the decline in social function.

Quantitative measurement of social functioning should be done so that it can be known whether an older adult has at least a minimum amount of activity, support, and interaction with others. In addition, social functioning should be measured qualitatively in order to discover whether an older adult has someone in whom to confide and to whom to turn in times of crises (Kane et al., 1985). Deciding the purpose for the assessment is the first step. The purpose of the measurement will determine which scale will be useful to gather the required information as well as what factors need assessment and the strategy for collecting the information (Kane & Kane, 1981). Clinicians and researchers also need to determine their older clients' social functioning expectations to know what interventions will be necessary (Kane, 1987). Noticing changes in activity levels and functioning is vital to identifying problems in older adults' social functioning. Thus, changes in social func-

**Table 6.19.** Social Resources and Economic Resources Sections of the Assessment Older Americans Resources and Services

*Social Resources*

1. Are you single, married, widowed, divorced, or separated?
2. Who lives with you? (yes or no to the following)
   No one
   Husband or wife
   Children
   Grandchildren
   Parents
   Grandparents
   Brothers and sisters
   Other relatives
   Friends
   Nonrelated paid helper
   Others (specify) _____
3. How many people do you know well enough to visit with in their homes?
4. About how many times did you talk to someone — friends, relatives, or others — on the telephone in the past week?
5. How many times during the past week did you spend some time with someone who does not live with you, that is, you went to see them or they came to visit you, or you went out to do things together?
6. Do you have someone you can trust and confide in?
7. Do you find yourself feeling lonely quite often, sometimes, or almost never?
8. Do you see your relatives and friends as often as you want to, or are you somewhat unhappy about how little you see them?
9. Is there someone who would give you any help at all if you were sick or disabled, for example, your husband/wife, a member of your family, or a friend?
   If yes, (a) is there someone who would take care of you as long as needed, or only for a short time, or only someone who would help you now and then? (b) Who is this person? Relationship to you?

*Economic Resources*

1. Are you presently (check yes or no)
   Employed full-time
   Employed part-time
   Retired
   Retired on disability
   Not employed and seeking work
   Not employed and not seeking work
   Full-time student
   Part-time student
2. What kind of work have you done most of your life?
   Never employed
   Housewife
   Other (state the specific occupation in detail)
3. Does your husband/wife work or did he/she ever work?
   a. What kind of work did or does he/she do? (describe in detail)
4. Where does your income (money) come from (yours and your husband's/wife's)?
   Earnings from employment
   Income from rental property, interest from investments, etc.
   Social Security
   VA benefits such as GI Bill, and disability payments
   Disability payments not covered by Social Security, SSI, or VA
   Unemployment compensation
   Retirement pension from job
   Alimony or child support
   Scholarships, stipends
   Regular assistance from family members
   SSI payments

. *(continued)*

**Table 6.19.** Social Resources and Economic Resources Sections of the Assessment Older Americans Resources and Services — (Continued)

Regular financial aid from private organizations and churches
Welfare payments or Aid for Dependent Children
Other

5. How much income do you have a year?
6. How many people altogether live on this income?
7. Do you own your own home?
   a. How much is it worth?
   b. Do you own it outright, or are you still paying a mortgage?
8. Are your assets and financial resources sufficient to meet emergencies?
9. Are your expenses so heavy that you cannot meet the payments, or can you barely meet the payments, or are your payments no problem to you?
10. Is your financial situation such that you feel you need financial assistance or help beyond what you are already getting?
11. Do you pay for your own food, or do you get any regular help at all with costs of food or meals?
    a. From where?
12. Do you feel that you need food stamps?
13. Are you covered by any kinds of health or medical insurance?
    a. What kind?
14. Please tell me how well you think you (and your family) are now doing financially compared with other people your age — better, about the same, or worse?
15. How well does the amount of money you have take care of your needs — very well, fairly well, or poorly?
16. Do you usually have enough to buy those little "extras"; that is, those small luxuries?
17. Do you feel that you will have enough for your needs in the future?

Source: Pfeiffer (1975).

tioning may be more important than the actual measured value (Kane, 1987). An example is an individual who has had a great deal of social interaction throughout her lifetime who falls and breaks her hip and refuses to interact with anyone aside from her health care providers. This individual's social functioning has changed dramatically, and intervention is necessary. This change in social functioning should be noted and assessed to determine the underlying etiology and meaning of the behavior and interventions provided accordingly. On the other hand, an individual has always been reclusive and, after an acute illness, continues to have few social contacts, he or she will also probably score poorly on social functioning measures. This low score will not, however, represent an overall change in functioning, and, because social functioning is subjective for each individual, there should be no alarm or need for further assessment or intervention. We also need to respect privacy. If older adults do not want people to see them disabled or in a frail state until they have recovered, it may be better to think of implications of such a role and how it affects social functioning.

## REFERENCES

Antonucci, T. C. (1990). Social supports and social relationships. In R. H. Binstock & L. K. George (Eds.), *Handbook of aging and the social sciences*, Third Edition. San Diego: Academic Press, pp 205–226.

Antonucci, T. C., Sherman, A. M., & Vandewater, E. A. (1997). Measures of social support and caregiver burden. *Generations*, 21, 48–51.

Atchley, R. C. (1997). *Social forces and aging: An introduction to social gerontology* (8th ed.). Belmont, CA: Wadsworth Publishing Company.

Barrabee, P., Barrabee, E. L., & Finesinger, J. E. (1995). A normative social adjustment scale. *American Journal of Psychiatry, 112*, 252–259.

Barrera, M., Sandler, I. N., & Ramsay, T. B. (1981). Preliminary development of a scale of social support: Studies on college students. *American Journal of Community Psychology, 9,* 435–447.

Berkman, L. F., & Syme, S. L. (1979). Social networks, host resistance and mortality: A year follow-up study of Alameda County residents. *American Journal of Epidemiology, 109,* 186–204.

Cassel, J. (1976). The contribution of the social environment to host resistance. *American Journal of Epidemiology, 104*(2), 107–123.

Cecil, H., Stanley, M. A., Carrion, P. G., & Swann, A. (1995). Psychometric properties of the MSPSS and NOS in psychiatric outpatients. *Journal of Clinical Psychology, 51,* 593–602.

Cohen, S., & Wills, T. A. (1985). Stress, social support, and the buffering hypotheses. *Psychological Bulletin, 98,* 310–357.

Cumming, E., & Henry, W. E. (1961). *Growing old: The process of disengagement.* New York: Basic Books.

Dahlem, N. W., Zimet, G. D., & Walker, R. R. (1991). The Multidimensional Scale of Perceived Social Support: A confirmation study. *Journal of Clinical Psychology, 47,* 756–761.

De-Nour, A. K. (1982). Psychosocial Adjustment to Illness Scale (PAIS): A study of chronic hemodialysis patients. *Journal of Psychosomatic Research, 26,* 11–22.

Derogatis, L. R. (1986). The Psychosocial Adjustment to Illness Scale (PAIS). *Journal of Psychosomatic Research, 30,* 77–91.

Eker, D., Arkar, H. (1995). Perceived social support: psychometric properties of the MSPSS in normal and pathological groups in a developing country. *Social Psychiatry and Psychiatric Epidemiology, 30,* 121–126.

Fillenbaum, G. (Ed.). (1975). *The OARS methodology.* Durham, NC: Duke University.

Froland, C., Brodsky, G., Olson, M., & Steward, L. (1979). Social support and social adjustment: Implications for mental health professionals. *Community Mental Health Journal, 15,* 82–93.

Gallo, J. J., Reichel, W., & Andersen, L. M. (1995). *Social assessment. Handbook of geriatric assessment* (2nd ed.). Gaithersburg, MD: Aspen Publishers.

Glass, T. A., & Maddox, G. L. (1992). The quality and quantity of social support: Stroke recovery as psycho-social transition. *Social Science and Medicine, 34*(11), 1249–1261.

Graney, M. J. (1975). Happiness and social participation in aging. *Journal of Gerontology, 30*(6), 701–706.

Graney, M. J., & Graney, E. E. (1974). Communications activity substitutions in aging. *Journal of Communication, 24*(4), 88–96.

Heitzmann, C. A., & Kaplan, R. M. (1988). Assessment of methods for measuring social support. *Health Psychology, 7,* 75–109.

Henderson, A. S., & Brown, G. W. (1988). Social support: The hypothesis and the evidence. In A. S. Henderson & G. D. Burrows (Eds.), *Handbook for social psychiatry.* Amsterdam: Elsevier, pp 73–85.

Henderson, S. (1981). Social relationships, adversity, and neuroses: An analysis of prospective observations. *British Journal of Psychiatry, 138,* 391–399.

Henderson, S., Duncan-Jones, P., Byrne, D. G., & Scott, R. (1980). Measuring social relationships: The interview schedule for social interaction. *Psychological Medicine, 10,* 723–734.

House, J. S., Landis, K. R., & Umberson, D. (1988). Social relationships and health. *Science, 241,* 540–545.

Kane, R. A. (1987). Assessment of social function. *Clinics in geriatric medicine, 3*(1), 87–98.

———. (1995). Assessment of social functioning: Recommendations for comprehensive geriatric assessment. In L. Rubenstein, R. Bernabei, & D. Wieland (Eds.), *Geriatric Assessment Technology: State of the Art.* Milano: Editrice Kurtis.

Kane, R. A., & Kane, R. L. (1981). Measures of social functioning in long-term care, *Assessing the elderly: A practical guide to measurement.* Lexington, MA: DC Heath, pp 133–208.

Kane, R. A., Kane, R. L., & Arnold, S. (1985). *Measuring social functioning in mental health studies: Concepts and instruments* (DHHS Pub. No. [ADM]85–1384). Washington, DC: National Institutes of Mental Health, Series DN, No. 5, Superintendent of Documents, U.S. Government Printing Office.

Lindsey, A. M. (1997). Social support: Conceptualization and measurement instruments. In M. Frank-Stromborg & S. J. Olsen (Eds.), *Instruments for Clinical Health-Care Research.* Sudbury, MA: Jones and Bartlett Publishers, pp 149–176.

Lindsey, A. M., & Hughes, E. M. (1981). Social support and alternatives to institutionalization for the at-risk elderly. *Journal of American Geriatrics Society, 29,* 308–315.

Linn, M. W. (1988). Social Dysfunction Rating Scale (SDRS). *Psychopharmacology Bulletin, 24,* 801–802.

Linn, M. W., Sullthorpe, W. B., Evje, M., Slater, P. H., & Goodman, S. P. (1969). A social dysfunction rating scale. *Journal of Psychiatric Research, 6,* 299–306.

Litwin, H. (1998). Social network type and health status in a national sample of elderly Israelis. *Social Science and Medicine, 46*(4–5), 599–609.

Lubben, J. E. (1988). Assessing social networks among elderly populations. *Family Community Health, 11,* 45–52.

McDowell, I., & Newell, C. (1996). Social health. *Measuring health: A guide to rating scales and questionnaires.* New York: Oxford University Press.

Morrow, G. R., Chiarello, R. J., & Derogatis, L. R. (1978). A new scale for assessing patients' psychosocial adjustment to medical illness. *Psychological Medicine, 8,* 605–610.

Newsom, J. T., Bookwala, J., & Schulz, R. (1997). Social support measurement in group residences for older adults. *Journal of Mental Health and Aging, 3*(1), 47–66.

Norbeck, J. S., Lindsey, A. M., & Carrieri, V. L. (1981). The development of an instrument to measure social support. *Nursing Research, 30*(5), 264–269.

———. (1983). Further development of the Norbeck Social Support Questionnaire: Normative data and validity testing. *Nursing Research, 32,* 4–9.

O'Reilly, P. (1988). Methodological issues in social support and social network research. *Social Science and Medicine, 26,* 863–873.

Pfeiffer, E. (Ed.). (1975). *Multidimensional functional assessment: The OARS methodology.* Durham, NC: Center for the Study of Aging and Human Development.

Procidano, M. E., & Heller, K. (1983). Measures of perceived social support from friends and from family: Three validation studies. *American Journal of Community Psychology, 11,* 1–24.

Rushing, B., Ritter, C., & Burton, R. P. D. (1992). Race differences in the effects of multiple roles on health: Longitudinal evidence from a national sample of older men. *Journal of Health and Social Behavior, 33,* 126–139.

Sarason, I. G., Levin, H. M., Basham, R. B., & Sarason, B. R. (1983). Assessing social support: The social support questionnaire. *Journal of Personality and Social Psychology, 44*(1), 127–139.

Weissman, M. M. (1975). The assessment of social adjustment: A review of techniques. *Archives of General Psychiatry, 32,* 357–375.

Winemiller, D. R., Mitchell, E., Sutliff, J., & Cline, D. J. (1993). Measurement strategies in social support: A descriptive review of the literature. *Journal of Clinical Psychology, 49,* 638–649.

Zimet, G. D., Dahlem, N. W., Zimet, S. G., & Farley, G. K. (1988). The Multidimensional Scale of Perceived Social Support. *Journal of Personality Assessment, 52*(1), 30–41.

# 7

# Assessment of Qualty of Life in Older Adults

JENNIFER R. FRYTAK

Quality of life (QOL) means different things to different people. For some researchers and clinicians, QOL measurement effectively means anything beyond mortality data; for others it is a subjective valuation made by the individual. The concept of overall QOL can include perceptions about almost every aspect of daily existence: standard of living, housing and neighborhood, work, health, marriage, friendships, national life, leisure, government, and education (Andrews & Withey, 1976; Campbell, Converse, & Rodgers, 1976). Work in the health sciences has narrowed the definition to health-related quality of life (HRQL), which limits medical responsibility for outcomes by emphasizing deviations from normal functioning in areas that clinicians deem amenable to medical intervention. When assessing QOL in older adults, the challenge for providers and researchers is to avoid measures of QOL/HRQL that exclude or ineffectively explore areas that are important to an elderly population or worse yet are used in a manner that disadvantages older adults in health resource allocation decisions. In the absence of adequate measures, work should focus on succinctly delineating the domains of QOL that have meaning to older adults. These may or

may not correspond to existing measures of QOL that typically focus on younger and healthier populations.

This chapter provides a framework for conceptualizating QOL and explores the implications of choices among QOL definitions and instruments when measuring QOL in older adults and in general. Several questions are salient:

- Is a QOL instrument measuring what it purports to measure?
- Are the domains of QOL and the weights attached to the domains consistent across the life course?
- Whose valuation of QOL should be used in existing measures?
- Do existing QOL measures disadvantage older adults?
- Should a multiple or single measure approach for gathering QOL information be used?

## IMPORTANCE OF QUALITY OF LIFE (QOL) IN HEALTH-RELATED RESEARCH AND CLINICAL PRACTICE

Before the 1970s, there was little mention of QOL in the social science and medical literature (Katz & Gurland, 1991), but that has changed dramatically over the past two decades (Gill & Feinstein, 1994). There has been an ongoing debate in gerontology about the trade-off that increasing life expectancy at the cost of increasing morbidity represents. While one view is that there will be a compression of morbidity and disability (Fries, 1980), another view is that increasing life expectancy may lead to people living longer but with more disabilities (Verbrugge, 1984) and in less than ideal environments (Kemper & Murtaugh, 1991). For frail older adults, the prospect of extended periods of disability, institutionalization, and shrinking social networks and decision-making capacity in later life have prompted an intense interest in using QOL measures to assess the unintended consequences of long-term care environments. In the context of an acute illness, bombardment by an ever increasing number of life-extending treatments with variable levels of intrusiveness and efficacy has complicated decision-making for both older adults and clinicians. The concept of QOL has been sought as a gold standard for weighing the benefits and costs of life-extending treatments and long-term care environments.

Changing demographics and medical inflation have focused attention on the distribution of scarce social resources and the sustainability of current spending levels for health care (Newhouse, 1993). A proliferation of new medical technology, procedures, and pharmaceuticals has prompted the need to determine the cost-effectiveness of these advances. To keep costs from spiraling, private and public insurers are keenly interested in avoiding coverage of treatments with little or no medical benefit. The result has been to introduce the concept of economic efficiency into the health care system. Measures of effectiveness often take the form of quality-adjusted life years (QALYs), which attempts to combine quantity and quality (weighted by consumer preferences for health states) of life. Quality-adjusted life years are a product of life expectancy or

survival over a set time period (quantity) and an aggregate health score (quality) calculated as illness-related deviations from normal functioning. Quality-adjusted life years are discussed later in the section on implications of choice of QOL measures.

Although not entirely congruous with a cost-effectiveness emphasis, providers and policy makers have shifted their thinking about health from strictly a disease and mortality focus to one emphasizing health, functioning, QOL, and well-being (Greenfield & Nelson, 1992). The World Health Organization (WHO, 1948) defines health as a "state of complete physical, mental, and social well-being and not merely the absence of disease or infirmity." Health-related quality of life measures have proliferated in the health sciences literature (Gill & Feinstein, 1994) and in the increasing role of the federal government in advocating use of HRQL information (Steinwachs, Wu, & Cagney, 1996). The Agency for Health Care Policy and Research was legislated in 1989 to conduct and fund research on medical care effectiveness, including QOL. The Food and Drug Administration encourages inclusion of QOL in trials of experimental drugs before final approval, and the National Institutes of Health has at least an unofficial mandate for inclusion of QOL measures in randomized controlled trials.

An ongoing movement to include the consumer's point of view in health-related measures of medical effectiveness and health plan and provider effectiveness is underway. Because HRQL is generally recognized as a subjective measure, it is seen as a good vehicle for the consumer's point of view in clinical trials, program evaluations, outcomes research, and so forth. Understandably, some blurring of the concepts of satisfaction and QOL has taken place in practice. Treating the two concepts as equivalent may, however, limit the potential of QOL instruments. Distinctions between the two concepts are discussed in a later section.

## CONCEPTUALIZATION OF QUALITY OF LIFE

No consensus exists on a universal definition of QOL. Ongoing debates focus on how broad or narrow, subjective or objective, negative or positive, and so forth one's conceptualization of QOL is. Researchers with subjective conceptualizations of QOL believe that the individual's perception of his or her well-being is most important to understanding QOL. Researchers with objective conceptualizations of QOL believe that the existence of selected conditions evident to all observers that impinge on or bolster well-being is most important to measuring QOL. Early work on QOL (Andrews & Withey, 1976; Campbell et al., 1976) has relied on purely subjective conceptualizations of QOL that were based on the concepts of satisfaction, expectations, and affect. Overall well-being measures, which were aggregations of items based on life satisfaction and affect and life experience domains, were evaluated by degree of satisfaction with the domain.

Quality of Life could be treated as satisfaction with various domains, but it is difficult to divorce the concept from social norms. Many researchers interested in QOL and HRQL believe that poor health is a normatively undesirable state regardless of one's current health status and that institutional environments often have unintended negative consequences for well-being. Moreover, it is possible that expectations for QOL domains decrease with age (Campbell et al., 1976), resulting in older adults being highly satisfied with situations that are socially unacceptable to younger persons. Thus, it is important both to know the perceptions of the individual and to have objective indicators of the phenomenon.

Most clinical and gerontological researchers, however, differentiate the concept of QOL from purely subjective unidimensional concepts such as happiness, morale, and life satisfaction (Gentile, 1991; McDowell & Newell, 1996; Patrick

& Erickson, 1993), which have been used widely in gerontological research (Kozma & Stones, 1980; Lawton, 1975; Neugarten, Havighurst, & Tobin, 1961).

Currently, many clinical and gerontological researchers are advocating a combination of subjective and objective indicators for assessing QOL in older adults and the general population (George & Bearon, 1980); (Lawton, 1991); (Stewart, Sherbourne, & Brod, 1996). For example, researchers may be interested in measuring physical functioning objectively (e.g., ability to dress) and also in measuring pain and discomfort, which are generally viewed as subjective concepts.

In social research, health is only one aspect of QOL. Overall QOL encompasses an individual's subjective assessment of an amalgamation of possible life domains that largely reflect social roles and institutions in people's lives, including marriage, family, friendships, job, housing, self, health, leisure, community, and government (Andrews & Withey, 1976; Campbell et al., 1976). In clinical research, QOL is rarely conceptualized overtly (Gill & Feinstein, 1994). It is generally called *health-related quality of life* (HRQL) and is synonymous with general health status (Greenfield & Nelson, 1992; Guyatt, Feeny, & Patrick, 1993; Ware et al., 1995). Health-related quality of life conceptualizations are often based on the WHO definition of health and emphasize physical, psychological, and social functioning but may take on a disease-specific focus.

Measuring QOL reflects essentially an interest in broadening one's perspective, and that, of course, depends on where one starts. Quality of life for a particular field is an extension of the previous paradigm in the field and incorporates multiple domains that are important to the field's research or clinical agenda. Early work on QOL in the 1970s by social researchers was focused on developing social indicators that moved beyond standard economic indicators to measure social well-being in the United States (Andrews &

Withey, 1976; Campbell et al., 1976), resulting in broad subjective conceptualizations of QOL. Clinical researchers began from a disease-based focus and have attempted to move beyond that to incorporate health-related functioning into their focus. Given the starting point, it is not surprising that HRQL focused on negative aspects of health (wellness), while work in the social sciences was focusing on positive aspects of well-being.

### General Population

A growing number of health researchers are suggesting that the gold standard for HRQL measures at least includes physical, psychological, and social health as well as global perceptions of health and well-being (Berzon, Mauskopf, & Simeon, 1996; Ware, 1995), but considerable variation exists in the literature.

"Narrow" definitions of HRQL reject the WHO conceptualization of health. Kaplan and Anderson (1996) define HRQL as "the impact of health conditions on function." Narrower still, Feeny, Torrance, and Furlong (1996) focus on only physical and emotional dimensions of health. An example of a broader definition of HRQL is supplied by Patrick and Erickson (1993), who define HRQL as "the value assigned to the duration of life as modified by impairments, functional states, perceptions, and social opportunities that are influenced by disease, injury, treatment, or policy." Schipper, Clinch, and Olweny (1996) provide a clinical perspective whereby HRQL is defined as "the functional effect of an illness and its consequent therapy upon a patient, as perceived by the patient." For Berzon and coworkers (1996), citing Cella and Tulsky (1990), "Quality of life refers to patients' appraisal of and satisfaction with their current level of functioning as compared to what they perceive to be possible or ideal," suggesting the importance of health expectations and individual weighting in HRQL constructs.

### Older Adults

Researchers with a gerontological focus prefer a broader definition of QOL and argue for greater attention to the environment and positive measures of well-being not based completely on functioning. Katz and Gurland (1991) propose that the QOL of older adults should be a combination of the older adult (mind, body, and spirit), the older adult's animate and inanimate environment, and the older adult's life experiences. George and Bearon (1980) view QOL as "both an objective and subjective phenomenon, including both the conditions and the experience of life. The suggested components of quality of life are: life satisfaction, self-esteem, general health and functional status, and socioeconomic conditions."

Lawton (1991) also rejects the restrictive ideas of HRQL and provides a broad conceptualization of QOL as "the multidimensional evaluation by both intra personal and social–normative criteria of the person–environment system of an individual in time past, current, and anticipated." This definition emphasizes both a subjective and an objective approach to QOL and implies the centrality of expectations in QOL assessment. One's evaluation of the current situation relies on some internal standard or ideal.

### Nursing Home Residents

Quality of life can take on special meaning for older persons in constricted circumstances. In a study now in progress to define and measure QOL for nursing home residents, Kane and colleagues (1999) posited 11 outcome domains that would constitute psychosocial QOL: autonomy/choice, dignity, privacy, individuality, enjoyment, meaningful activity, relationships, sense of sincerity/safety/order, comfort, spiritual well-being, and functional competence. The researchers have provided further definitions of each domain as well as thoughts about how each domain relates to people with dementia (Table 7.1). The

**Table 7.1.**
Specification of Quality of Life Domains

| Definition of resident outcome | Associated nursing facilities policies and practices | Implications for dementia |
|---|---|---|
| **Autonomy.** Residents take initiative and make choices for their lives and care | Facility policies, practices, and staff permit and encourage residents to take initiative and make choices to direct their lives | Autonomy and choice imply some level of cognitive processing and will not be measured for residents falling below that level |
| **Individuality.** Residents express their preferences and pursue their past and current interests while living at the nursing home, maintaining a sense of their own personal identify and continuity with their past | Facility staff are aware of residents' preferences and interests, and facility policies and practices and staff behavior promote each resident's individuality. Staff behavior and resident's immediate environments show markers of the residents' backgrounds and present interests | Individuality as a resident outcome implies some level of cognitive processing and will not be measured for residents falling below that level. For all residents, however, staff are measured on how aware they are of that person's unique nature and history |
| **Dignity.** Residents perceive that their dignity is intact and respected and do *not* experience feelings of being belittled, devalued, or humiliated | Facility policies and practices and staff behavior maintain and promote residents' sense of dignity and do not belittle, devalue, or humiliate residents | Sense of dignity as a resident outcome implies some level of cognitive processing and will not be measured for residents falling below that level. All residents are however, monitored for whether they are treated with dignity or the converse |
| **Privacy.** Residents experience a sense of bodily privacy, have the ability to keep personal information confidential, and have sufficient opportunities to be alone and to communicate and interact with others in private | Facility policies and practices and staff behavior show sensitivity to residents' modesty, desires to determine how and to whom their information and feelings are disclosed, to be alone, or to be unobserved by others. | A sense of appropriate or inappropriate privacy as a resident outcome implies some level of cognitive processing and is not measured for residents falling below that level |
| **Enjoyment.** Residents express or exhibit pleasure and enjoyment, verbally and nonverbally. Conversely, they do not express or exhibit unhappiness, distress, and lack of enjoyment. | Facility policies, practices, and staff behavior promote resident enjoyment | Measured for all residents. Family and staff reports and observations are used when residents cannot report |
| **Meaningful activity.** Residents engage in discretionary behavior, either active activity or passive observation, that they find interesting, stimulating, worthwhile. Conversely, they tend not to be bored with their lives | Facility policies and practices and the behavior of staff encourage residents to engage in tasks and activities that interest or stimulate them | Applies to all but standard shifts with resident competence. For some residents, upper level includes making a contribution to others inside or outside the facility. For very low functioning residents, having interest engaged satisfies this domain. Family and staff report used when residents cannot report |
| **Relationships.** Residents engage in meaningful person-to-person interchange where the purpose is social | Facility policies and practices promote and do not deter residents' ability to have meaningful person-to-person interchanges with other residents, staff, and family and friends outside the facility | Applies to all residents although standard shifts based on competence. Family and staff reports and observations used when residents cannot report |
| **Security/safety.** Residents feel secure and confident about their | The facility does all possible to produce the perception of safety | Applies to all residents although standard shifts based on compe- |

*(continued)*

**Table 7.1.**— Continued

| | | |
|---|---|---|
| personal safety and security of their possessions and have clarity about rules and practices | and security, to enable residents to move about freely, to keep their possessions intact, to present expectations clearly, and to apply them fairly and flexibly | tence. Family and staff reports and observations used when residents cannot report |
| **Comfort.** Residents experience minimal physical discomfort, including symptoms such as pain, aches, nausea, dizziness, constipation, and itching, and no discomfort from being cold, hot, thirsty, or in an uncomfortable position. They perceive that staff notice and attend to their physical comfort | Staff notice and attend to resident's physical comfort, including attempting to discover and assist those who cannot easily express themselves | Applies to all residents although standard shifts based on competence. Family and staff reports and observations used when residents cannot report |
| **Spiritual well-being.** Residents perceive that their needs and concerns for religion, prayer, meditation, moral values, and meaning in life are met | Policies, practices, and staff behavior show respect for each resident's religious beliefs and practices and moral values and facilitate their needs for religious observation, prayer, and meditation. | This domain not measured for people with minimal cognitive functioning |
| **Functional competence.** Residents function independently in the nursing home in keeping with their abilities and preferences | Policies, practices, and staff behavior encourage and do not discourage residents from being independent around self-care, care of their environment, or mobility | Applies to all residents although standard shifts based on competence. Family and staff reports and observations used when residents cannot report |

Source: Kane et al. (1999).

middle column suggests ways in which nursing home policies and procedures might affect residents' QOL in each domain. Because of the wide range of cognitive and physical capabilities of nursing home residents, we expect a wide spread in QOL on most of these domains and that the theoretical upper threshold for QOL will depend on resident characteristics. For example, meaningful activity at one end of cognitive abilities refers to making a meaningful contribution and being interested and stimulated intellectually and in other ways. At the very lowest level of cognitive abilities, perhaps the most that can be achieved is that the resident is actively engaged in observing the world around him or her. The investigators intend to empirically examine whether each of these domains can be independently measured.

The third column of Table 7.1 shows the way QOL domains are conceptualized for people with the highest levels of cognitive impairment. At the extreme lowest level of cognitive functioning (e.g., comatose or vegetative state), none of these QOL domains has meaning, or at least current abilities to measure and discern do not allow us to interpret them. Also at very low levels of cognitive functioning, several of these domains—namely, autonomy, individuality, privacy, dignity, and spiritual well-being—may cease to be relevant in the way that we have defined them. To make choices and to experience a sense of identity, a sense of privacy, of dignity, or of spiritual well-being, some minimal cognitive processing is needed. Therefore, the researchers do not intend to measure spiritual well-being, privacy, or autonomy at all for residents who fall below a threshold where no interview is possible. They do, however, intend at the facility level to measure the extent to which staff are aware of the individual characteristics and background of each resident (individuality) and respect the dignity of each resident in the sample. In a setting where dignity of all residents is respected and treatment of all residents is individualized, the QOL for all residents is expected to be better. Even for those whose with minimal cognitive functioning, some domains (i.e., relationships, activity, enjoyment, comfort, functional competence) are likely to be sensitive to whether the resident is individualized and treated with dignity. Privacy as a value is also interesting in relation to cognitive impairment. Although one can speculate that being in a private room will enhance the well-being of some residents with advanced dementia (allowing them territorial space and mitigating anxiety), it may increase the anxiety of others. For residents with advanced dementia, a sense of privacy may be less important than other outcomes, like enjoyment or security.

This formulation of QOL for nursing home residents is at an early stage of development. A variety of other formulations have also been developed that are either dementia-specific or dementia-friendly. These are reviewed in detail in Chapter 17.

## POTENTIAL QUALITY OF LIFE DOMAINS FOR OLDER ADULTS

Numerous researchers have questioned the suitability of HRQL measures for assessing frail older adults (Birren, Lubben, Rowe, & Deutchman, 1991). Although generic HRQL measures make the assumption that the underlying HRQL construct is stable across populations differing by age and disease burden (McHorney, 1996), the real issue is what domains are included. If the domains of interest for assessing older adults are excluded, the QOL concept would certainly be misspecified for this population. Quality of life as a concept should be contemporaneous in that researchers should use measures focused on the life and functioning domains most salient for older adults.

Birren and Dieckmann (1991) mention

the following domains for a frail elderly population: physical health; physical, psychological, social, and cognitive functioning; economic status; environment; health perceptions; life satisfaction; self-esteem; sense of control; autonomy; and choice. A focus-group study by Abt Associates Inc. (1996) found that for institutionalized older adults QOL included the following dimensions: dignity, privacy, interactions with staff, physical features and decor of the nursing home facility, nursing home services and adequacy of staff, and relationships with friends, residents, and staff. Residents were most concerned with retaining some semblance of their lifestyle in the community after institutionalization. Exploratory work by Cohn and Sugar (1991) described six domains of QOL for institutionalized older adults: care, physical environment, social–emotional environment, ability, autonomy, and morale. Many of the psychosocial dimensions mentioned are usually excluded from general instruments designated to measure HRQL.

Table 7.2 lists potential domains for assessing QOL in older adults. The domains in the right-hand column should be considered for inclusion in QOL measures for assessing older adults. Most of the domains covered separately in this book can be considered potential QOL domains.

Incorporating additional psychosocial and environmental domains into QOL conceptualizations is important for several reasons. Frail older adults are faced with a diminishing circle of social involvement and have less control over their environment and daily routines in ways that are unfamiliar to a healthy general population. For instance, meaningful social roles for older adults are limited in U.S. society, control over decision making is reduced in the face of physical and cognitive limitations, dependency on others or mechanical devices may become a part of daily life, attending social and other events may be hindered by transportation difficulties and health, and the quality of one's physical

**Table 7.2.** Health-Related Quality of Life (HRQL) and Quality of Life (QOL) Domains

| General population HRQL | Older adults HRQL + QOL |
| --- | --- |
| Physical functioning | Time use |
| Psychological functioning | Environment |
| Cognitive functioning | Autonomy |
| Social functioning | Self-efficacy |
| Role functioning | Satisfaction with care and environment |
| Sexual functioning | |
| Symptoms/pain | |
| Energy/fatigue | |
| General health perceptions | |
| Overall QOL | |
| Survival | |

environment may decrease substantially in the event of relocation from one's home. Because these circumstances are uncharacteristic of the general population, they are often not considered in general HRQL and QOL life measures. Arguably, because they are subject to radical restructuring, features of the physical and social environment take on increased importance in the lives of older adults.

Residents of institutions have often commented on the boredom and loneliness of everyday life (Wilkin & Hughes, 1987; Thomas, 1994). For example, Degenholtz, Kane, and Kivnick (1997) found that about one-fourth of community dwelling frail older people reported that they had nothing to look forward to. Work by Rowe and Kahn (1998) on successful aging stresses continued engagement in productive activity as a key feature, and Lawton (1983) stresses inclusion of how much time is spent on enriching activities such as creative innovation, exploration, recreation, curiosity, and stimulus variation in QOL measures. We must be careful, however, when inferring what meaningful social involvement is to an individual.

The onset of cognitive and physical disabilities generally diminishes the scope of one's environment and control over decision-making regarding the environment. Formally, the issue of control in discussions of QOL in older adults has been labeled *autonomy* and specifically refers to the ability of an individual to control deci-

sion-making and other activities (Collopy, 1988). Institutional environments generally run counter to the idea of autonomy. Stringent regulations and routine erode the ability of residents to make decisions over the most basic matters of life. Even in the community, family members often take an active role in decision making, and home environments may be poorly designed to accommodate deficits in functioning.

Finally, tension exists between quality of care and QOL as defined by the older adult. For many frail older adults, the home and the care setting have become one. Older adults expect more than technical quality of care; they are interested in the quality of the relationship as well. Inevitably, provider interaction with the resident takes on an element of social functioning because the providers generally have more contact with residents than do family members. Moreover, older adults and providers may have different conceptions of what constitutes quality of care. Providers may focus on the safety of the older adult, while the older adult may be focused on autonomy issues. Curtailment of the older adult's autonomy by the provider has implications for the older adult's QOL.

The work of Lawton (1983, 1991) offers the most systematic attempt to conceptualize QOL in frail older adults. Building on his definition discussed previously, Lawton has developed a model of QOL (previously labeled *The Good Life*) composed of four main sectors: behavioral competence, psychological well-being, perceived QOL, and objective environment. The sectors are presented as overlapping because they are not conceptualized to be independent from one another. Behavioral competence is described as "the social-normative evaluation of the person's functioning in the health, cognitive, time-use, and social dimensions" (Lawton, 1991). Many of these behavioral competence categories overlap with HRQL domains. Perceived QOL is a function of an individual's subjective evaluation of performance in each of the areas of behavioral competence as well as other subjective domains such as pain, self-rated health, cognitive self-efficacy, quality of spare time, and quality of relationships with spouse and children (Lawton, 1991). Operationalizing QOL is left largely to the individual researcher, allowing the specific measures of the QOL sectors to be chosen to suit the stated research objective. Lawton, Moss, Fulcomer, & Kleban (1982) have, however, developed the Multi-level Assessment Instrument (MAI), which measures behavioral competence (physical health, cognition, activities of daily living, time use, social relations), psychological well-being, and perceived environmental quality. This measure is discussed in more detail at the end of this chapter.

## ISSUES ARISING FROM THE CHOICE OF QOL MEASURE FOR ASSESSING OLDER ADULTS

There has been a movement toward using function-based HRQL measures in effectiveness measures such as quality-adjusted life years (QALY). Benefits of programs and interventions are expressed in terms of QALYs produced. Quality-adjusted life years attempt to combine health quality and mortality into a single aggregate measure that takes into account consumer preferences for various health states. Quality-adjusted life years are a product of life expectancy or survival over a set time pe-

riod and an aggregate health score calculated as illness-related deviations from normal functioning. A QALY can take a value from 0 to 1, reflecting the amount of QOL it contains.

Several techniques have been used to calculate QALYs in the literature: (1) the use of life tables (an average level of HRQL is calculated for each age interval in a life table); (2) cohort analysis (the mortality and duration of health states are followed over time in a cohort, and the number of years survived for each member is weighted by the HRQL measure and then aggregated into a single score); and (3) simple estimation (an average value of HRQL is available for a group, and it is multiplied by the life expectancy for that group to obtain a crude measure of QALYs (Patrick & Erickson, 1993). A cost utility/effectiveness ratio is obtained by dividing QALYs by program costs (appropriately discounted).

Table 7.3 summarizes the scales that have been commonly used estimate QALYs. The first three measures have been widely used in the United States. A European Consortium has developed a simple 5 item scale called the EUROQOL (Brooks, 1996). A fifth measure, years of healthy life (YHL), was developed to take advantage of information available in the National Center for Health Statistic's National Health Interview Survey (Erickson, Wilson, & Shannon, 1995).

The use of QALYs as a resource allocation tool for health services raises the possibility of an age disability bias through several avenues: (1) the goals of health maximization (allocate resources efficiently, not equitably); (2) the use of only negative valuations of health; (3) insensitivity of HRQL to change in disabled adults; and (4) the treatment of optimal health and health values over the life course as fixed concepts. Wagstaff (1996) notes that health maximization through the use of QALYs "leads to the conclusion that resources ought to be redeployed away from people (or groups of people) who have a low capacity to benefit from

**Table 7.3.**

Characteristics of Measures Commonly Used in Quality-Adjusted Life Years*

| | SIP | QWB | HUI3 | EUROQOL† | YHL‡ |
|---|---|---|---|---|---|
| Number of items | 136 | 3 attributes; 27 symptoms | 8 attributes | 5 | 2 |
| **Domains** | | | | | |
| Mobility | X | X | X | | |
| Ambulation | X | X | X | X | |
| Self-care | X | | | X | X (Ages 65+) |
| Dexterity | | | X | | |
| Communication | X | X§ | X | | |
| Vision | | X§ | X | | |
| Hearing | | | X | | |
| Cognitive function | X | X§ | X | | |
| Psychological function | X | X§ | X | X | |
| Social/role activities | X | X | X | X | X (Ages 5–64) |
| Sexual function | X | X§ | | | |
| Pain | X | X§ | X | X | |
| Sleep | X | X§ | | | |
| Leisure time use | X | | | | |
| Global health rating | | | | | X |
| Sample for value weights | Convenience sample, n = 25 health care professionals & students; random sample, n = 108 prepaid group practice enrollees | Probability sample, n = 867 San Diego residents | Random sample, n = 504 Ontario adults | In process; probability sample, n = 3395 in Britain | National Health Interview Survey probability sample, non-institutional population, n = 50,000+ |
| Aggregation of items | Percent score: sum of scale values for individuals divided by total possible score multiplied by 100 | Negative value weights subtracted from 1 | Multiplicative utility function | Negative value weights subtracted from 1 or visual analog global health rating 0–100 | Multiplicative utility function |

*SIP, Sickness Impact Profile; QWB, Quality of Well-Being Scale; HUI3, Health Utilities Index Mark 3; EUROQOL, European standardized Quality of Life measure; YHL, Years of Healthy Life.

†Source: Brooks (1996).

‡Source: Erickson et al. (1995).

§Contained in the QWB symptom and problem complex list.

treatment. If A and B are identical in other respects, the impact of medical care on their quality of life will be the same, but the productivity of medical care in terms of QALYs will be higher for B than A, simply because B is younger" (Wagstaff, 1996, pp. 431–432).

Not all QALYs are created equal. One should be keenly aware of what is going into the Q, or, in other words, how we are adjusting for quality and what the upper bound for quality is. Generally measures that generate a single health status score and are scaled from 0 (death) to 1 (normal/perfect health) are used in the calculation of QALYs, but it has become common in the literature to use absence of a particular condition instead of excellent health. One should be wary of results from QALYs calculated in such a manner because the amount of QALYs gained from a program or intervention will be inflated because the measure is not taking into account other comorbid conditions (Fryback & Lawrence, 1997).

Quality-adjusted life years may be deflated for older adults by treating the upper bound of quality as having no functional limitations. For example, gerontologists have created a measure (similar to QALYs), years of active life expectancy, using life table techniques and activities of daily living measures to calculate remaining years of functional well-being (lack of dependence) in older adults (Katz et al., 1983). Dysfunction is treated as a dichotomous state. Under this system, once people become dependent, they have no QOL because no more remaining years of functional well-being are left. Needless to say, this method is relatively insensitive to changes in disability among older adults.

The inclusion of only negative valuations of functioning may further the age/disability bias in resource allocation for health care because for older adults there may be little hope for improvement in the physical domains, but improvements in some psychosocial domains may offset the negative functioning values. A study of

QOL in the last year of life found that two-thirds of the sample were living quality lives based on the following indicators: experiencing pain seldom or never; enjoying mental clarity all or most of the time; needing no functional help at all or less than once a week; having an average of one to three social contacts a month; spending 5 hours or less during the waking day doing nothing; satisfied with time use always or most of the time; seldom or never depressed; expressing some or very much interest in the world; and feeling somewhat or very much that there was something to live for (Lawton, 1991). Failure to capture areas where older adults are improving puts them at a disadvantage in assessments of the relative benefits of programs targeted toward them. In fact, positive aspects of health and well-being seem to be areas that older adults often score higher in compared with younger adults; U.S. males and females over age 65 years have higher mean levels of mental health on the SF-36 subscale than do males and females under 65 years (Ware, Snow, Kosinski, & Gandek, 1993).

Valuation of life and health states is implicit in discussions of HRQL. Most HRQL measures assign weights to health states that are assumed to be equal for everyone regardless of age, sex, race, income, disability, and so forth. Judges rate items in terms of either preferences for expressed health states or degree of dysfunction expressed (Ware & Keller, 1996). In existing HRQL measures, judges have been members of the general public as well as clinicians and preprofessional students (Bergner, Bobbit, Carter, & Gilson, 1981; Feeny et al., 1996; Kaplan & Anderson, 1988).

Two points are important here. First, the valuations of health states are not necessarily equal for everyone. Second, the valuation of health states is not the same as individual valuation of life. Expectations play a crucial role here—at what level do they matter, for example, individual, subgroups, population? Do expectations of optimal health (what it is possible to achieve) change for the very old or disabled? Should optimal health be scaled differently for inclusion in QALY calculations for those 85 years and older than for those 45 to 55 years old? Or should weights be more personal and self-normed by the individual who has his or her own expectations about his or her ideal level of functioning and the most important domains? Kaplan (1995) argues that preferences for health states of the general population can be used in specific populations because freedom from disability is universally preferred by all groups. Studies comparing general population weights to condition-specific populations such as rheumatoid arthritis (Balaban, Sagi, Goldfarb, & Nettler, 1986) and long-term care residents (Hays et al., 1996) found almost perfect agreement in ratings. On the other hand, some researchers argue that there may be differential valuation of health states over the life course if QOL was conceptualized as part of an ongoing process of balancing negative aspects of health with positive nonhealth sources of QOL (Lawton, 1997). Studies of persons with and without serious chronic illness indicate that those with the disease are much less motivated to get rid of it than are those without it to avoid it (Sackett & Torrance, 1978).

Valuation of health is not the same as the valuation of life. Lawton (1997) conceptualized valuation of life (VOL) as a function of hope, personal goals, meaning of life, wish to live, sense of future, and self-motivation and found that there was not an independent relationship between health condition and VOL. Furthermore, analyses revealed that few QOL domains (including health) were independently associated with years of desired life in frail older adults, while VOL was independently associated with years of desired life for several groups of older adults (Lawton, 1997). Moreover, a study of hospitalized cognitively intact patients 80 years or older using time trade-off techniques found that most patients (69%) were unwilling give up more than 1 month out of

a year for excellent health even though only one-third of the sample rated their QOL as excellent (Tsevat et al., 1998).

When assessing QOL, some researchers may use measures that are not reported by the individual but rather by proxies such as health professionals or family members. At the objective level, we are observing external behavior and features of environment but we should keep in mind that we are also making judgments about what constitutes "normal or desirable" levels of these attributes. Assessing QOL relies on being able to tap the subject's response to specific conditions. Observers interpreting behavior may have a hard time determining the person's real response. Use of proxies may be necessitated by factors such as severe cognitive impairment, but this is not always the case. The Minimum Data Set uses ratings of nursing home residents made by health professionals to determine QOL dimensions such as social engagement for both cognitively intact and demented individuals (Mor et al., 1995) (see Chapter 16).

Use of proxies may introduce bias into one's measures (Rubenstein, Schairer, Wieland, & Kane, 1984; Magaziner, Simonsick, Kashner, & Hebel, 1988; Grootendorst, Feeny, & Furlong, 1997; Wu et al., 1997). For example, proxies overestimated how much time hospitalized patients 80 years and older would trade for better health (Tsevat et al., 1998). Because QOL is largely subjective by definition, QOL information should be elicited from the older adult whenever possible. Moreover, recent research suggests that "objective indicators of quality of life correlate poorly with patient perceptions of their global quality of life" (Pearlman & Uhlmann, 1991). Recent evidence is promising for obtaining information from individuals not previously considered capable of providing it; administration of the SF-36 to cognitively impaired participants in the Medical Outcomes Study found comparable psychometric scale results between the cognitively impaired and the cognitively intact (McHorney, 1996). Chapter 17 provides an in-depth discussion of strategies for and implications of assessing older adults with cognitive limitations.

Finally, when selecting domains, one should also take note of varying perspectives. Providers and consumers will likely have differing conceptions of what is important for QOL. Providers will probably choose to define QOL in terms of what they believe they can affect. For example, QOL measures based on the Minimum Data Set are operationalized as the prevalence of daily restraints and the prevalence of little or no activity (Zimmerman et al., 1995), a very restricted definition. Conversely, residents typically list domains that are more under their control as the most important, for example, psychosocial domains (Abt Associates Inc., 1996; Cohn & Sugar, 1991).

## CHOOSING A QOL INSTRUMENT

### Conceptualizing the Measure

First, what is to be measured and how the information will be used must be determined clearly. Here, theory and the conceptual model for the study should serve as guides. The domains of QOL must be decided as well as the data collection strategy. For example, a researcher interested in psychological functioning should be aware that mental health is conceptualized differently in different measures claiming to measure HRQL. Ware and Sherbourne (1992) conceptualize mental health as a distinct domain of health that should be measured separately, whereas Kaplan and Anderson (1988) do not. Thus, mental health can be used as a subscale in one situation and treated as a separate dependent or independent variable in another instance.

Well-articulated study goals for the use of the chosen measure will help ensure the quality of the data obtained. For example, it should be clear whether one is interested in capacity of an individual versus functional performance of an individual. Likewise, specific instruments may contain content inappropriate for certain populations. Quality of data is poorer when items do not directly apply to the respondent's situation (McHorney, 1996). A scale developed to measure QOL in a younger developmentally disabled population may include items addressing work force issues that are not applicable to retired older adults. Too often scales take on an artificial reality after they have been in use for a while and people assume that they are interchangeable for any study. Finally, it is important to be aware of the analysis requirements of the study before data collection of the measures is undertaken and to select HRQL measures with desirable scaling properties.

After the researcher has decided what dimensions of HRQL are most relevant to the treatment/intervention, the researcher must decide how the QOL data are to be collected. Should a prepackaged QOL measure be used that provides a sampling of the domains of interest, or should each of the domains be collected separately using measures discussed throughout the book that capture individual domains in depth? The advantages of the former strategy are brevity and the possibility of generating a single score, while the latter approach allows more in-depth coverage of each domain.

Researchers selecting a prepackaged HRQL instrument must generally make a choice between a health profile and a utility measure. Health profiles attempt to measure all-important dimensions of HRQL, but each dimension of the profile is scored separately. Profiles may or may not be able to be aggregated to obtain an overall score. Utility measures incorporate consumer preference, morbidity, and mortality into a single index ranging from death (0) to perfect health (1). These measures are useful for conducting cost-utility analyses, but they cannot be broken down into separate health domains. The main differences between the two types of measures is the weighting of health states; these differences are discussed in more detail in the descriptions of the selected measures.

Researchers or clinicians interested in a specific disease must decide whether to use a generic or a disease-specific measure of HRQL. For instance, an investigator may be interested in HRQL in a nursing home population. Initially, a generic measure may seem to serve the study well. If the study question specifically deals with HRQL of arthritis patients in nursing homes, however, a disease-specific measure may also be considered. Disease-specific instruments may be more sensitive to change attributable to the treatment of interest, but they are limited to specific diseases and interventions (Guyatt et al., 1996). Currently, most researchers favor a combination of generic and disease specific measures in clinical research (Atherly, 1997; Essink-Bot, et al., 1997; Ware, 1996).

The necessary precision of the QOL measure should be specified. This involves checking for the susceptibility of the measure to floor and ceiling effects. For example, using the Sickness Impact Profile (SIP) to capture changes in functioning in a well older adult population may be a mistake because the SIP has been shown to differentiate well between those with poor health but not well between healthy older adults (Andresen, et al., 1995). This represents a ceiling effect. A floor effect occurs when the measure cannot differentiate well between unhealthy individuals. In general, short measures of general health are subject to floor and ceiling effects because they do not include a broad range of items in any single domain.

## COMMONLY USED MEASURES OF QUALITY OF LIFE

Although much of the initial interest in assessing QOL stemmed from the dynamics of scarce resources, an aging population, and increased prevalence of chronic condi-

tions, the bulk of the existing measures were not developed for general use in an elderly population. Many of the early QOL prepackaged measures were developed for use with specific diseases such as cancer and arthritis, and those used to assess HRQL generally and more recently in older adults (McHorney, 1996) were developed as generic health status measures.

The QOL measures chosen for discussion are well known in the HRQL literature. Only one of the measures selected (the Multi-level Assessment Instrument), however, was designed specifically for use with older adults. Many instruments purporting to measure QOL have been developed by provider organizations. These instruments are, however, almost entirely measures of satisfaction and purposely excluded from this chapter.

Measures of generic health status assume that the underlying health concepts are invariant for populations differing in age, race, socioeconomic status, and disease burden (McHorney, 1996), but little work has been done to confirm this assumption. Moreover, as suggested earlier in this chapter, current HRQL may lack coverage of domains important in an older adult population. The use of each HRQL measure in older adult populations is discussed. Table 7.4 compares the domains covered by each instrument. Table 7.5 compares the aggregation and implementation factors of the selected instruments. Table 7.6 compares the reliability and validity of the selected instruments.

## GENERAL POPULATION MEASURES

### Sickness Impact Profile (SIP)
### (Bergner et al. 1976)

The Sickness Impact Profile, shown in Table 7.7, measures overall health status as a function of changes in an individual's behavior in relation to a period of illness. Developed in the 1970s, the SIP was designed to meet the research community's need for a generic outcome-based health

**Table 7.4.**
Selected Domains of Commonly Used Quality of Life Measures*

|  | SIP | SF-36 | QWB | COOP | NHP | HUI3 | MAI |
|---|---|---|---|---|---|---|---|
| Physical functioning | x | x | x | x | x | x | x |
| Impairment | x | x | x | x | x | x | x |
| Psychological functioning | x | x | x | x | x | x | x |
| Cognitive functioning | x |  |  |  |  | x | x |
| Social support | x |  |  | x |  |  | x |
| Social activities | x | x | x | x | x |  | x |
| Role functioning | x | x | x |  | x |  | x |
| Sexual functioning | x |  | x |  | x |  |  |
| Pain | x | x | x | x | x | x |  |
| Energy/fatigue | x | x | x |  | x |  |  |
| Time use | x |  |  |  | x | x |  |
| Environment |  |  |  |  |  | x |  |
| Quality of life |  |  |  | x |  |  |  |
| General health perception |  | x |  | x |  |  | x |
| Quality of care |  |  |  |  |  |  |  |
| Satisfaction with health |  |  |  |  |  |  |  |
| Survival |  |  | x |  |  | x |  |

*SIP, Sicknesss Impact Profile; SF-36, Medical Outcomes Study 36 Item Short Form Health Survey; QWB, Quality of Well-Being Scale; COOP, Dartmouth Cooperative; NHP, Nottingham Health Profile; HUI3, Health Utilities Index Mark 3; MAI, Multi-level Assessment Instrument.

**Table 7.5.**
Selected Aspects of Commonly Used Quality of Life Measures*

|  | SIP | SF-36 | QWB | COOP | NHP | HUI3 | MAI |
|---|---|---|---|---|---|---|---|
| Population intended | Adults | Adults | General | General | Adults | General | Older Adults |
| Administration method† | I/S | I/S | I | I/S | S | I/S | I |
| Administration time (min)‡ | 20–30 OA: 20–65 | 5–10 OA: 15+ | 7+ OA: 17.4 | <5 | 10–15 | 5–10 | 50 |
| Weighting§ | T | L | U | L | T | U | L |
| Scoring‖ | P/SI/SS | P/SS | SI | P | P | SI | P |
| Time period | That day | 4 week 1 week | That day | 4 week | That day | 1 week 2 weeks 4 weeks Usual and customary | That day and past year |
| Floor (F)/Ceiling (C) effects | C | C/F | Cluster Middle | F/C | F | C | ? |

*SIP, Sicknesss Impact Profile; SF-36, Medical Outcomes Study 36 Item Short Form Health Survey; QWB, Quality of Well-Being Scale; COOP, Dartmout Cooperative; NHP, Nottingham Health Profile; HUI3, Health Utilities Index Mark 3; MAI, Multi-level Assessment Instrument.

†I = interviewer; S = self.

‡OA = older adults.

§T = Thurstone; L = Likert; U = Utility.

‖P = profile; SI = summary index; SS, summary score.

Source: Adapted from McDowell & Newell (1996).

**Table 7.6.** Reliability and Validity of Commonly Used Quality of Life Measures*

| | SIP | SF-36 | QWB | COOP | NHP | HUI3 | MAI |
|---|---|---|---|---|---|---|---|
| | | | Reliability | | | | |
| Internal consis-tency | $\alpha = 0.94^{a,b}$ overall score | $\alpha = 0.78$–$0.93^{c}$ domains | | $\alpha = 0.78$–$0.93^{d,t}$ charts | $\alpha = 0.68$–$0.87^{e}$ domains | | $\alpha = 0.71$–$0.93^{f}$ domains |
| Test–retest | 24 hour $\alpha$ $= 0.92^{a,b}$ overall score | 2 week $\alpha =$ $0.60$–$0.81^{e}$ domains | $\alpha = 0.94^{g}$ weights | 2 week $\alpha =$ $0.42$–$0.88^{b}$ charts | 4 week, part I, $\alpha =$ $0.75$–$0.88^{i}$; part II, $\alpha =$ $0.55$–$0.89^{i}$ domains | 1 month $\alpha$ $= 0.77^{i}$ | 3 week $\alpha =$ $0.73$–$0.95^{f}$ domains |
| Inter-rater | $\alpha = 0.92^{b}$ overall score | | | $\alpha = 0.50$–$0.98^{b}$ charts | | | $\alpha = 0.58$–$0.88^{f}$ domains |
| | | | Validity‡ | | | | |
| | DBG,$^{a}$ SAH,$^{a,b}$ OHM,$^{a,b}$ PR$^{a,b}$ | DBG,$^{k}$ OHM,$^{l}$ PR$^{m}$ | DBG,$^{n}$ OHM,$^{o}$ SAH$^{p}$ | DBG,$^{d}$ OHM,$^{b}$ SAH$^{b}$ | DBG,$^{q,r}$ OHM,$^{e,r}$ PR$^{s}$ | DBG$^{i}$ | DBG,$^{f}$ PR$^{f}$ |

*SIP, Sickness Impact Profile; SF-36, Medical Outcomes Study 36 Item Short Form Health Survey; QWB, Quality of Well-Being Scale; COOP, Dartmouth Cooperative; NHP, Nottinham Health Profile; HUI3, Health Utilities Index Mark 3; MAI, Multi-level Assessment Instrument.

†Lower bound.

‡DBG = distinguishes between clinical subgroups; SAH = correlates with self-assessed measures of health; OHM = correlates with other health measures; PR = correlates with provider ratings.

Sources: a, Bergner et al. (1981); b, de Bruin, et al. (1992); c, McHorney et al. (1994); d, McHorney et al. (1992). e, Brazier et al. (1991); f, Lawton et al. (1982); g, Balaban et al. (1986); h, Nelson et al. (1990); i, Hunt et al. (1985); j, Boyle et al. (1995); k, McHroney et al. (1993); l, Ware et al. (1993); m, Nerenz et al. (1992); n, Kaplan & Anderson (1996); o, Fryback et al. (1997), Andresen et al. (1995); p, Kaplan et al. (1976); q, Hunt et al. (1980), Jenkinson et al. (1988); r, Essink-Bot et al. (1997); s, Martini & McDowell (1976); t, Feeny et al. (1996).

status measure for use in evaluation, program planning, and policy formulation (Bergner et al., 1981). The goal was a measure that could discriminate well among different subgroups (e.g., illness, cultural) and be sensitive enough to detect change over time in order to monitor a patient's progress (Bergner et al., 1976, 1981).

Conceptually, the measure focuses on interruptions in social role functioning due to illness (i.e., dysfunction), and, in keeping with a clinical focus, the measure includes only items on deviations from normal functioning. Employing sickness-related behavior as the scale's foundation was considered useful by developers for several reasons: (1) behavior could be re-ported directly by individuals or indirectly by others' observations of the individual; (2) behavior may be affected by medical treatment (positively or negatively) even though the disease seems unaffected; (3) behaviors can be measured in individuals not currently in the health care system; and (4) measuring sickness-related behavioral changes provides a common ground for discussion of illness between patients and health care providers (Damiano, 1996).

From the existing literature on illness-related behavior and survey information from over 1100 open-ended surveys completed by patients, health care professionals, caregivers, and healthy individuals, an all-inclusive list of 312 unique

**Table 7.7.**
The Sickness Impact Profile

| Dimension | Category | Items describing behavior related to | Selected items |
|---|---|---|---|
| Independent categories | SR | Sleep and Rest | I sit during much of the day<br>I sleep or nap during the day |
| | E | Eating | I am eating no food at all; nutrition is taken through tubes or intravenous fluids<br>I am eating special or different food |
| | W | Work | I am not working at all<br>I often act irritable toward my work associates |
| | HM | Home management | I am not doing any of the maintenance or repair work around the house that I usually do<br>I am not doing heavy work around the house |
| | RP | Recreation and pastimes | I am going out for entertainment less<br>I am not doing any of my usual physical recreation or activities |
| Physical | A | Ambulation | I walk shorter distances or stop to rest often<br>I do not walk at all |
| | M | Mobility | I stay within one room<br>I stay away from home only for brief periods of time |
| | BCM | Body care and movement | I do not bathe myself at all, but am bathed by someone else<br>I am very clumsy in body movements |
| Psychosocial | SI | Social interaction | I am doing fewer social activities with groups of people<br>I isolate myself as much as I can from the rest of the family |
| | AB | Alertness behavior | I have difficulty reasoning and solving problems, for example, making decisions, learning new things<br>I sometimes behave as if I were confused or disoriented in place or time, for example, where I am, who is around, directions, what day it is |
| | EB | Emotional behavior | I laugh or cry suddenly<br>I act irritable and impatient with myself, for example, talk badly about myself, swear at myself |
| | C | Communication | I blame myself for things that happen<br>I am having trouble writing or typing<br>I do not speak clearly when I am under stress |

illness behaviors was compiled (Bergner et al., 1976). Three field trials of the SIP were conducted on a wide range of sample populations to assess content, reliability, validity, and administration methods. The final version of the SIP contains 136 items in 12 categories of illness-related behavior: sleep and rest, eating, work, home management, recreation and pastimes, ambulation, mobility, body care and movement,

social interaction, alertness behavior, emotional behavior, and communication (Bergner et al., 1981). Respondents are asked to respond only to items that describe their behavior on the day of the interview and that are related to their health (Bergner et al., 1976).

Several options are available for scoring the SIP. The SIP can be scored as a profile, an index, or summary scores. Scale values for the SIP were carefully developed in a two stage process employing the method of equally appearing intervals (Bergner et al., 1976). Twenty-five health care professionals and students rated the items in each category according to relative severity on an interval scale. Next, the least and most dysfunctional items in each category were rated on an interval scale to establish end points for each category so that items could be combined into a single overall score ranging from 0 (no dysfunction) to 100 (maximal dysfunction). Each category may be scored separately, or summary scores can be created for a physical dimension (ambulation, mobility, and body care and movement) and a psychosocial dimension (communication, alertness behavior, emotional behavior, and social interaction) (Damiano, 1996). The SIP can be administered by an interviewer or can be self-administered; administration time is 20–30 minutes (Bergner et al., 1981). The best method of administration is for a trained interviewer to give instructions and answer questions and then have respondents fill out the questionnaire themselves (Bergner et al., 1981).

The reliability and validity of the SIP have been thoroughly tested (Bergner et al., 1981; de Bruin, de Witte, Stevens, & Diederiks, 1992; McDowell & Newell, 1996). For overall scores of the final version of the SIP, internal consistency was 0.94 and test–retest reliability was 0.92. Concurrent validity and discriminant validity of the SIP have been established. The SIP correlates well with other health measures and clinical and self-assessments, and it discriminates well among illness groups. Questions concerning the SIP's sensitivity to change have been raised. Some evidence suggests that the SIP may be somewhat insensitive to clinical or self assessments of change as well as to small daily changes or improvements in health status (de Bruin et al., 1992; McDowell & Newell, 1996). Using behaviors as the basis for the instrument may be somewhat limiting for assessing change.

A short form of the SIP (68 items) has been developed, and initial reliability and validity results are promising (McDowell & Newell, 1996). Attempts have been made to determine the feasibility of using the SIP with nursing home patients (Gerety et al., 1994; Rothman, Hedrick, & Inui, 1989). Gerety and colleagues (1994) have developed another short version of the SIP (66 items) for this population. Investigators generally exclude the work and home management categories for this population, but Rothman and colleagues (1989) note that home management is an area of severe impairment for residents and should be included. Moreover, defining what is meant by health seems to be necessary for this population because many residents did not see functional impairment due to their health but rather to their age, and attention should be given to simplifying the response task (Rothman et al., 1989). Work in this area is still ongoing because modifications to the SIP require the re-establishment of psychometric properties. In a sample of nursing home patients, Gerety and colleagues (1994) report an alpha of 0.95 for the general SIP and an alpha of 0.92 for the SIP-NH.

### Medical Outcomes Study 36 Item Short Form Health Survey (MOS SF-36) (Ware & Sherbourne, 1992)

The Medical Outcomes Study 36 Item Short Form Health Survey was designed as a multipurpose survey of general health status for use in clinic practice and research and in health policy evaluations. Developed for use in the RAND Corporation's Medical Outcomes Study, the SF-36 was an attempt to "fill the gap between lengthy health surveys used successfully in research projects and the relatively coarse single-item measures used in national surveys and numerous clinical investigations" (Ware & Sherbourne, 1992, p. 474). Table 7.8 shows a formatted version of the SF-36.

Conceptually, the SF-36 items are adapted from health instruments used in

**Table 7.8.**

**The Short-Form-36 Health Survey**

**General Health**

In general, would you say your health is: (Select one)
☐ Excellent
☐ Very Good
☐ Good
☐ Fair
☐ Poor

Compared to one year ago, how would you rate your health in general now?
(Select one)
☐ Much better now than one year ago
☐ Somewhat better now than one year ago
☐ About the same
☐ Somewhat worse now than one year ago
☐ Much worse now than one year ago

**Limitations of Activities**

The following items are about activities you might do during a typical day. Does your health now limit you in these activities? If so, how much? (Select one on each line)

| | Yes, Limited A Lot | Yes, Limited A Little | No, Not Limited At All |
|---|---|---|---|
| a. Vigorous activities, such as running, lifting heavy objects, participating in strenuous sports | 1 | 2 | 3 |
| b. Moderate activities, such as moving a table, pushing a vacuum cleaner, bowling, or playing golf | 1 | 2 | 3 |
| c. Lifting or carrying groceries | 1 | 2 | 3 |
| d. Climbing several flights of stairs | 1 | 2 | 3 |
| e. Climbing one flight of stairs | 1 | 2 | 3 |
| f. Bending, kneeling, or stooping | 1 | 2 | 3 |
| g. Walking more than a mile | 1 | 2 | 3 |
| h. Walking several blocks | 1 | 2 | 3 |
| i. Walking one block | 1 | 2 | 3 |
| j. Bathing or dressing yourself | 1 | 2 | 3 |

**Physical health problems**

During the past 4 weeks, have you had any of the following problems with your work or other regular daily activities as a result of your physical health? (Select Yes or No)

| | Yes | No |
|---|---|---|
| a. Cut down the amount of time you spent on work or other activities | 1 | 2 |
| b. Accomplished less than you would like | 1 | 2 |
| c. Were limited in the kind of work or other activities | 1 | 2 |
| d. Had difficulty performing the work or other activities (for example, it took extra effort) | 1 | 2 |

**Emotional health problems**

During the past 4 weeks, have you had any of the following problems with your work or other regular daily activities as a result of any emotional problems (such as feeling depressed or anxious)? (Select Yes or No)

| | Yes | No |
|---|---|---|
| a. Cut down the amount of time you spent on work or other activities | 1 | 2 |
| b. Accomplished less than you would like | 1 | 2 |
| c. Didn't do work or other activities as carefully as usual | 1 | 2 |

**Social activities**

During the past 4 weeks, to what extent has your physical health or emotional problems interfered with your normal social activities with family, friends, neighbors, or groups? (Select one)
☐ Not at all
☐ Slightly
☐ Moderately

(continued)

**Table 7.8.** — Continued

☐ Quite a bit
☐ Extremely

**Pain**

How much bodily pain have you had during the past 4 weeks? (Select one)
☐ None
☐ Very Mild
☐ Mild
☐ Moderate
☐ Severe
☐ Very Severe

During the past 4 weeks, how much did pain interfere with your normal work (including both work outside the home and housework)? (Select one)
☐ Not at all
☐ A little bit
☐ Moderately
☐ Quite a bit
☐ Extremely

**Energy and Emotions**

these questions are about how you feel and how things have been with you during the past 4 weeks. For each question, please give the one answer that comes closest to the way you have been feeling. (Select one on each line)

| How much of the time During the past 4 weeks.... | All of the Time | Most of the Time | A Good Bit of the Time | Some of the Time | A Little of the Time | None of the Time |
|---|---|---|---|---|---|---|
| a. Did you feel full of pep? | 1 | 2 | 3 | 4 | 5 | 6 |
| b. Have you been a very nervous person? | 1 | 2 | 3 | 4 | 5 | 6 |
| c. Have you felt so down in the dumps that nothing could cheer you up? | 1 | 2 | 3 | 4 | 5 | 6 |
| d. Have you felt calm and peaceful? | 1 | 2 | 3 | 4 | 5 | 6 |
| e. Did you have a lot of energy? | 1 | 2 | 3 | 4 | 5 | 6 |
| f. Have you felt downhearted and blue? | 1 | 2 | 3 | 4 | 5 | 6 |
| g. Did you feel worn out? | 1 | 2 | 3 | 4 | 5 | 6 |
| h. Have you been a happy person? | 1 | 2 | 3 | 4 | 5 | 6 |
| i. Did you feel tired? | 1 | 2 | 3 | 4 | 5 | 6 |

**Social activities**

During the past 4 weeks, how much of the time has your physical health or emotional problems interfered with your social activities (like visiting with friends, relatives, etc.)?
☐ All of the time
☐ Most of the time
☐ Some of the time
☐ A little of the time
☐ None of the time

**General Health**

How true or false is each of the following statements for you? (Select one on each line)

| | Definitely True | Mostly True | Don't Know | Mostly False | Definitely False |
|---|---|---|---|---|---|
| I seem to get sick a little easier than other people | 1 | 2 | 3 | 4 | 5 |
| I am as healthy as anybody I know | 1 | 2 | 3 | 4 | 5 |
| I expect my health to get worse | 1 | 2 | 3 | 4 | 5 |
| My health is excellent | 1 | 2 | 3 | 4 | 5 |

the RAND Health Insurance Experiment and represent an amalgamation of several conceptions of health, including physical functioning, psychological distress and well-being, and general health perceptions (Ware & Sherbourne, 1992). Overall, eight health concepts are measured: *(1)* physical functioning, *(2)* role limitations due to physical problems, *(3)* social functioning, *(4)* bodily pain, *(5)* general mental health, *(6)* role limitations due to emotional problems, *(7)* vitality, and *(8)* general health perceptions (Ware & Sherbourne, 1992). A question about changes in overall health status over the past year is also asked but is not included in the eight categories. Questions cover respondents' behaviors as well as feeling states in the past 4 weeks. An acute version of the questionnaire is available with a 1 week recall period (Ware, 1996).

The SF-36 can be scored as a profile or as summary scores. The SF-36 was not designed to be aggregated into a single score. Scale values for SF-36 are based on the method of summated ratings that allows items in each category to be aggregated without score standardization or item weighting (Ware, 1996). All items in each category were designed to represent equivalent amounts of the underlying health concept. Two scoring methods exist that aggregate items in each category and transform the items to a 0 to 100 scale with high values oriented to good health (Rand Health Sciences Program, 1992; Ware et al., 1993). Based on factor analytic studies, summary scores can be created for physical health and mental health dimensions (Ware et al., 1995). Physical functioning, role limitations due to physical problems, bodily pain, and general health form the basis for the Physical Component Summary. General mental health, role limitations due to emotional problems, social functioning, and vitality form the basis for the Mental Component Summary. The SF-36 can be self-administered or administered by a computer or a trained interviewer in person or by telephone (Ware, 1996). Average administration time of the SF-36 across all age groups is 10 minutes (McHorney, 1996). Extensive use of the SF-36 has resulted in published norms for many different populations (Ware, 1996).

The reliability and validity of the SF-36 have been thoroughly tested (Brazier et al., 1992; McDowell & Newell, 1996; McHorney, Ware, & Raczek, 1993; McHorney, Ware, Lee, & Sherbourne, 1994; Ware, 1995). Internal consistencies of the eight scales exceed 0.75, and most exceed 0.80 and are even higher for the summary scores. The empirical validity of the SF-36 has been established. The SF-36 correlates well with longer health surveys such as the SIP and moderately with other health surveys such as the Nottingham Health Profile. The SF-36 discriminates well between types and levels of disease. Overall, some components of the SF-36 appear to be sensitive to change. Although the physical function scale performs well over time, the mental health scale seems to be rather insensitive to change (Katz, Larson, Phillips, Fossel, & Liang, 1992). As a general measure, the SF-36 lacks some of the scope necessary for assessing the impact of interventions in some populations. Ware (1996) recommends using the SF-36 as a generic core in outcomes studies and then supplementing with appropriate disease-specific measures. The SF-36 does not include health concepts such as cognition or instrumental activities of daily living that are relevant to an older population, and the coverage of activities of daily living is limited.

Several features of the SF-36 should be considered when using the measure with older populations. In a study of older adults, Hayes, Morris, Wolfe, and Morgan (1995) found almost half unable to self-administer the SF-36. For older respondents (65–75 + years), floor effects were problematic for the role functioning scales and ceiling effects were problematic for pain, social functioning, and role-emotional (McHorney, 1996). Moreover, the sensitivity to change of the SF-36 for this population has not been demonstrated (McHorney, 1996).

A 12 item version (the SF-12) is also available. It provides summary scores for physical and mental functioning but not the subscores (Ware, Kosinski, & Keller, 1996; Jenkinson et al., 1997).

### Quality of Well Being Scale (QWB) (Kaplan & Anderson, 1988)

The Quality of Well-Being Scale was designed as a general health status measure for use in population monitoring, program evaluation, clinical research, and policy analysis. Development of the QWB in the 1970s (initially called the Health Status Index [Fanshel & Bush, 1970]) coincides with the development of several other health status measures, for example, the SIP and the predecessors to the SF-36 (Kaplan & Anderson, 1996). The scale is part of a General Health Policy Model that focuses on the allocation of health care resources (Kaplan & Anderson, 1988).

Conceptually, the QWB is different from the other scales discussed thus far. Early on, researchers conceptualized health status as "the product of the social preferences assigned to levels of function and the probabilities of transition among the levels over the life expectancy of an individual or a group" (Patrick, Bush, & Chen, 1973, p. 7). Function was defined in terms of deviations from usual/normal social role functioning as well as deviations (e.g., symptoms and pain) from normal well-being (Patrick et al., 1973). After an exhaustive and mutually exclusive set of functional levels were defined, scale items were culled from existing survey instruments such as the Health Interview Survey (Patrick et al., 1973). Three dimensions defined as Physical Activity, Mobility, and Social Activity cover the spectrum of dysfunction in role performance (Patrick et al., 1973). A list of symptoms and problems that can inhibit function has also been developed; there are currently 25 symptoms with the inclusion of four mental health symptoms that were previously excluded for conceptual reasons (Kaplan & Anderson, 1996; Patrick et al., 1973). Items refer to health on the given day. Contrary to many conceptualizations of health, Kaplan and Anderson (1988, 1996) argue that mental health and social support should not be included as separate categories of health status. They argue that defining an optimal level of social support/resources is problematic, as is making it a target for the health care system, and that separating mental and physical health results in an artificial dichotomy because both components can affect functioning similarly.

Table 7.9 lists the symptom and problem complexes for the QWB scale. Table 7.10 lists the weights for the other components. The QWB is scored as a single index ranging from 0 (death) to 1 (total well-being). Scale values are derived by developing negative weights for functional levels and symptoms based on relative desirability through the method of equally appearing intervals (McDowell & Newell, 1996). Raters were a random sample of San Diego community members. (Kaplan et al., 1976). To obtain the QWB score for a point-in-time estimate of well-being (W), W = 1 − (symptom weight) − (mobility weight) − (physical activity weight) − (social activity weight). To incorporate prognosis, well-life expectancy is calculated as the product of QWB times the expected duration of stay in each function level over a standard life period (Kaplan & Anderson, 1988). In program evaluations, well years or QALYs are calculated from the QWB score and used to describe program effectiveness. The QWB can be administered in roughly 7 minutes or more (McDowell & Newell, 1996). A trained interviewer should administer the scale; a self-administration version is under development (McDowell & Newell, 1996).

The stability of the preference weights has been established (McDowell & Newell, 1996). Recent work on long-term care residents' preference weights for health

**Table 7.9.**

Symptom and Problem Complexes (CPX) for the Quality of Well-Being Scale

| CPX No. | CPX description | Weight |
|---|---|---|
| 1 | Death [not on respondent's card] | −0.727 |
| 2 | Loss of consciousness such as seizure (fits), fainting, or coma (out cold or knocked out) | −0.407 |
| 3 | Burn over large areas of face, body, arms, or legs | −0.387 |
| 4 | Pain, bleeding, itching, or discharge (drainage) from sexual organs — does not include normal menstrual bleeding | −0.349 |
| 5 | Trouble learning, remembering, or thinking clearly | −0.340 |
| 6 | Any combination of one or more hands, feet, arms, or legs either missing, deformed (crooked), paralyzed (unable to move), or broken — includes wearing artificial limbs or braces | −0.333 |
| 7 | Pain, stiffness, weakness, numbness, or other discomfort in chest, stomach (including hernia or rupture), side, neck, back, hips, or any joints or hands, feet, arms, or legs | −0.299 |
| 8 | Pain, burning, bleeding, itching, other difficulty with rectum, bowel movements, or urination (passing water) | −0.292 |
| 9 | Sick or upset stomach, vomiting or loose bowel movement, with or without chills, or aching all over | −0.290 |
| 10 | General tiredness, weakness, or weight loss | −0.259 |
| 11 | Cough, wheezing or shortness of breath, *with* or *without* fever, chills, or aching all over | −0.257 |
| 12 | Spells of feeling upset, being depressed, or of crying | −0.257 |
| 13 | Headache, or dizziness, or ringing in ears, or spells of feeling hot, nervous, or shaky | −0.244 |
| 14 | Burning or itching rash on large areas of face, body, arms, or legs | −0.240 |
| 15 | Trouble talking, such as lisp, stuttering, hoarseness, or being unable to speak | −0.237 |
| 16 | Pain or discomfort in one or both eyes (such as burning or itching) or any trouble seeing after correction | −0.230 |
| 17 | Overweight for age and height or skin defect of face, body, arms, or legs, such as scars, pimples, warts, bruises or changes in color | −0.188 |
| 18 | Pain in ear, tooth, jaw, throat, lips, tongue; several missing or crooked permanent teeth — includes wearing bridges or false teeth | −0.170 |
| 19 | Took medication or stayed on a prescribed diet for health reasons | −0.144 |
| 20 | Wore eyeglasses or contact lenses | −0.101 |
| 21 | Breathing smog or unpleasant air | −0.101 |
| 22 | No symptoms or problems [not on respondent's card] | −0.000 |
| 23 | Standard symptom/problem | −0.257 |
| 24 | Trouble sleeping | −0.257 |
| 25 | Intoxication | −0.257 |
| 26 | Problems with sexual interest or performance | −0.257 |
| 27 | Excessive worry or anxiety | −0.257 |

Reproduced from an original supplied by Dr. Robert M. Kaplan, University of California, San Diego. With permission.

states on the QWB found that long-term care residents and younger adults did not vary significantly on rated preferences for health states (Hays et al., 1996). Convergent and discriminant validity are exhibited by the QWB. The measure is able to discriminate between types and levels of illness (Kaplan & Anderson, 1996) and correlates well with chronic health problems and physician visits (Kaplan et al., 1976) and with the SIP (Read, Quinn, & Hoefer, 1987). The QWB has been sensitive to treatment effects in clinical trials

(Kaplan & Anderson, 1996; McDowell & Newell, 1996). Less work has, however, been done on the reliability and validity of the QWB than on the measures previously discussed.

The instrument has been used in elderly populations but not extensively (Andresen et al., 1995). The ability of the scale to assess change and discriminate between groups of frail older adults is unproved. Kaplan and Anderson (1988) note that the QWB was able to detect treatment benefits in older adult patients with chronic ob-

**Table 7.10.** Dimensions, Function Levels, and Weights or the Quality of Well-Being Scale

| Step definition | Weight |
| --- | --- |
| **Mobility Scale (MOB)** | |
| No limitations for health reasons | 5 |
| Did not drive a car, health related; did not ride in a car as usual for age (younger than 15 years), health related, *and/or* did not use public transportation, health related; *or* had or would have used more help than usual for age to use public transportation, health related | 4 |
| In hospital, health related | 2 |
| **Physical Activity Scale (PAC)** | |
| No limitations for health reasons | 4 |
| In wheelchair, moved or controlled movement of wheelchair without help from someone else, or had trouble or did not try to lift, stoop, bend over, or use stairs or inclines, health related; and/or had any other physical limitation in walking, or did not try to walk as far as or as fast as others the same age are able, health related | 3 |
| In wheelchair, did not move or control the movement or wheelchair without help from someone else, or in bed, chair, or couch for most or all of the day, health related | 1 |
| **Social Activity Scale (SAC)** | |
| No limitations for health reasons | 5 |
| Limited in other (e.g., recreational) role activity, health related | 4 |
| Limited in major (primary) role activity, health related | 3 |
| Performed no major role activity, health related, but did not perform self-care activities | 2 |
| Performed no major role activity, health related, and did not perform or had more help than usual in performance of one or more self-care activities, health related | 1 |

Reproduced from an original supplied by Dr. R.M. Kaplan, University of California, San Diego. With permission.

structive pulmonary disease, although there was no change in pulmonary function. Moreover, recent work derived long-term care residents' preference weights for the following 11 new symptom/problem complexes: incontinent, restrained in bed or chair, unable to control one's behavior, disturbed sleep, agitated, hallucinating, lonely, feeding tube through the nose or stomach, urinary catheter, sit-to-stand requires maximal effort, and walking a short distance causes extreme fatigue (Hays et al., 1996).

### COOP Charts (Nelson et al., 1987)

The COOP Charts are the screening component of the Dartmouth Primary Care Cooperative Information Project's model to assess patient's functional health in routine office visits. The developers of the COOP Charts believe that physicians should be managing and treating functional health as well as the traditional domain of biologic health (Nelson et al., 1987). Nelson, Wasson, Johnson, and Hays (1996, p. 161) describe the Charts as a "simple, easily administered, self-scoring system for screening, assessing, monitoring, and maintaining patient function." Figure 7.1 shows elements of the COOP charts.

Although, the COOP Charts were designed as a clinical rather than a research tool, their conceptual design draws heavily on prior work done by clinical and health status researchers such as Sidney Katz and John Ware (Nelson et al., 1987). The design principles for the COOP Charts required demonstration of reliability, validity, integration into office practice, applicability to a wide range of problems and diagnoses, face validity, ease of inter-

# PHYSICAL FITNESS

During the past 4 weeks . . .
What was the hardest physical activity
you could do for at least 2 minutes?

| | | |
|---|---|---|
| Very heavy (for example)<br>• Run, fast pace<br>• Carry a heavy load upstairs or uphill<br>(25lb/10kg) | | 1 |
| Heavy (for example)<br>• Jog, slow pace<br>• Climb stairs or a hill moderate pace | | 2 |
| Moderate (for example)<br>• Walk, medium pace<br>• Carry a heavy load level ground<br>(25lb/10kg) | | 3 |
| Light (for example)<br>• Walk, medium pace<br>• Carry a light load on level ground<br>(10lb/5kg) | | 4 |
| Very Light (for example)<br>• Walk, slow pace<br>• Wash dishes | | 5 |

A

# FEELINGS

During the past 4 weeks . . .
How much have you been bothered by
emotional problems such as feeling anxious,
depressed, irritable or downhearted and blue?

| | | |
|---|---|---|
| Not at all | | 1 |
| Slightly | | 2 |
| Moderately | | 3 |
| Quite a bit | | 4 |
| Extremely | | 5 |

B

# DAILY ACTIVITIES

During the past 4 weeks . . .
How much difficulty have you had doing your
usual activities or task, both inside and outside
the house because of your physical and
emotional health?

| | | |
|---|---|---|
| No difficulty at all | | 1 |
| A little bit of difficulty | | 2 |
| Some difficulty | | 3 |
| Much difficulty | | 4 |
| Could not do | | 5 |

C

**Figure 7.1.** A. Physical fitness; B. Feelings; C. Daily activities; Dartmouth COOP function and health status measures (A–I) for adults. Copyright © Trustees of Dartmouth College/COOP project 1989. Support provided by the Henry J. Kaiser Family Foundation.

## SOCIAL ACTIVITIES

During the 4 past weeks . . .
Has your physical and emotional health limited
your social activities with family, friends,
neighbors or groups?

| | |
|---|---|
| Not at all | 1 |
| Slightly | 2 |
| Moderately | 3 |
| Quite a bit | 4 |
| Extremely | 5 |

D

## PAIN

During the past 4 weeks . . .
How much bodily pain have you
generally had?

| | |
|---|---|
| No pain | 1 |
| Very mild pain | 2 |
| Mild pain | 3 |
| Moderate pain | 4 |
| Severe pain | 5 |

E

## CHANGE IN HEALTH

How would you rate your overall health
now compared to 4 weeks ago?

| | |
|---|---|
| Much better | 1 |
| A little better | 2 |
| About the same | 3 |
| A little worse | 4 |
| Much worse | 5 |

F

**Figure 7.1** — Continued. D. Social activities; E. Pain; F. Change in health; Dartmouth COOP function and health status measures (A–I) for adults. Copyright © Trustees of Dartmouth College/COOP project 1989. Support provided by the Henry J. Kaiser Family Foundation.

**SOCIAL SUPPORT**

During the past 4 weeks . . .
Was someone available to help you if you
needed and wanted help? For example if you

– felt very nervous, lonely, or blue     – needed help with daily chores
– got sick and had to stay in bed          – needed help just taking care
– needed someone to talk to                    of yourself

| | | |
|---|---|---|
| Yes, as much as I wanted | | 1 |
| Yes, quite a bit | | 2 |
| Yes, some | | 3 |
| Yes, a little | | 4 |
| No, not at all | | 5 |

H

**OVERALL HEALTH**

During the past 4 weeks . . .
How would you rate your health in general?

| | | |
|---|---|---|
| Excellent | | 1 |
| Very good | | 2 |
| Good | | 3 |
| Fair | | 4 |
| Poor | | 5 |

G

**QUALITY OF LIFE**

How have things been going for you during
the past 4 weeks?

| | |
|---|---|
| Very well: could hardly be better | 1 |
| Pretty good | 2 |
| Good & bad parts about equal | 3 |
| Pretty bad | 4 |
| Very bad: could hardly be worse | 5 |

I

**Figure 7.1**—Continued.    G. Overall health; **H**. Social support; **I**. Quality of life; Dartmouth COOP function and health status measures (A–I) for adults. Copyright © Trustees of Dartmouth College/COOP project 1989. Support provided by the Henry J. Kaiser Family Foundation.

pretation, and usefulness to physicians (Nelson et al., 1987). Nine single item charts measure health status in the previous 4 weeks. The charts cover physical fitness, feelings, daily activities, social activities, change in health, overall health, social support, and quality of life. Along with a question, each chart contains simple illustrations representing each level of the health concept. The COOP Charts are scored as a profile, because each chart is a five-point ordinal scale. No summary score is calculated. Higher scores represent worse health, and scores of 4 or 5 should be considered abnormal (Nelson et al., 1996). Charts can be self-administered or administered by a health professional. Completion of the Charts takes less than 5 minutes (McDowell & Newell, 1996).

The reliability and validity of the COOP Charts have been explored in collaboration with researchers on the Medical Outcomes Study (McHorney, et al., 1992) and through multitrait–multimethod techniques (Nelson et al., 1987; see also see McDowell & Newell, 1996). Lower bound estimates of reliabilities of the single items were much lower than multi-item measures of the same concept as well as nonillustrated Medical Outcomes Study global ratings, which causes some concern (McHorney et al., 1992). The inter-rater reliabilities and test–retest reliabilities of the COOP Charts are good (McDowell & Newell, 1996). In terms of validity, the COOP Charts were substantially correlated with longer forms of concepts that they were trying to measure, and they were successful in detecting moderate to large differences between clinically different groups (McHorney et al., 1992). Use of illustrations in single item measures seemed to improve validity, but use of identical illustrations across different health concepts appeared to increase sensitivity to mental health problems in several of the physical domains (McHorney et al., 1992). Relatively low levels of precision for the Charts suggest that their ability to detect minor change in individual patients

is doubtful. Physicians seem to find the information useful, however, in uncovering problems, and patients like the pictures (Nelson et al., 1987).

The COOP Charts have been used successfully with elderly patients (Nelson et al., 1987; Nelson et al., 1990). The Charts have the potential advantage of avoiding the issues of poor literacy and readability of surveys for this population. The inclusion of social support may also be useful for those interested in assessing an elderly population, although cognition is not included.

### Nottingham Health Profile (NHP)

The Nottingham Health Profile was developed in the 1970s as a general health status measure that could be used in community studies to compare health in different populations, to evaluate health interventions, and to identify areas of unmet health need. The NHP was not intended for use in clinical trials, although it has been widely used in this capacity. Developed in England, the NHP is the most widely used general health status measure in Europe (McEwen & McKenna, 1996).

Conceptually, the NHP draws on the work of other heath status measures being developed at the time, but it is unique in its emphasis on the patient's subjective assessment of health status given the growing understanding of importance of this concept in a patient's decision to seek medical care (McEwen & McKenna, 1996). The design principles for the NHP were similar to the COOP charts described earlier: ease of administration and scoring, unambiguous response categories, literacy levels compatible with most of the population, reliability, face and biologic validity and sensitivity to change in individuals over time, and ability to discriminate between illness states (McEwen & McKenna, 1996). Items for the NHP were taken from 768 acute and chronically ill patients describing the effects of ill health and supplemented by items from other health indices (McDowell & Newell, 1996). Items refer to departures from "normal" functioning because it is difficult to specify a norm itself (Hunt, McKenna, & McEwen, 1980). Part I of the NHP has 38 items in six categories: energy level, pain, emotional reaction, sleep, social isolation, and physical abilities. Part II of the NHP has seven items regarding how health affects daily life: work, leisure activities, home management, holidays, sex life, social activities, and family life. All items are answered in a yes/no format.

Developers of the NHP recommend scoring the scale as a profile (McEwen & McKenna, 1996). The six profile scores in Part I are weighted for severity by Thurstone's method of paired comparison. The items are aggregated to form a 0–100 scale. In Part II, the items are not weighted and are simply summed to yield a count of yes responses. Other researchers have attempted to produce overall scores for the NHP (O'Brien, Buxton, & Ferguson, 1987). The NHP is self-administered and takes 10–15 minutes to complete (McDowell & Newell, 1996).

The instrument was initially validated on a sample of four groups of adults over age 60 years with varying levels of health status because these groups were likely to have the greatest problems with self-administration (Hunt et al., 1980). The NHP was able to discriminate between the different groups of older adults. In this study, other demographic factors were not found to affect the scores significantly. Other studies have also demonstrated the NHP's validity by assessing the ability of the instrument to discriminate between clinically distinct groups (Hunt, McEwen, & McKenna, 1985; McDowell & Newell, 1996). Test–retest reliability and other forms of reliability are adequate (McDowell & Newell, 1996). A floor effect has been noted in the NHP due to its initial design focus on those with health care needs (Hunt et al., 1980; McDowell & Newell, 1996). It is not sensitive to change in well populations or those with minor ailments.

The NHP seems to work well in older adults and chronically ill populations because it is sensitive to dysfunction, is written at a reading level of 9 years, and has a simple yes/no response format (McEwen & McKenna, 1996). Cognitive functioning and positive aspects of well-being are not included in the measure.

### Health Utilities Index Mark 3 (HUI) (Feeny et al., 1996)

The Health Utilities Index was developed as a generic HRQL measure for use in clinical studies and population health surveys. The HUI derives from an ongoing stream of research that has resulted in three HUI systems—Mark 1, Mark 2, and Mark 3—over the past 20 years (Boyle et al., 1995). The system has moved from evaluating outcomes of specific populations to use in general population surveys: Mark 1, low-birth-weight infants, Mark 2, survivors of childhood cancer; and Mark 3, general population (Feeny et al., 1996). The Mark 3 is discussed here.

In its conceptualization of health, the HUI is similar to other multidimensional measures discussed earlier. Methodologically, the HUI is unique; its closest relative is the QWB. The HUI has a narrow definition of HRQL, including only physical and emotional dimensions of health status that are "within the skin" of an individual, therefore excluding dimensions such as social interaction (Feeny et al., 1996). The developers have chosen to focus on functional capacity rather than on performance in terms of how deficits from health status inhibit or prohibit the normal functioning of an individual (Feeny et al., 1996).

The Mark 3 includes eight attributes or dimensions of health—vision, hearing, speech, ambulation, dexterity, emotion, cognition, and pain—and each attribute has five to six levels. There are 972,000 possible unique health states. The HUI system ties a multiattribute theory of health status with multiattribute utility theory to value health states and estimate a scoring function (Feeny et al., 1996). The developers note that two types of preferences, either values or utilities, can be used for determining preferences for health states. Only utilities, based on Von Neumann and Morgenstern's utility theory (1944), however, take into account uncertainty in decision making and therefore are more appropriate for use in determining health preferences that are necessarily made under uncertainty (Feeny et al., 1996). To measure preferences for health states, the visual analog scale, the time trade-off technique, and the standard gamble technique can be used, although the standard gamble is the only method that produces the utilities. The scoring system for the HUI Mark 3 (third version) uses a combination of measurements obtained from visual analog scale and standard gamble; the visual analog scale scores are converted to utilities using power curves (Feeny et al., 1996). Table 7.11 shows the items that are included in the Mark 3 version.

Moreover, the investigators are in the process of determining whether the utility function is additive, multiplicative, or multilinear. Determining the form of the utility function is important because it describes the nature of the interactive relationships between the different attributes and their levels. For example, an additive form assumes that there is no preference interactions among attributes or, for example, "a change from level 1 mobility to level 3 mobility would reduce the overall utility by .2 regardless of the health status on the other attributes" (Feeny et al., 1996). Whereas the QWB uses values to determine health state preferences and assumes an additive model, the developers of the HUI contend that model assumptions seem to matter in multiattribute models of health status because their empirical applications reject the assumption of an additive model, and they found substantial differences between utility and value preference scores (Feeny et al., 1996). Value scores tend to place greater weight on minor disability than utility scores (Feeny et al., 1996). The HUI overall score ranges from 0 (dead) to 1

(healthy); one state judged worse than death has a negative utility of 0.03 (Feeny et al., 1996).

Reliability of the scoring formula as well as the instrument is important in these types of measures. The scoring formula for Mark 3 is still in process and is using a random sample of adults, but the scoring formula for Mark 2, which is based on the same principles, was redeveloped on a second population that produced nearly identical scores (Feeny et al., 1996). One month test–retest reliability of the Mark 3 overall scores, using provisional index scores based on Mark 2, was assessed in the 1991 cycle 6 Canadian General Social Survey Health Questionnaire; an intraclass correlation coefficient of 0.767 was obtained (Boyle et al., 1995). Validity assessment of the HUI Mark 3 is ongoing. The HUI Mark 3 has been successfully used in the 1990 Ontario health survey to discriminate health differences by socioeconomic status (Roberge, Berthelot, & Wolfson, 1995). Moreover, all of the possible health states suggested by the HUI system have shown up at least once in population health surveys (Feeny et al., 1996).

The HUI Mark 3 has been successfully used with older adults in Canada in population health surveys. The measure has a potential ceiling effect because it does not capture health beyond "normal" functioning, where many people may be categorized. This is probably not a problem in an elderly population, however, where one is more concerned with floor effects.

## OLDER ADULTS POPULATION

The *Multi-level Assessment Instrument* (MAI) was designed to assess overall well-being or the "good life" in community dwelling older adults (Lawton et al., 1982). The MAI builds on the work of existing assessment instruments such as the OARS and is intended to fill the gaps in existing instruments in the area of well-being (Lawton et al., 1982).

**Table 7.11.**
**Mark 3 Health Status Classification System**

| Attribute | Level | Level description |
|---|---|---|
| Vision | 1 | Able to see well enough to read ordinary newsprint and recognize a friend on the other side of the street, without glasses or contact lenses |
| | 2 | Able to see well enough to read ordinary newsprint and recognize a friend on the other side of the street, but with glasses |
| | 3 | Able to read ordinary newsprint with or without glasses but unable to recognize a friend on the other side of the street, even with glasses |
| | 4 | Able to recognize a friend on the other side of the street with or without glasses but unable to read ordinary newsprint, even with glasses |
| | 5 | Unable to read ordinary newsprint and unable to recognize a friend on the other side of the street, even with glasses |
| | 6 | Unable to see at all |
| Hearing | 1 | Able to hear what is said in a group conversation with at least three other people, without a hearing aid |
| | 2 | Able to hear what is said in a conversation with one other person in a quiet room without a hearing aid, but requires a hearing aid to hear what is said in a group conversation with at least three other people |
| | 3 | Able to hear what is said in a conversation with one other person in a quiet room with a hearing aid, and able to hear what is said in a group conversation with at least three other people with a hearing aid |
| | 4 | Able to hear what is said in a conversation with one other person in a quiet room without a hearing aid, but unable to hear what is said in a group conversation with at least three other people even with a hearing aid |
| | 5 | Able to hear what is said in a conversation with one other person in a quiet room with a hearing aid, but unable to hear what is said in a group conversation with at least three other people even with a hearing aid |
| | 6 | Unable to hear at all |
| Speech | 1 | Able to be understood completely when speaking with strangers or friends |
| | 2 | Able to be understood partially when speaking with strangers but able to be understood completely when speaking with people who know the respondent well |
| | 3 | Able to be understood partially when speaking with strangers or people who know the respondent well |
| | 4 | Unable to be understood when speaking with strangers but able to be understood partially by people who know the respondent well |
| | 5 | Unable to be understood when speaking to other people (or unable to speak at all) |
| Ambulation | 1 | Able to walk around the neighborhood without difficulty, and without walking equipment |
| | 2 | Able to walk around the neighborhood with difficulty, but does not require walking equipment or the help of another person |
| | 3 | Able to walk around the neighborhood with walking equipment, but without the help of another person |
| | 4 | Able to walk only short distances with walking equipment and requires a wheelchair to get around the neighborhood |
| | 5 | Unable to walk alone, even with walking equipment; able to walk short distances with the help of another person and requires a wheelchair to get around the neighborhood |
| | 6 | Cannot walk at all |
| Dexterity | 1 | Full use of two hands and ten fingers |
| | 2 | Limitations in the use of hands or fingers, but does not require special tools or help of another person |
| | 3 | Limitations in the use of hands or fingers, is independent with use of special tools (does not require the help of another person) |
| | 4 | Limitations in the use of hands or fingers, requires the help of another person for some tasks (not independent even with use of special tools) |
| | 5 | Limitations in use of hands or fingers, requires the help of another person for most tasks (not independent even with use of special tools) |

*(continued)*

**Table 7.11.— Continued**

| | | |
|---|---|---|
| | 6 | Limitations in use of hands or fingers, requires the help of another person for all tasks (not independent even with use of special tools) |
| Emotion | 1 | Happy and interested in life |
| | 2 | Somewhat happy |
| | 3 | Somewhat unhappy |
| | 4 | Very unhappy |
| | 5 | So unhappy that life is not worthwhile |
| Cognition | 1 | Able to remember most things, think clearly, and solve day to day problems |
| | 2 | Able to remember most things, but have a little difficulty when trying to think and solve day to day problems |
| | 3 | Somewhat forgetful, but able to think clearly and solve day to day problems |
| | 4 | Somewhat forgetful and have a little difficulty when trying to think or solve day to day problems |
| | 5 | Very forgetful and have great difficulty when trying to think or solve day to day problems. |
| | 6 | Unable to remember anything at all and unable to think or solve day to day problems |
| Pain | 1 | Free of pain and discomfort |
| | 2 | Mild to moderate pain that prevents no activities |
| | 3 | Moderate pain that prevents a few activities |
| | 4 | Moderate to severe pain that prevents some activities |
| | 5 | Severe pain that prevents most activities |

Conceptually, assessment of four sectors represents quality of life in older adults: behavioral competence, psychological well-being, perceived QOL, and objective environment (Lawton et al., 1982). The MAI is a measure of behavioral competence, perceived environmental quality, and psychological well-being; the measure contains a total of 152 items. The following domains and subdomains are measured in the MAI: behavioral competence; physical health (self-rated health, use of health services, health conditions, mobility, use of assistive devices); cognition (mental status, cognitive symptoms), activities of daily living, (instrumental activities of daily living personal maintenance activities); time use (social activities, sports, hobbies); social relations and interaction (family and friends); psychological well-being (morale, psychiatric symptoms); and perceived quality of environment (housing quality, neighborhood quality, personal security). Table 7.12 indicates the number of questions given to each domain. Domain indices and subindices can be scored by summing the items. Lawton (1997) has been expanding on the MAI in

**Table 7.12. Multi-level Assessment Instrument: Numbers of Items in Each Domain**

| | No. of items |
|---|---|
| 1. Physical health | |
| Self-rated health | 4 |
| Use of health services | 3 |
| Health conditions | 24 |
| Mobility | 3 |
| Use of mobility aids | 13 |
| 2. Cognition | |
| Mental status | 11 |
| Cognitive symptoms | 4 |
| 3. Activities of daily living | |
| Instrumental activities of daily living scale | 9 |
| Physical self-maintenance activities | 7 |
| 4. Time use | |
| Social activities, hobbies | 19 |
| 5. Social relations and interactions | |
| Family | 10 |
| Friends | 6 |
| 6. Personal adjustment | |
| Morale | 9 |
| Psychiatric symptoms | 5 |
| 7. Perceived environment | |
| Housing quality | 9 |
| Neighborhood quality | 12 |
| Personal security | 4 |
| Total | 152 |

Source: Adapted from Lawton et al. (1982).

his current work. Measures of friends quality, family quality, and time quality have been developed.

The MAI scale was developed and tested using samples of independently living older people (n = 426), high-intensity in-home service recipients (n = 99), and institutional waiting-list clients (n = 65) (Lawton et al., 1982). Administration of the MAI takes roughly 50 minutes (Lawton et al., 1982). Inter-rater reliability ranged from 0.88 to 0.58 on the seven scales; internal consistency reliability was above 0.7 for all the domain scales and ranged from a low of 0.39 to 0.91 for the subdomains. Test–retest reliabilities for the subdomains ranged from 0.65 to 0.99 except for physical self-maintenance, which had a correlation of 0.36 (Lawton et al., 1982). The MAI showed a weak ability to discriminate between the samples described, and there was weak agreement between MAI scores and independent determinations made by a clinical psychologist and a housing administrator (Lawton et al., 1982). Lawton and colleagues (1982) noted that the social interaction, environment, and time use scales require improvement.

## CONCLUSION

Researchers and clinicians have advanced the idea of QOL into clinical practice and research and onto the national policy agenda. We must, however, be careful to not make the mistake of hubris in this difficult area. Measurement is always an abstraction; and QOL can be seen as an evanescent concept, given that a large part of it rests with the perception of the individual.

Most widely used QOL measures represent aggregations of QOL, which are useful for research and policy purposes. Several issues, however, remain unresolved. Lack of consistency of definition remains a problem. Also, to effectively quantify this concept, there must be a rational basis for the measure's weighting system. Finally,

this research begs the question of whether a single value can convey enough information to accurately measure QOL.

The same QOL measures may be used for different purposes. Quality of Life measures are used at a population level to inform policy, at a clinical level to inform quality of care, and at an individual level to inform personal treatment decisions. A potential conflict, however, exists in preferences for individual versus policy level allocation of health care resources. Using aggregations of QOL based on group norms is most constructive when making inferences at a group level. At the level of the individual treatment decision, however, QOL considerations are critical, but it is more reasonable to apply individual weights to quality of life domains unless one is allocating resources on the basis of public policy where societal values form the basis for allocation decisions.

## REFERENCES

Abt Associates Inc. (1996). *Evaluation of the long term care survey process* (final report). Cambridge, MA: Abt Associates Inc.

Andresen, E. M., Patrick, D. L., Carter, W. B., & Malmgren, J. A. (1995). Comparing the performance of health status measures for older adults. *Journal of the American Geriatrics Society, 43*(9), 1030–1034.

Andrews, F. M., & Withey, S. B. (1976). *Social indicators of well-being: Americans' perceptions of life quality.* New York: Plenum Press.

Atherly, A. (1997). Condition-specific measures. In R. L. Kane (Ed.), *Understanding health care outcomes research* (pp. 51–63). Gaithersburg, MD: Aspen Publishing.

Balaban, D. J., Sagi, P. C., Goldfarb, N. I., & Nettler, S. (1986). Weights for scoring the quality of well-being instrument among rheumatoid arthritics. A comparison to general population weights. *Medical Care, 24*(11), 973–980.

Bergner, M., Bobbit, R. A., Carter, W. B., & Gilson, B. S. (1981). The Sickness Impact Profile: Development and final revision of a health status measure. *Medical Care, 19*(8), 787–805.

Bergner, M., Bobbitt, R. A., Kressel, S., Pollard, W. E., Gilson, B. S., & Morris, J. R. (1976). The sickness impact profile: Conceptual formulation and methodology for the development of a health status measure. *International Journal of Health Services, 6,* 393–415.

Berzon, R. A., Mauskopf, J. A., & Simeon, G. P. (1996). Choosing a health profile (descriptive) and/or a patient-preference (utility) measure for a clinical trial. In B. Spilker (Ed.), *Quality of life and pharmacoeconomics in clinical trials* (2nd ed., pp. 375–380). Philadelphia: Lippincott-Raven.

Birren, J. E., & Dieckmann, L. (1991). Concepts and content of quality of life in the later years: An overview. In J. E. Birren, J. E. Lubben, J. C. Rowe, & D. E. Deutchman (Eds.), *The concept and measurement of quality of life in the frail elderly* (pp. 344–360). San Diego: Academic Press.

Birren, J. E., Lubben, J. E., Rowe, J. C., & Deutchman, D. E. (Eds.). (1991). *The concept and measurement of quality of life in the frail elderly.* San Diego: Academic Press.

Boyle, M. H., Furlong, W., Feeny, D., Torrance, G. W., & Hatcher, J. (1995). Reliability of the Health Utilities Index—Mark III used in the 1991 cycle 6 Canadian General Social Survey Health Questionnaire. *Quality of Life Research, 4,* 249–257.

Brazier, J. E., Harper, R., Jones, N. M., O'Cathain, A., Thomas, K. J., Usherwood, T., & Westlake, L. (1992). Validating the SF-36 health survey questionnaire: New outcome measure for primary care. *British Medical Journal, 305*(6846), 160–164.

Brooks, R. (1996). EUROQOL: The current state of play. *Health Policy, 37*(1), 53–72.

Campbell, A., Converse, P. E., & Rodgers, W. L. (1976). *The Quality of American Life: Perceptions, Evaluations, and Satisfactions.* New York: Russell Sage Foundation.

Cella, D. F., & Tulsky, D. S. (1990). Measuring quality of life today: Methodological aspects. *Oncology, 5*(4), 29–38.

Cohn, J., & Sugar, J. A. (1991). Determinants of quality of life in institutions: Perceptions of frail older residents, staff, and families. In J. E. Birren, J. E. Lubben, J. C. Rowe, & D. E. Deutchman (Eds.), *The concept and measurement of quality of life in the frail elderly* (pp. 28–49). San Diego: Academic Press.

Collopy, B. (1988). Autonomy in long-term care: Some crucial distinctions. *Gerontologist, 28,* 10–17.

Damiano, A. M. (1996). The Sickness Impact Profile. In B. Spilker (Ed.), *Quality of life and pharmacoeconomics in clinical trials*

(2nd ed., pp. 347–354). Philadelphia: Lippincott-Raven.

de Bruin, A. F., de Witte, L. P., Stevens, F., & Diederiks, J. P. (1992). Sickness Impact Profile: The state of the art of a generic functional status measure. *Social Science & Medicine, 35*(8), 1003–1014.

Degenholtz, H. D., Kane, R. A., & Kivnick, H. Q. (1997). Care-related preferences and values of elderly community-based LTC consumers: Can case managers learn what's important to clients? *Gerontologist, 37*(6), 767–777.

Erickson, P., Wilson, R., & Shannon, I. (1995). *Years of healthy life* (Healthy People 2000 Statistical Notes, Number 7). Washington, DC: US Department of Health and Human Services, Public Health Service, Centers for Disease Control and Prevention, National Center for Health Statistics.

Essink-Bot, M. L., Krabbe, P. F., Bonsel, G. J., & Aaronson, N. K. (1997). An empirical comparison of four generic health status measures. The Nottingham Health Profile, the Medical Outcomes Study 36-item Short-Form Health Survey, the COOP/WONCA charts, and the EuroQol instrument. *Medical Care, 35*(5), 522–537.

Fanshel, S., & Bush, J. W. (1970). A Health-Status Index and its application to health-services outcomes. *Operations Research, 18,* 1021–1065.

Feeny, D. H., Torrance, G. W., & Furlong, W. J. (1996). Health utilities index. In B. Spilker (Ed.), *Quality of life and pharmacoeconomics in clinical trials* (2nd ed., pp. 239–252). Philadelphia: Lippincott-Raven.

Fries, J. F. (1980). Aging, natural death, and the compression of morbidity. *New England Journal of Medicine, 303,* 130–136.

Fryback, D. G., & Lawrence, W. F. J. (1997). Dollars may not buy as many QALYs as we think: A problem with defining quality-of-life adjustments. *Medical Decision Making, 17*(3), 276–1284.

Fryback, D. G., Lawrence, W. F., Martin, P. A., Klein, R., & Klein, B. E. (1997). Predicting Quality of Well-being scores from the SF-36: Results from the Beaver Dam Health Outcomes Study. *Medical Decision Making, 17*(1), 1–9.

Gentile, K. M. (1991). A review of the literature on interventions and quality of life in the frail elderly. In J. E. Birren, J. E. Lubben, J. C. Rowe, & D. E. Deutchman (Eds.), *The concept and measurement of quality of life in the frail elderly* (pp. 74–88). San Diego: Academic Press, Inc.

George, L. K., & Bearon, L. B. (1980). *Quality*

*of life in older persons.* New York: Human Sciences Press.

Gerety, M. B., Cornell, J. E., Mulrow, C. D., Tuley, M., Hazuda, H. P., Lichtenstein, M., Kanten, D. N., Aguilar, C., Kadri, A. A., & Rosenberg, J. (1994). The Sickness Impact Profile for nursing homes (SIP-NH) [published erratum appears in J Gerontol 1994 49(2):M43]. *Journal of Gerontology, 49*(1), M2–8.

Gill, T. M., & Feinstein, A. R. (1994). A critical appraisal of the quality of quality-of-life measurements. *Journal of the American Medical Association, 272,* 619–626.

Greenfield, S., & Nelson, E. C. (1992). Recent developments and future issues in the use of health status assessment measures in clinical settings. *Medical Care, 30*(5), MS23–MS41.

Grootendorst, P. V., Feeny, D. H., & Furlong, W. (1997). Does it matter whom and how you ask? Inter- and intra-rater agreement in the Ontario Health Survey. *Journal of Clinical Epidemiology, 50,* 127–135.

Guyatt, G. H., Feeny, D. H., & Patrick, D. L. (1993). Measuring health-related quality of life. *Annals of Internal Medicine, 118,* 622–629.

Guyatt, G. H., Jaeschke, R., Feeny, D. H., & Patrick, D. L. (1996). Measurements in clinical trials: Choosing the right approach. In B. Spilker (Ed.), *Quality of life and pharmacoeconomics in clinical trials* (2nd ed., pp. 41–48). Philadelphia: Lippincott-Raven.

Hayes, V., Morris, J., Wolfe, C., & Morgan, M. (1995). The SF-36 health survey questionnaire: Is it suitable for use with older adults? *Age & Ageing, 24*(2), 120–125.

Hays, R. D., Siu, A. L., Keeler, E., Marshall, G. N., Kaplan, R. M., Simmons, S., el Mouchi, D., & Schnelle, J. F. (1996). Long-term care residents' preferences for health states on the quality of well-being scale. *Medical Decision Making, 16*(3), 254–261.

Hunt, S. M., McEwen, J., & McKenna, S. P. (1985). Measuring health status: A new tool for clinicians and epidemiologists. *Journal of the Royal College of General Practitioners, 35*(273), 185–188.

Hunt, S. M., McKenna, S. P., & McEwen, J. A. (1980). A quantitative approach to perceived health status: A validation study. *Journal of Epidemiology and Community Health, 34,* 281–285.

Jenkinson, C., Fitzpatrick, R., & Argyle, M. (1988). The Nottingham Health Profile: An analysis of its sensitivity in differentiating illness groups. *Social Science & Medicine, 27*(12), 1411–1414.

Jenkinson, C., Layte, R., Jenkinson, D., Lawrence, K., Petersen, S., Paice, C., & Stradling, J. (1997). A shorter form health survey: Can the SF-12 replicate results from the SF-36 in longitudinal studies? *Journal of Public Health Medicine, 19*(2), 179–186.

Kane, R. A., Giles, K., Lawton, M. P., & Kane, R. L. (1999). *Development of measures and indicators of quality of life in nursing homes: Wave I* (Report to the Health Care Financing Administration ). Minneapolis: University of Minnesota School of Public Health.

Kaplan, R. M. (1995). Utility assessment for estimating quality-adjusted life years. In F. A. Sloan (Ed.), *Valuing health care* (pp. 31–60). New York: Cambridge University Press.

Kaplan, R. M., & Anderson, J. P. (1988). A general health policy model: Update and applications. *Health Services Research, 23*(2), 203–235.

Kaplan, R. M., & Anderson, J. P. (1996). The general health policy model: an integrated approach. In B. Spilker (Ed.), *Quality of life and pharmacoeconomics in clinical trials* (2nd ed., pp. 309–322). Philadelphia: Lippincott-Raven.

Kaplan, R. M., Bush, J. W., & Berry, C. C. (1976). Health status: Types of validity and the index of well-being. *Health Services Research, 11*(4), 478–507.

Katz, J. N., Larson, M. G., Phillips, C. B., Fossel, A. H., & Liang, M. H. (1992). Comparative measurement sensitivity of short and longer health status instruments. *Medical Care, 30*(10), 917–925.

Katz, S., Branch, L. G., Branson, M. H., Papsidero, J. A., Beck, J. C., & Greer, D. S. (1983). Active life expectancy. *New England Journal of Medicine, 309*(20), 1218–1224.

Katz, S., & Gurland, B. J. (1991). Science of quality of life in elders: Challenge and opportunity. In J. E. Birren, J. E. Lubben, J. C. Rowe, & D. E. Deutchman (Eds.), *The concept and measurement of quality of life in the frail elderly* (pp. 335–343). San Diego: Academic Press.

Kemper, P., & Murtaugh, C. M. (1991). Lifetime use of nursing home care. *New England Journal of Medicine, 324,* 595–600.

Kozma, A., & Stones, M. J. (1980). The measurement of happiness: Development of the Memorial University of Newfoundland Scale of Happiness (MUNSH). *Journal of Gerontology, 35*(6), 906–912.

Lawton, M. P. (1975). The Philadelphia geriatric center morale scale: A revision. *Journal of Gerontology, 30*(1), 85–89.

Lawton, M. P. (1983). Environment and other determinants of well-being in older people. *Gerontologist, 23*(4), 349–357.

Lawton, M. P. (1991). A multidimensional view of quality of life in frail elders. In J. E. Birren, J. E. Lubben, J. C. Rowe, & D. E. Deutchman (Eds.), *The concept and measurement of quality of life in the frail elderly* (pp. 3–27). San Diego: Academic Press.

Lawton, M. P. (1997) *Quality of life in health and illness.* Paper presented at the American Psychological Association, Section on Aging of the Division of Health Psychology, Chicago, August 15, 1997.

Lawton, M. P., Moss, M., Fulcomer, M., & Kleban, M. H. (1982). A research and service oriented multilevel assessment instrument. *Journal of Gerontology, 37*(1), 91–99.

Magaziner, J., Simonsick, E., Kashner, E., & Hebel, J. (1988). Patient-proxy response comparability on measures of patient health and functional status. *Journal of Clinical Epidemiology, 41*(11), 1065–1074.

Martini, C. J., & McDowell, I. (1976). Health status: Patient and physician judgments. *Health Services Research, 11*(4), 508–515.

McDowell, I., & Newell, C. (1996). *Social health. Measuring health: A guide to rating scales and questionnaires.* (2nd ed.). New York: Oxford University Press.

McEwen, J., & McKenna, S. P. (1996). Nottingham Health Profile. In B. Spilker (Ed.), *Quality of life and pharmacoeconomics in clinical trials* (2nd ed., pp. 281–286). Philadelphia: Lippincott-Raven.

McHorney, C. A. (1996). Measuring and monitoring general health status in elderly persons: Practical and methodological issues in using the SF-36 health survey. *Gerontologist, 36*, 571–583.

McHorney, C. A., Ware, J. E. Jr., Lee, J. F. R., & Sherbourne, C. D. (1994). The MOS 36-item short-form health survey (SF-36): III. Tests of data quality, scaling assumptions, and reliability across diverse patient groups. *Medical Care, 32*(1), 40–66.

McHorney, C. A., Ware, J. E. Jr., & Raczek, A. E. (1993). The MOS 36-Item Short-Form Health Survey (SF-36): II. Psychometric and clinical tests of validity in measuring physical and mental health constructs. *Medical Care, 31*(3), 247–263.

McHorney, C. A., Ware, J. E. Jr., Rogers, W., Raczek, A. E., & Lu, J. F. (1992). The validity and relative precision of MOS short- and long-form health status scales and Dartmouth COOP charts. Results from the Medical Outcomes Study. *Medical Care, 30*(5 Suppl), MS253–MS265.

Mor, V., Branco, K., Fleishman, J., Hawes, C., Phillips, C., Morris, J., & Fries, B. (1995). The structure of social engagement among nursing home residents. *Journal of Gerontology Psychological Sciences, 50B*(1), P1–P8.

Nelson, E., Wasson, J., Kirk, J., Keller, A., Clark, D., Dietrich, A., Stewart, A., & Zubkoff, M. (1987). Assessment of function in routine clinical practice: Description of the COOP chart method and preliminary findings. *Journal of Chronic Diseases, 40 Suppl 1*, 55S–69S.

Nelson, E. C., Landgraf, J. M., Hays, R. D., Wasson, J. H., & Kirk, J. W. (1990). The functional status of patients: How can it be measured in physicians' offices? *Medical Care, 28*(12), 1111–1126.

Nelson, E. C., Wasson, J. H., Johnson, D. J., & Hays, R. D. (1996). Dartmouth COOP functional health assessment charts: Brief measures for clinical practice. In B. Spilker (Ed.), *Quality of life and pharmacoeconomics in clinical trials* (2nd ed., pp. 161–168). Philadelphia: Lippincott-Raven.

Nerenz, D. R., Repasky, D. P., Whitehouse, F. W., & Kahkonen, D. M. (1992). Ongoing assessment of health status in patients with diabetes mellitus. *Medical Care, 30*(5 Suppl), MS112–MS124.

Neugarten, B. L., Havighurst, R. J., & Tobin, S. S. (1961). The measurement of life satisfaction. *Journal of Gerontology, 16*, 134–143.

Newhouse, J. P. (1993). An iconoclastic view of health cost containment. *Health Affairs* (Suppl), 12, 152–171.

O'Brien, B. J., Buxton, M. J., & Ferguson, B. A. (1987). Measuring the effectiveness of heart transplant programmes: Quality of life data and their relationship to survival analysis. *Journal of Chronic Diseases, 40 (Suppl 1)*, 137S–158S.

Patrick, D. L., Bush, J. W., & Chen, M. M. (1973). Toward an operational definition of health. *Journal of Health & Social Behavior, 14*(1), 6–23.

Patrick, D. L., & Erickson, P. (1993). *Health Status and health policy: Quality of life in health care evaluation and resource allocation.* New York: Oxford University Press.

Pearlman, R. A., & Uhlmann, R. F. (1991). Quality of life in elderly, chronically ill outpatients. *Journal of Gerontology, 46*(2), M31–38.

Rand Health Sciences Program (1992). *RAND 36-item Health Survey 1.0.* Santa Monica, CA: RAND Corporation.

Read, J. L., Quinn, R. J., & Hoefer, M. A. (1987). Measuring overall health: An evaluation of three important approaches.

*Journal of Chronic Diseases, 40 Suppl*(1), 7S–26S.

Roberge, R., Berthelot, J.-M., & Wolfson, M. (1995). The Health Utility Index: Measuring health differences in Ontario by socioeconomic status. *Health Reports, 7*(2), 25–32.

Rothman, M. L., Hedrick, S., & Inui, T. (1989). The Sickness Impact Profile as a measure of the health status of noncognitively impaired nursing home residents. *Medical Care, 27*(3 Suppl), S157–S167.

Rowe, J. W., & Kahn, R. L. (1998). *Successful Aging.* New York: Random House.

Rubenstein, L., Schairer, C., Wieland, G., & Kane, R. (1984). Systematic biases in functional status of assessment of elderly adults: Effects of different data sources. *Journal of Gerontology, 39*(6), 686–691.

Sackett, D. L., & Torrance, G. W. (1978). The utility of different health states as perceived by the general public. *Journal of Chronic Diseases, 31,* 697–704.

Schipper, H., Clinch, J. J., & Olweny, C. L. M. (1996). Quality of life studies: Definitions and conceptual issues. In B. Spilker (Ed.), *Quality of life and pharmacoeconomics in clinical trials* (2nd ed., pp. 11–24). Philadelphia: Lippincott-Raven.

Steinwachs, D. M., Wu, A. W., & Cagney, K. A. (1996). Outcomes Research and Quality of Care. In Spilker (Ed.), *Quality of life and pharmacoeconomics in clinical trials* (2nd ed., pp. 747–752). Philadelphia: Lippincott-Raven.

Stewart, A., Sherbourne, C., & Brod, M. (1996). Measuring health-related quality of life in older and demented populations. In B. Spilker (Ed.), *Quality of life and pharmacoeconomics in clinical trials* (2nd ed., pp. 819–830). Philadelphia: Lippincott-Raven.

Thomas, W. H. (1994). *The Eden alternative: Nature, hope, and nursing homes.* Sherburne, NY: Eden Alternative Foundation.

Tsevat, J., Dawson, N. V., Wu, A. W., Lynn, J., Soukup, J. R., Cook, E. F., Vidaillet, H., & Phillips, R. (1998). Health values of hospitalized patients 80 years or older: HELP investigators. Hospitalized Elderly Longitudinal Project. *JAMA, 279*(5), 371–375.

Verbrugge, L. M. (1984). Longer life but worsening health? Trends in health and mortality of middle-aged and older persons. *Milbank Memorial Fund Quarterly, 62,* 475–519.

Von Neumann, J., & Morgenstern, O. (1944). *Theory of Games and Economic Behaviour.* Princeton, NJ: Princeton University Press.

Wagstaff, A. (1996). Health care: QALYs and the equity-efficiency tradeoff. In R. Layard & S. Glaister (Eds.), *Cost-benefit analysis* (2nd ed.). New York: Cambridge University Press.

Ware, J. E. (1995). The status of health assessment, 1994. *Annual Review of Public Health, 16,* 327–354.

Ware, J. E., Kosinski, M., & Keller, S. D. (1996). A 12-item short-form health survey: Construction of scales and preliminary tests of reliability and validity. *Medical Care, 34*(3), 220–233.

Ware, J. E. Jr. (1996). The SF-36 Health Survey. In B. Spilker (Ed.), *Quality of life and pharmacoeconomics in clinical trials* (2nd ed., pp. 337–346). Philadelphia: Lippincott-Raven.

Ware, J. E. Jr., & Keller, S. D. (1996). Interpreting General Health Measures. In B. Spilker (Ed.), *Quality of life and pharmacoeconomics in clinical trials* (2nd ed., pp. 445–460). Philadelphia: Lippincott-Raven.

Ware, J. E. Jr., Kosinski, M., Bayliss, M. S., McHorney, C. A., Rogers, W. H., & Raczek, A. (1995). Comparison of methods for the scoring and statistical analysis of SF-36 health profile and summary measures: Summary of results from the medical outcomes study. *Medical Care, 33*(4, Suppl), AS264–AS279.

Ware, J. E. Jr., & Sherbourne, C. D. (1992). The MOS 36-item short-form health survey (SF-36). I. Conceptual framework and item selection. *Medical Care, 30*(6), 473–483.

Ware, J. E. Jr., Snow, K. K., Kosinski, M., & Gandek, B. (1993). *SF-36 Health Survey: Manual and interpretation guide.* Boston: The Health Institute, New England Medical Center.

Wilkin, D., & Hughes, B. (1987). Residential care of elderly people: The consumers' view. *Ageing and Society, 7,* 175–201.

World Health Organization. (1948). *Constitution of the World Health Organization.* Geneva, Switzerland: WHO Basic Documents.

Wu, A., Jacobson, D., Berzon, R., Revicki, D., van der Horst, C., Fichtenbaum, C., Saag, M., L, L., Hardy, D., & Feinberg, J. (1997). The effect of mode of administration on Medical Outcomes Study health ratings and EuroQol scores in AIDS. *Quality of Life Research, 6,* 3–10.

Zimmerman, D. R., Karon, S. L., Arling, G., Clark, B. R., Collins, T., Ross, R., & Sainfort, F. (1995). Development and testing of nursing home quality indicators. *Health Care Financing Review, 16*(4), 107–127.

# 8

# Values and Preferences

ROSALIE A. KANE

In clinical settings, the preferences and values of older people are rarely assessed systematically. In research contexts, if a research project incorporates questions about preferences and values, an instrument tends to be designed ad hoc for that purpose, sometimes based on measures of specific values developed for studies with younger people and sometimes narrowly tailored to the particular preference being investigated—for example, to enter a nursing home (Mattimore et al., 1997), to participate in research (Sachs et al., 1994), to have (or decline) end-of-life-treatment (Sachs et al., 1994; Tsevat et al., 1988; Wetle et al., 1988; Zweibel & Cassel, 1989), or to have cash payments as opposed to in-kind home-care services (Mahoney & Simon-Rusinowitz, 1997). In contrast to the domains discussed in other chapters, for which many of the available instruments have long pedigrees and use histories, tools to measure the preferences and values of older people, particularly those with needs for care, are underdeveloped.

This chapter advances arguments to support the systematic assessment of the general preferences and values of older people to use in clinical settings and for research purposes. It also argues that preferences and values should be the focus of gerontological research that goes beyond the well-mined topic of end-of-life treatment preferences. Having made that general point, however, a host of questions remain about the degree of specificity and detail that should be sought in an assessment tool, the types of preferences and values that should be assessed, and what, if any, aggregations and scoring should be attempted. Even more basically, one can ask whether it is possible to develop tools that meet the tests of reliability and validity, and, indeed, how one validates a tool that assesses anything as individualized and subjective as a preference or value.

Thus, in the values domain, the number of caveats, questions, and nagging doubts varies inversely with the number of instruments available for inspection. The late 1980s and 1990s have, however, witnessed a particular interest in examining older people's values and preferences and incorporating such assessment into care management. The chapter concludes with an examination of some of the instruments still at the early testing stages.

## DEFINITIONS

The terms *preference* and *value* are sometimes used interchangeably. For the purpose of this chapter, we have adopted the view Ogletree (1995) put forward in the *Encyclopedia of Bioethics*. He described values as "concepts we use to explain how and why various realities matter . . . ideas, images, and notions that attract us. We aspire after the good they articulate. We expect to find our own good in relation to what they offer." Values, that is, deeply held views of what constitutes the good and desirable, are balanced by *disvalues* — concepts that explain what is undesirable, harmful, or unworthy and that relate to realities we resist or avoid.

Values are associated with both reasoning and feelings. We can argue rationally in favor of a particular value — be it moral, social, or aesthetic — but we also know it as our *own* value if it evokes positive emotion, makes us feel good or feel moved, or, in the case of disvalues, it evokes negative feelings and repugnance. As people clarify the connections and priorities that order their own values, they may be said to evolve a *values system*. But, as Ogletree (1995) points out, coherent sets of values are not easily achieved or sustained, and, "because of the complexity of experience, value syntheses can never fully overcome areas of ambivalence or wholly resolve internal strains." If values tend to be uncertain and conflicting rather than part of coherent personal value systems, then additional problems arise in interpreting information about the values of an older patient or client that is collected at any one point in time.

*Preferences* is used here to refer to specific choices that typically flow from values. Preferences may be important or trivial; they may be enduring or transitory. Consider the differences between a preference for vanilla ice cream most of the time (trivial and not necessarily consistent) and a preference for outdoor rural life (possibly important and likely consistent). The latter preference may, in turn, spring from a value for self-sufficiency, closeness to nature, or some other larger value. In practice, "values" and "preferences" are often used interchangeably, and distinctions made between them differ from author to author.

The economist's term *utility* is sometimes defined as "satisfaction of preferences." Much theoretical economic modeling is based on the assumption that people will act so as to maximize their utilities. Philosophers also use the concept of "utility" to apply utilitarian views that the good society acts so as to maximize the utilities (i.e., satisfy the preferences) of the majority. (Some ethicists, however, believe it important to distinguish between utility in terms of "that which is desired" and utility in terms of "that which is desirable" [Campbell, 1995].) If one believes, as do many economists, that people always act so as to maximize their utilities, then one could infer persons' values and preferences by observing their behavior. For reasons discussed in the next few sections, this chapter rejects the view that behavior provides an adequate and accurate lens into preferences. Rather, we propose that values and preferences be assessed directly and that research be conducted that describes the relationship between expressed preferences and behavior.

Values and preferences are linked to two other concepts: *personality,* on the one hand, and *beliefs* or *attitudes,* on the other (Ajzen, 1988). At some level, it is hard to distinguish whether a person's strong preferences — for example, to comply with authority, to take risks, to be innovative, to be contemplative — are more a function of personality traits than of preferences. Although values and preferences have an emotional dimension (people recognize them because they feel good and right), they also bear a relationship to cognitive understanding of the world and how it works and, therefore, are related to individuals' beliefs and attitudes.

## CONCEPTUAL FRAMEWORK

### Autonomy and Values and Preferences

Personal autonomy is considered important as an end in itself and as an instrumental goal related to maximizing a person's well-being. Some would say autonomy is necessary for human beings to enjoy fulfilled lives and to make moral decisions. Autonomy can be simply defined as "self-direction." Autonomous individuals control and shape their own lives and are the final arbitrators of their own choices. Ethicists worldwide, and even more particularly in the United States, tend to give great weight to the principle of respect for autonomy, a value that is also found in the ethical codes of many health professions. Autonomy is assigned such a pivotal position, in part, because in the pluralistic U.S. society, where one cannot assume cultural or religious commonality, the best means of ensuring the interest and welfare of each citizen seems to reside in respect for his or her autonomy. Thus, health professionals and social service professionals widely profess to support personal autonomy, sometimes called *self-determination,* for their clientele. The doctrine of informed consent also flows from this principle. Arguably, if health professionals are to do a good job of enhancing and respecting autonomy, they need to know something about older persons' preferences.

Philosophers (Agich, 1993) and sociologists (Lidz, Fischer, & Arnold, 1992) have eloquently attested to the short shrift that is given to the autonomy of older people needing long-term care, either in public policy or in current practice. This practice is particularly documented with nursing homes, but it is also apparent in the home care context (Clemens et al., 1994; Kane & Caplan, 1990, 1993).

An ongoing debate rages about the conditions under which autonomy can be said to exist. At a minimum, an autonomous choice is one made freely and without coercion, is made based on accurate information about the alternatives and their likely effects, and involves application of one's own values to the selection of alternatives. The latter condition is sometimes called *authenticity*—that is, choices made in accordance with values. To process information, weigh alternatives, and reflect on one's own values, some threshold of cognitive performance is needed. A decision that others widely disparage as foolish cannot be used as evidence that the decision-maker is decisionally incompetent because the competence of the decision-maker cannot be judged by the content of the choice or its results. Rather, the competent decision-maker needs to demonstrate some understanding of the available choices and the likely results of each, as well as reasons for the choice that comport with his or her values (Caplan, 1990). Figure 8.1 shows how preferences are related to autonomy.

The prerequisites to use to consider that an individual is informed are debatable. First, the human mind is typically incapable of retaining, computer-style, all the variables related to a decision. Second, even if these variables are reduced to a manageable number—no more than seven (Miller, 1956)—the way issues are framed can markedly influence choices. Profes-

Autonomous choice or action =

Freely made (uncoerced)
+
Informed regarding choices and their effects
+
Weighed against own *values/preferences*
+
Cognitive capability for decision-making

Figure 8.1.   Relationship of values to autonomy.

sionals may dwell on the negative versus the positive; some may offer mortality statistics, and others may offer some identical information in the form of survival statistics; and others may alter the order in which information is presented. Such slight differences in framing are associated with different choices in hypothetical situations (Kahneman & Tversky, 1982; Mazur & Merz, 1993; Tversky & Kahneman, 1981). This observation suggests that those who control the information also control the decision. Physicians and other health professionals may be unconscious of how influential casual framing of choices can be, or they may deliberately frame issues to attract what they consider the best decision.

Beyond the problems of unbiased framing of issues is the question of whether people can accurately express a value regarding a health state that they have not experienced. In Shakespeare's language, "present fears are less than horrible imaginings." Studies show that people are more likely to devalue a condition they do not have (e.g., blindness, paralysis, stroke) than one they have experienced. This is evidenced, for example, by their willingness to pay to avoid or cure the condition, or, even more notably, by the extent to which they judge the conditions as "worse than death" (Kane & Kane, 1982; Patrick et al., 1994). Typically such studies are cross-sectional so that information is not available from the *same* person before and after the condition (see Tsevat et al. [1998] and Danis et al. [1988] for examples that suggest that older people may seek more medical technology than others judge they want or need), but the differences are still alarming.

Given all these concerns, legitimate questions arise about the extent to which people are sufficiently informed about and able to take account of their values and preferences. Even more elemental is the question of whether values are sufficiently stable to form the basis for autonomy. Caplan (1990) argues that, all other things

being equal, older people have a greater likelihood of knowing with certainty their own values, beliefs, and preferences because a lifetime of experience has given them more opportunity for deliberation and choice. Therefore, age may be an advantage where autonomy is concerned.

Finally, is autonomy relevant to people with cognitive impairment? The enthusiasm for using advance directives such as living wills and durable powers of attorney for health to guide the care of those who cannot make decisions is based on respect for autonomy. The theory holds that the person expresses his or her values and preferences while cognitively intact and that following these directives constitutes respect for autonomy. To examine this contention requires undertaking the murky exploration of whether the self with dementia is the same self that made the advance directive. How should one regard a preference made while cognitively intact that enjoins health care providers to do nothing to sustain the person's life if he or she had dementia? The temporal binding is more difficult than the already knotty problem of understanding life with a physical disease. There at least information can be gathered directly from those who suffer from it. What if the person with Alzheimer's disease seems to be enjoying life? Perhaps the directive was based on a desire to preserve one's image and dignity in the minds of family and associates by preventing the physical and mental deterioration associated with advanced dementia. The question is whether such a preference carries weight given that no cognitively intact person can really enter into or comprehend the existential experience of a person with dementia.

## How Values and Preferences Are Shaped

As suggested, values and preferences are related to beliefs and attitudes, personality, and emotion. They tend to be shaped by cultural and religious forces, and people with common developmental experiences within an age cohort may share certain

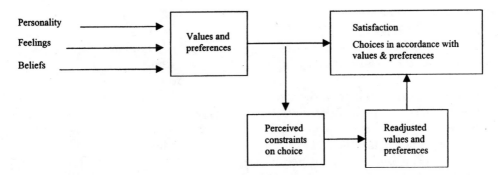

**Figure 8.2.** Schematic model for formation of values and preferences. Source: Adapted from Elster (1983).

values. Thus far, these determinants of values cause no problems in their measurement. It has also been noted, however, that people tend to shape their preferences by their understanding of the realistic constraints involved in realizing them, a relationship diagrammed in Figure 8.2. This phenomenon, which Elster (1983) calls "sour grapes," raises questions about whether "true" preferences can be measured if a constant adjustment of preferences takes place.

## WHY ASSESS VALUES AND PREFERENCES

### In Clinical Contexts

We have already suggested that autonomy is an important value, that health and social service professionals should respect people's desire to exercise autonomy. Exercising autonomy requires self-knowledge of one's own preferences, knowledge that is not as obviously available at one might expect (Gibson, 1990). Furthermore, professionals cannot act to support their clients' values and preferences unless they are aware of them, a truth that underlies the design of a quasiexperiment to try to enhance professional awareness of the preferences of older people (Kane, Degenholtz, & Kane, 1999).

Acting to support the preferences and values of people with cognitive impairment is, of course, more difficult, because those values and preferences are hard to discern. If one accepts the idea that advance directives are an expression of autonomy, then it makes sense to elicit and record a patient's preferences while he or she is still an autonomous agent capable of making decisions. The advance directive, however, is typically not applied to the full range of choices that might be made in the interests of someone with dementia, but rather to choices about end-of-life treatments. Although the importance of inquiring about end-of-life preferences has become a legal mandate in many contexts, it is equally or more important to systematically assess preferences regarding everyday life. Such an assessment is especially important for those who will be reshaping their lives in various ways in order to receive long-term care. Unfortunately, there is no reason to be sanguine that people who are cognitively intact can anticipate whether and how they would prefer to live if they had dementia and could not express their preferences.

To summarize, the following reasons for assessing values and preferences can be advanced:

- Health professionals should offer the older person a chance to express his or her values regarding care issues (both the place and the nature of care) so that the health professionals can take this information into account when making individual plans with and for the person. As with other areas of endeavor, the availability of systematic tools to make the inquiry enhances the likelihood that the assessments will be done consistently and systematically, and, for that matter, at all (Kane et al., 1999).

- Discussion of values and preferences will increase older people's awareness of their own values and preferences. People may have never carefully thought through how they feel about aspects of life that could be affected by their care decisions and may need to give some thought to deducing their own preferences. The process also provides a mechanism for discussion within families and for informing those who have an influence on the decisions of the older person (Gibson, 1990).

- Eliciting values and preferences may offer providers useful information to help them respond to the preferences of people who later develop dementia or other cognitive impairments. (One's view about this interpretation depends on one's theory about whether preferences carry forward from a predementia state.) Similarly, this information will fulfill legal requirements to act in accordance with previously expressed preferences when people cannot express their own preferences for life-sustaining treatments (e.g., because of being in a coma, in a persistent vegetative state, or unconscious).

- Currently, values and preferences are largely neglected in health care and long-term care practice. This omission is particularly stark when one considers the wide range of domains that are assessed in routine comprehensive assessments done by case managers (Kane, Penrod, & Kivnick, 1994). To omit values and preferences in such assessments seems to suggest that the area is unimportant. If any preference items are assessed clinically, they typically relate to end-of-life treatments. There is an irony here, however. On the one hand, professionals make great efforts, in Caplan's phrase (1990), "to fan the embers of autonomy" by respecting the previ-

ously expressed preferences of people who later develop dementia. On the other hand, the current preferences of people who are cognitively intact enough to express them are rarely even solicited.

- Arguably, professionals need not assess preferences because the older person is the one who applies his or her preferences to specific issues. The formal assessment, however, helps professionals to get to know the older person in much greater depth. In turn, this information should render them more sensitive to nuances in the older person's care. If clinicians come to recognize variation in the values and preferences of people in their caseload, they may become open to more individualized forms of care. Some argue that the exploration of values and preferences enhances trust between the older person and those offering help.

- Aggregated information about client values and preferences may illuminate the extent to which the dominant pattern of services conforms or fails to conform with predominant preferences of the clientele (Feldman, Gagen, & Putnam, 1988). Such extrapolations must, of course, be made with care, because preferences are individualized. "Average" preferences for a group may be statistical artifacts that end up reflecting no real person's views.

## In Research Contexts

There are many reasons for assessing values and preferences for studies of aging. For example, with values and preferences as independent variables, researchers could

- Study the relationships of various values and preferences to health status and well-being for people receiving specific forms of care.
- Study how older people order and prioritize their values and preferences.
- Study the relationship between preferences for certain aspects of care or environments and satisfaction with those en-

vironments. (As noted in Chapter 9, satisfaction is sometimes measured taking into account the importance of the various features on which satisfaction is tapped.)

- Study the stability of values and preferences through longitudinal approaches.
- Compare the preferences of older people with the preferences that family members and other proxy decision-makers and care providers have for the same people.

With values and preferences as dependent variables, one could

- Study demographic factors (e.g., age, gender, and ethnicity) and other factors (e.g., functional status, disease, and prognosis) associated with holding different preferences.
- Determine whether and how values and preferences change as a result of exposure to care environments or care conditions that differed from originally expressed preferences.

### Deterrents to Values Assessment

Some objections have been raised about routine assessment of values and preferences in clinical contexts, especially around everyday life matters.

- Asking about values and preferences encourages the idea that something can be done to honor them. What is the use, some wonder, of knowing that the home care client prefers to bathe in the evening or that a particular older person loathes the idea of entering a nursing home if there is no possibility of honoring that preference?
- Collecting information about an individual's values and preferences could become mechanistic and inaccurate if done hurriedly and without a backdrop of trust. Carefully eliciting this information takes time.
- If the information is handy, documented preferences and values may be inappropriately used in lieu of asking cognitively capable older people about their current views.

- Considerable hubris is involved in the effort to assess anything as personal and subtle as values and preferences. Some clinicians believe that inquiring about this domain is unnecessarily intrusive. Along the same lines, some critics worry that the assessment of values and preferences will lead to yet another set of simplistic formulations that will let professionals feel they are acting in accordance with values and preferences when, in fact, the assessment tool was so unsubtle or predetermined in its categories that it misses the point.

Taken together, these objections seem to be more related to the misuse of value assessments than to reasons to avoid the challenge.

### WHAT SHOULD BE ASSESSED

Of course, any value can be measured. Separate approaches have been developed to measure specific values such as "democracy," "friendship," "honor," and so on. These can tap the strength with which the value is held and classify different subtypes of those holding the value. It is beyond the scope of this chapter to examine this full range, nor is there much reason to think that there is anything different—beyond cohort effects—in measuring such values with older people. Similarly, questions can be devised to measure any specific preference that might be relevant to a policy option for older people—for example, the preference for cash versus in-kind services, the preference to participate or decline to participate in research, the preference to have a case manager or to manage the quality of one's own home care, and so on.

Many different approaches exist to measure values and preferences in a research context. As a series of comprehensive review articles suggests (Froberg & Kane, 1989 a–d), the methods should be tailored to the purpose. Strategies include rating how important something is to an individual; rating how much an individual likes various things or states; forced rankings among alternative things or states; choices after scenarios are presented or ratings of how much the respondent would like or dislike various scenarios; measures of how much a respondent would be willing to pay to avoid or to get rid of some condition; rating various conditions as to whether they are worse than death; standard gamble methods; and time trade-off methods (i.e., asking individuals how many years they would be willing to remove from the quantity of life in order to change some aspect of its quality).

Sometimes, measurement of preferences is an interim step on the road to developing multidimensional quality of life scales. For example, Kane, Bell, and Reigler (1989) conducted magnitude estimation studies whereby various groups of stakeholders rated how important certain outcome states (e.g., health status, functional status, cognitive status, social functioning, satisfaction) were to nursing home residents; this in turn permitted applying weights to summary measures of well-being. Another strategy is to develop a separate measure of importance of a variety of dimensions and a rating of satisfaction. Then, the *individual's* importance ratings can be used to weight the individual's satisfaction. In theory satisfaction with something that is unimportant should be viewed distinctly from dissatisfaction with something that is very important. Salmon and colleagues (1998) have suggested an approach whereby separate Likert-scale ratings of importance and satisfaction are combined and a four cell grid is constructed for each item: important and satisfied, important and not satisfied, unimportant and satisfied, and unimportant and not satisfied.

## TOPICS FOR VALUES ASSESSMENT

Although highly tailored assessments of values and preferences are feasible, certain preferences and values of older people seem worth measuring in clinical and research contexts, and there is merit for evolving common ways to do it so that studies may be compared. The following topics are among the many in which assessment of values and preferences may be needed:

- End-of-life preferences, which usually involve cardiopulmonary resuscitation, ventilator care, artificial nutrition and hydration, intubation, dialysis, and perhaps use of various medications and/or admissions to various kinds of health facilities. End-of-life preferences also involve for a proxy decision-maker when one cannot make decisions. A rather large literature exists on various ways to solicit end-of-life preferences.
- Preferences about outcomes associated with alternative discharge plans from the hospital. Skilled discharge planners can help patients and their families distinguish between the factors associated with different types of post-hospital care and those related to attributes of particular vendors or a given type of care (Potthoff, Kane, & Franco, 1995).
- Preferences about housing arrangements in latter years, including preferences related to types of congregate care settings: assisted living, nursing homes, small group homes, and continuing care retirement communities. The terminology and the definitions of these care settings are unlikely to be known to the older people being polled, and indeed some definitions vary depending on the state. Therefore, some effort would be needed to conduct a meaningful national study of these preferences. Preferences for various types of care settings will, in turn, be related to other preferences such as for proximity to professional care, risk aversion, and desire for privacy.
- Preferences for how the routines of everyday life are conducted, which could include basic care, household routines, and activities. The Preferences for Everyday Life (PELI) approach, being tested by the Visiting Nurse Service of New York (PGC & VNSNY, 1999), is

the most detailed example of such an approach. By the time a PELI is completed, the practitioner is aware of the most minute preferences in the individual's daily life, including care routines, diet, preferred activities, preferred colors, and decorative schemes.

- Preferences related to religious practices. (See Chapter 10 for measures of religiousness and spirituality; they point out the problem that existing measures of religious involvement seldom take into account individual preferences for such involvement.)

- Preferences related to privacy. A vigorous public policy debate is raging about whether federally certified nursing homes should be encouraged to move toward private rooms (except for those who truly make an unconstrained choice to share a room with someone they know) and whether states should require private rooms or apartments in assisted living as a condition of licensing and/or reimbursement. Various surveys and focus-group studies have been conducted to determine the importance of privacy in absolute terms and compared with other attributes of care settings (Hawes et al., 1997; Jenkens, 1997; Kane et al., 1998b; Lawton & Bader, 1970). Different approaches have been used to measure the preference. Privacy appears to be a particularly important value to older people, yet one that professionals are loath to recognize as important. Privacy itself, however, seems to be multidimensional. In a study in which we asked elderly home care clients to rate the importance of privacy and further asked them to describe what they meant by it, we found different meanings, independent of the ratings; some respondents viewed privacy as related to bodily privacy, some to privacy around their personal and business affairs, and some to the ability to be alone and unobserved (Degenholtz, Kane, & Kivnick, 1997).

- Preferences related to safety versus freedom. Professional preferences tend to govern long-term care (Kane, Kane, & Ladd, 1998a), and professionals tend to hold orthodox views about the importance of promoting safety and health and about ways to do so. The right to take risks has now been enshrined as a consumer-centered value (Kane, 1995). Consequently, measuring the preferences of older people on the trade-off between safety and protection versus freedom is a crucial endeavor. This is a hard concept to articulate and measure, however. The difficulty arises in part because the trade-offs are hard to articulate and in part because this issue is one about which both providers and consumers feel ambivalent.

- Preferences related to exercising control and choice over one's care. This particular issue is one that has received a great deal of attention in the 1990s. An entire research and demonstration initiative— Independent Choices—funded by the Robert Wood Johnson Foundation and managed by the National Council on Aging has been dedicated to increasing choice and control for long-term care consumers. In turn, these projects have multiplied efforts to measure both whether older people are exercising control and choice and, more pertinent for this topic, whether they want to do so.

## TYPES OF MEASURES

As with other domains, assessment of values can be approached in a variety of ways, and each has advantages for particular purposes. Table 8.1 summarizes some of the variations in methods, with examples of each kind of tool. When it comes to measuring preferences and values, however, choosing a tool is only one part of the problem. A general strategy must be devised for how to best ascertain the value or preference in question, which, in turn, should be sensitive to the particular use that will be made of the data. Table 8.2 summarizes different general approaches and, when possible, provides an example of an application of that method for older people.

The available approaches vary in their open endedness compared with the use of forced-response items, the depth with which they examine one or more values and preferences, and the extent to which they can be aggregated. Those that purport to measure the presence or absence of a particular value are easier to score than are those that attempt to determine which specific aspects of life and care are of value and importance to the individual. Those that use scenarios have the advantage of providing a common stimulus, but the disadvantage of possibly being too hypothetical for the judgment to be meaningful, too terse to be realistic or easily rated, or too long and complex to be easily understood.

## TECHNICAL ISSUES

The examples in Tables 8.1 and 8.2 foreshadow the technical issues described below.

### Selecting the Items

It is difficult to decide what items should be included in lists used to determine what is important to the older person. Issues also arise about the desired abstractness or concreteness—whether to explore broad topics like the importance of "friendship," "relationships," "financial security" such as is done in some classic studies of values (Rokeach, 1973; Rokeach & Ball-Rokeach, 1989; Simon, Hoew, & Kirschenbum, 1972) or very narrow preferences for specific food or activities such as those used in

**Table 8.1.**
Pros and Cons of Various Approaches to Values Assessment

| Type of instrument | Attributes | Examples |
| --- | --- | --- |
| Open ended | Creates a vehicle for a structured discussion of values. May be self-completed as an educational tool or administered in an interview. A useful heuristic tool but hard to aggregate and compare people on their values | Gibson's Values History (self-administered) (Gibson, 1990)<br><br>New York City Chronic Care Consortium (interview) (Feldman 1988) |
| Closed ended, using true–false items about general likes and dislikes or Likert-style ratings of importance on a variety of topics or items | Easy to administer and make comparisons; does not necessarily lend itself to a score because summing items may make little conceptual sense | Doukas & McCullough. True-false values items in their Values History (Doukas & McCullough, 1991a)<br><br>Kane Choice & Control in Nursing Homes (Kane et al., 1997) |
| Mixed closed ended and open ended | Permits recording some descriptive content and quantifying intensity of each preference | Kane & Degenholtz Values Baseline (Degenholtz et al., 1997) |
| Scale to measure a particular value | Good approach for an important value to assess clinically or for research; cumbersome to administer many | Measure of paternalism in families of the elderly (Cicirelli, 1992)<br><br>Siegaj Preferences for Consumer Direction (Sciegaj, 1997) |
| Multidimensional measure that could result in several scales | Tend to be very long instruments | Salmon & Polivka Preferences for Quality of Life (Salmon et al., 1998)<br><br>Choice and Decision Making in Everyday Care Survey for Persons with Cognitive Impairment (Friss-Feinberg, 1998) |

**Table 8.2.**
Strategies for Discerning Values and Preferences

| Type of strategy | Attributes | Example of use for seniors |
|---|---|---|
| Scenarios | A hypothetical situation is created, and respondents are asked to rate how likely it is that they would choose it. Alternatively, respondents may be asked to choose between or among scenarios | Emanuel and Emanuel advance directive protocol (Emanuel & Emanuel, 1989) Nursing home residents asked to rate various scenarios with different combinations of symptoms and problems, mobility limitations, social activity limitations, and physical activity limitations (Hays et al., 1996) |
| States worse than death | Using a visual analog or some other method, respondents rate given health states as to whether they are better or worse than death | States such as constant pain, dementia, and coma compared with death in a population of community elderly and nursing home residents (Patrick et al., 1994) |
| Willingness to pay | Respondents are asked how much they would pay (absolutely or as a fraction of income) to avoid getting or to get rid of a certain condition | Respondents asked how much they would pay to avoid or get rid of conditions like stroke, blindness, and so on (Thomson, 1986) |
| Time trade-off | Respondents are asked to make trade-offs between quantity of life and quality of life | Seriously ill hospitalized people over age 80 years were asked how much shortening of life they would accept in order to be pain free (Tvset et al., 1988) Staff raters are asked to imagine a cure for various dementia-related problems depicted in video scenarios and indicate how many years of life they think should be foregone to avoid these problems (Sano et al., 1999) |
| Standard gamble | Respondents are asked how much of a risk they are willing to assume to gain a defined improvement in their health status | |
| Magnitude estimation study | Respondents are asked to describe the relative importance of a value by locating it on a numerical scale such as 1–100. Alternatively, they may be asked to make choices between successive pairs of alternatives | Nursing home residents and other stakeholders were asked to rate the importance of various outcomes for nursing home residents, such as functional status, pain, emotions, activities, and so on (Kane et al., 1989) |

the Preferences for Everyday Life Measure (PGC & VNSNY, 1999), which is intended to be used to help frame the clinical interventions of visiting nurses. If too general, the list may be no more useful than the pilloried "motherhood and apple pie," and, if too specific, an interminable list is generated. Some investigators have taken a middle course, using categories that might be relevant to care (e.g., preferences for privacy, daily routines, behavior of health care professionals) and then asking the respondent to supply the details, such as were done in studies of case managers' clients in home and community-based care programs (Degenholtz et al., 1997; Kane et al., 1999).

## Anchoring the Inquiry

Like all other measures, those of preference and values can be gathered with reference to a particular time frame and context. Often, but not always, those being developed for use with older populations are anchored in relationship to long-term care or medical care, that is, the questions are framed in terms of "if you needed care or help because of a disability." Conversely, it is possible not to anchor the items at all or to anchor them by age, for example, "when you are over 65." Another way of anchoring the study is by selecting a particular population that is fairly homogeneous in terms of health status or residential characteristic or some other factors; it then becomes difficult to generalize those preferences to a different population.

## Absolute or Relative Importance

One approach quite widely used is to ask the respondent to rate the importance of a variety of items, perhaps on a 1–10 scale or a 1–5 scale. This strategy may lead to a large number of items being endorsed positively as important to the well-being of the individual. Another approach is to force rank-ordering in some way. Respondents can be asked to literally rank-order a list, although the lists are often too long to be kept in mind. Respondents can be asked to go over their previously rated list and select the top few, or they can be given a series of questions that keep forcing them to choose between two alternatives in a factorial design. The advantage of these forced-choice approaches is that the respondent ultimately is forced to offer a preference. The disadvantage is that it may be a time-consuming process to go through a series of choices.

## Considering the Important Without Being Biased by the Actual

Respondents find it difficult to state that something is important to them in a particular care program or setting if they deem it is unavailable or impractical. As in Elster's analysis (1983), mentioned earlier, older persons' preferences are tempered by their views of reality, perhaps to ward off disappointment. If they are already using a service or living in a care setting, it is even

harder for them to think in the abstract. In some studies, such as those of assisted living nationally and in the state of Oregon (Reinardy, Kane, & Huck, 1998), great effort is made to separate ratings of importance from rating of satisfaction within the interview. This avoids contaminating preference data with rating data, but it is a cumbersome process, lengthening an interview and requiring skilled interviewing to keep the respondent oriented to the question. Others ask about importance and actual experience in tandem; this speeds up the interview and makes it easier to do the exercise with people who are cognitively impaired (Friss-Feinberg, 1998). Still others insert preferences into questions about actual experience — for example, the respondent can be asked "how many times do you get a bath at this nursing home each week" followed by "how many times would you like to get a bath." Variants of this last strategy have been used by Simmons and colleagues (1997).

## Aggregating and Scoring

Sometimes individual items are scored on Likert scales in terms of their importance, the extent of agreement with various value statements, or the extent to which the individual "likes" or "dislikes" something. Simply summing all the items is likely to be meaningless, however, and it is by no means clear how to aggregate the information. Some factor analytic work is now being done with studies in progress to determine how certain preference items are correlated. This analysis may make it possible to speak of the strength of a preference or value around a particular issue (e.g., a value for solitary activities, or a preference for fixed routines, or a preference to control one's daily care).

## Dealing with the Hypothetical

Scenario approaches are common in the research literature and are also used clinically to determine treatment preferences. They have the advantage of standardizing the choices from which the person selects and, therefore, ensuring comparisons of "apples and apples." They have the disadvantage of being hypothetical and contrived. The respondent may not enter fully into the exercise, and the scenarios may appear unrealistic or irrelevant. There appear to be no studies that show whether people in real life would make the same choices they make in scenario studies, and indeed such research would be difficult to design. There would be enormous expense in developing and following a sample in order to find those later faced with the problems. Moreover, real life tends to be messier than the scenarios we create. Even if we do not use scenario approaches, however, a hypothetical component enters into all types of tools when used to ask respondents about the absolute or relative importance of features of programs they have not experienced — such as what attributes would be most important in a nursing home or a home-care worker.

### Values and Preference Measures with the Cognitively Impaired

If preferences are hard to measure in general, they are even more difficult to measure with cognitively impaired individuals. Some work has been done in both community settings (Friss-Feinberg, 1998) and nursing homes (Van Haitsma, 1999) to measure preferences held by people with dementia. In the second example, Van Haitsma developed the Pleasant Events Preference Inventory (PEPI) for use with people with dementia. She modeled the items to include many items in the Pleasant Events Schedule developed by Logsden and Teri (1997) and used a variety of sources to get information about preferences: residents were the preferred source, but family and staff were used otherwise. Van Haitsma argues that, at extremes of dementia, observers should use something like the Apparent Affect Rating Scale, discussed in another chapter, to judge preferences from reactions to stimuli. Relying on proxies to describe preferences of persons

with dementia is risky because several investigators show that the preferences expressed by family and staff differ from those of the person concerned or that families acknowledge that they are unfamiliar with daily preferences. This realization argues for tapping preferences at early stages of dementia. Then the problem arises, however, that perhaps preferences change as the disease advances.

### VALUES INSTRUMENTS

Tables 8.3 through 8.11 illustrate some of the approaches that have been attempted. Table 8.3 shows Sciegaj's approach (1997) to developing a measure of preference for consumer direction among home care clients. His tool was developed after meeting with focus groups of home care clients of different ethnicities and then was tested with 800 clients, divided about equally among Hispanic-American clients, Asian-American clients, African-American clients, and Caucasian clients of European ancestry.

Table 8.4 lists the items that were used for a study of preferences for control and choice in everyday life for nursing home residents (Kane et al., 1997). The items were generated from discussions with residents and professional experts, and the respondents were simply asked how important choice and control was in each area on a 3 point scale.

Table 8.5 presents the values statements contained in the Doukas and McCullough (1991b) Values History. This is a different approach from the previous illustrations in that it asks the respondent whether he or she subscribes to each of a group of values as well as (in the first question) to make a fixed choice between quantity and quality of life in a general way. There follows a directive section related to 11 specific treatments: *(1)* cardiopulmonary resuscitation; *(2)* ventilator; *(3)* endotracheal tube for cardiopulmonary resuscitation and ventilator; *(4)* parenteral nutrition; *(5)* intravenous medication and hydration; *(6)*

**Table 8.3.**

Sciegaj Preferences for Consumer Direction Measure

*Below is a list of activities related to your services. Please tell us whether you would like to have complete control over any of these activities. (Circle yes or no.)*

| | | |
|---|---|---|
| a. Choosing which services you receive | Yes | No |
| b. Making decisions about your services | Yes | No |
| c. Setting your services schedule | Yes | No |
| d. Finding and selecting your service workers | Yes | No |
| e. Hiring and firing your service workers | Yes | No |
| f. Training and supervising your service workers | Yes | No |
| g. Paying your service workers | Yes | No |

*Paying the service worker involves several tasks. Which of the following tasks would you like complete responsibility and control over?*

| | | |
|---|---|---|
| a. Negotiating the payment rate | Yes | No |
| b. Keeping track of hours worked per week | Yes | No |
| c. Handling paperwork associated with social security payments and taxes | Yes | No |
| d. Writing a check and paying the worker | Yes | No |

Source: From the questionnaire "Elder Preferences for Consumer Direction, 1997–1998" (Sciegaj, 1997).

**Table 8.4.** Desire for Choice and Control in Nursing Homes

*How important is it to you to have choice and control regarding*

| | |
|---|---|
| a. Leaving the facility for short trips | h. Time to get up in the morning |
| b. The telephone and mail | i. Time to go to bed at night |
| c. The timing and nature of personal care routines | j. Timing and identity of visitors |
| d. The nursing home activities | k. Calling or seeing a physician |
| e. Use of money | l. Entering a hospital |
| f. The timing and menus for eating | j. Being discharged from the nursing home |
| g. Selecting a roommate | |

Source: Kane et al. (1997).

**Table 8.5.**

Doukas and McCullough Quality of Life Values*

*Basic Life Values*

*Perhaps the most basic values in this context concern length of life versus quality. Which of the following statements is the most important to you?*

___ I want to live as long as possible regardless of the quality of life I experience.

___ I want to preserve a good quality of life even if this means that I may not live as long.

*Quality of Life Values*

*Many values help to define the quality of life we want to live. The following list contains some that appear to be the most common. Review this list (and feel free to elaborate on it or add to it), and circle those values that are most important to your definition of quality of life.*

1. I want to maintain my capacity to think clearly
2. I want to a feel safe and secure
3. I want to avoid unnecessary pain and suffering
4. I want to be treated with respect
5. I want to be treated with dignity when I can no longer speak for myself
6. I do not want to be an unnecessary burden on my family
7. I want to be able to make my own decisions
8. I want to experience a comfortable dying process
9. I want to be with my loved ones before I die
10. I want to leave good memories of me to my loved ones
11. I want to be treated in accord with my religious beliefs and traditions
12. I want respect shown for my body after I die
13. I want to help others by making a contribution to medical education and research
14. Other values or clarification of values above

*Meant to be contained within an advance directive.

Source: Doukas and McCullough (1991b).

continuation of all life sustaining medications; *(7)* nasogastric or other feeding tubes; *(8)* dialysis; *(9)* autopsy; *(10)* intensive care unit; and *(11)* (for long-term care facility residents) calling 911 in an emergency. Questions 2 through 8 have the following options: yes, yes for a specified trial period of _____, yet to determine medical effectiveness, and no. The others are yes/no questions. Questions 5 and 6 clarify that even if the person selects no intravenous or oral medications, this does not preclude pain medications or narcotics. It is hard to see how providers could use the value statements to help guide their actions although the very exercise of completing the instrument may be useful to consumers.

Table 8.6 contains a Values Baseline that is meant to be self-administered. It was developed in the 1980s by Joan Gibson (1990) to serve as a vehicle for reflection and for older people to discern and discuss their own values, and there is no intention that it be handed in to providers or used as a basis for analysis. As one of the earliest values assessment protocols, it has been extremely influential to others attempting assessment in this area.

Table 8.7 presents the instrument used to measure client values and preferences in two case-managed home care programs (Degenholtz et al., 1997). The items were developed in all-day workshops with case managers from the two participating programs who were asked what they thought was important to know about client values and preferences in order to make a care plan and how they would find out. The resultant form asks clients to rate the importance of each value on a 3 point scale but also to elaborate on what they mean by their answers. Thus, for example, by securing a rating of the importance of having routines flexible or fixed, but also the specific details of what the respondent preferred, allowed analyses that showed that, among more than 800 clients, those who preferred a fixed routine were more likely to attach high importance to that prefer-

ence than those who preferred a flexible routine and that those who preferred that certain family members be involved in their care were more likely to attach importance to the preference than were those who preferred that certain family members *not* be involved in their care. We also learned a great deal about the range of what clients mean when they say that they prefer privacy or pursuing activities. This approach is potentially useful clinically and was useful for exploratory research, but obviously the open-ended features are difficult to analyze in large-scale studies.

Table 8.8 presents the Preferences for Everyday Life Scale (PELI), under development by Philadelphia Geriatric Center and the Visiting Nurse Service of New York (PGC & VNSNY, 1999). It can be contrasted with the instrument in Table 8.7 by the sheer level of detail in the inquiry. If a PELI is completed, the home care providers would surely have a panoramic view of the individual's preferences at a single point in time.

Tables 8.9 and 8.10 present, for comparison, two approaches to gathering information about the importance of various features of care and the environment to long-term care consumers, especially those in assisted living. Table 8.9 presents the tool used by Salmon and colleagues (1998) to study the preferences of low-income long-term care consumers in a variety of settings, including assisted living, home care, and nursing homes. The items are grouped in conceptually linked topics, and the list is highly comprehensive. The investigators report that some subjects had trouble with the lead-in phrase: "how important is _____ to your quality of life." This may be abstract to some consumers; quality of life as a stand-alone term is professional jargon. If doing it again, they might have said: "how important is _____ to a good life" (Salmon, personal communication).

Table 8.10 presents the instrument that researchers at the University of Minnesota are using in a new study of services in as-

**Table 8.6.**
Gibson's Values Baseline*

---

*Section 1A*

Summary of any legal documents, including date of execution, document location, and content of: Living Will; Durable Power of Attorney; Durable Power of Attorney for Health; and/or Organ Donations.

*Section 1B*

Wishes regarding specific medical procedures, including to whom expressed (if oral), when (if written), and content regarding: organ donation; kidney dialysis, CPR, respirators; artificial nutrition; and artificial hydration.

*Section 2*

A. Your overall attitude toward your health
   1. How would you describe your current health status? If you have any medical problems how would you describe them?
   2. If you have current medical problems, in what way do they affect your ability to function?
   3. How do you feel about your current health status?
   4. How well are you able to meet the basic necessities of life — eating, food preparation, sleeping, personal hygiene, etc?
   5. Do you wish to make any general comments about your overall health?
B. Your perception of the role of your doctor & other health caregivers
   1. Do you like your doctors?
   2. Do you think your doctors should make the final decision concerning any treatment you might need?
   3. How do you relate to your caregivers, including nurses, therapists, chaplains, social workers, etc?
   4. Do you wish to make any general comments about your doctor and other health caregivers?
C. Your thoughts about independence and control
   1. How important is independence and self-sufficiency in your life?
   2. If you were to experience decreased physical and mental abilities how would that affect your attitude toward independence and self-sufficiency?
   3. Do you wish to make any general comments about the value of independence and control in your life?
D. Your personal relationships
   1. Do you expect that your friends, family, or others will support your decisions regarding medical treatment you may need now or in the future?
   2. Have you made any arrangements for your family or friends to make medical decisions on your behalf? If so, who has agreed to make decisions for you and in what circumstances?
   3. What, if any, unfinished business from the past are you concerned about (e.g., personal and family relationships, business and legal matters)?
   4. What role do your friends and family play in your life?
   5. Do you wish to make any general comments about the personal relationships in your life?
E. Your overall attitude toward life
   1. What activities do you enjoy (e.g., hobbies, watching TV)?
   2. Are you happy to be alive?
   3. Do you feel that life is worth living?
   4. How satisfied are you with what you have achieved in your life?
   5. What makes you laugh? Cry?
   6. What do you fear most? What upsets you?
   7. What goals do you have for the future?
   8. Do you wish to make any general comments about your attitude toward life?
F. Your attitude toward illness, dying, and death
   1. What will be important to you when you are dying (e.g., physical comfort, family members present, etc)?
   2. Where would you prefer to die?
   3. What is your attitude toward death?
   4. How do you feel about the use of life-sustaining measures in the face of terminal illness? In the face of permanent coma? In the face of irreversible chronic illness (e.g., Alzheimer's disease)?
   5. Do you wish to make any general comments about your attitude toward illness, dying, and death?
G. Your religious background and beliefs
   1. What is your religious background?
   2. How do your religious beliefs affect your attitude toward serious or terminal illness?
   3. Does your attitude toward death find support in your religion?

*(continued)*

**Table 8.6.**
Gibson's Values Baseline* (Continued)

 4. How does your faith, community, church, or synagogue view the role of prayer or religious sacraments in an illness?
 5. Do you wish to make any general comments about your religious background and beliefs?

H. Your living environment
 1. What has been your living situation over the past 10 years (e.g., alone, with others, etc)?
 2. How difficult is it for you to maintain the kind of environment for yourself that you find comfortable?
 3. Do you wish to make any general comments about your living environment?
 4. Do you wish to make any general comments concerning your finances and the cost of health care?

I. Your attitude concerning finances
 1. How much do you worry about having enough money to provide for your care?
 2. Would you prefer to spend less money on your care so that more money can be saved for the benefit of your relatives or friends?
 3. Do you wish to make any general comments concerning your finances and the cost of health care?

J. Your wishes concerning your funeral
 1. What are your wishes concerning your funeral, burial, or cremation?
 2. Have you made your funeral arrangements? If so, with whom?
 3. Do you have any general comments about how you would like your funeral or burial or cremation to be arranged or conducted?

*Optional Questions*

 1. How would you like your obituary (announcement of your death) to read?
 2. Write yourself a brief eulogy (a statement about yourself to be read at your funeral).

*Suggestions for Use*

After you have completed this form, you may wish to provide copies to your doctors and other health caregivers, your family, your friends, and your attorney. If you have a Living Will or Durable Power of Attorney for Health Care Decisions, you may wish to attach a copy of this form to those documents.

*Note: Plenty of room is contained for explanation on this 7-page form. Spaces have been omitted and reformatting done for space considerations.*
Source: Gibson (1990).


**Table 8.7.**
Values Assessment Protocol

*The next questions are about the kinds of choice that might be important to you as you plan your care now and in the future. I would like to know how important each topic is to you and more about what the topic means.*

*Thinking about your care, now and in the future, would it be very important, somewhat important, or not important to*

| | |
|---|---|
| 1. ". . . organize your daily routines in a particular way?" | v s n |
| 2. ". . . participate in particular activities, either in your home or outside your home?" | v s n |
| 3. ". . . involve or *not* involve particular family or friends with your care?" | v s n |
| 4. ". . . have the person helping you be or behave a certain way?" (What kind of a person would you want the helper to be?)* | v s n |
| 5. ". . . have the place where you live be a certain way?" (What makes a place a home to you?)* | |
| 7. ". . . have personal privacy?" | v s n |
| 8. ". . . take steps to avoid pain or discomfort?" | v s n |
| 9. Would it be more important to have the freedom to come and go and do as you please or would it be more important to be safe and accept some restrictions on your life? | Come & go _____ Restrictions _____ v s n |
| 10. If you could not make decisions about your care, whom would you want to make them? | |
| 11. What in your life (what activities or experiences) makes you feel most like yourself? | |

*Questions 4 and 5 were used in one version of the protocol and omitted in another. The parentheses contain the probes used.
Source: Degenholtz et al. (1997).

**Table 8.8.**
Preferences for Everyday Life Inventory (PELI)*

### Social Activities

1. I enjoy spending time by myself.
2. I enjoy spending time with small groups of people.
3. I enjoy spending time with large groups of people.
4. I like being a member of clubs, committees, or other organizations.
5. I enjoy being a group leader.
6. I would enjoy living in the same room as someone else.
7. I like to keep in weekly contact with my family.
8. I like to keep in frequent contact with my friends.
9. I enjoy physical contact with someone I care about (e.g., hugging, holding hands).
10. I enjoy contact with animals.
11. I like celebrating holidays and birthdays.
12. I enjoy meeting new people.

### Not Primarily Social Activities

1. I enjoy being physically active.
2. I like to participate in religious/spiritual activities.
3. I like to volunteer my time to help others.
4. I enjoy music.
5. I enjoy doing crafts/handiwork/hobbies.
6. I enjoy watching TV.
7. I enjoy reading.
8. I enjoy cultural activities (e.g., concerts, theatre, museums).
9. I like to eat at restaurants.
10. I enjoy traveling.

### ADL/IADL

1. I like to follow a routine when I go to bed and get up.
2. I like to nap.
3. I like to choose when I eat.
4. I like to choose what I eat.
5. I like to breakfast every morning.
6. I like to snack.
7. I like to decide when I get dressed.
8. I like to choose what I wear.
9. I like to bathe at a specific time.
10. I enjoy paying special attention to my appearance and dress.
11. I enjoy doing household tasks such as cooking, tidying up, and laundry.

### Staff

1. I like to discuss personal things with staff caring for me.
2. I like the people who care for me to have the same background.
3. I like to keep my relationship with someone providing care to me formal.
4. I like that direct care providers address me by my first name.

### Involvement of Family in Direct Care

1. I like having particular family members involved in my care.
2. I like having particular friends involved in my care.

### Environmental Features

1. I like to have the temperature where I live to be on the warm side.
2. I like the lighting where I live to be on the bright side.
3. I like to keep blinds/curtains open.
4. I like to keep certain personal mementos on display where I live.
5. I like to be where it is quiet.
6. I enjoy being in a lively, noisy place.
7. I like a colorful environment.
8. I enjoy spending time outside.
9. I like to have a place to lock my things.
10. I like being in a place that has ramps, hand rails, and things like that.
11. I like being in a place that has carpeting.

### Health Care Services

1. There are certain people I want to be involved in discussions of my care.
2. I'd like the chance to talk to a professional if I had an emotional problem or worry.
3. I would like to be able to decide whether to take medication for pain or other symptoms.
4. I like being able to use hearing aids/glasses/dentures.
5. I like to have routinely scheduled medical/dental exams.
6. I like to use herbs, vitamins, and supplements.
7. I like to have access to alternative medical providers—chiropractors, acupuncturists, etc.
8. I like to know about every aspect of my medical condition and treatment.
9. I like to receive my medical care from an MD rather than a physician assistant or nurse practitioner.

### Time

1. I like to be most active at the same time every day.
2. I like to have times during the day when I have nothing in particular to do.
3. I like to have a plan for my day.
4. I like to keep to a regular routine each day.
5. I like to keep busy.

### Individualization

1. I like to be given help to get motivated to do things.
2. I like having things to I do to make me feel better when I am upset.

*(continued)*

254

## Table 8.8.—Continued

*Individualization—continued*

| | |
|---|---|
| 3. I like doing new things. | 8. I like people to call me by a particular name. |
| 4. I like to be challenged. | 9. I like to feel in control of my life. |
| 5. I like to learn things in particular ways. | 10. I like being the center of attention. |
| 6. I like privacy. | 11. I like to stay around the house. |
| 7. I like reminiscing about the past. | 12. I like having people take care of me. |

ADL, activities of daily living; IADL, instrumental activities of daily living.

*Note: The actual version of this instrument is a lengthy booklet with factual follow-up questions and plenty of room for those who complete it to supply the client's detailed responses to each question (PGC & VNSNY, 1999). PELI, Preferences for Everyday Life Inventory. Usual response set is: not at all, a little, much, very much.*

## Table 8.9.
### Preferences for Quality of Life

*How important is _____ to your quality of life. (Choose 1–5 with 1 = not at all important and 5 = very important.)*

**Physical Health**

Your physical health?
Keeping your pain under control?
Having medical care available?
Eating healthy meals?
Getting physical exercise?

**Function and Self-Care**

Doing your own self-care, like bathing & dressing?
Getting around inside your home or unit?
Getting around in community & neighborhood?

**Relationships, Intimacy, & Reciprocity**

Visiting family & friends at their homes?
Helping family & friends in ways you are able?
Family & friends visiting you at your home?
Receiving help from family & friends?

**Privacy**

Living alone?
Sharing a home with others?
Having privacy?

**Mental Health**

Having your mind intact?
Feeling good about yourself?

**Religion and Spirituality**

Your religion?
Your spirituality?
Time for meditation and prayer?
Attending church or synagogue?

**Risk-Taking and Safety**

Taking financial risks?
Taking physical risks?
Having a security system in your place?
Having an alarm to push for an emergency?
Having someone nearby to help you if you fall & hurt yourself
Feeling protected from crime?
Going outside when you want?

**Financial and Material**

Having enough money for your lifestyle?
Having more money than you currently have?
Having your own furniture & belongings?
Leaving a financial legacy to your family?
Having money to pay for unexpected expenses?

**Transportation**

Having reliable transportation for medical appts., shopping?
Having reliable transportation for leisure activities?

**Choice and Control**

Having control over your time?
Helping those who help you?
Having order in your life?
Choosing the person who takes care of you if you need help?
Choosing what services are provided to you?
Choosing the day & time those services are provided?
Having lots of options to choose from?
Having professional advice when making decisions?
Participating in activities organized by other people?

**Work, Productivity, Interests**

Doing hobbies?
Having paid employment?
Volunteering in the community?
Having a pet in your home?
Having time to watch television?
Other activities not already mentioned?

**Community**

Making a difference in your community or the world?
Making a difference in your family?

**Meaning and Purpose**

Having a purpose to your life?
Having respect from people around you?
Leaving a legacy of your personal values & contributions?

**Table 8.10.**

Importance Ratings for Kane's Study of Assisted Living

| | | | | | |
|---|---|---|---|---|---|
| 1 | 2 | 3 | 4 | 5 | a. Having an apartment specifically designed for people with disabilities? |
| 1 | 2 | 3 | 4 | 5 | b. Having a comfortable and attractive apartment? |
| 1 | 2 | 3 | 4 | 5 | c. Having a refrigerator and <u>either</u> a stove or microwave in your own apartment? |
| 1 | 2 | 3 | 4 | 5 | d. Being able to lock your apartment door for privacy? |
| 1 | 2 | 3 | 4 | 5 | e. Meals that you like in the dining room? |
| 1 | 2 | 3 | 4 | 5 | f. Pleasant service and atmosphere in the dining room? |
| 1 | 2 | 3 | 4 | 5 | g. Having housekeeping done the way you like? |
| 1 | 2 | 3 | 4 | 5 | h. Having laundry done the way you like? |
| 1 | 2 | 3 | 4 | 5 | i. Having assistance available for bathing and other personal care? |
| 1 | 2 | 3 | 4 | 5 | j. Having a nurse in the building? |
| 1 | 2 | 3 | 4 | 5 | k. Someone on duty in the building at night? |
| 1 | 2 | 3 | 4 | 5 | l. Having help available for taking medicines? |
| 1 | 2 | 3 | 4 | 5 | m. Having the <u>same</u> people help you on a regular basis? [PROBE - FEW CHANGES] |
| 1 | 2 | 3 | 4 | 5 | n. Organized activities for the residents of the building? |
| 1 | 2 | 3 | 4 | 5 | o. Having physical rehabilitation programs, like physical therapy? |
| 1 | 2 | 3 | 4 | 5 | p. Having transportation arranged for the building? |
| 1 | 2 | 3 | 4 | 5 | q. Having religious services and programs right in the building? |
| 1 | 2 | 3 | 4 | 5 | r. Being able to decorate and arrange the apartment how you want? |
| 1 | 2 | 3 | 4 | 5 | s. Deciding how much or little care or help you receive? |
| 1 | 2 | 3 | 4 | 5 | t. Deciding who comes into your apartment and when? |
| 1 | 2 | 3 | 4 | 5 | u. Being able to refuse services that doctors or nurses recommend to you? |
| 1 | 2 | 3 | 4 | 5 | v. Being allowed to stay in the apartment even if your care needs are very high? |
| 1 | 2 | 3 | 4 | 5 | w. Having things in common with the other residents in the building? |
| 1 | 2 | 3 | 4 | 5 | x. Keeping the price reasonable? |

Source: Assisted Living/Home Care Connection, a study funded by the Robert Wood Johnson Foundation under its Home Care Research Initiative.

sisted living. This particular tool is a second-generation instrument and represents an elaboration and improvement over a similar tool used for a study in Oregon. The items reflect characteristics of the physical plant, characteristics of the services, and aspects of choice and control. There is an essentially arbitrary character to the selection of items, in that we could have had fewer or more to represent a concept. We are currently undertaking factor analysis to see how these items cluster together. In a related study, family members are also being asked the same questions regarding the assisted living of their relative, giving us an opportunity to see how family values and preferences differ from those of their own relatives in assisted living.

Finally, Table 8.11 presents an application specifically designed for Alzheimer's disease. It is based directly on the Pleasant

**Table 8.11.**

Preferences for Pleasant Events — Alzheimer's Disease

*Does this person like, dislike, or have no preference for each of the following?*

| | |
|---|---|
| *Music* | *Social Interaction* |
| Playing an instrument | Being left alone |
| Singing | Watching people |
| Listening to music | Joking |
| | Looking at photos |
| *Physical Exercise* | Visits by children |
| | Animals |
| Walking | Meeting new people |
| Exercise | Group socializing |
| Dancing | Writing cards |
| Watching dance | Receiving cards |
| Playing sports | Talking on the phone |
| Watching sports | Reminiscing |
| | Being told you're loved |
| *Sensory Stimulation* | Being read to |
| | Going to movies |
| Hugging | |
| Holding hands | *Activities of Daily Living* |
| Getting a back rub | |
| Sitting close | Putting on makeup |
| Hand massage | Getting a manicure |
| Smelling flowers | Wearing bright colors |
| Listening to nature | Brushing own hair |
| Touching fabrics | Having hair brushed |
| | Dressing up |
| *Crafts/Handiworks/Hobbies* | Receiving compliments |
| | Making bed |
| Working on crafts | Dusting |
| Sewing | Decorating |
| Painting/drawing | Eating snacks |
| Woodworking | Keeping tidy |
| Making collections | Organizing closets |
| Houseplants | Sorting drawers |
| Gardening | Folding clothes |

Source: Van Haitsma (1999).

Events Schedule — AD (see Chapter 17), but it eliminates and replaces items not deemed suited to a highly impaired nursing home population. The investigators left it open how the instrument would be completed: It could be done through an interview with the demented resident, through a self-administered questionnaire completed by a knowledgeable family caregiver, or completed as a questionnaire by a staff member, usually an activity therapist (Van Haitsma, 1999). Preliminary information is available on frequencies, and it has been used to select individual interventions that nurse's aides can perform that are linked to an individual resident's preferences. The most commonly selected intervention protocols are sing-a-long, active listening to music, reminiscing about housework, stretching, making a memory book, making a greeting card, and beauty time.

## SUMMARY AND CONCLUSIONS

In this chapter, the measures presented are in a much more developmental stage than are those described in other chapters. Even this tentative assessment of values and preferences, however, is a signal that researchers are paying attention to this topic. Painstaking methodological work is needed to advance this field.

# REFERENCES

Agich, G. C. (1993). *Autonomy and long-trm care.* New York: Oxford University Press.

Ajzen, I. (1988). *Attitudes, personality, and behavior.* Chicago: Dorsey Press.

Campbell, C. S. (1995). Utility. In W. Reich (Ed.), *Encyclopedia of bioethics,* (rev. ed. vol. 5, pp. 2509–2513). New York: McMillan.

Caplan, A. L. (1990). Can autonomy be saved? In A. L. Caplan (Ed.), *If I were a rich man, could I buy a pancreas? and other essays on the ethics of health care* (pp. 256–281). Bloomington: Indiana University Press.

Cicirelli, V. G. (1992). *Family caregiving: Autonomous and paternalistic decision-making.* Newbury Park, CA: Sage.

Clemens, E., Wetle, T., Feltes, M., Crabtree, B., & Dubitsky, D. (1994). Contradictions in case management: Client-centered theory and directive practice with the frail elderly. *Journal of Aging and Health, 6,* 70–88.

Danis, M., Patrick, D. L., Southerland, L. I., & Green, M. L. (1988). Patients' and families' preferences for medical intensive care. *Journal of the American Medical Association, 260,* 797–802.

Degenholtz, H. B., Kane, R. A., & Kivnick, H. Q. (1997). Care-related prferences and values of elderly community-based LTC consumers: Can case managers learn what's important to clients? *Gerontologist, 37,* 767–776.

Doukas, D. J., & McCullough, L. B. (1991a). The Values History: The evaluation of the patient's values and advance directives. *Journal of Family Practice, 32,* 145–153.

Doukas, D. J., & McCullough, L. B. (1991b). The Values History: The evolution of the values history. *Journal of Patient's Values and Advance Directives, 32,* 145–150.

Elster, J. (1983). *Sour Grapes: Studies in the Subversion of Rationality.* New York: Cambridge University Press.

Emanuel, L., & Emanuel, E. (1989). The medical directive. *Journal of the American Medical Association, 261,* 3288–3293.

Feldman, P., Gagen, D., & Putnam, P. (1988). *Information stratgies to support consumer- and family-centerd care in managed long-term care settings: Final report of an expert panel.* New York: Center for Home Care Policy and Research, Visiting Nurse Service of New York.

Friss-Feinberg, L. (1998). *Making Hard Choices: Respecting Both Voices: Choice and Decision-Naking in Everyday Care: Survey for Persons with Cognitive Impair-ments.* San Francisco: Family Caregiver Alliance, personal communication.

Froberg, D., & Kane, R. L. (1989a). Methodology for measuring health preferences—I: Measurement strategies. *Journal of Clinical Epidemiology, 42*(4), 345–354.

Froberg, D., & Kane, R. L. (1989b). Methodology for measuring health preferences—II: Scaling methods. *Journal of Clinical Epidemiology, 42*(5), 459–471.

Froberg, D., & Kane, R. L. (1989c). Methodology for measuring health preferences—III: Population and context effects. *Journal of Clinical Epidemiology, 42*(6), 485–592.

Froberg, D., & Kane, R. L. (1989d). Methodology for measuring health preferences—IV. Progress and a research agenda. *Journal of Clinical Epidemiology, 1989*(7), 675–685.

Gibson, J. I. (1990). National Values History project. *Generations, 14*(Suppl), 51–64.

Hawes, C., Greene, A., Wood, M., & Woodsong, C. (1997). *Family members' views: What is quality in assisted living facilities providing care to people with dementia.* Washington, DC: Alzheimer's Association.

Hays, R. D., Siu, A. L., Keeler, E., Marshall, G. N., Kaplan, R. M., Simmons, S., Mouchi, D. E., & Schnelle, J. F. (1996). Long-term care residents' preferences for health states on the quality of well-being scale. *Medical Decision Making, 16*(3), 254–261.

Jenkens, R. (1997). *Assisted living and private rooms. What people say they want.* Washington, DC: American Association of Retired Persons.

Kahneman, D., & Tversky, A. (1982). The psychology of preference. *Scientific American, 246,* 160–172.

Kane, R. (1995). *Quality, autonomy, and safety in home and community-based long-term care: Towards regulatory and quality assurance policy (report of a national miniconference officially recognized by the White House Conference on Aging).* Minneapolis: National LTC Resource Center, University of Minnesota School of Public Health.

Kane, R., Kane, R., & Ladd, R. (1998a). *The heart of long-term care.* New York: Oxford University Press.

Kane, R. A., Baker, M., Salmon, J., & Veazie, W. (1998b). *Consumer perspectives on private versus shared accommodations in assisted living settings.* Washington, DC: American Association of Retired Persons.

Kane, R. A., & Caplan, A. L. (Eds.) (1990). *Everyday ethics: Resolving dilemmas in nursing home life.* New York: Springer.

Kane, R. A., & Caplan, A. L. (Eds.). (1993).

*Ethical issues in the management of home care: The case manager's dilemma.* New York: Springer.

Kane, R. A., Caplan, A. L., Urv-Wong, E. K., Freeman, I. C., Aroskar, M. A., & Finch, M. (1997). Everyday matters in the lives of nursing home residents: Wish for and perception of choice and control. *Journal of the American Geriatrics Society, 45*(9), 1086–1093.

Kane, R. A., Degenholtz, H. B., & Kane, R. L. (1999). Adding values: An experiment in systematic attention to values and preferences of community long-term care clients. *Journal of Gerontology Social Sciences, 54B*(2), S109–S119.

Kane, R. A., Penrod, J. D., & Kivnick, H. Q. (1994). Case managers discuss ethics: Dilemmas of an emerging occupation in long-term care in the United States. *Journal of Case Management, 3,* 3–12.

Kane, R. L., Bell, R. M., & Reigler, S. L. (1989). Value preferences for nursing home outcomes. *Gerontologist, 26,* 303–308.

Kane, R. L., & Kane, R. A.. (Eds.) (1982). *Values and long-term care.* Lexington, MA: D. C. Heath.

Lawton, M., & Bader, J. (1970). Wish for privacy by young and old. *Journal of Gerontology, 25*(1), 48–54.

Lidz, C. W., Fischer, L., & Arnold, R. M. (1992). *The erosion of autonomy in long-term care.* New York: Oxford University Press.

Logsdon, R. G., & Teri, L. (1997). The Pleasant Events Schedule—AD: Psychometric properties and relationship to depression and cognition in Alzheimer's disease patients. *Gerontologist, 37,* 40–45.

Mahoney, K. J., & Simon-Rusinowitz, L. (1997). Cash and counseling demonstration and evaluation: Start-up activities. *Journal of Case Management, 6*(1), 25–31.

Mattimore, T., Wenger, N., Cesbiens, N., Teno, J., Hamel, M., Liu, H., Carliff, R., Connors, A., Lynn, J., & Oye, R. (1997). Surrogate and physicain understanding of patients' preferences for living permanently in a nursing home. *Journal of the American Geriatrics Society, 45,* 818–824.

Mazur, D. J., & Merz, J. F. (1993). How the manner of presentation of data influences older patients in determining their treatment preferences. *Journal of the American Geriatrics Society, 41*(3), 223–228.

Miller, G. (1956). The magical number seven plus or minus two: Some limits on your capacity to process information. *Psychological Review, 63,* 81–97.

Ogletree, T. (1995). Values and valuation. In W. Reich (Ed.), *Encyclopedia of Bioethics* (rev. ed., vol. 5, pp. 2525–2520). New York: McMillan.

Patrick, D. L., Straks, H. E., Cain, K. C., Uhlmann, R., & Pearlman, R. (1994). Measuring preferences for health states worse than death. *Medical Decision-Making, 14*(1), 9–18.

PGC & VNSNY (1999). *Preferences for everyday living: A survey for the Visiting Nurse Service of New York.* Philadelphia Geriatric Center and Visiting Nurse Service of New York. Version 6/99, mimeo.

Potthoff, S. J., Kane, R. L., & Franco, S. J. (1995). *Hospital discharge planning for elderly patients: Improving decisions, aligning incentives* (Final report to Health Care Financing Administration). Minneapolis: University of Minnesota.

Reinardy, J., Kane, R., & Huck, S. (1998). *Destination assisted living versus destination nursing home in Oregon: Factors accounting for location decisions.* Paper presented at the Gerontological Society of America Annual Meeting, Philadelphia, November 21, 1998.

Rokeach, M. (1973). *The nature of human values.* New York: McMillan.

Rokeach, M., & Ball-Rokeach, S. (1989). Stability and change in American value priorities. *American Psychologist, 44,* 775–584.

Sachs, G. A., Stocking, C. B., Stern, P., Cox, D. M., Hougham, G., & Sachs, R. (1994). Ethical aspects of dementia research: Informed consent and proxy consent. *Clinical Research, 42,* 403–412.

Salmon, J. R., Weber, S. M., Perry, J. L., Stetka, K. A., & Polivka, L. (1998). *Exploring quality of life in long-term care: A pilot study.* Paper presented at the Gerontological Association of America, Annual Conference, Philadelphia, November 22, 1998.

Sano, M., Albert, S., Tractenberg, R., & Schittini, M. (1999). Developing utilities: Quantifying quality of life for stages of Alzheimer's disease as measured by the Clinical Dementia Rating. *Journal of Mental Health and Aging, 5*(1), 59–68.

Sciegaj, M. (1997). Elder Preferences for Consumer Direction. Questionnaires and early results made available by the author. Waltham MA: Florence Heller Graduate School of Advanced Studies in Social Welfare, Brandeis University.

Simmons, S., Schnelle, J., Uman, G., Kulvicki, A., Lee, K.-O., & Ouslander, J. (1997). Selecting nursing home residents for satisfaction surveys. *Gerontologist, 37,* 543–550.

Simon, S., Hoew, L., & Kirschenbum, H.

(1972). *Values clarification*. New York: Hart Publishing Company.

Thomson, M. (1986). Willingness to pay and accept risks to cure chronic disease. *American Journal of Public Health, 76,* 195–215.

Tsevat, J., Dawson, N. V., Wu, A. W., Lynn, J., Soukup, J. R., Cook, E. F., Vidaillet, H., & Phillips, R. (1998). Health values of hospitalized patients 80 years or older: HELP investigators. Hospitalized Elderly Longitudinal Project. *JAMA, 279,* 371–375.

Tversky, A., & Kahneman, D. (1981). The framing of decisions and the psychology of choice. *Science, 211,* 453–458.

Van Haitsma, K. (1999). The Assessment and Integration of Preferences into Care Practices for Persons with Dementia Residing in the Nursing Home: Unpublished manuscript. Philadelphia: Philadelphia Geriatric Center.

Wetle, T., Levkoff, S., Cwikel, J., & Rosen, A. (1988). Nursing home residents' participation in medical decisions: Perceptions and preferences. *Gerontologist, 28*(Suppl), 53–58.

Zweibel, N. R., & Cassel, C. K. (1989). Treatment choices at the end of life: A comparison by older patients and their physician-selected proxies. *Gerontologist, 29,* 615–621.

# 9

# Satisfaction

## MAUREEN A. SMITH

The role of the client in the health care
and social services system is evolving. In
recent years, previously unquestioned beliefs in professional omnipotence and beneficence have given way to discussions of
patient autonomy and consumerism (Deber, 1994; Kravitz, 1996). "Patients/cli-
ents" became "consumers" and are now
often referred to as "customers." This emphasis on the consumer's perspective has
created a demand for information on consumers' experiences and satisfaction with
health and social services.

This evolution toward a consumer focus
has also increased the importance of measuring satisfaction with care for older
adults. Older adults often experience transitions from acute care to rehabilitative
care to long-term care. Several characteristics distinguish long-term care from more
acute care, including a slower pace, lower
level of technology, heterogeneous population with disparate goals, and continuing
patterns of transitions over time (Kane &
Kane, 1988). These characteristics imply
that satisfaction with services can become
increasingly important in long-term care
settings relative to other measures of quality. It may even be considered the major
outcome of interest.

## WHO MEASURES SATISFACTION?

Accurate assessment of patient satisfaction
is important for patients, clinicians, policy-
makers, researchers, and health care organizations. For both *clinicians* and *patients,*
fulfilling a patient's perceived needs may
be viewed as a direct goal of health care
(Cleary & McNeil, 1988). Satisfied patients may be more likely to comply with
therapy (Sherbourne et al., 1992) and be
less likely to sue for malpractice (Hickson
et al., 1994). Understanding a patient's expectations can help one to identify the
value a patient places on an outcome,
which is critical for patient care decisions
(Hornberger, Habraken, & Bloch, 1995).
The very process of eliciting patient expectations also increases the participation of
patients in their own health care, which
may provide intrinsic benefit and promote
better outcomes (Greenfield, Kaplan, &
Ware, 1985).

For *policy-makers,* measurement of patient satisfaction can provide useful information on current policy initiatives. Many
policies involve the design and implementation of programs to increase or decrease
the utilization of health care services, contain the costs of care, or improve quality.

261

High levels of patient dissatisfaction with a program may be an early indicator of problems with program design or implementation. *Researchers* may wish to identify factors that influence patient satisfaction, including the impact of interventions specifically designed to improve satisfaction with care. Other studies could examine the influence of satisfaction on subsequent patient behaviors or clinical outcomes and enhance our understanding of the quality improvement process.

Finally, *health care organizations* assess patient satisfaction for a variety of reasons. Satisfaction data often support continuous quality improvement or program evaluation efforts. Regular measurement of patient satisfaction assists organizations in meeting regulatory requirements or the requirements of third-party payors. Finally, many health care organizations use satisfaction data for the purposes of customer relations or marketing.

## WHAT IS SATISFACTION?

Pascoe (1983) defined patient satisfaction as "a health care recipient's reaction to salient aspects of the context, process, and result of their service experience." According to this definition, patients evaluate a directly received service by comparing their personal experience to a subjective standard, which is closely related to their expectations regarding their health care. Understanding older adults' expectations is crucial to assessing and interpreting measures of patient satisfaction. Finally, measures of satisfaction should be distinguished from measures of quality of life, life satisfaction, and preferences for care, which are discussed elsewhere in this volume.

## CONCEPTUAL FRAMEWORK

Conceptual models provide a useful framework for interpreting the results of a satisfaction survey. Research in patient satisfaction lacks a universally accepted conceptual or theoretical framework, although several models have been proposed. Two of these models and their implications for surveying satisfaction among older adults are discussed in this chapter.

Client satisfaction usually refers to satisfaction with directly received care (Geron, 1998). The term *satisfaction* implies an emotional or affective response, but there has been substantial debate over whether satisfaction also incorporates a cognitively based evaluation of the service based on the client's expectations (Pascoe, 1983). A model incorporating both of these aspects of satisfaction relies on the theory of disconfirmation of expectations (Rust & Oliver, 1994). In this model, the client cognitively evaluates the perceived quality of the service attributes compared with expectations of those attributes and also has an affective response to that evaluation. When actual performance disconfirms the expectations of performance, the result is satisfaction (or dissatisfaction) with the service. This model helps us to interpret the results of satisfaction surveys by emphasizing the importance of identifying and understanding client expectations regarding their care. For example, institutionalized older adults may become habituated to lowered expectations over time (Kane & Kane, 1988). As a result, truly unsatisfactory care may be rated as satisfactory by survey respondents who have substantially lower expectations as a result of this "learned dependency" (Geron, 1991). In addition, measuring satisfaction with care over time becomes problematic. Greater satisfaction over time may be due to lowered expectations, not to changes in the actual care delivered.

A second model focuses on the ways in which attitudes are formed (Strasser, Aharony, & Greenberger, 1993). Based on the theory of satisfaction attitude formation, client satisfaction is seen as an attitudinal response to the value judgments that clients form about their health care experience (Fig. 9.1). By definition, satisfaction is assumed to be an attitude; it combines

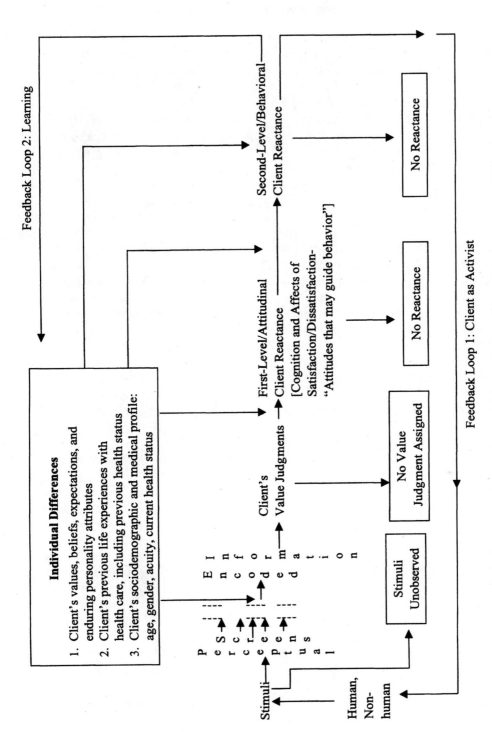

Figure 9.1. A model of client satisfaction. Source: Adapted from Strasser (1993).

cognition and affect but excludes behavior. Client behaviors may, however, influence the formation of subsequent satisfaction attitudes (Feedback Loop 1). Clients are also viewed as learners who develop a database of information and expectations used to influence future health care encounters (Feedback Loop 2). This second model is helpful because it emphasizes the importance of client perceptions, value judgments, and feedback loops in influencing the results of a satisfaction survey. Because there are multiple points of influence along these pathways, it seems clear that the results of most satisfaction surveys should be interpreted cautiously. In particular, older clients may differ in how they perceive and encode information, make value judgments, incorporate their own individual differences, and interpret feedback information. Another advantage of this model is its explicit recognition of client behavior as a consequence of satisfaction/dissatisfaction attitudes. Research on the relationship of satisfaction ratings to subsequent client behaviors has, however, been limited (Aharony & Strasser, 1993).

## COMPONENTS OF SATISFACTION

Satisfaction with care appears to be simultaneously a unidimensional and a multidimensional construct. Clients appear to make unique summary judgments about their overall experiences with care, implying that a global measure of satisfaction is an appropriate measure (Aharony & Strasser, 1993). There is also substantial evidence that satisfaction is multidimensional (Abramowitz, Cote, & Berry, 1987; Meterko, Nelson, & Rubin, 1990). Consequently, separate scales measure satisfaction with more specific aspects of medical care, such as access to services, technical quality, and the provider's interpersonal skills. (Hulka et al., 1970). The ability of clients to distinguish completely all of the dimensions of satisfaction has been questioned, however, particularly for the distinction between technical competence and interpersonal skills (Ben-Sira, 1976).

The lack of a widely accepted conceptual framework complicates attempts to examine the structure of client satisfaction. As a result, the dimensions of satisfaction may vary from study to study, as different satisfaction measures are developed to deal with different aspects of health care (Pascoe, 1983). For example, in the acute care setting, Ware and associates (1983) identified seven dimensions of satisfaction with physician and other medical services, including interpersonal manner, technical quality/competence, accessibility/convenience, finances/cost, continuity, availability, and general satisfaction. In contrast, satisfaction with in-home supportive services has recently been postulated to include the dimensions of humaneness, competence, dependability, continuity of care, adequacy of services, advocacy from the home care worker, accessibility of services, and choice (Geron, 1995).

## FACTORS RELATED TO SATISFACTION

Numerous factors have been related to patient satisfaction (Aharony & Strasser, 1993). These include sociodemographic characteristics, prior health status, expectations about care, and the structure, process, and outcomes of care (Cleary & McNeil, 1988). For most of these factors, there are many inconsistencies across studies and no consensus about which are most strongly related to satisfaction with care. Conflicting conclusions may be due to the type of care examined, the specific context of the study, or differences in survey methodologies (Aharony & Strasser, 1993; Pascoe, 1983).

Among sociodemographic characteristics, patient age and gender are most consistently associated with satisfaction, with both female and older patients being more satisfied (Locker & Dunt, 1978; Nelson-Wernick et al., 1981; Pascoe, 1983; Strasser, 1992). Prior health status may also be related to satisfaction separately from the outcomes of care (Rubin, 1990), suggesting that controlling for preexisting differences in health may be important when examining the relationships between outcomes and satisfaction. Patient expectations also play a role, although much previous research has been conducted with little consistency in the way expectations are studied (Aharony & Strasser, 1993; Cleary & McNeil, 1988). In general, patients with lower expectations tend to be more satisfied (Swan et al., 1985; Ware, Davies-Avery, & Stewart, 1978).

The structure of care includes both the organization and financing arrangements, as well as issues of accessibility and continuity of care (Cleary & McNeil, 1988). Patients were more satisfied with organizations that had greater autonomy and communication with other organizations (Greenley & Schoenherr, 1981). Patients were also less satisfied as the cost of care rose, and health maintenance organization patients tended to be more satisfied with their financial arrangements for care (Cleary & McNeil, 1988). Provider characteristics that influence satisfaction include nursing care, medical care, food quality, noise levels, and physical surroundings, with nursing and physician care generally being the most important determinants (Cleary et al., 1983; Doering, 1983). Finally, many studies have suggested that greater accessibility, availability, and continuity of care are positively related to satisfaction (Cleary & McNeil, 1988; Weiss & Ramsey, 1989).

The process of care includes both the technical and interpersonal aspects of care. Although technical quality may be difficult for patients to judge, the quality of physician–patient interaction can be judged more easily. As a result, although patient perceptions of the technical quality of care have been related to satisfaction, interpersonal and communication skills usually explain more variation in satisfaction ratings (Cleary & McNeil, 1988; Doering, 1983). Satisfaction with communication tends to be one of the most important elements of overall satisfaction, and patients are often the least satisfied with physician communi-

cation (Cleary & McNeil, 1988; Doering, 1983; Nelson-Wernick et al., 1981).

The relationship of the outcomes of medical care to satisfaction is poorly understood. Perceived improvement in health has been shown to be a predictor of patient satisfaction (Carmel, 1985; Fleming, 1981), but satisfaction has been shown to be more highly related to patients' absolute outcomes (i.e., their state of current health) rather than to the extent of their improvement in outcome (Kane, Maciejewski, & Finch, 1997).

## HOW DOES SATISFACTION DIFFER IN AN AGING POPULATION?

Older adults are more likely than younger adults to be satisfied with health care services (Pope & Mays, 1993). The reasons for this are unclear, although they may relate to different expectations or experiences with the health care system (Kasper & Riley, 1992). Older adults who use health care services differ in a variety of ways from younger populations, and these differences have the potential to influence both the measurement of satisfaction and the interpretation of the results.

Chronic disabling conditions and poor health are more prevalent among older adults. As a result, this group has higher utilization of health care services and may have more need for continuing care. Three mechanisms have been postulated by which older age and poorer health might influence judgments regarding satisfaction. Increased exposure to the health care system could provide more experience with which to judge access or quality, and satisfaction measures may reflect this increased experience (Kasper & Riley, 1992). The overwhelming importance of health care providers to older adults with chronic illness could also, however, a more favorable view of those provider–patient relationships (Owens & Batchelor, 1996). Many older adults may view their transitions to poor health as normal, and their relative satisfaction with medical care may reflect lower expectations of the effects of treatment (Kasper & Riley, 1992).

Aging is also associated with a high prevalence of major life changes related to health. These changes often involve an alteration in living arrangements (e.g., a move to a nursing home or assisted living facility). As a result, satisfaction must be measured in a variety of settings (e.g., hospitals, nursing homes, home care, or outpatient services). Compared with the acute care setting or a physician office visit, long-term care provided in the home or nursing home is often "low-technology" care from personnel with limited training (Kane & Kane, 1988). Consequently, issues for satisfaction measurement may differ substantially for acute and long-term care services, but few adequately tested measures are available for long-term care (Geron, 1998). Because older adults are more likely to receive these services, this lack of measurement tools leaves older adults at a disadvantage.

The redefinition of the patient as a consumer may be especially problematic for vulnerable older adults (Owens & Batchelor, 1996). A good consumer has been defined as "someone who can adequately assimilate information on the costs and quality of health care, and, on the basis of such information, has an ability and a desire to make health care choices and is then prepared to search for the best 'package' of health care in terms of cost and quality" (Shackley & Ryan, 1994). This role may be difficult to achieve for many older adults, particularly those frail elderly patients with severe physical, mental, or cognitive impairments.

Assessing satisfaction for patients with impairments also requires modifications in survey design and administration (Henry & Capitman, 1995). Modifications may need to be made for patients with hearing, vision, or speech disorders or for those with cognitive or physical impairments. Patients with dementia or other types of cognitive impairments are often completely excluded from satisfaction surveys.

The rationale for these exclusions is often weak, however, given that people with dementia vary substantially in their ability to communicate their preferences and expectations. There is also evidence that many cognitively impaired nursing home residents can accurately answer simple yes or no questions about their daily care (Simmons et al., 1997). Some surveys include patients with cognitive impairments by interviewing caregivers or family members as proxies. Unfortunately, there can be substantial problems with this approach, as the perceptions of the patient and the caregiver/family member may not always be the same (see Chapter 17).

## METHODOLOGIC DILEMMAS IN CHOOSING A SATISFACTION MEASURE

The methodologicl dilemmas involved in measuring patient satisfaction are substantial (Aharony & Strasser, 1993). To develop a reliable and valid satisfaction measure, researchers must overcome a variety of conceptual and operational problems.

The *reliability* of a satisfaction measure is crucial. Two main types of reliability are at issue, including the interitem reliability or internal consistency of multi-item scales (e.g. Cronbach's $\alpha$) and test–retest reliability. Interobserver reliability may also be relevant for surveys that are administered by in-person interview. Unfortunately, most studies examining patient satisfaction do not report the reliability of their measures. When internal consistency has been tested, scales have been developed that meet the traditional psychometric standards for group comparisons (Aharony & Strasser, 1993). Test–retest reliability is reported even less frequently, perhaps because it is unclear whether test–retest correlations are a function of poor recall or changing perceptions over time.

Most measures of patient satisfaction have not been *validated* against either internal or external criteria. The ability of patients to discriminate among different features of care (discriminant validity) is often used as an internal test. These tests do not, however, show whether or not patients make externally valid discriminations; patient ratings of different features of care are rarely compared with independent ratings of the same features (Aharony & Strasser, 1993). There are several approaches to external validation of satisfaction ratings, including experiments that manipulate features of care and measure subsequent satisfaction, comparison of patient ratings with ratings of care from other sources, and comparison of patient ratings with other variables that should theoretically be related to patient satisfaction (e.g., construct validation) (Rubin, 1990). Unfortunately, very few measures of satisfaction have been tested extensively for validity, perhaps because researchers have lacked well-developed conceptual models to guide their efforts. This raises particular concern for aspects of satisfaction measurement that may have poor face validity, such as patient ratings of the technical quality of care (Ben-Sira, 1976; Davies & Ware, 1988; DiMatteo & Hays, 1980). Finally, even validated measures have usually been tested in only one population or setting of care.

Satisfaction measures are subject to a host of potential *biases*. Three types of bias are relevant, including bias from nonresponse, acquiescent responses, and social–psychological artifacts. Nonresponse bias is a substantial problem, and satisfaction survey response rates are often well below 50% (Aharony & Strasser, 1993). Given evidence that nonrespondents evaluate care less favorably than do patients who respond (Eisen & Grob, 1979; Ley et al., 1976), survey results must be interpreted with extreme caution when response rates fall below an acceptable level (usually 80%). Acquiescent response bias is the tendency to agree with a statement regardless of content. For example, positively worded items may result in higher ratings of satisfaction, whereas negatively worded items may result in lower ratings.

This increases the correlation between similarly worded items. Acquiescent response bias may significantly influence satisfaction ratings, and recent evidence suggests that this bias operates most strongly for the oldest and sickest patients (Ross, Steward, & Sinacore, 1995). Finally, social–psychological artifacts can also bias satisfaction measures. Examples include social desirability response bias and bias due to fear of retribution. Social desirability is the tendency to offer answers that are consistent with the normative expectations of the interviewer and may be responsible for the universally high approval ratings found in many satisfaction surveys. Bias due to fear of retribution is closely related to social desirability and can be partially addressed with guarantees of confidentiality. These two potential biases may also be reduced if the survey is administered by an independent external group in a neutral location.

Satisfaction measures incorporate a personal or general reference for the survey items. A personal referent asks patients how satisfied they are with their own medical care, whereas a general referent asks patients to rate the care received by people in general. Items with a personal referent have been seen as more acceptable, less ambiguous, and more useful for program evaluation than are items with a general referent (Pascoe, Attkisson, & Roberts, 1983). It is also well known that patients are consistently more satisfied with their own medical care than when they rate care received by people in general, which contributes to skewed results (Pascoe et al., 1983; Ware et al., 1983). The more favorable ratings of medical care using a personal referent may, however, be due in part to bias from a tendency to give socially desirable responses and potentially explains the more highly skewed response distributions (Hays & Ware, 1986).

The *timing of survey administration* can influence the results. A patient's perceived satisfaction with care may change over time, as well as in response to external shocks (Aharony & Strasser, 1993). Few studies have examined this issue directly. A U-shaped curve has been described for the relationship between length of time after discharge and patient satisfaction with communication in the hospital; patients expressed greater satisfaction during their hospitalization or several months post-discharge compared with a few weeks post-discharge (Ley et al., 1976). Others have found no relationship between timing of the questionnaire and response rate for a 2 to 12 week time frame between hospitalization and survey (Meterko et al., 1990).

Most measures must determine an explicit *time reference* for the survey items, although it is not clear how meaningful this time reference is to the patient. Usually, the patients are asked for a summary evaluation of their satisfaction with care over a specific time period (e.g., 6 months or 1 year) (Ware & Hays, 1988). The resulting data may be used in a variety of ways, including to assess the quality of care and assist purchasers in making contracting decisions with selected providers. The second approach focuses on satisfaction with care for a single medical visit or a single episode of care (e.g., a hospitalization). By examining patient perceptions of specific aspects of care during a particular encounter, this approach may provide more useful information for quality improvement efforts (Seibert, Strohmeyer, & Carey, 1996).

The *utilization patterns* of the respondents may also influence the results. To address this, some satisfaction surveys separate users from nonusers of care. This is often accomplished by the use of a skip pattern. For example, an initial question may ask whether respondents have received care in the last 12 months. A "yes" response allows the respondent to continue with that section of the survey, whereas a "no" response skips that section and moves to the next section. A related approach separates low users from high users of care. For example, many studies of satisfaction with ambulatory care report

high ratings because they are conducted on random samples of adults, most of whom are healthy. Future reporting of consumer satisfaction is likely to focus more critically on the analysis of sicker subpopulations, whose satisfaction may differ from that of the generally healthy random sample (Allen & Rogers, 1997; Cleary et al., 1997).

The *response format* for individual items can have a substantial impact on the reliability and validity of the results. Satisfaction surveys often use statements of opinion about doctors and a 5 point Likert "agree/disagree" response scale. This indirect approach usually requires relatively long items and many items per dimension to achieve validity. It has also been suggested that this scale may generate acquiescent response bias, although this bias can be reduced if both positively and negatively worded items are included throughout the survey (LaMonica et al., 1986). The "satisfied/dissatisfied" option is simpler and more direct, but both the "satisfied/dissatisfied" and the "agree/disagree" scale can produce highly skewed response distributions. An "excellent/poor" response scale may have several advantages. Ware and Hays (1988) compared a 6 point "very satisfied/very dissatisfied" scale and a five-point "excellent/poor" scale for measuring satisfaction with a specific medical encounter. The "excellent/poor" format produced responses that were less skewed, had greater variability, and performed better on validity tests.

The relationship of *mode of administration* (e.g., self-administered, telephone, in-person interview) to patient ratings has not been well studied. Some evidence suggests that the administration method can influence the results, with telephone surveys producing higher response rates and slightly higher ratings (Casarreal, Mills, & Plant, 1986; Walker & Restuccia, 1984). In contrast, a literature review suggested that response rates were relatively similar for interviews and self-administered surveys (French, 1981). An important caveat is that the characteristics of nonrespondents may differ depending on the mode of administration (Walker & Restuccia, 1984).

The use of *proxies* to rate satisfaction with care may be necessary for older adults with severe disabilities. Proxy satisfaction should always be distinguished from patient satisfaction. The perceptions of the patient and the caregiver/family member may not always be the same. For example, patients' relatives, or proxies, may rate care more negatively than the patients do (Strasser & Schweikhart, 1992; Walker & Restuccia, 1984). The use of proxies should be determined based on prespecified criteria and with the recognition that results do not necessarily represent the same scores that would have been provided by the patient.

## SATISFACTION SURVEYS

This section provides an overview of surveys potentially useful in assessing the satisfaction of older adults with health and social services but is not restricted solely to tools developed for older adults because few such tools are available. Whenever possible, widely used surveys were included that offer evidence of their reliability and validity. Some surveys still in the process of development are described, usually because no comparable well-tested instruments are available. Surveys are examined for a wide variety of settings, including ambulatory, hospital, long-term care, home care, assisted living, and adult day care. Given the increasing enrollment of older adults in health maintenance organizations, we also describe several surveys developed to measure health plan member satisfaction. The surveys included in this chapter are not an exhaustive list of all the instruments available. Several more extensive reviews of consumer satisfaction surveys are available for ambulatory, hospital and health plan care (Allen & Rogers, 1996; McDaniel & Nash, 1990;.

McGee et al., 1997; Rubin, 1990; van Campen et al., 1995).

### Ambulatory Care Satisfaction Surveys

There are several widely used surveys of satisfaction with ambulatory care. These surveys generally ask patients for either a summary evaluation of their satisfaction with care over a specific time period (e.g., 6 months or 1 year) or their satisfaction with care for a single medical encounter. Most of the instruments we review focus on a patient's summary evaluation, although the last two measures focus on satisfaction with a specific medical visit.

### Patient Satisfaction Questionnaire (PSQ)

The development of the Patient Satisfaction Questionnaire (PSQ) began in the 1970s, and it has since become one of the most commonly used measures of patient satisfaction (Table 9.1, Fig. 9.2) (Ware & Karmos, 1976; Ware, Snyder, & Wright, 1976a; Ware, Wright, & Snyder, 1976b; Ware et al., 1983; Ware & Young, 1976). During its development, an initial large pool of 900 items was constructed from extensive literature reviews, focus groups, analyses of responses to open-ended questions, and analyses of complaints, grievances, and reasons for disenrollment. A five-point Likert response scale was chosen (from Strongly Agree to Strongly Disagree). The survey was administered in person by trained interviews, and subsequent psychometric analyses were used to reduce the number of items in the original PSQ to 80 and to classify them into a wide range of concepts measuring consumer satisfaction with care. Further revision resulted in a 68 item version (PSQ-II) and a short-form version with 43 items that was administered in the RAND Health Insurance Experiment and other national studies. In a third phase, a 50 tem version was developed for the Medical Outcomes Study (PSQ-III) (Marshall et al., 1993).

The PSQ is based on the assumption that satisfaction is a multidimensional construct requiring multiple scales designed to

**Table 9.1.**
Ambulatory Care Satisfaction Surveys

| Survey | Description | Dimensions | Data collection | Reliability | Validity |
|---|---|---|---|---|---|
| Patient Satisfaction Questionnaire—Form III (PSQ-IIII) (Marshall et al., 1993) | Patient satisfaction with medical care | Interpersonal manner, communication, technical competence, time spent with doctor, financial aspects, access to care, general satisfaction | Item number: 50 Item type: 5 point "strongly agree" to "strongly disagree" Administration: Mailed questionnaire | $\alpha$ = 0.82–0.89 for subscales | Construct validity established using factor analysis. Discriminant validity questioned for some subscales, particularly technical and interpersonal care |
| Client Satisfaction Questionnaire (CSQ-8) (Larsen et al., 1979) | General patient satisfaction with health care services | General satisfaction | Item number: 8 Item type: Various Administration: Self-administered | $\alpha$ = 0.90 | Construct validity established using factor analysis. Predictive validity established |
| Service Quality Instrument (SERVQUAL) (Parasuraman et al., 1988) | General quality of services from the customer's perspective | Tangibles, reliability, responsiveness, assurance, empathy | Item number: 22 Item type: 7 point "strongly agree" to "strongly disagree" Administration: Self-administered | $\alpha$ = 0.87–0.90 overall, 0.52–0.84 for subscales | Content validity established. Convergent validity established |

| Instrument | Purpose | Dimensions | Item characteristics | Reliability | Validity |
|---|---|---|---|---|---|
| Risser Patient Satisfaction Scale (PSS) (Risser, 1975.) | Outpatient satisfaction with nursing care | Technical–professional, trusting relationship, educational relationship | Item number: 25 Item type: 5 point "strongly agree" to "strongly disagree" Administration: Self-administered | $\alpha$ = 0.91 overall, 0.64–0.89 for subscales | Content validity established. Discriminant validity questioned due to high interscale correlations |
| Visit-Specific Satisfaction Questionnaire (VSQ) (Ware and Hays, 1988) | Outpatient satisfaction at the conclusion of a specific medical care visit | General satisfaction, technical care, interpersonal care, waiting time | Item number: 7 Item type: 5 point "excellent" to "poor" Administration: Self-administered | $\alpha$ = 0.82–0.94 for subscales | Construct validity established |
| Physician Office Quality of Care Monitor (PQCM) (Seibert et al, 1996) | Outpatient satisfaction with care focusing on the most recent office visit | Physician care, nursing care, front office services, accessibility, billing, testing services, facility characteristics | Item number: 56 Item type: 5 point "excellent" to "poor" Administration: Mail | $\alpha$ = 0.67–0.95 for subscales | Construct validity established by factor analysis. Predictive validity established. Discriminant validity questioned due to high interscale correlations |

*General Satisfaction*

I am very satisfied with the medical care I receive.
There are some things about the medical care I receive that could be better.
All things considered, the medical care I receive is excellent.
There are things about the medical system I receive my care from that need to be improved.
The medical care I have been receiving is just about perfect.
I am dissatisfied with some things about the medical care I receive.

*Technical Quality*

When I go for medical care, they are careful to check everything when treating and examining me.
Doctors need to be more thorough in treating and examining me.
I think my doctor's office has everything needed to provide complete care.
Sometimes doctors make me wonder if their diagnosis is correct.
The medical staff that treats me knows about the latest medical developments.
Some of the doctors I have seen lack experience with my medical problems.
My doctors are very competent and well trained.
I have some doubts about the ability of the doctors who treat me.
Doctors never expose me to unnecessary risk.
Doctors rarely give me advice about ways to avoid illness and stay healthy.

*Interpersonal Aspects*

Doctors act too businesslike and impersonal toward me.
Doctors always do their best to keep me from worrying.
When I am receiving medical care, they should pay more attention to my privacy.
The doctors who treat me have a genuine interest in me as a person.
Sometimes doctors make me feel foolish.
My doctors treat me in a very friendly and courteous manner.
The doctors who treat me should give me more respect.

*Communication*

Doctors are good about explaining the reason for medical tests.
Sometimes doctors use medical terms without explaining what they mean.
During my medical visits, I am always allowed to say everything that I think is important.
Doctors sometimes ignore what I tell them.
Doctors listen carefully to what I have to say.

*Financial Aspects*

I feel confident that I can get the medical care I need without being set back financially.
I worry sometimes about having to pay large medical bills.
Regardless of the health problems I have now or develop later, I feel protected from financial hardship.
Sometimes it is a problem to cover my share of the cost for a medical care visit.
I feel insured and protected financially against all possible medical problems.
I have to pay for more of my medical care than I can afford.
The amount I have to pay to cover or insure my medical care needs is reasonable.
Sometimes I go without the medical care I need because it is too expensive.

*Time Spent with Doctor*

Doctors usually spend plenty of time with me.
Those who provide my medical care sometimes hurry too much when they treat me.

(*continued*)

**Figure 9.2.** Patient Satisfaction Questionnaire (PSQ-III) items. Source: Adapted from Marshall (1993).

---

*Accessibility and Convenience*

If I need hospital care, I can get admitted without any trouble.
It is hard for me to get medical care on short notice.
It is easy for me to get medical care in an emergency.
The office where I get medical care should be open for more hours than it is.
Places where I can get medical care are very conveniently located.
Where I get medical care, people have to wait too long for emergency treatment.
If I have a medical question, I can reach a doctor for help without any problem.
I find it hard to get an appointment for medical care right away.
The office hours when I can get medical care are convenient (good) for me.
I am usually kept waiting for a long time when I am at the doctor's office.
I have easy access to the medical specialists I need.
I am able to get medical care whenever I need it.

---

**Figure 9.2.** — Continued

tap different dimensions. Although there is evidence that the seven subscales of the PSQ measure distinct dimensions of patient satisfaction, there are also relatively high interscale correlations between the subscales measuring the interpersonal and technical skills of providers (Marshall et al., 1993; Ware et al., 1983). As a result, the discriminant validity of these scales is doubtful. This is consistent with arguments that patients may not be able to make fine distinctions between the different dimensions of satisfaction, particularly between the interpersonal aspects of care and the technical quality dimensions (Ben-Sira, 1976). Consequently, the practical utility of some of the subscales in the PSQ is an unsettled question.

*Client Satisfaction Questionnaire (CSQ)*

The Client Satisfaction Questionnaire (CSQ) is a widely used unidimensional scale assessing general patient satisfaction with health care services (Table 9.1, Fig. 9.3) (Larsen et al., 1979). It was developed in the 1970s as a collection of 81 items from published and unpublished sources. Thirty-two mental health professionals reduced the number of items to 31 by assessing the degree to which each item tapped one of eight hypothesized dimensions. The resulting survey was administered to outpatient mental health clients and analyzed using principal components factor analysis. Because the analysis generated only one factor explaining 75% of the common variance, it was concluded that the instrument was unidimensional. Several different versions of the CSQ have been developed in addition to the original 8 item version and include scales with 3, 4, 7, and 18 items (Daly & Flynn, 1985; Greenfield, 1983; LeVois, Nguyen, & Attkisson, 1981; Pascoe et al., 1983; Roberts, Pascoe, & Attkisson, 1983).

Because the CSQ items ask patients to rate their satisfaction with the services provided for them personally (i.e., a personal referent), the validity of the CSQ has been questioned (Hays & Ware, 1986). Surveys with personal referents tend to have higher satisfaction ratings than do surveys with general referents (Pascoe et al., 1983; Ware et al., 1983), and these more favorable ratings of medical care may be due in part to bias from a tendency to give socially desirable responses (Hays & Ware, 1986).

*Service Quality Instrument (SERVQUAL)*

The Service Quality Instrument (SERV-QUAL) is one of few instruments developed from an explicit model of consumer satisfaction (see Table 9.1) (Parasuraman, Zeithaml, & Berry, 1985). A 22 item survey was constructed and refined based on this conceptual model (Parasuraman, Zeithami, & Berry, 1988). The SERV-QUAL, however, measures perceptions of service quality from the perspective of the

How would you rate the quality of the care you receive?

| Excellent | Good | Fair | Poor |

Did you get the kind of service you wanted?

| No, definitely not | No, not really | Yes, generally | Yes, definitely |

To what extent has our program met your need?

| Almost all of my needs have been met | Most of my needs have been met | Only a few of my needs have been met | None of my needs have been met |

If a friend were in need of similar help, would you recommend our program to him/her?

| No, definitely not | No, I don't think so | Yes, I think so | Yes, definitely |

How satisfied are you with the amount of help you received?

| Quite dissatisfied | Indifferent or mildly dissatisfied | Mostly satisfied | Very satisfied |

Have the services you received helped you to deal more effectively with your problems?

| Yes, they helped a great deal | Yes, they helped somewhat | No, they really didn't help | No, they seemed to make things worse |

In an overall, general sense, how satisfied are you with the service you received?

| Very satisfied | Mostly satisfied | Indifferent or mildly dissatisfied | Quite dissatisfied |

If you were to seek help again, would you come back to our program?

| No, definitely not | No, I don't think so | Yes, I think so | Yes, definitely |

**Figure 9.3.** Client Satisfaction Questionnaire (CSQ). Source: Adapted from Larsen (1979).

consumer, not necessarily a patient. Although there are similarities between the five dimensions of SERVQUAL and the dimensions of many patient satisfaction instruments, the validity of SERVQUAL has been questioned with regard to measuring major aspects of patient satisfaction (van Campen, Friele, & Kerssens, 1992). Nonetheless, this instrument has been adapted for use with physiotherapy patients (de Haan et al., 1993), hospital patients (Babakus & Mangold, 1992), and long-term care (Kleinsorge & Koenig, 1991).

### Risser Patient Satisfaction Scale (PSS)

In 1975, Risser designed and tested the Patient Satisfaction Scale (PSS) to examine specifically patient satisfaction with nurses and nursing care in a primary care setting (see Table 9.1). This approach was based on a conceptualization of satisfaction that included three dimensions: technical–professional, trusting relationship, and educational relationship. Fifty-eight items for a preliminary questionnaire were devel-

oped from interviews with patients, literature reviews, judgments of experts, other patient satisfaction questionnaires, and critical review by nursing staff. A five-point Likert response format was chosen. The item number was reduced to 25 based on pretesting and eventually to 22 based on the final results of the study. The instrument has also been adapted to use with inpatients (Hinshaw & Atwood, 1982; LaMonica et al., 1986).

Several issues should be considered when using the PSS (Ventura et al., 1982). The discriminant validity of the PSS subscales is doubtful due to high correlations between the subscales. As is common with measures of satisfaction, there is also little variability in scale scores, and the results are skewed. As a result, it is questionable whether the measure is sensitive to potential differences between types of care modalities. Adaptations of this instrument have attempted to address these issues (Hinshaw & Atwood, 1982; LaMonica et al., 1986).

## Visit-Specific Satisfaction Questionnaire (VSQ)

The Visit-Specific Satisfaction Questionnaire (VSQ) was developed to measure satisfaction with care at the time of a specific medical care visit (see Table 9.1) (Ware & Hays, 1988). Initially, a 51 item version was based on previous visit-specific satisfaction instruments. Because the ultimate goal was a very short and simple form, items were reworded to focus on satisfaction with a specific feature of care, and two other response sets (a six-point "very satisfied/very dissatisfied" and a five-point "excellent/poor") were used instead of a more traditional five-point "strongly agree/strongly disagree" scale. The type of response scale had a substantial impact on the psychometric properties of the VSQ, and the "excellent/poor" format was recommended over the "very satisfied/very dissatisfied" format. A 7 item version was developed and tested along with the 51 item version. The authors concluded that both versions had adequate reliability and validity. A 9 item version of this survey was also developed for use in the Medical Outcomes Study (Davies & Ware, 1991).

## Physician Office Quality of Care Monitor (PQCM)

The Physician Office Quality Care Monitor (PQCM) was designed specifically to measure physician office issues for quality improvement (see Table 9.1) (Seibert et al., 1996). A pool of 60 potential survey items was developed based on published questionnaires, literature review, and interviews with physicians and administrators. The survey was revised on the basis of interviews with patients and pilot-testing. The final instrument had 56 items addressing patient experiences before, during, and after their most recent office visit. The survey identifies seven dimensions of physician office care (physician care, nursing care, front office services, accessibility, billing, testing services, and facility characteristics).

There are several issues to consider when using the PQCM. Several of the sub-scales had high intercorrelations, suggesting poor discriminant validity and potentially limiting the usefulness of this measure for quality improvement efforts. A 47% response rate may also limit the generalizability of the results. Although the authors argue that the response rate was sufficient to obtain a psychometric assessment of the survey tool, an adequate response rate is critical when assessing patient satisfaction. The results of satisfaction surveys should be interpreted cautiously when response rates fall below a satisfactory level.

## Health Plan Satisfaction Surveys

Surveys measuring satisfaction with health plans are closely related to (and in some cases derived directly from) ambulatory care satisfaction surveys. There are several major lines of health plan survey development. The Consumer Satisfaction Survey (CSS) is probably the most widely used instrument and has contributed heavily to several other surveys, including the Annual Member Health Care Survey, the Employee Health Care Value Survey, and the Consumer Health Plan Value Survey (Allen & Rogers, 1996) .We also briefly describe the Consumer Assessment of Health Plans Survey (CAHPS), which constitutes a second major line of survey development. Although information is currently limited on the properties of the CAHPS instrument, we discuss both the CSS and CAHPS lines to illustrate how satisfaction surveys evolve and contribute to the development of other instruments over time. In addition, we describe one survey developed specifically for use with older health plan members and another set of surveys that are designed to separate the measurement of health plan member expectations and satisfaction with care.

## Consumer Satisfaction Survey (CSS)

The first version of the Consumer Satisfaction Survey (CSS) was developed in 1988 by the Group Health Association of America (Table 9.2) (Davies & Ware, 1991). Its purpose was to allow employers and busi-

**Table 9.2.  Health Plan Satisfaction Surveys**

| Survey | Description | Dimensions | Data collection | Reliability | Validity |
|---|---|---|---|---|---|
| Consumer Satisfaction Survey (CSS) (Davies & Ware, 1991) | Member satisfaction with services, providers, and the plan | Multi-item scales: Access, finances, technical quality, communication, choice and continuity, interpersonal care, services covered, information, paperwork, costs of care, general satisfaction<br><br>Single-item scales: overall care, time spent, outcomes, overall quality, overall plan, plan satisfaction | Item number: 47<br>Item type: 5 point "excellent" to "poor"<br><br>Administration: Self-administration, telephone interview, or face-to-face interview | $\alpha$ = 0.80–0.97 for subscales | Content validity claimed<br><br>Predictive validity established |
| Consumer Assessment of Health Plans Survey (CAHPS) (Hays et al., 1997) | Satisfaction with health plan performance for groups of consumers (e.g., private insurance, Medicaid, Medicare) | Global rating items: Health plan, quality of care, personal doctor, specialist<br><br>Multi-item scales: Getting care you need, getting care without long wait, communication, enough time spent, office staff, customer service, reasonable paper work<br><br>Single-item scales: Prevention, finding personal doctor, referral to specialists | Item number: 28<br>Item type: 11 point, "worst health care possible" to "best health care possible"; 4 point "never" to "always"; and 2 point, "yes" or "no"<br><br>Administration: Mail self-administration or telephone | Medicaid: $\alpha$ = 0.48–0.79 for subscales<br><br>Private insurance: $\alpha$ = 0.48–0.88 for subscales | Predictive validity established<br><br>Discriminant validity questioned for some subscales due to high interscale correlations |
| Older Patient Satisfaction Survey (OPSS) (Cryns et al., 1989) | Patient satisfaction among older health maintenance organization (HMO) members | Undifferentiated positive regard for health care providers, complaints about waiting time, concern about quality of care, appreciation of financial arrangements at HMO, appreciation of treating physician, ease of access, special care for serious problems, doctor informs about tests, Continuity of physician–provider relationship, good value for money, physician–provider access difficulties, HMO is for routine care, availability of regular provider, general appreciation of the HMO | Item number: 60<br>Item type: 5 point "strongly agree" to "strongly disagree"<br><br>Administration: Self-administered | $\alpha$ = 0.41–0.86 for subscales | Construct validity established using factor analysis |

ness coalitions to compare satisfaction across health plans and other employee health benefit options. The CSS relied heavily on the PSQ-III for items and on the advice and input of health plans and employers. A major change from the PSQ surveys, however, was the use of the "excellent" to "poor" response scale for all rating items. This was based on the earlier work by Ware and Hays (1988) suggesting that the "excellent" to "poor" scale had superior psychometric properties; this change would also allow comparison of ratings across different features of care (e.g., access vs. quality) and reduce the number of items needed. The second version of the CSS was released in 1991 (Davies & Ware, 1991). The satisfaction battery was expanded to add items rating certain features of the health plan in addition to the ratings of medical care and services found in the first version. These health plan–specific features include the range of services covered, availability of information, paperwork, and costs. The CSS has been extensively fielded by both mail and telephone procedures, and national norms for several items are available. As a result, it has essentially set the de facto standard for health plan satisfaction surveys.

The CSS contributed substantially to the Annual Member Health Care Survey (AMHCS) developed by the National Committee on Quality Assurance (NCQA) (Kippen, Strasser, & Joshi, 1997; National Committee for Quality Assurance, 1995). The AMHCS resulted from an effort by the NCQA to create a standardized consumer survey instrument for evaluating and comparing plan performance. Since its release in 1995, the AMHCS has been chosen for use in a large number of studies sponsored by health plans and employer groups, and the survey has been one of the most widely used instruments in the private sector (Allen & Rogers, 1996).

## Consumer Assessment of Health Plans Survey (CAHPS)

Consumer Assessment of Health Plans Survey (CAHPS) instruments have been developed in accordance with three national, 5 year, cooperative agreements with consortia headed by the RTI, RAND Corporation, and Harvard University and sponsored by the Agency for Health Care Policy and Research (AHCPR) (Table 9.2, Fig. 9.4) (Agency for Health Care Policy and Research, 1996; Consumer Assessment of Health Plans Survey, 1997). These surveys expand on earlier work from the Survey Design Project completed in 1995 for AHCPR (Lubalin et al., 1995). CAHPS instruments are being developed for a wide range of potential users, including adult and pediatric populations, Medicare and Medicaid beneficiaries, and persons with chronic conditions. CAHPS has also been included the Health Plan Employer Data Information Set.

CAHPS has several characteristics that distinguish it from previous surveys like the CSS (Agency for Health Care Policy and Research, 1996). It is specifically designed to provide information to consumers, rather than purchasers or health plans, and to focus on assessing health care experiences where consumers are the best or only source of information. As a result, developers relied far less on previous surveys like the CSS to identify items and domains of interest. Items were generated mainly through extensive cognitive testing and focus groups. Cognitive testing assesses potential survey items through feedback from interviews in which people are asked to react to the survey questions. These two approaches to item generation resulted in a substantially higher concentration of items on access, interpersonal skills, and communication issues and far fewer items on provider technical skills. CAHPS also de-emphasizes information that can be obtained through other sources such as claims data and assessments of plan features such as design and benefit provisions. It requires (through a skip pattern) that respondents have received care in the last 6 months in order to complete the sections on evaluation of care. Unlike the CSS, it frequently employs a "don't

*Single items*

0–10 scale, worst possible to best possible:
- Global rating of health plan
- Global rating of quality of care
- Global rating of personal doctor
- Global rating of specialists

*Composites*

Getting the care you need (4 items, never to always):
- How often did you have to see someone else when you wanted to see your personal doctor or nurse?
- How often did you see a specialist when you thought you needed one?
- How often did you get the medical help or advice you needed when you phoned the doctor's office or clinic during the day Monday to Friday?
- How often did you get the tests or treatment you thought you needed?

Getting care without long waits (4 items, never to always):
- How often did you get that help or advice during the day Monday to Friday without a long wait?
- When you tried to be seen for an illness or injury, how often did you see a doctor or other health professional as soon as you wanted?
- When you needed regular or routine health care, how often did you get an appointment as soon as you wanted?
- How often did you wait in the doctor's office or clinic more than 30 minutes past your appointment time to see the person you went to see?

Easy to find a personal doctor you are happy with (1 item, yes/no):
- With the choices your health insurance plan gives you, was it easy to find a personal doctor or nurse you are happy with?

Doctors who communicate well with their patients (4 items, never to always):
- How often did doctors or other health professionals listen carefully to you?
- How often did doctors or other health professionals explain things in a way you could understand?
- How often did doctors or other health professionals show respect for what you had to say?
- How often were you involved as much as you wanted in decisions about your health care?

Doctors who spend enough time with their patients and know their medical history (2 items, never to always):
- How often did doctors or other health professionals spend enough time with you?
- How often did doctors or other health professionals know what you thought they should know about your medical history?

Being encouraged to exercise or eat a healthy diet (1 adult item, yes/no):
- Has a health insurance professional or your health insurance plan encouraged you to exercise or eat a healthy diet?

Courtesy, respect, and helpfulness of medical office staff (2 items, never to always):
- How often did office staff at a doctor's office or clinic treat you with courtesy and respect?
- How often were office staff at a doctor's office or clinic as helpful as you thought they should be?

Health plan's customer service: efficiency and helpfulness (3 items, never to always):
- How often were your calls to the health insurance plan's customer service taken care of without a long wait?
- How often did you get all the information or other help you needed when you called the health insurance plan's customer service?
- How often were the people at the health insurance plan's customer service as helpful as you thought they should be?

Reasonable paperwork, handling of approvals and payments (2 items, never to always):
- How often did you have more forms to fill out than you thought was reasonable?
- How often did your health insurance plan deal with approvals or payments without taking a lot of your time and energy?

Easy to get referrals to specialists (1 item, yes/no):
- Was it always easy to get a referral when you needed one?

**Figure 9.4.** Consumer Assessment of Health Plans Survey (CAHPS) items. Source: Adapted from Hays (1997).

know" or "does not apply" option. Finally, because of the focus on the consumer perspective, differences in the wording of the questions will make future comparisons with the CSS and other instruments more difficult.

## Older Patient Satisfaction Survey (OPSS)

The Older Patient Satisfaction Survey (OPSS) was designed to measure patient satisfaction among older (65 years and over) subscribers to health maintenance organizations (HMOs) (Table 9.2, Fig. 9.5) (Cryns et al., 1989). Survey items were constructed from discussions with four focus groups of elderly HMO enrollees. The substantive content of these interviews was systematically analyzed, and 60 attitudinal statements were created with the same proportion of ideas in the statements as the number of transcribed lines from the discussion devoted to each idea. The resulting survey was mailed to 229 elderly HMO enrollees. Factor analysis of the results identified 14 primary dimensions of satisfaction. Two additional scales were identified that represented general positive attitude (5 items) and general negative attitude (7 items). An overall global satisfaction scale was also generated.

The OPSS has advantages for surveying older populations. Seven of the OPSS primary factors did not correlate with other satisfaction surveys, indicating that previous surveys may miss some important dimensions of satisfaction. These included three factors pertaining specifically to HMOs and two factors that might represent specific concerns of geriatric patients (special care for serious problems and difficulty traveling for health care). The remaining two factors may represent neglected areas of measurement in other patient satisfaction surveys (waiting time and prompt feedback from tests).

## Picker/Commonwealth Surveys of HMO Member Expectations and Satisfaction (PCHMO)

The Picker/Commonwealth Project for Patient Centered Care has developed two surveys that, when used together, attempt to bridge the gap between member expectations and experiences (Fig. 9.6) (McGee et al., 1997). The first is the HMO Member Expectations Survey, and a companion questionnaire is the Member Satisfaction Survey. Because data on the psychometric properties of these instruments are not available, they are excluded from Table 9.2. They are described here, however, because of the growing recognition that collecting data on consumer expectations is an important step in understanding the results of satisfaction surveys.

Item pools for both surveys were based on literature reviews and focus groups with HMO staff and members. The 42 item Expectations Survey asks members to think about what is important to them when arranging health care for themselves or their family. Expectations about the following topics are included: access to care; convenience, quality, and cost of care; technical skills and thoroughness of providers; interpersonal manner of providers and staff; and continuity of care. Most questions use a five-point response scale from "a little important" to "essential." The 82 item Satisfaction Survey uses factual reports and rating scales to ask HMO members about the care they have received. There is one version for staff model HMOs and another version for independent practice association model HMOs. Topics include appointment scheduling, examinations and treatment, prescriptions, laboratory tests, telephone help referrals, and responsiveness to members' concerns. The survey uses a variety of response scales, including yes/no; "yes, very" to "no, not at all"; and options based on frequency (e.g., "within the past 3 months").

## Hospital Satisfaction Surveys

Satisfaction with inpatient care represents another area in which several widely used surveys are available. We discuss two general surveys of hospital services, one additional survey that focuses specifically on

**Undifferentiated Positive Regard for Health Care Providers**
Doctors are honest; they tell you both the good and the bad about your health condition.
Everyone of the medical staff—doctors and nurses alike—give you really good care.
Most doctors make you really feel good.
I do not find it hard to get through to my doctor on the phone.
The eye examinations are really good.
Practically without exception, the medical staff is very helpful.
The medical staff always gives you an explanation of what is going on in your body.

**Complaints about Waiting Time**
You sometimes have to wait a long time before the doctor sees you.
I have to wait a long time before the doctor sees me.
I think the doctor has too many patients scheduled at the same time.
According to my experience, you only have to wait a few minutes when you have a doctor's appointment.

**Concern about Quality of Care**
Despite the care I get, my problems or symptoms tend to persist.
There should be a greater choice of hospitals for us.
Sometimes I worry that I cannot get the right kind of care exactly when I need it.
The doctors here seem so young compared with those you see elsewhere.

**Appreciation of Financial Arrangements at HMO**
When you are really sick, all bills are automatically taken care of.
Al hospital costs are automatically being paid for you.

**Appreciation of the Treating Physician**
The doctors I get treated by impress me as being competent.
I like my doctor.
All I can say is that I am satisfied with the health care services I receive.

**Ease of Access**
When I have a problem needing attention, I can get an appointment to be seen right away.

**Special Care for Serious Problems**
I like the hospitals I am being sent to when I require hospitalization.

**Doctor Informs about Tests**
Although he does not have to do it, my doctor tends to call me to give the results of my tests.
Although they promise to do so, some doctors do not call you to give the results of your tests.

**Continuity of Physician-Provider Relationship**
I have one complaint: they change doctors on you too often here.

**Good Value for Money**
Whatever you may say, other insurance plans cost more.
Our health insurance plans cover more services than other plans.
The medicines I get from the pharmacy are making me feel better.
I am too old to do all the driving to different doctors' offices, so I prefer a group health care plan such as this one.

**Physician-Provider Access Difficulties**
It is often a real problem to be referred to a specialist who practices in a hospital.

**HMO is for Routine Care**
The physical check-ups you get should really be given by your regular doctor.
The health care classes we get are really informative.

**Availability of Regular Provider**
You have to wait a long time for your appointments.
If you have to go in for an urgent visit, you'll never know who is going to attend to you.

**General Appreciation of the HMO**
I get better care now than I did with my old doctor.
The medical care I am receiving now is better than I got elsewhere.
I like the emphasis they place here on prevention and maintenance.

**Figure 9.5.** Older Patient Satisfaction Survey (OPSS) items. Source: Adapted from Cyrns (1989).

*Picker Commonwealth Survey of HMO Member Expectations*

**How important is it to you to. . . .**
Get answers to the questions you ask, in words you understand?
Pay no more than a few dollars out of your own pocket for care of a new problem?
Have the provider greet you in a friendly way?
Be able to choose which hospital you go to for a planned admission?
Pay no more than a few dollars out of your own pocket for laboratory tests?
Have the provider tell you what to do is certain problems or symptoms occur?
Not be interrupted by the provider?
Pay no more than a few dollars out of your own pocket to see a specialist?
Have the reception and nursing staff treat you warmly?
See your regular provider, rather than someone else, for care of a new problem?
Feel confident that the provider has the technical skills to provide high quality medical care?
See your regular provider, rather than someone else, for a routine check-up or physical exam?
Have an emergency or severe problem taken care of where you usually go for medical care without having to go to
    a hospital?
Know that you can count on skilled treatment in an emergency?
Speak with your regular provider, rather than someone else, when you call with a medical problem?
See a doctor, rather than a nurse practitioner or a physician's assistant, for a routine check-up or physical exam?
Not feel embarrassed during your examination?
Keep the cost of health insurance premiums that you pay low compared to your other health plan choices?
Get a thorough examination for the problem you came in for?
Pay no more than a few dollars out of your own pocket for a hospitalization?
See doctor at each routine visit for an ongoing problem (like diabetes), rather than a nurse practitioner or
    physician's assistant?
Pay no more than a few dollars out of your own pocket for prescriptions?
Get information from the provider about what you can expect with your medical problem in the future?
Get your test results explained, in words you understand?
Get solid facts about the benefits and risks of treatment?
See a doctor for care of a new problem, rather than a nurse practitioner or physician's assistant?
Be placed in an exam room within a reasonable amount of time after your appointment time?

*Picker Commonwealth HealthCarePlan Member Satisfaction Survey*

**Access to Your Provider**
In general, if you need to see your provider for a current problem, how long do you usually have to wait for an
    appointment?
In general, if you need to see your provider for a routine checkup, how long do you usually have to wait for an
    appointment?
How did you make the appointment for your most recent visit?
How long did it take for reception to give you an appointment for your most recent visit?
How many days before your scheduled appointment did you make the appointment for your most recent visit?
What prompted you to make the appointment for your last visit?
When was this appointment?
Was the time of this appointment convenient?
Did the nursing and reception staff treat you warmly on your most recent visit?
De you feel the reception and nursing staff took your concerns seriously?
About how long after your appointment time did you wait before you were placed in an examination room?
About how long after you were placed in an examination room did it take before your provider came to see you?
While you were in the examination room did a staff person keep you informed if the provider was running late?

**The Provider You Saw At Your Most Recent Visit**
What kind of provider did you see at your most recent visit? (If you saw more than one provider, who was your
    appointment with?)
Did your provider address you in a friendly way?
Do you feel your provider seemed familiar with your recent medical history?

*(continued)*

**Figure 9.6.** Picker/Commonwealth survey of HMO members (PCHMO) items. Source: Adapted from
McGee (1997).

Did your provider seem to ask the right questions?

Do you feel your provider took your concerns seriously?

Do you feel your provider genuinely cared about your situation?

Do you feel your provider understood the problems affecting your health?

Did you feel comfortable enough to ask your provider questions?

Did your provider explain what he or she was going to do during your examination?

Considering the reason you came to see your provider, do you feel your examination was thorough?

Did your provider explain what you can expect with this medical problem in the future?

Was this visit long enough to talk about your concerns and ask questions?

About how long did your provider spend in the examination room with you?

How much did your provider involve you in making decisions about your health care at your last visit?

How confident do you feel that your provider has the technical skills to provide you with high quality medical care?

Please grade your primary care provider on the following aspects of care:

How would you grade the ability of your provider to explain treatment, tests, and health problems to you?

> How would you grade the medical care your provider offers?
> How would you grade your provider's medical skill and knowledge?
> How would you grade your provider's "bedside manner"?
> Overall, how would you grade your provider?

### Prescriptions

When was the last time a HealthCarePlan provider prescribed medication for you?

Was this for a new prescription?

Please grade the pharmacy on the following aspects of care:

> How would you grade the pharmacy cashier's courtesy?
> How would you grade the pharmacist's courtesy?
> How would you grade the ability of the pharmacist to explain the dosage, scheduling, and side effects?
> Overall, how would you grade your experience filling your prescription(s)?

About how long did it take between the time you handed the pharmacy your prescription and the time you picked up your medication?

Did you know that you can purchase over-the-counter medications from the HealthCarePlan pharmacies at a discount?

### Laboratory Tests

When was the last time a HealthCarePlan provider ordered any laboratory tests for you?

About how long did it take for you to get the results of your tests back?

Was this wait acceptable to you?

How did you get the results of your tests?

How would you prefer to get the results of your laboratory tests?

### Telephone Help For Health Problems

When was the last time you called your provider to get help for your health problem over the telephone?

About how long did it take between the time you first called and the time you spoke to somebody about your problem?

Was this wait acceptable to you?

Who helped you with your medical problem when you called?

Were you confident that the person you spoke to about your problem had the technical skills to decide what you needed?

Do you feel the person you spoke to took your concerns seriously?

What was the outcome of this phone call for your health problem?

### Referrals

During the past year, did you have an appointment with a specialist?

How long a wait was it from when the referral was made and you were actually seen by the specialist?

How confident do you feel that the specialist had the technical skills to provide you with high quality medical care?

Do you feel that your care was well coordinated between your provider and the specialist?

### Prevention

How much influence do you feel that preventive care has on your health?

Overall, how attentive is HealthCarePlan in assisting you with preventive care?

*(continued)*

**Figure 9.6.** Picker/Commonwealth survey of HMO members (PCHMO) items. — Continued

Did your provider give you advice about ways to improve your health (for example, about diet, exercise, smoking, drugs, alcohol, or stress)?

During the past year, did you receive a reminder to have a periodic checkup, screening test, or other preventive care (such as a flu vaccination, mammography, pap smear, asthma check, or cholesterol check)?

Did the reminder you received lead you to obtain preventive services?

During the past year, did you have a periodic checkup, screening test, or other preventive care (such as a flu vaccination, mammography, pap smear, asthma check, or cholesterol check)?

**Member Services**

Do you understand your covered benefits and services?

How much input do you feel you have in choosing a regular primary provider?

How many times have you contacted the HealthCarePlan Member Services in the past 6 months?

With your most recent contact in mind, why did you contact HealthCarePlan Member Services?

Were you confident that the Member Services representative was knowledgeable and had the skills to solve your problem?

Did the HealthCarePlan Member Services representative behave in a professional manner?

With your most recent contact in mind, how many times did you speak with Member Services regarding the same question or concern?

During the past year, did you have any complaints about the medical care or the services you received through HealthCarePlan?

Was your complaint handled quickly?

Was your complaint handled fairly?

Which of the following statements explains why you didn't report your complaints about your medical care or service?

Overall, how would you grade your experience with the HealthCarePlan Member Services Department?

**Agree or Disagree**

Joining HealthCarePlan was a good decision

I would suggest joining HealthCarePlan to my family and friends

I am satisfied with the medical care I receive

I am satisfied with HealthCarePlan

I intend to leave HealthCarePlan at the next opportunity

My health is excellent

I expect my health to improve

**Figure 9.6.** — Continued

hospital nursing services, and another survey that examines patient reports of specific problems with hospital care.

### Patient Judgments of Hospital Quality (PJHQ)

The Patient Judgments of Hospital Quality (PJHQ) measures patients' judgments of the key attributes of hospital quality and does not focus exclusively on the measurement of satisfaction (Table 9.3, Fig. 9.7; Nelson et al., 1989). Its development has been described at length in an eight-article supplement to the journal *Medical Care* (Meterko et al., 1990). The survey items were constructed from literature reviews, preexisting questionnaires, focus groups with patients, and interviews with hospital administrators, physicians, and nurses. The original 1000 item pool was reduced to 106 items. Forty-six of these items were considered key evaluations of eight hypothesized aspects of hospital care. Most items used a five-point "poor" to "excellent" scale. Factor analysis of the first pilot test suggested six dimensions of hospital quality, along with one large general factor. The dimensions supported a conceptual framework based on staff and service categories (e.g., admissions, nursing and daily care, medical care, hospital environment, discharge). A short-form version of the questionnaire with 69 items was also developed (Hays et al., 1991).

The PJHQ system has been used extensively in non-poor populations with adult patients and the parents of pediatric pa-

**Table 9.3.**
Hospital Satisfaction Surveys

| Survey | Description | Dimensions | Data collection | Reliability | Validity |
|---|---|---|---|---|---|
| Patient Judgments on Hospital Quality (PJHQ) (Meterko et al., 1990) | Patient's perceptions of the quality of hospital care and services | Admissions, nursing and daily care, medical care, hospital environment, information, discharge | Item number: 46<br><br>Item type: 5 point "excellent" to "poor"<br><br>Administration: Mail or telephone survey | α = 0.87–0.95 for subscales | Content validity claimed. Construct validity established using factor analysis and correlations. Convergent validity established using multitrait multimethod analysis. Discriminant and predictive validity established |
| Hospital Quality of Care Monitor (HQCM) (Carey & Seibert, 1993) | Perceptions of the quality of hospital services for inpatients and outpatients (emergency room and ambulatory surgery patients) | Inpatient QCM: Courtesy, nursing care, food service, comfort and cleanliness, physician care, admission and billing, religious care, Medical outcome<br><br>Outpatient QCM: Physician care, nursing care, medical outcome, facility characteristics, waiting time, testing services, registration process | Item number: 44 (inpatient) or 32 (outpatient)<br><br>Item type: Not reported<br><br>Administration: Mailed survey | α = 0.44–0.92 for subscales (inpatient) and 0.52–0.95 (outpatient) | Construct validity established using factor analysis. High degree of scale independence. Predictive validity established using regression |
| LaMonica-Oberst Patient Satisfaction Scale (LOPSS) (LaMonica et al., 1986) | Satisfaction with nursing care for hospitalized cancer patients | Dissatisfaction, interpersonal support, good impression | Item number: 42<br><br>Item type: 7 point "strongly agree" to "strongly disagree"<br><br>Administration: Self-administered | α = 0.95 overall, 0.84–0.90 for subscales | Content validity claimed. Construct validity established using factor analysis. Moderate discriminant validity |

**Admission: Entering the Hospital**

PREPARATION FOR ADMISSION: How clear and complete the information was about how to prepare for your stay in the hospital and what to expect once you got there

EFFICIENCY OF THE ADMITTING PROCEDURE: Ease of getting admitted, including the amount of time it took

HELPFULNESS AND CONCERN OF THE ADMITTING STAFF: Their courtesy and concern for your comfort and feelings

ATTENTION OF ADMITTING STAFF TO YOUR INDIVIDUAL NEEDS: Their flexibility in handling your personal needs and wants

**Your Care in the Hospital**

MEDICAL FACILITIES: How complete and up-to-date the medical equipment was

OVERALL EFFICIENCY OF HOSPITLAL: How smoothly things ran

RECOGNITION OF YOUR OPINIONS: Asking you what you think is important and giving you choices

CONSIDERATION OF YOUR NEEDS: Willingness to be flexible in meeting your needs

INFORMATION YOU WERE GIVEN: How clear and complete were the explanations about tests, treatments, and what to expect

INSTRUCTIONS: How well doctors, nurses, and other staff explained how to prepare for tests and operations

COORDINATION OF CARE: The teamwork of all the hospital staff who took care of you

THE DAILY ROUTINE OF THE DOCTORS, NURSES, AND HOSPITAL STAFF: How well they adjusted their schedules to your needs

INFORMING FAMILY OR FRIENDS: How well they were kept informed about your condition and needs

INVOLVING FAMILY OR FRIENDS IN YOUR CARE: How much they were allowed to help in your care

EASE OF GETTING INFORMATION: Willingness of hospital staff to answer your questions

SPECIALISTS AND SPECIAL THERAPY: Availability of getting the specialized tests, medicines, or treatments you needed

HELPFULNESS: Ability of hospital staff to make you comfortable and reassure you

SAFETY AND SECURITY: The provisions for your safety and the security of your belonging

**Your Nurses**

SKILL AND COMPETENCE OF NURSES: How well things were done, like giving medicine and handling IVs

ATTENTION OF NURSES TO YOUR CONDITION: How often nurses checked on you and how well they kept track of how you were doing

NURSING STAFF RESPONSE TO YOUR CALLS: How quick they were to help

CONCERN AND CARING BY NURSES: Courtesy and respect you were given; friendliness and kindness

INFORMATION GIVEN BY NURSES: How well nurses communicated with patients, families, and doctors

**Your Doctor**

ATTENTION OF DOCTOR TO YOUR CONDITION: How often doctors checked on you and how well they kept track of how you were doing

AVAILABILITY OF DOCTOR: How easy it was to get your doctor when needed

CONCERN AND CARING BY DOCTOR: Courtesy and respect you were given; friendliness and kindness

SKILL OF DOCTORS: Ability to diagnose problems, thoroughness of examinations, skill in treating your condition, and scientific knowledge

RESPECT FOR YOU: How well the doctor listened to what you had to say, how well the doctor understood what you thought was important

**Other Hospital Staff**

HOUSEKEEPING STAFF: How well they did their job and how they acted towards you

LABORATORY WORKERS: How well they and their jobs and how they acted towards you

X-RAY STAFF: How well they did their jobs and how they acted towards you

**Living Arrangements**

CONDITION OF YOUR ROOM: Cleanliness, comfort, lighting, and temperature

SUPPLIES AND FURNISHINGS: Completeness of supplies, condition of the furniture, and how well things worked

*(continued)*

**Figure 9.7.** Patient Judgments of Hospital Quality (PJHQ) items. Source: Adapted from Meterko (1990).

RESTFUL ATMOSPHERE: Amount of peace and quiet
PRIVACY: Provisions for your privacy
QUALITY OF FOOD: Overall, how well it tasted, serving temperature, and variety available
HOSPITAL ENVIRONMENT: Other than your room, how comfortable, quiet, and pleasant it was
SIGNS AND DIRECTIONS: Ease of finding your way around the hospital
HOSPITAL BUILDING: How you would rate the hospital building overall
PARKING: Number of spaces available, convenience of location, and cost
PROVISIONS FOR FAMILY AND FRIENDS: Adequacy of visiting hours and facilities for them; visitors
   treated like welcome guests

**Discharge: Leaving the hospital**
DISCHARGE PROCEDURES: Time it took to be discharged from the hospital and how efficiently it was
   handled
DISCHARGE INSTRUCTION: How clearly and completely you were told what to do and what to expect
   when you left the hospital
COORDINATION OF CARE AFTER DISCHARGE: Hospital staff's efforts to provide for your needs after you left the hospital

**Billing by hospital**
EXPLANATIONS ABOUT COSTS AND HOW TO HANDLE YOUR HOSPITAL BILLS: The complete-
   ness and accuracy of information and the willingness of hospital staff to answer your questions about
   finances
EFFICIENCY OF BILLING: How fast you got your bill, how accurate and understandable it was

**Looking back on your care**
Overall quality of care and services you received
How good a job the hospital did in meeting your expectations for your stay
Amount of information you were given about your illness and treatment
Teamwork among doctors who cared for you
Competence and skill of the nurses
Courtesy and friendliness of the nurses
The outcome of your hospital stay: How much you were helped by the hospitalization

**Figure 9.7.** Patient Judgments of Hospital Quality (PJHQ) items. Source: Adapted from Meterko
(1990)–Continued

tients (McGee et al., 1997). There is less information about its use with inpatients who have psychiatric or organic brain syndrome diagnoses or in poor populations.

### Hospital Quality of Care Monitor (HQCM)

The Hospital Quality of Case Monitor (HQCM) was designed specifically to measure the results of quality improvement efforts (see Table 9.3) (Carey & Seibert, 1993). Unlike the PJHQ system, the HQCM does not focus exclusively on acute care hospital inpatients, but developed two additional questionnaires for hospital outpatient populations (emergency room and ambulatory surgery). These three questionnaires were revised over a 7 year period based on patient focus groups and feedback from partici-

pating hospitals. Additional items were incorporated to supplement traditional questions covering hospital services, including items on perceived outcome, guest relations, and religious care.

The scales of the HQCM are more independent than those of the PJHQ, and the authors argue that the items comprising the scales are easier to interpret. This may make the HQCM more useful for quality improvement efforts. The overall response rates for each of the three surveys ranged from 33% to 54%, however, which may limit the generalizability of the results.

### LaMonica-Oberst Patient Satisfaction Scale (LOPSS)

In 1986, LaMonica and coworkers adapted Risser's PSS to examine cancer patients' satisfaction with nurses and nursing care in a hospital setting (see Table 9.3). The items were revised to incorporate nursing behaviors expected in the acute care setting, particularly for issues dealing with physical care and comfort measures. Factor analysis failed to confirm the subscales initially conceptualized by Risser (1975), but three other factors were identified: dissatisfaction, interpersonal support, and good impression. The reliabilities of these new subscales were higher than the reliabilities of the original subscales.

One of the goals in developing the LaMonica-Oberst Patient Satisfaction Scale (LOPSS) was to develop a more sensitive measure of patient satisfaction. Comparison of the LOPSS with the PSS suggests that the LOPSS was not substantially more sensitive. A possible advantage of the measure, however, lies in the general nature of the items. Because the LOPSS does not contain items specifically related to cancer, it may be valid for other hospitalized patients with life-threatening illnesses. Additional research must be undertaken to assess this potential generalizability.

### Picker/Commonwealth Hospital Satisfaction Survey (PCHSS)

The Picker/Commonwealth Hospital Satisfaction Survey (PCHSS) was designed to focus on specific actions taken by hospital staff as opposed to rating general aspects of care (Fig. 9.8) (Cleary et al., 1991; Delbanco et al., 1995). Because no information was available on the psychometric properties of the survey, it is not included in Table 9.3. The survey focused on events in several clinical areas where patients were thought to be the best judges of quality: communication, financial information, patients' needs and preferences, emotional support, physical comfort, pain management, education, family participation, and discharge preparation/continuity of care. Items were developed based on interviews with patients, their families and friends, and health care providers. Most responses were coded as yes/no, with additional follow-up questions if more information was required. Summary scores were created for each clinical area by calculating the percentage of items that had responses indicating a problem.

One of the advantages of the PCHSS is the precise nature of the items. Patient reports that identify specific problems with their care may be more useful for quality improvement efforts. The survey has limitations, however, including a poor response rate, which may compromise the generalizability of the results.

### Long-Term Care Satisfaction Surveys

There are no widely used instruments with proven reliability and validity that measure consumer satisfaction for the institutionalized elderly. The surveys described here represent some initial efforts to develop instruments for use in these settings.

### Long-Term Care Satisfaction Survey (LTCSS)

The Long-Term Care Satisfaction Survey (LTCSS) was developed to guide quality improvement efforts, and measure global performance, and monitor organizational change (Table 9.4) (Norton et al., 1996). Parallel resident and family questionnaires were constructed. An initial pool of 100 items in seven domains was developed based on literature reviews, qualitative data sets of interviews with long-term care residents (including interviews with cognitively impaired residents), and focus groups. The questionnaire was shortened to 60 items by removing redundant topics. Several response options were tested in pilot interviews, and the final version utilized a three-point scale of "yes," "sometimes," and "no" with Chernoff faces* to assist in interpretation.

The LTCSS has both advantages and disadvantages. It was specifically developed to include cognitively impaired residents among survey respondents. Although the response rate for the

---

* Chernoff faces are simple diagrams that indicate smiling or frowning to reflect positive or negative feelings.

### Communication
Not told about daily routine
Not told whom to ask for help, if needed
No doctor in charge of care or doctor in charge not available to answer questions
Doctor or nurse did not explain, before a test, how much pain or discomfort to expect
Not told before or shortly after admission things patient should have been told
Did not get understandable answers from nurses in response to important questions
Did not get understandable answers from doctors in response to important questions
Not given enough privacy while receiving important information about condition
Information about condition given in a way that upsets patient

### Financial Information
Not knowing how much would have to be paid worried patient
Needed help figuring out how to pay hospital bills and did not get it

### Patients Needs and Preferences
Hospital staff did not go out of their way to meet patient's needs
Something was not done that patients thought should have been done
Not involved in decisions about care as much as patient wanted
Did not have enough say about medical treatment
Thought hospital staff put own needs first
Something done to patients in hospital that he or she thought should not have been done
Doctors sometimes talked in front of patients as if he or she weren't there
Religious practices or preferences not respected
Not given enough privacy while being examined

### Emotional Support
Did not have relationship of trust with any hospital staff other than doctor in charge of care
No one at hospital went out of way to make patient feel better
Difficult to find someone on staff to talk to about personal concerns
Did not have relationship of confidence or trust with doctor in charge of treatment at hospital

### Physical Comfort
Nurses were overworked and too busy to take care of patient
Awakened for no reason by hospital staff
Needed, but did not get, help going to bathroom in time
Needed, but did not get, help bathing
On average, waited more than 15 minutes for help after pushing call button

### Pain Management
Had moderate or severe pain that could have been eliminated by prompt attention by hospital staff
Pain experienced in hospital greater that patient was told to expect
Waited, on average, more than 15 minutes fore pain medicine
Received too little pain medicine

### Education
Important side effects of medicines not explained in a way patient could understand
Test results not explained in a way patient could understand
Why important tests were being done not explained in a way patient could understand
Purposes of medicines patient was getting in hospital not explained in a way patient could understand

### Family Participation
Family or care partner not given all information needed to help patient recover at home
Family given too little information about care

### Discharge Preparation/Continuity of Care
Not told which foods patients should or should not eat
Not told about important side effects of medicines
Not told what danger signals to watch for at home

*(continued)*

**Figure 9.8.** Picker/Commonwealth Hospital Satisfaction Survey (PCHSS). Source: Adapted from Cleary (1991).

Not told when patient could resume normal activities
Not told what activities patient should or should not do
Not told what to do to help recover
Not told when patient could go back to work
No hospital staff tried to help patient with worries about returning home
Hospital did not assist patient prior to discharge in finding help needed after leaving hospital
Purposes of discharge medicines not explained in a way patients could understand
Not told when and how to take medications at home

**Figure 9.8.** — Continued

cognitively impaired patients was low (28%), the authors concluded that these patients were able to give meaningful answers. On the other hand, the reliabilities for some of the scales were poor, and no tests of validity were reported. Future work on the reliability and validity of this instrument should help address its suitability for broader use.

### Nursing Home Resident Satisfaction Scale (NHRSS)

The Nursing Home Resident Satisfaction Scale (NHRSS) was designed to be easily administered to nursing home residents for use as an indicator of nursing home quality and to provide feedback to nursing home administrators (Table 9.4, Fig. 9.9) (Zinn et al., 1993). Twenty-six items were initially selected based on a review of the literature. A pilot study suggested that the ability of the residents to make meaningful distinctions deteriorated over the length of the interview. Consequently, the number of items was reduced to 10, with eliminated items being either redundant or deemed less critical to the assessment of satisfaction. Pilot study participants also gave more detailed responses when first asked a question with a yes/no response. This yes/no question was followed with an item asking the participant to rate the services on a four-point scale from "very good" to "not so good."

The NHRSS has several advantages. It is short, easy to administer, and was not compromised by mild levels of cognitive impairment among respondents. The survey was, however, administered only to residents who comprehended English and had a family member who could also participate. This potential bias may affect the generalizability of the survey to other populations. A small sample size also limited the ability to test the sensitivity of the instrument to detect differences among facilities. Additional research is necessary to establish instrument validity.

### Nursing Home Customer Satisfaction Survey (NHCSS)

The NHCSS was designed to provide ongoing feedback to nursing home administrators about the satisfaction of nursing home residents or their surrogates (family members, appointed custodians, or concerned friends; see Table 9.4) (Kleinsorge & Koenig, 1991). This instrument was adapted from the SERVQUAL tool developed to measure quality in service industries (Parasuraman et al., 1988). Items were developed from focus groups with nursing home residents and their surrogates. Focus-group discussions were directed using the service quality dimensions identified by the SERVQUAL, as well as dimensions identified by the states in their annual inspection of nursing homes. These discussions were used to develop a 32 item survey with six hypothesized dimensions.

There are several issues to consider when using the NHCSS. The reliability of some of the scales needs to be improved, although the results provided some preliminary evidence of validity. The response rate for the survey was not reported but appeared to be low. Complete control of the survey process was also maintained by the participating nursing home administrators. As a result, no information was avail-

**Table 9.4.**
Long-Term Care Satisfaction Surveys

| Survey | Description | Dimensions | Data collection | Reliability | Validity |
|---|---|---|---|---|---|
| Long-Term Care Satisfaction Survey (LTCSS) (Norton et al., 1996) | Patient and family satisfaction with long-term care | Autonomy, living area, laundry, food, activity, staff, dignity, global satisfaction | Item number: 65<br><br>Item type: 3 point, "yes," "sometimes," "no"; and 5 point, "excellent" to "terrible"<br><br>Administration: In-person interview (patient) or mailed questionnaire (family) | $\alpha = 0.39-0.81$ for subscales | Not reported |
| Nursing Home Resident Satisfaction Scale (NHRSS) (Zinn et al., 1993) | Nursing home residents' satisfaction with care | Physician services, nursing services, environment, global satisfaction | Item number: 10<br><br>Item type: 4 point "very good" to "not so good"<br><br>Administration: In-person interview | $\alpha = 0.69-0.74$ for subscales<br><br>Test–retest and inter-rater reliability: Pearson product moment correlations = 0.64–0.79 for subscales | Not reported |
| Nursing Home Customer Satisfaction Scale (NHCSS) (Kleinsorge & Koenig, 1991) | Customer satisfaction in nursing homes for residents and surrogates | Nurse/aide, administration, staff empathy, food, housekeeping, home issues | Item number: 32 (resident), 36 (surrogates)<br><br>Item type: 5 point "strongly agree" to "strongly disagree"<br><br>Administration: Self-administered (resident) or mailed (surrogates) | $\alpha = 0.51-0.73$ for subscales (resident) | Convergent, discriminant, and nomologic validity established for several subscales using correlations (resident survey only) |

**Physician Services**
Do the doctors treat you well? (yes/no)
  How well do they treat you?
Do the doctors come quickly when you ask to see them? (yes/no)
  How would you rate the time it takes to come to see you?
Do you have confidence in the doctors' abilities? (yes/no)
  How would you rate your confidence?

**Nursing Services**
Do the nurses treat you well? (yes/no)
  How well do they treat you?
Do the nurses come quickly when you call them? (yes/no)
  How would you rate the time it takes to come to you?
Do you have confidence in the nurses' abilities? (yes/no)
  How would you rate your confidence?

**Other Services**
  Do you enjoy mealtime (presentation, service, choices, taste)? (yes/no)
  How would you rate mealtime?
Do you like your room (cleanliness, roommate, space, temperature)? (yes/no)
  How would you rate your room?
Do you get enough quiet and privacy? (yes/no)
  How would you rate the amount of quiet and privacy?
Do you like the daily schedule (visitation, mealtime, bedtime, wake-up time)? (yes/no)
  How would you rate the daily schedule?

**General Services**
Considering everything how would you rate your overall satisfaction (doctor, nursing care facilities, etc.)?

**Figure 9.9.** The Nursing Home Resident Satisfaction Scale (NHRSS). Source: Adapted from Zinn (1993).

able on how the pool of potential respondents was selected or whether any of the respondents was cognitively impaired. This implies that the generalizability of conclusions is extremely limited. Finally, the sample size for the surrogate survey was too small to analyze fully, and substantially more research is needed to define its potential use.

*American Health Care Association Satisfaction Assessment Questionnaires (SAQs)*

The American Health Care Association has developed measures of satisfaction with care for nursing home residents and family members based on six guiding principles identified as appropriate for the long-term care industry (Case, 1996). Separate Satisfaction Assessment Questionnaires (SAQs) have been developed for cognitively intact residents, rehabilitation residents, medically complex residents, family members of cognitively intact and mildly demented residents, and residents of assisted living facilities. Because there is no information on the psychometric properties of these tools, they are not included in Table 9.4. These questionnaires are lengthy (ranging from 87 to 113 items each) and cover a variety of domains. For example, the survey for cognitively intact residents examines overall satisfaction, family and community involvement, independence and respect, programs, facility setting, meals and dining, health care, doctor's care, staff, safety and security, roommates and other residents, and moving in or out. A 5 point "excellent" to "poor" rating scale is used, and the surveys are designed to be administered either in person or by telephone interview. A major caveat to the use of these tools is their lack of reliability and validity testing. The results of these surveys must be interpreted very cautiously until their reliability and validity are confirmed.

## Satisfaction Surveys for Other Care Settings

There are also no widely used reliable and valid satisfaction measures available for the growing number of other care settings (e.g., home care, hospice care, assisted living, adult day care). Characterization of existing measures is difficult for several reasons, including the broad array of potential issues (from satisfaction with terminal care to grocery services) and the lack of a widely accepted conceptual framework for examining satisfaction across a variety of health care settings. We describe several tools that have been developed to measure satisfaction with home care, adult day care, and assisted living services, although extensive work remains to be done in this area.

### Home Care Satisfaction Measure (HCSM)

The Home Care Satisfaction Measure (HCSM) was designed to assess the satisfaction of frail older adults with five common home care services: homemaker, home health aide, home-delivered meals, grocer, and case management services (Table 9.5, Fig. 9.10) (Geron, 1997). Focus groups were held with older adults who use home care services and included separate focus groups for several ethnic minorities: African-American, Hispanic, and non-Hispanic white (Jewish, Italian-American, and Irish-American). Item pools were developed from themes identified from the focus group discussions, preexisting satisfaction measures for acute care and other types of health care services, and by reviews of individual quotes from focus-group participants. The survey was refined based on two pretests.

The HCSM has several advantages. It directly incorporates the perspective of frail elderly service recipients, including ethnic minorities. Because it measures satisfaction with specific services (e.g., case

management, home health aide), it may provide useful guidance for quality improvement efforts. This measure is also based on a conceptual model of home care satisfaction that has identified different dimensions from models of satisfaction with acute medical care. However, all sampled participants received case management services, and subjects were excluded if their case manager indicated that the client could not complete a structured interview or had significantly impaired memory. As a result, the generalizability is limited, particularly for frail elders with more severe impairments (as evidenced by their inability to be interviewed). Finally, the reliabilities of some of the subscales were low, and results should be interpreted cautiously.

### Home Care and Terminal Care Satisfaction Scales (HCTC)

The Home Care and Terminal Care Satisfaction Scales were designed to measure satisfaction with care and preferences for the location and style of care for chronically and terminally ill patients and their families (see Table 9.5) (McCusker, 1984). Three instruments were developed, including a measure to evaluate home care for chronically and terminally ill homebound patients, a companion measure for the caretakers of these patients, and a post-bereavement version administered to caretakers after the death of the patient. Items were adapted from previous satisfaction measures of acute medical care, and new items were added as suggested by project investigators and staff. Pretesting was used to identify and delete items that were ambiguous, had low variability, or did not correlate with other items in the hypothesized direction.

A major advantage of these instruments is the characteristics of the samples: Each sample had significant experience with chronic or terminal illness. Several of the subscales did not perform well, however, and were not recommended for use. Thought should also be given to the timing

**Table 9.5. Satisfaction Surveys for Other Care Settings**

| Survey | Description | Dimensions | Data collection | Reliability | Validity |
|---|---|---|---|---|---|
| Home Care Satisfaction Measure (HCSM) (Geron, 1997) | Older adult satisfaction with five types of home care services: Homemaker, home health aide, case management, home-delivered meal, grocery | Homemaker and home health aide: Competency, system Adequacy, positive interpersonal, negative interpersonal<br><br>Case management: Competency, service choice, positive interpersonal, negative interpersonal<br><br>Home-delivered meal: Service quality, service adequacy, service Dependability<br><br>Grocery: Service quality, service adequacy, service convenience | Item number: 61 (homemaker, home health aide, and case management each have 13 items; home-delivered meal and grocery each have 11 items)<br><br>Item type: 5 point "yes, definitely" to "no, definitely not"<br><br>Administration: In-person interview | Homemaker: α = 0.46–0.87 for subscales<br><br>Home health aide: α = 0.26–0.83 for subscales<br><br>Case management: α = 0.54–0.88 for subscales<br><br>Home-delivered meal: α = 0.58–0.88 for subscales<br><br>Grocery: α = 0.49–0.79 for subscales | Construct validity established by factor analysis and Pearson correlations |
| Home Care and Terminal Care Satisfaction Scales (HCTC) (McCusker, 1984) | Patient and caretaker satisfaction with (1) home care for chronically and terminally ill homebound patients and (2) terminal care in last 6 months of life for cancer patients who died | General satisfaction, availability of care, continuity of care, physician availability, physician competence, personal qualities of physician, communication with physician, involvement of patient and family in treatment decisions, freedom from pain, pain control | Item number: 58 (home care) or 34 (terminal care)<br><br>Item type: 5 point "strongly agree" to "strongly disagree"<br><br>Administration: In-person interview (home care patient), self-administered (caretaker), or in-person interview with surviving relative (terminal care) | Home care: α = 0.10–0.75 for patient subscales; α = 0.50–0.85 for caretaker subscales<br><br>Terminal care: α = 0.59–0.90 for subscales | Face validity claimed. Convergent validity established for several subscales. Discriminant validity established for several subscales. Several subscales not recommended |
| Program of All-Inclusive Care for the Elderly Satisfaction Survey (PACE) (Kane & Atherly, 1996) | Patient and proxy satisfaction with services for frail older adults in adult day care | Patient survey: Access, concern, decision making<br><br>Proxy survey: Perceived technical quality, family pressure, ease of access, affective | Item number: 14 (patient) or 18 (proxy)<br><br>Item type: 5 point "strongly agree" to "strongly disagree"<br><br>Administration: In-person interview with patient or proxy | α = 0.54–0.88 for subscales | Construct validity established by factor analysis |

> I know I can contact my case manager if I need to
> My case manager ignores what I tell her about what things I need
> My case manager has become a friend
> I need more help from my case manager than I get
> My case manager is very knowledgeable about the services that are available
> I would like more choices about the types of services I get
> My case manager is kind to me
> My case manager has failed to get me the services I need
> On the whole, my case manager does a good job setting up care for me
> My case manager is rude to me
> My case manager does extra things for me
> I wish my case manager could do more things for me that I need to have done
> It would be a waste of time to call my case manager if I had a problem

**Figure 9.10.** Home Care Satisfaction Measure: Case Management Service (HCSM-CM13) items. Source: Adapted from Geron (1997).

of the interviews. The period of bereavement may be associated with substantial bias in perceptions of care received before death.

### Program of All-Inclusive Care for the Elderly (PACE) Satisfaction Survey

The Program of All-Inclusive Care for the Elderly (PACE) Satisfaction Survey was developed as part of an effort to design an ongoing quality assurance program for the PACE program (see Table 9.5) (Kane & Atherly, 1996). PACE is a program of capitated acute and long-term care for frail elderly (nursing home eligible) patients based mainly on adult day care services. Separate surveys were developed for patients and their proxies. The original patient survey contained 23 items believed to tap different dimensions of satisfaction, whereas the original proxy survey had 27 items. Items were excluded if they had high numbers of missing responses or did not load onto a single factor in the factor analysis. The final version of the patient survey has 14 items, whereas the proxy survey retains 18 items.

One advantage of the PACE survey is the incorporation of items specific to the adult day care setting. The analysis was complicated by high numbers of missing responses, however, which may limit validity. In addition, the originally hypothesized dimensions of satisfaction were not

completely confirmed by the factor analysis. Both of these issues suggest that the conceptualization of satisfaction with adult day care services could benefit from further development and testing.

### Oregon Assisted Living Project (OALP) Satisfaction Survey

At the University of Minnesota, a survey was developed to examine satisfaction with services for residents of assisted living facilities in Oregon. Because information on the reliability and validity of the instrument is not available, it is not included in Table 9.5. A distinctive feature of the Oregon Assisted Living Project is its separate measurement of the importance of the item to the resident and the resident's rating of the facility quality in that area.

## CONCLUSIONS AND FUTURE DIRECTIONS

There is currently an inadequate array of validated satisfaction measures for older adults, particularly for nonhospital and nonambulatory care settings. This lack of adequate tools limits our ability to draw conclusions from research on satisfaction and constrains efforts to use the results for practical purposes such as quality improvement. Future research needs to address the development of additional tools, as well as a variety of remaining issues such as the responsiveness of satisfaction measures, the relationship of importance and expectations to satisfaction, and the need to coordinate survey efforts.

Do we have the capacity to influence the results of satisfaction measures? If measures are not responsive to attempts to improve satisfaction ratings, they will be far less useful for tracking the results of quality improvement and marketing efforts. Examining responsiveness could take the form of experimental studies that manipulate variables to determine whether they have an influence on satisfaction or longitudinal studies that track changes in satisfaction over time.

The relationship of item importance and patient expectations to satisfaction measurement needs to be delineated. For example, a nursing home patient may be very satisfied with her nursing home's policy on plants, but if she does not rate plants as particularly important, the relative value of this item should presumably be downweighted. The relationship of expectations to satisfaction also requires further study, particularly for changing expectations over time. For example, nursing home residents may become habituated over time to a certain level of care. It is important to recognize that a high satisfaction rating may be a function of lowered expectations and that our current understanding of the relationship between expectations and satisfaction is relatively crude.

More attention in general needs to be devoted to testing whether the current measures of satisfaction with managed care work with older recipients who are enrolled in Medicare risk products. With Medicare's clear intention to make managed care more accessible to its beneficiaries, this examination is even more salient. In the context of long-term care, satisfaction needs to define who is the prime target. Because most of the marketing of long-term care products is directed toward family members, their satisfaction may be of greater interest to the mar-keters. On the other hand, if one is evaluating the effectiveness of long-term care, the recipients' satisfaction should be at least as important as that of their family members.

Finally, we also need to begin thinking about coordinating our efforts. Many health care institutions undertake some type of satisfaction survey, and patients who receive services in a variety of settings may be swamped. Coordinated efforts could have several benefits (besides reducing respondent burden), including the opportunity to link surveys over time and to use standardized instruments so that the results are comparable across institutions.

## REFERENCES

Abramowitz, S., Cote, A. A., & Berry, E. (1987). Analyzing patient satisfaction: a multianalytic approach. *Quality Review Bulletin, 13*(4), 122–130.

Agency for Health Care Policy and Research (1996). Technical Overview of Consumer Assessment of Health Plans (CAHPS) (AHCPR Pub. No. 97–R013). Rockville, MD: Public Health Service, Agency for Health Care Policy and Research.

Aharony, L., & Strasser, S. (1993). Patient satisfaction: What we know about and what we still need to explore. *Medical Care Review, 50*(1), 49–79.

Allen, H. M. Jr., & Rogers, W. H. (1996). Consumer surveys of health plan performance: A comparison of content and approach and a look to the future. *Joint Commission Journal on Quality Improvement, 22*(12), 775–794.

Allen, H. M., & Rogers, W. H. (1997). The Consumer Health Plan Value Survey: round two. *Health Affairs, 16*(4), 156–166.

Babakus, E., & Mangold, W. G. (1992). Adapting the SERVQUAL scale to hospital services: An empirical investigation. *Health Services Research, 26*(6), 767–786.

Ben-Sira, Z. (1976). The function of the professional's affective behavior in client satisfaction: A revised approach to social interaction theory. *Journal of Health and Social Behavior, 17*(1), 3–11.

Carey, R. G., & Seibert, J. H. (1993). A patient survey system to measure quality improvement: Questionnaire reliability and validity. *Medical Care, 31*(9), 834–845.

Carmel, S. (1985). Satisfaction with hospitalization: A comparative analysis of three types of services. *Social Science and Medicine, 21*(11), 1243–1249.

Casarreal, K. M., Mills, J. I., & Plant, M. A. (1986). Improving service through patient surveys in a multihospital organization. *Hospital and Health Services Administration, 31*(2), 41–52.

Case, T. (1996). A quality assessment and improvement system for long-term care. *Quality Management in Health Care, 4*(3), 15–21.

Cleary, P. D., Edgman-Levitan, S., Roberts, M., Moloney, T. W., McMullen, W., Walker, J. D., & Delbanco, T. L. (1991). Patients evaluate their hospital care: A national survey. *Health Affairs, 10*(4), 254–267.

Cleary, P. D., Keroy, L., Karpanos, G., & McMullen, W. (1983). Patient assessment of hospital care. *Quality Review Bulletin, 15*(5), 172–179.

Cleary, P. D., Lubalin, J., Hays, R. D., Short, P. F., Edgman-Levitan, S., & Sheridan, S. (1997). Debating survey approaches. *Health Affairs, 17*(1), 265–266.

Cleary, P. D., & McNeil, B. J. (1988). Patient satisfaction as an indicator of quality care. *Inquiry, 25*(1), 25–36.

Consumer Assessment of Health Plans Survey (1997). CAHPS 1.0 Survey and Reporting Kit (AHCPR Publication No. 97–0063). Washington, DC: U.S. Department of Health and Human Services, Public Health Service, Agency for Health Care Policy and Research.

Cryns, A. G., Nichols, R. C., Katz, L. A., & Calkins, E. (1989). The hierarchical structure of geriatric patient satisfaction. An Older Patient Satisfaction Scale designed for HMOs. *Medical Care, 27*(8), 802–816.

Daly, R., & Flynn, R. J. (1985). A brief consumer satisfaction scale for use in inpatient rehabilitation programs. *International Journal of Rehabilitation Research, 8*(1985), 335–338.

Davies, A. R., & Ware, J. E., Jr. (1988). Involving consumers in quality of care assessment. *Health Affairs, 7*(1), 33–48.

Davies, A. R., & Ware, J. E. (1991). *GHAA's consumer satisfaction survey and user's manual* (2nd ed.). Washington, DC: Group Health Association of America.

Deber, R. B. (1994). Physicians in health care management: 7. The patient–physician partnership: Changing roles and the desire for information. *Canadian Medical Association Journal, 151*(2), 171–176.

de Haan, R., Aaronson, N., Limburg, M., Hewer, R. L., & van Crevel, H. (1993). Measuring quality of life in stroke. *Stroke, 24*(2), 320–327.

Delbanco, T. L., Stokes, D. M., Cleary, P. D., Edgman-Levitan, S., Walker, J. D., Gerteis, M., & Daley, J. (1995). Medical patients' assessments of their care during hospitalization: Insights for internists. *Journal of General Internal Medicine, 10*(12), 679–685.

DiMatteo, M. R., & Hays, R. (1980). The significance of patients' perceptions of physician conduct: A study of patient satisfaction in a family practice center. *Journal of Community Health, 6*(1), 18–34.

Doering, E. R. (1983). Factors influencing inpatient satisfaction with care. *Quality Review Bulletin, 9*(10), 291–299.

Eisen, S. V., & Grob, M. C. (1979). Assessing consumer satisfaction from letters to the hospital. *Hospital and Community Psychiatry, 30*(5), 344–347.

Fleming, G. V. (1981). Hospital structure and consumer satisfaction. *Health Services Research, 16*(1), 43–63.

French, K. (1981). Methodological considerations in hospital patient opinion surveys. *International Journal of Nursing Studies, 18*(1), 7–32.

Geron, S. M. (1991). Assessment of subjective well-being and client satisfaction. Minneapolis: University of Minnesota Long-Term Care DECISIONS Resource Center.

Geron, S. M. (1995). *Utilizing elder focus groups to develop client satisfaction measures for home-based services.* Paper presented at the 41st Annual Meeting of the American Society on Aging, Atlanta, GA.

Geron, S. M. (1997). *The Home Care Satisfaction Measures (HCSM): Study design and initial results of item analyses.* Boston: Boston University School of Social Work.

Geron, S. M. (1998). Assessing the satisfaction of older adults with long-term care services: Measurement and design challenges for social work. *Research on Social Work Practice, 8*(1), 103–119.

Greenfield, S., Kaplan, S., & Ware, J. E. Jr. (1985). Expanding patient involvement in care. Effects on patient outcomes. *Annals of Internal Medicine, 102*(4), 520–528.

Greenfield, T. K. (1983). The role of client satisfaction in evaluating university counseling services. *Evaluation and Program Planning, 6*(3–4), 315–327.

Greenley, J. R., & Schoenherr, R. A. (1981). Organization effects on client satisfaction with humaneness of service. *Journal of Health and Social Behavior, 22*(1), 2–18.

Hays, R. D., Larson, C., Nelson, E. C., & Batalden, P. B. (1991). Hospital quality trends. A short-form patient-based measure. *Medical Care, 29*(7), 661–668.

Hays, R. D., Shaul, J. A., Williams, V. S., Lubalin, J. S., Harris-Kogjetin, L. D., Sweeny, S. F., & Cleary, P. D. (1997). Psychometric properties of the CAHPS 1.0 survey measures. Consumer Assessment of Health Plans Study. *Medical Care, 37*(3 Suppl).

Hays, R. D., & Ware, J. E. Jr. (1986). My medical care is better than yours. Social desirability and patient satisfaction ratings. *Medical Care, 24*(6), 519–524.

Henry, M. E., & Capitman, J. A. (1995). *Assessing consumer satisfaction (A provider's guide).* Waltham, MA: Brandeis University.

Hickson, G. B., Clayton, E. W., Entman, S. S., Miller, C. S., Githens, P. B., Whetten-Goldstein, K., & Sloan, F. A. (1994). Obstetricians' prior malpractice experience and patients' satisfaction with care. *JAMA, 272*(20), 1583–1587.

Hinshaw, A. S., & Atwood, J. R. (1982). A patient satisfaction instrument: Precision by replication. *Nursing Research, 31*(3), 170–175.

Hornberger, J. C., Habraken, H., & Bloch, D. A. (1995). Minimum data needed on patient preferences for accurate, efficient medical decision making. *Medical Care, 33*(3), 297–310.

Hulka, B. S., Zyzanski, S. J., Cassel, J. C., & Thompson, S. J. (1970). Scale for the measurement of attitudes toward physicians and primary medical care. *Medical Care, 8*(5), 429–436.

Kane, R. A., & Kane, R. L. (1988). Long-term care: Variations on a quality assurance theme. *Inquiry, 25*(1), 132–146.

Kane, R. L., & Atherly, A. J. (1996). Analysis of Satisfaction Survey for PACE (HCFA Contract No. 500-92-0014). Minneapolis: University of Minnesota School of Public Health.

Kane, R. L., Maciejewski, M., & Finch, M. (1997). The relationship of patient satisfaction with care and clinical outcomes. *Medical Care, 35*(7), 714–730.

Kasper, J. D., & Riley, G. (1992). Satisfaction with medical care among elderly people in fee-for-service care and an HMO. *Journal of Aging and Health, 4*(2), 282–302.

Kippen, L. S., Strasser, S., & Joshi, M. (1997). Improving the quality of the NCQA (National Committee for Quality Assurance) Annual Member Health Care Survey Version 1.0. *American Journal of Managed Care, 3*(5), 719–730.

Kleinsorge, I. K., & Koenig, H. F. (1991). The Silent Customers: measuring customer satisfaction in nursing homes. *Journal of Health Care Marketing, 11*(4), 2–13.

Kravitz, R. L. (1996). Patients' expectations for medical care: An expanded formulation based on review of the literature. *Medical Care Research and Review, 53*(1), 3–27.

LaMonica, E. L., Oberst, M. T., Madea, A. R., & Wolf, R. M. (1986). Development of a patient satisfaction scale. *Research in Nursing and Health, 9,* 43–50.

Larsen, D. L., Attkisson, C. C., Hargreaves, W. A., & Nguyen, T. D. (1979). Assessment of client/patient satisfaction: Development of a general scale. *Evaluation and Program Planning, 2*(3), 197–207.

LeVois, M., Nguyen, T. D., & Attkisson, C. C. (1981). Artifact in client satisfaction assessment: Experience in community mental health settings. *Evaluation and Program Planning, 4*(2), 139–150.

Ley, P., Bradshaw, P. W., Kincey, J. A., & Atherton, S. T. (1976). Increasing patients' satisfaction with communications. *British Journal of Social and Clinical Psychology, 15*(4), 403–413.

Locker, D., & Dunt, D. (1978). Theoretical and methodological issues in sociological studies of consumer satisfaction with medical care. *Social Science and Medicine, 12*(4A), 283–292.

Lubalin, J., Schnaier, J., Forsyth, B., Gibbs, D., McNeill, A., Lynch, J., & Ardini, M. (1995). *Design of a survey to monitor consumers' access to care, use of health services, health outcomes and patient satisfaction.* Final report (AHCPR95-N003). Rockville, MD: Agency for Health Care Policy and Research, Department of Health and Human Services.

Marshall, G. N., Hays, R. D., Sherbourne, C. D., & Wells, K. B. (1993). The structure of patient satisfaction with outpatient medical care. *Psychological Assessment, 5*(4), 477–483.

McCusker, J. (1984). Development of scales to measure satisfaction and preferences regarding long-term and terminal care. *Medical Care, 22*(5), 476–493.

McDaniel, C., & Nash, J. G. (1990). Compendium of instruments measuring patient satisfaction with nursing care. *Quality Review Bulletin, 16,* 182–188.

McGee, J., Goldfield, N., Riley, K., & Morton, J. (1997). *Collecting information from health care consumers: A resource manual of tested questionnaires and practical advice.* Gaithersburg, MD: Aspen Publishers, Inc.

Meterko, M., Nelson, E. C., & Rubin, H. R. (1990). Patient judgments of hospital quality: Report of a pilot study. *Medical Care, 28*(9 Suppl), S1–S56.

National Committee for Quality Assurance (1995). *Annual Member Health Care Survey Manual,* Version 1.0. Washington, DC: National Committee for Quality Assurance.

Nelson, E. C., Hays, R. D., Larson, C., & Batalden, P. B. (1989). The patient judgment system: Reliability and validity. *Quality Review Bulletin, 15*(6), 185–191.

Nelson-Wernick, E., Currey, H. S., Taylor, P. W., Woodbury, M., & Cantor, A. (1981). Patient perception of medical care. *Health Care Management Review, 6*(1), 65–72.

Norton, P. G., van Maris, B., Soberman, L., & Murray, M. (1996). Satisfaction of residents and families in long-term care: I. Construction and application of an instrument. *Quality Management in Health Care, 4*(3), 38–46.

Owens, D. J., & Batchelor, C. (1996). Patient satisfaction and the elderly. *Social Science and Medicine, 42*(11), 1483–1491.

Parasuraman, A., Zeithaml, V. A., & Berry, L. L. (1985). A conceptual model of service quality and its implications for future research. *Journal of Marketing, 49*(Fall 1985), 41–50.

Parasuraman, A., Zeithami, V. A., & Berry, L. L. (1988). SERVQUAL: A multiple-item scale for measuring consumer perceptions of service quality. *Journal of Retailing, 64*(1), 12–40.

Pascoe, G. C. (1983). Patient satisfaction in primary health care: A literature review and analysis. *Evaluation and Program Planning, 6*(3–4), 185–210.

Pascoe, G. C., Attkisson, C. C., & Roberts, R. E. (1983). Comparison of indirect and direct approaches to measuring patient satisfaction. *Evaluation and Program Planning, 6*(3–4), 359–371.

Pope, C., & Mays, N. (1993). Opening the black box: an encounter in the corridors of health services research. *BMJ, 306*(6873), 315–318.

Risser, N. L. (1975). Development of an instrument to measure patient satisfaction with nurses and nursing care in primary care settings. *Nursing Research, 24*(1), 45–52.

Roberts, R. E., Pascoe, G. C., & Attkisson, C. C. (1983). Relationship of service satisfaction to life satisfaction and perceived well-being. *Evaluation and Program Planning, 6*(3–4), 373–383.

Ross, C. K., Steward, C. A., & Sinacore, J. M. (1995). A comparative study of seven measures of patient satisfaction. *Medical Care, 33*(4), 392–406.

Rubin, H. R. (1990). Can patients evaluate the quality of hospital care? *Medical Care Review, 47*(3), 267–326.

Rust, R. T., & Oliver, R. L. (1994). *Service quality: New direction in theory and practice.* Thousand Oaks, CA: Sage.

Seibert, J. H., Strohmeyer, J. M., & Carey, R. G. (1996). Evaluating the physician office visit: In pursuit of a valid and reliable measure of quality improvement efforts. *Journal of Ambulatory Care Management, 19*(1), 17–37.

Shackley, P., & Ryan, M. (1994). What is the role of the consumer in health care? *Journal of Social Policy, 23,* 518.

Sherbourne, C. D., Hays, R. D., Ordway, L., DiMatteo, M. R., & Kravitz, R. L. (1992). Antecedents of adherence to medical recommendations: Results from the Medical Outcomes Study. *Journal of Behavioral Medicine, 15*(5), 447–468.

Simmons, S. F., Schnelle, J. F., Uman, G. C., Kulvicki, A. D., Lee, K. O., & Ouslander, J. G. (1997). Selecting nursing home residents for satisfaction surveys. *Gerontologist, 37*(4), 543–550.

Strasser, S., Aharony, L., & Greenberger, D. (1993). The patient satisfaction process: Moving toward a comprehensive model. *Medical Care Review, 50*(2), 219–248.

Strasser, S., & Schweikhart, S. (1992). *Who is more satisfied with medical care? Patients or family members and friends?* (Working Paper Series #92024.) Columbus, OH: The Ohio State University, College of Medicine, Division of Hospital and Health Services Administration.

Strasser, S. A. A. (1992). *The patient satisfaction measurement project.* Columbus, OH: The Ohio State University, College of Medicine, Division of Hospital and Health Services.

Swan, J. E., Sawyer, J. C., Van Matre, J. G., & McGee, G. W. (1985). Deepening the understanding of hospital patient satisfaction: Fulfillment and equity effects. *Journal of Health Care Marketing, 5*(3), 7–18.

van Campen, C., Friele, R. D., & Kerssens, J. J. (1992). *Methods for assessing patient satisfaction with primary care: Review and annotated bibliography.* Utrecht, the Netherlands: NIVEL.

van Campen, C., Sixma, H., Friele, R. D., Kerssens, J. J., & Peters, L. (1995). Quality of care and patient satisfaction: A review of measuring instruments. *Medical Care Research and Review, 52*(1), 109–133.

Ventura, M. R., Fox, R. N., Corley, M. C., & Mercurio, S. M. (1982). A patient satisfaction measure as a criterion to evaluate primary nursing. *Nursing Research, 31*(4), 226–230.

Walker, A. H., & Restuccia, J. D. (1984). Obtaining information on patient satisfaction with hospital care: Mail versus telephone. *Health Services Research, 19*(3), 291–306.

Ware, J. E. Jr., Davies-Avery, A., & Stewart, A. L. (1978). The measurement and meaning of patient satisfaction. *Health and Medical Care Services Review, 1*(1), 3–15.

Ware, J. E. Jr., & Hays, R. D. (1988). Methods for measuring patient satisfaction with specific medical encounters. *Medical Care, 26*(4), 393–402.

Ware, J. E. Jr., & Karmos, A. H. (1976). *Development and validation of scales to measure patient satisfaction with health care services,* Volume II. Perceived Health and Patient Role Propensity. Final Report, June 30, 1972 to March 31, 1976, Carbondale, IL: Southern Illinois University, p. 274.

Ware, J. E. Jr., Snyder, M. K., & Wright, W. R. (1976a). *Development and validation of scales to measure patient satisfaction with health care services,* Volume I. Part B. Results of Scales Constructed from the Patient Satisfaction Questionnaire and Other Health Care Perceptions. Final Report, June 30, 1972 to March 31, 1976, Carbondale, IL: Southern Illinois University, p. 447.

Ware, J. E. Jr., Snyder, M. K., Wright, W. R., & Davies, A. R. (1983). Defining and measuring patient satisfaction with medical care. *Evaluation and Program Planning, 6*(3–4), 247–263.

Ware, J. E. Jr., Wright, W. R., & Snyder, M. K. (1976b). *Development and validation of scales to measure patient satisfaction with health care services,* Volume IV. Key Health Concepts: Methodological Appendix. Final Report, June 30, 1972 to March 31, 1976, Carbondale, IL: Southern Illinois University, p. 245.

Ware, J. E. Jr., & Young, J. (1976). *Development and validation of scales to measure patient satisfaction with health care services,* Volume III. Conceptualization and Measurement of Health as a Value. Final Report. June 30, 1972 to March 31, 1976, Carbondale, IL: Southern Illinois University, p. 203.

Weiss, G. L., & Ramsey, C. A. (1989). Regular source of primary medical care and patient satisfaction. *Quality Review Bulletin, 15*(6), 180–184.

Zinn, J. S., Lavizzo-Mourey, R., & Taylor, L. (1993). Measuring satisfaction with care in the nursing home setting: The nursing home resident satisfaction scale. *Journal of Applied Gerontology, 12*(4), 452–465.

# 10

# Spiritual Assessment

DOUGLAS M. OLSON AND ROSALIE A. KANE

Increasingly gerontologists perceive the spiritual lives of older people as important to their well-being. Practitioners are urged to consider spiritual well-being as an aspect of health. They are urged to act and design programs to enhance (and certainly to avoid harming) the spiritual lives of elderly people. Some programs, such as hospice, include spiritual care as a built-in service and view spiritual well-being as a sought-after outcome, however elusive to measure.

Spirituality and aging have taken on currency as a linked topic. The Forum on Religion, Spirituality, and Aging (FORSA) within the American Society on Aging has grown to 600 members since its founding in 1989 (Ellor, McFadden, & Sapp, 1999). A growing number of researchers are studying the relationship between religiousness and spirituality on the one hand and health on the other. In those research endeavors, however, investigators are hampered by a paucity of standardized tools to examine a phenomenon that is complex, clearly multidimensional, hard to define, and potentially overlapping with other concepts. A group of investigators acting under the aegis of the National Institute of Aging and the Fetzer Institute, a founda-

tion in Kalamazoo, Michigan, have undertaken a Working Group collaborative process to develop tools that might effectively and efficiently permit study of the relationships between spirituality and health among older people; the efficiency ideal relates to the practicality of inserting the measures into large-scale studies (Fetzer Institute, 1999; Koenig & Futterman, 1995). Because that work has entailed extensive reviews of definitions and measures in a large number of domains related to spirituality and religiousness, we draw on it heavily in this chapter.

Some underlying questions guide our consideration of this area.

1. Is measurement of spiritual domains feasible and desirable? Is spiritual well-being an outcome that can and *should* be assessed in clinical contexts, much as we assess other functional abilities and depression? Or, is it, as some suggest, an arena best left untouched by measurement tools and unprobed in a secular society (Sherril, Larson, & Greenwold, 1993)?

2. If we decide affirmatively that we should assess religion and spirituality, then how do we further characterize

the concepts and domains of interest? How are spiritual outcomes to be understood, and how do they relate to other concepts considered in this book, such as social and psychological well-being?

3. Can spiritual activities and processes be assessed and tabulated to determine whether the elements of a meaningful spiritual life are present or lacking for a given individual? What, if anything, does organized religion have to do with spiritual well-being, and can we develop the tools to help us find out?

Certainly religious activity (sometimes called "religiosity" and, more recently by the Fetzer investigators, "religiousness") and its role in a good old age has been of interest to a small handful of empirical researchers for decades (Fetzer Institute, 1999; Payne, 1982). More importantly, philosophers, theologians, and psychologists have written a great deal about wisdom, meaning in life, and inner tranquility, all of which are sometimes associated with being able to face loss, suffering, and the prospect of one's own death while holding the view that life is meaningful (Cole & Gadow, 1986; Frankl, 1959; Moody, 1986). Moody, a philosopher and gerontologist, has described the development stages associated with searching for and finding meaning in life (Moody & Carroll, 1997), and Atchley, a well-known sociologist and gerontologist, has examined mysticism and the search for the transcendent among older people (Atchley, 1999). With some exceptions, however, measurement is usually far from the scholarly agenda of those interested in religion, spirituality, and aging.

Without doubt, religion and spirituality are salient to many older people. According to a Gallop Poll, 76% of persons over age 65 years state that religion is very important to them (Princeton Religious Research Center, 1994). Older adults are more likely than younger ones to be members of religious congregations and to par-

ticipate in groups associated with prayer (Levin, 1996; Levin & Taylor, 1997). This participation is correlated with better social functioning and psychological well-being; of 27 studies, 22 found a positive relationship between religiousness and well-being (Levin & Vanderpool, 1987a). Cause and effect relationships are seldom delineated, however, and it is possible that social well-being leads to religious participation rather than the opposite. To complicate things further, religious participation could be seen as an element of good social functioning. Indeed it is embedded, along with marital status and other social activities, in Berkman and Syme's well-known brief measure of social functioning (1979), and religious ways of coping are embedded as two items in Lazarus and Folkman's Ways of Coping Scale (1984).

Although spirituality is poorly defined, the link between an entity that people recognize as spirituality and a quality that makes life meaningful or sustains people faced with its vicissitudes is widely acknowledged. Some see religiousness or spirituality as more of a personality trait than a state. Religiousness and spirituality seem to take on increasing importance in old age, however, making them appear more amenable to change than most personality traits. Perhaps this increase with age occurs because older people, retired from the labor force and no longer actively engaged in child-rearing, have more time for reflection. Perhaps it occurs because they experience more hardship during and preceding death and rely on their spirituality because of an increased sense of their own mortality and losses of people or things important to them. Their spiritual world may be something they can depend on to be there and to be theirs, and spirituality is often viewed as a life strength. In some psychological theories of the life cycle, notably Erikson's, the task of old age is to achieve a higher integration and understanding of human life and the world so as to temper despair with wisdom (Erikson, Erikson, & Kivnick, 1989). All this being said, one cannot study spirituality and religiousness or try to develop programs to enhance psychological well-being without clear concepts and measures to depict the phenomena.

Sectarian religious organizations, these days often dubbed "faith-based organizations," have been at the forefront of providing long-term care, and clergy are a common presence at nursing homes and hospitals, yet it is unclear whether and how the effectiveness of pastoral counseling or organizational missions directed at spiritual well-being could or should be measured. Congregations have been encouraged to develop outreach to older people (Tobin, Ellor, & Anderson-Ray, 1986), but, again, how to formally assess such activities is not part of the prescription.

## DEFINING TERMS

The terms *religion, religiosity/religiousness, spirituality,* and *spiritual well-being* are used inconsistently and are sometimes carelessly interchanged. Although related, each term can have distinct definitions, as described below.

### Religion

Religion is a viewpoint, usually derived from outside the self, that offers meaning in the face of the unknown and guidelines for living. Religions are typically characterized by doctrine and beliefs, moral principles, and external forms of expression that are practiced in community, in private, or both (e.g., liturgy, worship, rites, ceremony, and prayer). These characteristics of organized religion have stabilizing effects on social groups. A question about one's religion or "religious preference" invites the respondent to name one of the world's major religious groups or a denomination or sect within it. As such, religion is a categorical classification. As Ellison (1999) points out, classifying religious preference is by no means easy. In answer to the question "what is your religion" and a further probe for specification

of Protestant and Jewish denominations, he provides a coding list of 56 choices within Christian groups, 4 within Jewish groups, 7 that are neither Christian nor Jewish (including "Wiccan and other ritual magic"), and several for "no religion," "Christian, no further information" and "Protestant, no further information." The coding system also allows for members of particular denominations—for example, Baptist, Presbyterian—to signify their general Protestant affiliation and indicate that they do not know which subgroups apply. Clearly, one would seldom incorporate this level of detail into the analysis plan for a study, but there is much merit in finding an agreed on classification for coding religious preference.

Some would extend the term *religion* to personally constructed belief systems about the divine and the supernatural (McFadden, 1996). This conceptual approach views having a religion as an end in itself and is closely associated with spirituality. Examples of a personally constructed belief system might include faith in the goodness of human kind or belief in the power of good deeds. For clarity, however, we would argue against coding such personal belief systems as a religion.

### Religiousness

Religiousness refers to religious practice, which can be defined as the activities or behaviors reflecting religious commitment, such as participation in religious organizations, attending public worship, and participating in private practices associated with one's faith (e.g., prayer meetings, reading scripture, observing rituals).

### Spirituality

Spirituality has been defined as the motivational and emotional foundation of a quest for meaning, which may be lifelong (Frankl, 1959). Thus, the "spiritual" person is one who seeks out these understandings. Among the many definitions of spirituality, one with the benefit of succinctness is "subjective experience of the sacred" (Zinnbauer et al., 1996). The concept could be viewed as multidimensional, connected, for example, to experiences with God or the creator, with nature, with other human beings, or with self-awareness (Kimble et al., 1995). Religion may play a role, but it is not a necessary element of spirituality. In their detailed exploration of how people understand religiousness and spirituality, Zinnbauer and colleagues found that a higher proportion of people considered themselves to be religious than to be spiritual. The uncoupling of spirituality from religion, moreover, is an increasing trend.

### Spiritual Well-being

Spiritual well-being is perhaps the most elusive concept of all because it implies a normative idea of a good spiritual state. It was introduced into the gerontological world by the 1971 White House Conference on Aging. According to Ellor (1999), one of its first documented uses was at a 1969 meeting at national Lutheran headquarters, which was attended by officials of the aging network. An often-quoted definition, first advanced by leaders of the National Interfaith Coalition on Aging in 1975 is as follows:

Spiritual well-being is the affirmation of life in a relationship with God, self, community, and environment that nurtures and celebrates wholeness (Moberg, 1984). This definition emphasizes integration of internal and external forces in the individual's life and is often equated with a good quality of life. Early attempts to measure spiritual well-being were patterned after the early life satisfaction indexes; that is, they included multiple facets of life experience as dimensions of the phenomenon. The terms *vertical* and *horizontal* are sometimes used to distinguish between spiritual well-being in relation to God and spiritual well-being in relation to general life satisfaction. Some might include *transcendental experiences* or *self-transcendence* (i.e., getting beyond narrower preoccupations with self) as an aspect of spiritual well-being (Walton, Beck, Shultz, & Smith, 1990).

## CONCEPTUAL MODEL

No accepted, time-tested universal theory of the relationship between spirituality and religion is available, in part because of varying disciplinary approaches. Each of the concepts defined above can itself be seen as multidimensional. Relationships among the constructs and with other constructs such as psychological and social well-being are unclear.

Thibault, Ellor, and Netting (1991) have put forward a theoretical framework to help clarify spiritual functioning and integration that has heuristic value. Figure 10.1 shows an adaptation of this model.

The outer circles in the diagram represent, in descending order, the outer boundaries of the known universe, the outer boundaries of the individual's influence, and the individual's sphere of personal life and social involvement. Within the latter, the three intersecting circles in the Venn diagram show the interior life, which entails a consciousness of self in relation to others and the world (affective); the life of knowledge and beliefs, which entails assignment of meaning and value to events by a religion or philosophy (cognitive); and "external/institutional life," which entails the relationship of the individual to the organization of his or her ascribed belief system (social). Where the circles overlap are elements of spiritual functioning: prayer, meditation, and introspection are at the juncture between cognitive and affective life; group study, education, and preaching are at the intersection of the cognitive and social spheres; and public worship, public ritual, and acts of charity are at the juncture of the affective and social spheres. In the inner circle, faith is depicted as the heart of spirituality, with "vectors" that radiate out beyond the boundaries of the known universe. Faith is defined as the confidence an individual has in a story that gives meaning and value to life and creation.

The authors propose that an individual's spirituality is the way faith activates the

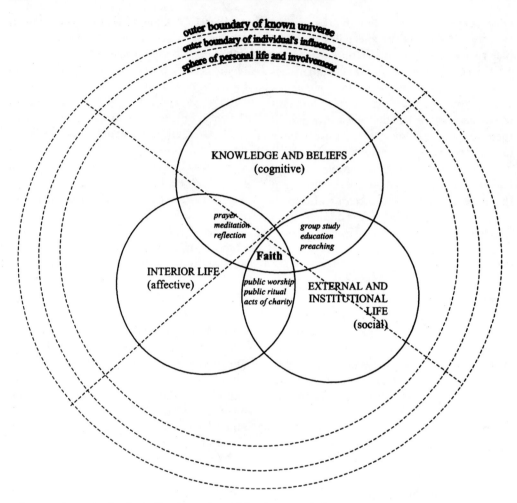

**Figure 10.1.** A theologically derived model of spiritual functioning. Source: Adapted from Thibault et al. (1991).

integration of all of the circles of personal life. This model, which has its roots in Protestant theology, is obviously difficult to make completely operational, evoking the comment that spiritual well-being is a concept "designed to be imprecise" (Marty, 1999) because to speak of the spirit is "to reach beyond the immediate, the tangible, the bounded, the containable." On the other hand, attempts have been made to measure many of the elements in the model.

Psychologists' approaches, as distinguished from the theological approaches just presented, are often built on the work of Allport (1960) and Allport and Ross (1967) and on subsequent work by Gorusch (1991, 1994). In psychology, the nature of religious commitment has largely been viewed as a question of motivation. The major focus of Allport's efforts is to examine intrinsic (as opposed to extrinsic) religious motivation. Intrinsic motivation breaks down into two different sets of theories needed to help explain this phenomenon. One group of theories claims that religious motivation developed originally for extrinsic reasons, including unconscious habit (Gorusch, 1991), misattribution of source, multiple complex sources, or social norms. The other theoretical position claims that a direct intrinsic religious motivation exists.

A sociological perspective on spirituality is also plausible. The theological and psychological approaches, however, seem to offer a greater understanding of a difficult topic. How the various constructs we have identified relate to each other is unclear. Initial work suggests that they are not fully independent (Zinnbauer et al., 1996). Empirical work is insufficient, however, to present a continuum or a hierarchy of well-tested constructs.

## RELATIONSHIP TO HEALTH

Efforts have been made to identify pathways that link religion, religiousness, spirituality, and spiritual well-being to health outcomes. These include behavioral, social, psychological, and physiological pathways (Fetzer Institute, 1999; Koenig & Futterman, 1995). A behavioral focus posits that those inclined toward religion lead healthier, more positive lives. For instance, people who use alcohol to excess are more likely not to have a religious background (Cochran, Beeghley, & Bock, 1992). A social explanation might suggest that involvement in a religious group or setting plays a buffering role against difficult life events in later life. Membership in a religious group has been associated with reduced mortality as the number of social ties increases (House, Landis, & Umberson, 1988; Zuckerman, Kasl, & Ostfelt, 1984). Psychological issues are particularly easily connected with religiosity and spirituality, and empirical support for that connection is substantial. For example, relationships have been observed between religiosity and spirituality, on the one hand, and coping (Koenig, George, & Siegler, 1988a), depression (Idler & Kasl, 1992), and anxiety (Koenig et al., 1993) on the other. More specific pathways are under exploration, such as how prayer affects emotion and how emotion affects health. Regarding physiological impact, hypertension and heart disease have both been empirically studied, showing moderate, positive relationships between them and religion (Koenig, Moberg, & Kvale, 1988b; Williams, 1989; Levin & Vanderpool, 1987b). It has also been proposed that religion influences health outcomes through a multifactorial combination of psychological, social, and physiological factors (McFadden & Levin, 1996). More recently, investigators have begun examining the relationship between religiousness and the ability to sustain both formal and informal caregiving, a phenomenon that has been noted in qualitative work on nursing assistants (Kane & Caplan, 1990) and family caregivers (Kane et al., 1999). For example, a recent study that compared the perceived rewards of family caregiving among black and white caregivers found that the former perceived greater rewards but that those positive perceptions were mediated by comfort from religion and prayer (Picot et al., 1997).

Note that the spiritual dimension in these studies is seen as the independent variable, which is linked to health as a dependent variable. The reverse relationships, namely, how health status affects spiritual outcomes, have not been studied. Such study might be interesting because the stressors associated with illness and loss could increase religiousness, spirituality, and faith or diminish them.

## DOMAINS

A long list of domains and subdomains that someone has sometime attempted to measure related to religion and spirituality could be compiled. Below we provide a list that is drawn from a variety of general writings (McFadden, 1996; Kimble et al., 1995) and, in particular, the framework developed by the cooperative researchers working in collaboration with the National Institute on Aging (NIA) and the Fetzer Institute (1999). The latter group took as a mission specifying the relationships between religion and health and, to that end, identified domains that required measurement. Their list thus far developed includes religious preference, religious and spiritual history, organizational religiousness, private religious practices, religious support, religious/spiritual coping, beliefs, values, meaning, forgiveness, commitment, and daily spiritual experiences. The domains we list below include all of these but draw on other work as well. We list the domains in order from an outer, extrinsic religious perspective to a more internal, spiritual perspective. Note that a number of different names have been used to designate essentially the same construct.

- *Religious preference (affiliation)* would appear to be a straightforward classification that respondents select from a list provided or that is later post-coded (somewhat the way occupation is post-coded). Developing a classification of religions is by no means simple, and, because of similarities in the names of Protestant denominations, error is likely. Furthermore, some commentators suggest that a time dimension be introduced so that religious preference be measured not only for the current period but also for other formative periods, for example, adolescence (Ellison, 1999).

- *Relationship (religious support)* is the degree of connectedness felt to other individuals or collectives in a religious context. This domain focuses on a sense of belonging and support drawn from religion. Krause (1999) has suggested that such measures might be modeled after more general social support scales; for example, the same properties of reciprocity and intensity could be measured and the same functions of a support network could be measured, but the reference point would be co-religionists or congregations. Essentially, that strategy uses tools that are already developed, changing only a few phrases to incorpo-

rate the religious context of the relationships.

- *Religious or spiritual history* is the past life experience in the context of religion. Approaches to measure this area may entail tabulating years of active participation or of individual religious practice of different types, both of which are hard to recall and count. A simpler approach, recommended by the Fetzer group, asks the individual to rate involvement in religious activities and the strength of his or her faith during different periods in his or her life, as well as eliciting a self-report on whether the individual has had a significant life-changing religious experience (George, 1999).

*Organizational practice* or *organizational religiousness* is the degree of formal individual participation within an organized setting. In the measure recommended by the Fetzer group, attendance at church and other related attendance, perceived fit with the religious organization, and worship experience are suggested components of organizational religiousness (Idler, 1999c).

- *Commitment* is how beliefs are translated into actions, behaviors, or decisions by individuals. Time, effort, monetary contributions, and sacrifice are all ways to measure commitment. There are examples of concrete measures of commitment, but more typically it is measured through the respondents rating the importance of their religious beliefs and involvement or, as in Hoge's approach (1972), asking respondents to agree or disagree with statements that reveal the salience of religion in their lives (Williams, 1999).

- *Religious/spiritual coping* is a process domain that enumerates religious or spiritual methods that might be used to cope with a specific crisis, life event, or stressor or to cope more generically. Pargament (1999b) reviewed the rather large number of measures of this type for the Fetzer Working Group; he himself contributed to the development of many of them. Positive and negative contributions of religion to coping have been identified, as have different substantive religious coping and different styles of religious problem solving (deferring, collaborative, or self-directing, depending on the extent to which the individual places responsibility with God (Pargament, 1999b).

*Private daily experience* is spiritual activity that takes place in private settings or outside the formal context of religious observation. Items recommended by the Fetzer Group include private prayer, watching or listening to religious programming on television or radio, reading the Bible or religious literature, and saying grace over meals (Levin, 1999).

*Values* can be assessed by asking about the importance of a wide range of values in an individual's life. Much of the work in this area stems from the seminal research of Rokeach (1969, 1973), who himself was interested in the relationship of religion and values. The Fetzer Group provides long lists of values that can be both rated and ranked in terms of their importance (or, if not ranked, the most and least important can be identified) (Idler, 1999d). In the approach suggested by the Fetzer Group, the values espoused need not be derived from religion. Another approach calls for ratings of the extent to which the respondent's values are derived from his or her religion.

*Spiritual and religious beliefs* include specific beliefs such as belief in the existence of God, belief in a personal relationship with God, belief in life after death, and belief in free will. The items in the short battery suggested by the Fetzer Group (Idler, 1999a) are rather generic, but clearly it is possible to develop scales to measure the extent to which an individual subscribes to the beliefs of a particular religion.

• *Spiritual development/spiritual maturity* is the strength and comfort gained from personal religious maturity over the course of a lifetime, or spiritual self-actualization. Although this would depend on self-perception, measurement requires a historical context or reference point. Ideally, a longitudinal data set would allow for spiritual development to be most fully subscribed. Many different names are found for tools that attempt to measure spiritual maturity, including *transcendence*. Transcendence is conceptually related to Abraham Maslow's well-known concept of "self-actualization"; he considered the need for self-actualization to be the highest need, satisfied only after more basic needs for security and affiliation are satisfied (Maslow, 1962).

## MEASUREMENT CHALLENGES

The challenges of assessment in this arena are similar to those that occur in any area of assessment, exacerbated by the recency of work (and, therefore, absence of norms) and the "interior" nature of the phenomenon, which makes external validation virtually impossible.

As stated, religiousness and spirituality are both multidimensional constructs. Little formal scale construction has been done to examine the independence or correlation among the various domains. Construct development is often done through convening focus groups, conducting in-depth interviews, and eliciting views in an open-ended way. The items derived from this process are, however, bound to reflect the backgrounds and experiences of the groups that participate. It appears that much of the work has been done within somewhat cohesive religious communities.

When religious or spiritual practices are used as independent variables to examine relationship to health status, quality of life, or some other outcome, aggregating those practices and deciding how to weight them is difficult. As age or illness makes attendance at organized services or study groups and performing acts of charity difficult, it may be necessary to develop a different way of measuring intensity. It is possible that more private pursuits such as contemplation, Bible reading, and prayer increase as more social aspects of religion decrease.

Little attention has yet been given to development, classification, and study of specific lists of activities that are plausible in long-term care facilities. These could include, for example, going out to a religious activity, attending a religious service in the facility, hearing a facility religious service broadcast on close circuit television, listening to religious services or music on the radio or television, private study, religious discussion with lay people such as staff, volunteers, and residents, and visits with clergy. In one direct long-term care example, Cohen-Mansfield and Rabinovich (1990) attempted to find out about the religious pasts and beliefs of a group of residents in a Jewish nursing home to draw conclusions about the adequacy of programming. Even with this homogeneous group, differences in religious lives were found, some of which were correlated with gender and age cohorts.

In areas such as beliefs, values, perceived comfort in beliefs, and transcendental experiences, there is simply no external validation for what the respondents report. It is hard to conceive of another source besides self-report. There are, however, examples in the literature where a rater, such as a spiritual counselor, asks questions in a semistructured interview format and then makes summary ratings of an individual's spiritual well-being (Leetun, 1996). How to validate such ratings is uncertain.

Given the difficulty of validating self-report, measuring spiritual dimensions for people with Alzheimer's disease is particularly difficult. Conventional practice wisdom holds that many people with early and moderate dementia seem to benefit from religious participation, religious music, and the presence of religious symbols. Whether such benefits reflect a spiritual process or rather pleasure in the familiar and intrinsic enjoyment of the activities is hard to judge. Little work has been done even to examine the test–retest reliability of various spiritual measures for people with cognitive impairment. Proxy informants such as a family member or staff member could, perhaps, report on participation in a variety of practices, but they are hardly able to speak to issues such as comfort with self and meaning in life.

Religious customs and observations are, of course, specific to different major religions and their branches, and they also have different manifestations in different national or cultural groups. It is quite challenging to develop generic measures of religious practices that permit comparisons that can be properly interpreted across such vastly different groups. For the most part, the work that is available to Western gerontologists is based on the Judeo-Christian tradition, and even there the applicability of scales is unclear. Scales developed and tested in one Protestant denomination may not apply well to another, and the problem is exacerbated when moving across religions (from Catholicism to Protestantism to Judaism) or incorporating a quite idiosyncratic group such as Mormons. Once departing from the Judeo-Christian tradition, the difficulties increase. The United States is still a nation of immigrants, and it is likely that U.S. care providers will encounter clientele with unfamiliar religious traditions. (Excluding new immigrants, the United States now contains many people who profess Islam, a religion that is expected to supplant Judaism as the second most popular religion by early in the new millennium [Sapp, 1996], although little attention is paid to the latter in scale development.) Given the number of religious beliefs, practices, and affiliations in U.S. secular society, it may be useful to build into religious participation measures whether the participation is in a tradition that is meaningful to the individual and consistent with his or her beliefs. In general, interpretation of existing tools calls for heightened cultural sensitivity.

Many of the instruments available to measure aspects of religiousness and spirituality are long. It was partly with this in mind that the Fetzer Working Group set out to examine existing measures in selected domains and recommend preferred forms. For most of the Fetzer domains, both a longer and a shorter format are recommended. What is unknown, however, is whether these measures will behave the same way when abbreviated, grouped together, and embedded in a health study as they behave in a study of religion itself. At least in the United States, religion is often considered a private matter. People are often reluctant to disclose religious preference on a survey, let alone more specific and personal religious values and practices.

Related to the point above, there may be a social desirability to give certain responses on measures of religious practices such as church attendance and charitable behavior and in religious attitudes such as the meaning of religion in one's life.

## EXAMPLES OF MEASURES

Although we have characterized measures of spirituality and religion as underdeveloped from the viewpoint of psychometric work or even clear constructs, there are, nonetheless, a large number of measures from which to choose.

Table 10.1 illustrates approaches to measuring private religious practices on the one hand and organizational religious practices on the other. Both are derived from the Fetzer Working Group. Taken together, these give some sense of religious involvement.

One of the most established ways to gage religious commitment is through Hoge's short form (1972) for measuring intrinsic religious motivation (Table 10.2). Also, as Williams (1999) points out, a single item to measure commitment has been

used in various research studies: "In general, how important are religious or spiritual beliefs in your day to day life? Would you say very important, fairly important, not too important, or not at all important?" Also possible is a method of measuring religious conviction in a way that has been used for a variety of opinions or attitudes. Emotional commitment to the view is approached by two items: "My beliefs about X express the real me," and "I can't imagine ever changing my mind about X." "Ego preoccupation" is tested by three items: "I think about X often"; "I hold my views very strongly"; "my belief is very important to me." Finally, "cognitive elaboration" is explored by two items: "I've held my views a long time compared to most people"; and "Several other issues could come up in a conversation about X." This technique would seem helpful if the point of the study was to identify the effects of strongly held religious views.

For the Fetzer Group, Williams (1999) proposed a 3 item set of questions to measure commitment, also shown in Table 10.2. This measure is appealing because it is simple to administer and has face validity; it consists of a Likert rating of how much the respondent carries his or her religious beliefs into his or her life, a dollar amount for spending on or because of religion, and a time expenditure on religious or spiritual matters. No psychometric work is yet available for this measure, however, and Williams (1999) does not explain how one would apply and interpret the interval scales on money and hours spent. Furthermore, an absolute dollar amount is meaningless unless considered as a proportion of income.

A historical approach is needed to better understand the impact and role of religion and spirituality among the old. George (1999) recommends an approach for the Fetzer Working Group (Table 10.3). She recognizes that no psychometric properties are available but suggests that we will never learn about how religious histories affect elderly people without asking and

Table 10.1.

Measures of Private and Organizational Religious Practices

*Private Religious Practices**

*Responses for 1–3: Several times a day, once a day, a few times a week, once a week, a few times a month, once a month, less than once a month*

1.  How often do you pray privately in places other than at church or synagogue?
2.  How often do you watch or listen to religious programs on TV or radio?
3.  How often do you read the Bible or other religious literature?
4.  How often are prayers or grace said before or after meals in your home? (all meals, once a day, at least once a week, only on special occasions, never)

*Organizational Religiousness†*

1.  How often do you attend religious services? (1–9 scale from never to several times a week)‡
2.  Besides religious services, how often do you take part in other activities at a place of worship? (1–9 scale)‡
3.  How well do you feel you fit in your church/synagogue? (extremely well, very well, slightly, not very well, not at all)§
    (*Responses for items 4–7 are Strongly agree, Agree, Not sure, Disagree, Strongly disagree*)
4.  If I had to change churches/synagogues, I would feel a great sense of loss.§
5.  I feel at home in this church/synagogue.§
6.  I would change my church/synagogue if it developed major leadership or financial problems.§
7.  The church/synagogue I attend matters a great deal to me.§
8.  How often do you do the following things when attending services and how important are they to you? (*Two response sets: five-point scale from more than once per service to never; five-point scale from extremely important to not important at all*)
    a.  Listening to others perform music?**
    b.  Singing or performing music yourself?**
    c.  Praying?**
    d.  Reading or listening to Scripture or Torah?**
    e.  Listening to the sermon?**
    f.  Participating in rituals or sacraments?**
    g.  Thinking about the beauty of the building?**
    h.  Sitting in silence?**
    i.  Being part of a healing ritual, like the laying on of hands?**
    j.  Receiving gifts of the spirit, like speaking in tongues?**

*Source: Levin (1999).

†Source: (Idler, 1999c).

‡Recommended for short form.

§Taps religious fit domain. Based on Pargament et al. (1979).

**Taps worship experience domain.

that a consistent format for asking would be advisable. She recommends highly that a question be included to determine whether the individual has had a transforming religious experience at any time. Otherwise, the measure asks about childhood and teenage religious practices and then asks the respondent to rate religious involvement in terms of both activity and meaning during each decade in the life cycle. This seems to be a systematic and efficient approach to get a descriptive overview of religion throughout the life cycle.

Table 10.4 presents a measure of religious support—that is, religion as a source of support. It is modeled after general social support measures in the literature and has the advantage of being relatively brief yet exploring multiple domains, including

**Table 10.2.**

Measures of Commitment

*Intrinsic Religious Motivation Scale**

1. My faith involves all of my life
2. In my life I experience the presence of the Divine
3. One should seek God's guidance when making every important decision
4. My faith sometimes restricts my actions
5. Nothing is as important to me as serving God as best I know how
6. I try hard to carry my religion over into all my other dealings in life
7. My religious beliefs are what really lie behind my whole approach to life
8. It doesn't matter so much what I believe as long as I lead a moral life
9. Although I am a religious person, I refuse to let religious considerations influence my everyday affairs
10. Although I believe in my religion, I feel there are many more important things in life than religion

*Commitment — Short Form†*

1. I try hard to carry my religious beliefs over into all my other dealings in life.
   a. Strongly agree
   b. Agree
   c. Disagree
   d. Strongly disagree
2. During the last year about how much was the average monthly contribution of your household to your congregation or to religious causes:
   $ _____   OR   $ _____
   Contribution per year             Contribution per month
3. In an average week, how many hours do you spend in activities on behalf of your congregation or activities that you do for religious or spiritual reasons?

*Source Hoge (1972).

†Source Williams (1999).

the opposite of support, that is, negative relationships with religion. Table 10.5 presents a selection of measures recommended by the Fetzer Working Group that relate to specific domains, including beliefs, forgiveness, and meaning.

Table 10.6 includes tools that assess spiritual well-being on various dimensions. Although the one by Underwood (1999) is labeled Daily Spiritual Practices, it seems to relate to experiences of transcendence and relationships with the divine and is similar to the other measures grouped together. The Spiritual Well-Being Scale presented in Table 10.6 contains some items that tap religious well-being and others that tap what the investigators call existential spiritual well-being; the latter items have no reference to God.

We identified many other measures in the course of doing this review, but have

limited the full presentation to a few. Moreover, given the extensive summarizing work done by the Fetzer Working Group, many of whose members developed the earlier iterations of measures in the published literature, we emphasize the Working Group's recommendations in the scales presented for illustration. Furthermore, we have illustrated only self-report measures. A number of other measures exist that require ratings on various spiritual dimensions after a conversation with the individual, or ratings based on observation and knowledge of the person. Although any well-trained interviewer should be able to administer many of the tools presented here, some people suggest that professional nursing staff or clergy be the ones to use the more open-ended structured interviews (Ellor & Bracki, 1995). These rating approaches may be more common

**Table 10.3.**
Measure of Religious/Spiritual History*

1. a. Have you had a religious or spiritual experience that changed your life?
   b. If yes, how old were you when it occurred?
2. Were you raised in a religious household?
   No   Yes *(If yes, answer questions 2a–2e)*
   a. When you were a young child, how often did you attend religious services?
   b. When you were a young child, how often did you participate in religious practices at home, either by yourself or with your family?
   c. When you were a teenager, how often did you attend religious services?
   d. When you were a teenager, how often did you participate in religious practices at home, either by yourself or with your family?
   e. Do you currently practice the same religion in which you were raised?
      No, I no longer practice any religion
      No, I have changed my religious affiliation
      Yes
3. Rate your religious involvement in the areas below for each age period listed:

| Age (Years) | Involvement in religious services | Involvement in private religious practices — prayer, meditation, study | Strength of your spiritual faith |
|---|---|---|---|
| | Low Medium High NA | Low Medium High NA | Low Medium High NA |
| 20–29 | | | |
| 30–39 | | | |
| 40–49 | | | |
| 49–50 | | | |
| 50–60 | | | |
| 65 | | | |

*Note: In another variant, depending on the population, the respondent would also be asked if he or she was a born-again Christian and at what age that conversion had occurred. Only if he or she said no would he or she be asked about a life-changing religious or spiritual experience. NA, not applicable.

Source: George (1999).

than we had originally thought. In response to a request for materials, the first author collected tools used by pastoral counseling programs serving older people to take a systematic spiritual history and identify spiritual needs. Although these are not published instruments or formally developed tools, any trend toward gathering information in a standardized way would seem positive.

## CLINICAL USES

As with other sometimes neglected areas, measurement can call attention to the need for better programming to meet needs — in this case, spiritual needs. The very act of assessment may produce a good result for the user of care. A provider's statement that "we provide holistic care" is greatly reinforced when a process ensues whereby the provider attempts to learn about sources of meaning in the client's life. Staff in many caregiving organizations, including frontline paraprofessional staff, have a strong religiously derived motivation to be of service. Attention to the spiritual dimension may enhance satisfaction and morale among staff. It should also permit evaluation of practices that staff believe are comforting and enhancing of spiritual well-being, helping to elucidate whether the practices work and for whom they work.

Organizational program decisions may be guided by the assessment of religion

Table 10.4.

Measure of Religious Support*

*How often do the people in your congregation . . . (Responses: very often, fairly often, once in a while, never)*

1.   . . . make you feel loved and cared for?†
2.   . . . listen to you talk about your private problems and concerns?†
3.   . . . express interest in your well being?

*How often do you . . .*

4.   . . . make the people in your congregation feel loved and cared for?†
5.   . . . listen to the people in your congregation talk about their private problems and concerns?†
6.   . . . express interest in the well-being of people you worship with?

*How often do the people in your congregation . . .*

7.   . . . make too many demands on you?†
8.   . . . criticize you and the things you do?†
9.   . . . try to take advantage of you?

*Responses for 10–12: a great deal, some, a little, none*

10.  If you were ill, how much would the people in your congregation be willing to help out?†
11.  If you had a problem or were faced with a difficult situation, how much comfort would the people in your congregation be willing to give you?†
12.  If you needed to know where to go to get help with a problem you were having, how much would the people in your congregation be willing to help out?

*The following domains are included: emotional support received from others (1–3), emotional support given to others (4–6), negative interaction (7–9), and anticipated support (10–12).

†Retained in the short version.

Source: Krause (1999).

and religious well-being. A recent application in point has been establishing the value of a pastoral care program in an organization. Financial pressures in the health care environment have spurred a desire to quantify the value gained from having pastoral care included. Furthermore, energy is currently going into exploring and clarifying the faith-based dimensions of sectarian organizations serving the elderly. The question is whether there really is a difference in performing caregiving tasks among sectarian and nonsectarian organizations (leaving aside for-profit/nonprofit distinctions). This inquiry goes beyond the current debate on the legitimacy of charitable tax status and focuses on defining and implementing religious values. Catholic Charities, the Association of Jewish Homes for the Aging, and, more recently, Lutheran Services in America have explored this area in an effort to articulate their "mission."

## CONCLUSION

Tools to measure religiousness and spirituality have become more plentiful in the 1990s. This should facilitate further explorations at the nexus of aging, spirituality, and health care. Finally, there seems to be a critical mass of researchers interested in studying this arena and practitioners (beyond clergy) interested in acknowledging it. Even the Nursing Home Minimum Data Set in its latest iteration has relevant items to be rated at admission under the

**Table 10.5.**
Selected Measures from the Fetzer Working Group

*Meaning (Responses: strongly agree, agree, neutral, disagree, strongly disagree)* \*

1. My spiritual beliefs give meaning to my life's joys and sorrows
2. The goals of my life grow out of my understanding of God
3. Without a sense of spirituality, my daily life would be meaningless
4. The meaning in my life comes from feeling connected to other living things
5. My religious beliefs help me find a purpose even in the most painful and confusing events in my life.
6. When I lose touch with God, I have a harder time feeling there is purpose and meaning in life
7. My spiritual beliefs give my life a sense of significance and purpose
8. My mission in life is guided by my faith in God
9. When I am disconnected from the spiritual dimension of my life, I lose my sense of purpose
10. My relationship with God helps me find meaning in the ups and downs of life
11. My life is significant because I am part of God's plan
12. What I try to do in my day to day life is important to me from a spiritual point of view
13. I am trying to fulfill my God-given purpose in life
14. Knowing that I am part of something greater than myself gives meaning to my life
15. Looking at the most troubling or confusing events from a spiritual perspective adds meaning to my life
16. My purpose in life reflects what I believe God wants for me
17. Without my religious foundation, my life would be meaningless
18. My feelings of spirituality add meaning to the events of my life
19. God plays a role in how I chose my path in life
20. My spirituality helps define the goals I set for myself

*A 2-item short form is under consideration with the neutral point dropped for a four-point response.*

1. The events in my life unfold according to a divine or greater plan
2. I have a sense of mission or calling in my own life

*Beliefs*†

1. How much is religion a source of strength and comfort to you? (None, a little, a great deal)‡
2. Do you believe there is a life after death? (yes, no, undecided)‡
   *(Responses for 3 to 7: agree strongly, agree somewhat, can't decide, disagree somewhat, disagree strongly)*
3. God's goodness and love are greater than we can possibly imagine
4. Despite all the things that go wrong, the world is still moved by love
5. When faced with a tragic event, I try to remember that God still loves me and that there is hope for the future
6. I feel that it is important for my children to believe in God
7. I think that everything that happens in life has a purpose

*Forgiveness (Responses: always, often seldom, never)*§

1. It is easy for me to admit that I am wrong
2. If I hear a sermon, I usually think of things I have done wrong
3. I believe that God has forgiven me for things I have done wrong
4. I believe there are times when God has punished me
5. I believe that when people say they forgive me for something I did they really mean it
6. I often feel that no matter what I do now I will never make up for the mistakes I have made in the past
7. I am able to make up pretty easily with friends who have hurt me in some way
8. I have grudges which I have held onto for months or years
9. I find it hard to forgive myself for some things that I have done
10. I often feel like I have failed to live the right kind of life

Forgiveness short form
1. I have forgiven myself for things that I have done wrong
2. I have forgiven those who hurt me
3. I know that God forgives me

\*Source: Pargament (1999a).

†Source: Idler (1999a).

§Source: Idler (1999b).

‡Recommended for 2 item short form.

## Table 10.6.
## Measures of Spiritual Well-Being

*Spiritual Well-Being Scale**

*For each statement, circle the choice that best indicates the extent of your agreement or disagreement as it describes you personal experience. (Choices: Strongly agree, moderately agree, agree, disagree, moderately disagree, strongly disagree)*

1. I don't find much satisfaction in private prayer with God
2. I don't know who I am, where I come from, or where I am going
3. I believe that God loves and cares about me
4. I feel that life is a positive experience
5. I believe that God is impersonal and not interested in my daily situations
6. I feel unsettled about my future
7. I have a personally meaningful relationship with God
8. I feel very fulfilled and satisfied with life
9. I don't get much personal strength and support from my God
10. I feel a sense of well-being about the direction my life is headed in
11. I believe that God is concerned about my problems
12. I don't enjoy much about life
13. I don't have a personally satisfying relationship with God
14. I feel good about my future
15. My relationship with God helps me not to feel lonely
16. I feel that life is full of conflict and unhappiness
17. I feel most fulfilled when I am in close communion with God
18. Life doesn't have much meaning
19. My relation with God contributes to my sense of well-being
20. I believe there is some real purpose for my life

*Daily Spiritual Experiences†*

*(Answer many times a day, every day, most days, some days, once in a while, never, or almost never)*

1. I feel God's presence‡
2. I experience a connection to all of life
3. During worship or at other times when connecting with God, I feel joy that lifts me out of my daily concerns
4. I find strength in my religion or spirituality§‡
5. I find comfort in my religion or spirituality§‡
6. I feel deep inner peace or harmony‡
7. I ask for God's help in the midst of daily activities
8. I feel guided by God in the midst of my daily activities
9. I feel God's love for me, directly**‡
10. I feel God's love for me, through others**‡
11. I am spiritually touched by the beauty of creation‡
12. I feel thankful for my blessings
13. I feel a selfless caring for others
14. I accept others even when they do things I think are wrong
15. I desire to be closer to God or in union with him
16. In general how close do you feel to God—not at all close, somewhat close, very close, as close as possible

*The Spiritual Experience Scale††*

1. I often feel closely related to a power greater than myself
2. I often feel that I have little control over what happens to me
3. My faith gives my life meaning and purpose
4. My faith is a way of life
5. Ideas from faiths different from my own may increase my understanding of spiritual truth
6. One should not marry someone of a different faith
7. My faith is an important part of my individual identity
8. My faith helps me to confront tragedy and suffering

*(continued)*

**Table 10.6.**

Measures of Spiritual Well-Being — Continued

9. My faith is often a deeply emotional experience
10. It is difficult for me to form a clear, concrete image of God
11. I believe faith is only one true faith
12. It is important that I follow the religious beliefs of my parents
13. Leaning about different faiths is an important part of my spiritual development
14. I often think about issues concerning my faith
15. If my faith is strong enough, I will not experience doubt
16. Obedience to religious doctrine is the most important aspect of my faith
17. My relationship to God is experienced as unconditional love
18. My spiritual beliefs change as I encounter new ideas and experiences
19. I am sometimes uncertain about the best way to resolve a moral conflict
20. I often fear God's punishment
21. Although I sometimes fall short of my spiritual ideals, I am still basically a good and worthwhile person
22. A primary purpose of prayer is to avoid personal tragedy
23. I can experience spiritual doubts and still remain committed to my faith
24. I believe that the world is basically good
25. My faith enables me to experience forgiveness when I act against my moral conscience
26. It is important that my spiritual beliefs conform with those of persons closest to me
27. Persons of different faiths share a common spiritual bond
28. I gain spiritual strength by trusting a higher power
29. There is usually only one right solution to any moral dilemma
30. I make a conscious effort to live in accordance with my spiritual values
31. I feel a strong spiritual bond with all humankind
32. My faith is a private experience that I rarely, if ever, share with others
33. Sharing my faith with others is important for my spiritual growth
34. I never challenge the teachings of my faith
35. I believe that the world is basically evil
36. Religious scriptures are best interpreted as symbolic attempts to convey ultimate truths
37. My faith guides my whole approach to life
38. Improving the human community is an important spiritual goal

*Source Ellison (1983).

†Items tap the following dimensions: connection with the transcendent (1–2), transcendent sense of self (3), sense of support from the transcendent (4–5), sense of wholeness or integration (6), sense of divine inspiration (7–8), perception of God's love (9–10), awe (11), gratitude (12), compassion (13), mercy (14), and longing for the transcendent (15–16). Source: Underwood (1999).

‡Used as an item in the 5 item recommended short form.

§Combined into a single item (I find strength and comfort in my religion or spirituality) and used in the 5 item recommended short form.

**Combined into a single item (I feel God's love for me, directly or through others) and used in the 5-item recommended short form.

††Source: Genia (1991).

heading of "customary routines." This includes a yes/no rating on "usually attends church, temple, synagogue, etc [AC1t]" and "finds strength in faith [AC1u]." The interviewer is instructed to code the former based on any of the respondent's spontaneous comments and is given no instruction for how to deduce the latter (Morris, Murphy, & Nonemaker, 1995). This bow to religious issues in a complex, multifaceted, mandated assessment is both good and bad. It is good that some systematic attention is being given to the spiritual domain, but it is odd to assume that even the more objective item on usual attendance at religious services will be reliably assessed, especially with the stress surrounding a nursing home admission, or that it will mean much given that the health status of this population might have led to less attendance lately. It hardly seems that there is a prayer (pun intended) that the tool can capture anything as subtle as "finds strength in faith."

In sum, considerable obstacles need to be overcome to develop creditable measures of religiousness and spirituality. On the clinical side, few pastoral counselors or clergy have the opportunity, time, or skills to pursue credible measurement development, yet, among them, there seems to be an interest in developing tools that will help guide individual practices and program development. Similarly, researchers are also coming together to tackle the technical problems. The "spiritual" dimension is still not well distinguished from the psychological and the social aspects of life, nor is the "spiritual" distinguished well from the "religious." Yet there is a strong societal sense that important ideas and ideals are grouped under what we tend to call "spiritual" and that this dimension takes on increasing importance for those who are nearer to death. In the twentieth century in industrialized countries, those near death are predominately older people. It is encouraging that some academic researchers are taking the subject seriously enough to wish to measure the concept and that some practitioners are perceiving more advantages than disadvantages in working with social scientists to articulate spiritual factors and to make them operational.

## REFERENCES

Allport, G. (1960). *Personality and Social Encounter*. Boston: Beacon Press.

Allport, G., & Ross, J. (1967). Personal religious orientation and prejudice. *Journal of Personality and Social Psychology, 5*, 432–443.

Atchley, R. C. (1999). Mystical experience and aging: Diverse pathways and experiences. In J. Ellor, S. McFadden, & S. Sapp (Eds.), *Aging and spirituality: The first decade* (pp. 9–12). San Francisco: American Society on Aging.

Berkman, L. F., & Syme, S. L. (1979). Social networks, host resistance, and mortality: A nine-year follow-up study of Alameda County residents. *American Journal of Epidemiology, 10*(2), 186–204.

Cochran, J., Beeghley, L., & Bock, E. (1992). The influence of religious stability and homogamy on the relationship between religiosity and alcohol use among Protestants. *Journal of Scientific Study of Religion, 31*, 441–456.

Cohen-Mansfield, J., & Rabinovich, B. A. (1990). Religious beliefs and practices of elderly Jewish nursing home residents. *Journal of Aging and Judaism. 5*(2), 87–94.

Cole, T. R., & Gadow, S. (Eds.) (1986). *What does it mean to grow old? Reflections from the humanities*. Durham, NC: Duke University Press.

Ellison, C. (1999). Religious preference. In Fetzer Institute (Ed.), *Multidimensional measurement of religiousness/spirituality for use in health research* (pp. 81–84). Kalamazoo, MI: The Fetzer Institute.

Ellison, C. W. (1983). Spiritual well-being: Conceptualization and measurement. *Journal of Psychology and Theology, 11*(4), 330–338.

Ellor, J. W., & Bracki, M. A. (1995). *Development of an assessment of older persons using a structured interview*. Wheaton, IL: National-Louis University.

Ellor, J. W., McFadden, S., & Sapp, S. (Eds.) (1999). *Aging and spirituality: The first decade*. San Francisco: American Society on Aging.

Ellor, J. W. (1999). Spiritual well-being defined. In J. W. Ellor, S. McFadden, & S. Sapp (Eds.), *Aging and spirituality: The first decade* (pp. 40–43). San Francisco: American Society on Aging.

Erikson, E. H., Erikson, J. M., & Kivnick, H. Q. (1989). *Vital involvement in old age*. New York: W. W. Norton & Company.

Fetzer Institute. (1999). *Multidimensional measurement of religiousness/spirituality for use in health research*. Kalamazoo, MI: John E. Fetzer Institute.

Frankl, V. (1959). *From death-camp to existentialism*. Boston: Beacon Press.

Genia, V. (1991). The Spiritual Experience Index: A measure of spiritual maturity. *Journal of Religion and Health, 30*(4), 337–347.

George, L. K. (1999). Religious/spiritual history. In Fetzer Institute (Ed.), *Multidimensional measurement of religiousness/spirituality for use in health research* (pp. 65–69). Kalamazoo, MI: John E. Fetzer Institute.

Gorusch, R. (1991). *Exploration of the intrinsic/extrinsic distinction across cultures*. Paper presented at the Annual Meeting of the Society for the Scientific Study of Religion and Religious Research Association, Pittsburgh, PA.

Gorusch, R. (1994). Toward motivational theories of intrinsic religious commitment. *Journal for the Scientific Study of Religion, 33*(4), 315–325.

Hoge, D. (1972). A validated intrinsic religious motivation scale. *Journal for the Scientific Study of Religion, 11*, 369–376.

House, J. S., Landis, K. R., & Umberson, D. (1988). Social relationships and health. *Science, 241,* 540–545.

Idler, E. (1999a). Beliefs. In Fetzer Institute (Ed.), *Multidimensional measurement of religiousness/spirituality for use in health research* (pp. 31–33). Kalamazoo, MI: John E. Fetzer Institute.

Idler, E. (1999b). Forgiveness. In Fetzer Institute (Ed.), *Multidimensional measurement of religiousness/spirituality for use in health research* (pp. 35–37). Kalamazoo, MI: John E. Fetzer Institute.

Idler, E. (1999c). Organizational religiousness. In Fetzer Institute (Ed.), *Multidimensional measurement of religiousness/spirituality for use in health research* (pp. 75–80). Kalamazoo, MI: John E. Fetzer Institute.

Idler, E. (1999d). Values. In Fetzer Institute (Ed.), *Multidimensional measurement of religiousness/spirituality for use in health research* (pp. 19–29). Kalamazoo, MI: John E. Fetzer Institute.

Idler, E., & Kasl, S. (1992). Religion, disability, depression and the timing of death. *American Journal of Sociology, 97*(4), 1052–1079.

Kane, R. A., & Caplan, R. (Eds.) (1990). *Everyday ethics: Resolving dilemmas in nursing home life.* New York: Springer.

Kane, R. A., Reinardy, J., Penrod, J. D., & Huck, S. (1999). After the hospitalization is over: A different perspective on family care of older people. *Journal of Gerontological Social Work, 31*(1&2), 119–142.

Kimble, M., McFadden, S., Ellor, J., & Seeber, J. (Eds.) (1995). *Aging, spirituality and religion: A handbook.* Minneapolis: Fortress Press.

Koenig, H., & Futterman, A. (1995). *Religion and health outcomes.* Paper presented at the NIH Conference on Methodological Approaches to the Study of Religion, Health and Aging, Bethesda, MD.

Koenig, H., George, L., Blazer, D., & Pritchett, J. (1993). The relationship between religion and anxiety in a sample of community-dwelling older adults. *Journal of Geriatric Psychiatry, 26,* 65–93.

Koenig, H., George, L., & Siegler, I. (1988a). The use of religion and other emotion-regulating coping strategies among older adults. *Gerontologist, 28,* 303–310.

Koenig, H., Moberg, D., & Kvale, J. (1988b). Religious activities and attitudes of older adults in a geriatric assessment clinic. *Journal of the American Geriatric Society, 36,* 362–374.

Krause, N. (1999). Religious support. In Fetzer Institute (Ed.), *Multidimensional measurement of religiousness/spirituality for use in health research* (pp. 57–64). Kalamazoo, MI: John E. Fetzer Institute.

Lazarus, R. S., & Folkman, S. (1984). *Stress, appraisal, and coping.* New York: Springer.

Leetun, M. C. (1996). Wellness spirituality in the older adult. *Nurse practitioner, 21*(8), 60–70.

Levin, J. (1999). Private religious practices. In Fetzer Publication (Ed.), *Multidimensional measurement of religiousness/spirituality for use in health research* (pp. 39–42). Kalamazoo, MI: John E. Fetzer Institute.

Levin, J. S. (1996). How religion influences morbidity and health: Reflections on natural history, salutogenesis and host resistance. *Social Science and Medicine, 43*(5), 849–864.

Levin, J. S., & Taylor, R. J. (1997). Age differences in patterns and correlates of the frequency of prayer. *Gerontologist, 37*(1), 75–88.

Levin, J. S., & Vanderpool, H. (1987a). Is frequent religious attendance really conducive to better health? Toward an epidemiology of religion. *Social Science Medicine, 24,* 589–600.

Levin, J. S., & Vanderpool, H. Y. (1987b). Is frequent religious attendance really conducive to better health? Toward an epidemiology of religion. *Social Science and Medicine, 24*(7), 589–600.

Marty, M. (1999). Designed to be imprecise. In J. W. Ellor, S. McFadden, & S. Sapp (Eds.), *Aging and spirituality: The first decade* (pp. 44–46). San Francisco: American Society on Aging.

Maslow, A. H. (1962). *Towards a psychology of being.* Princeton, NJ: Van Nostrand.

McFadden, S. H. (1996). Religion, spirituality and aging. In Birren J. E. & Schaie, K. W. (Eds.), *Handbook of the psychology of aging* (4th ed., pp. 162–173). San Diego: Academic Press.

McFadden, S. H., & Levin, J. (1996). Religion, emotions, and health. In Magai, C. M. & McFadden, S. H. (Eds.), *Handbook of emotion: Adult development and aging* (pp. 349–365). San Diego: Academic Press.

Moberg, D. O. (1984). Spiritual well-being: Background and issues. *Review of Religious Research, 25*(4).

Moody, H. R. (1986). The meaning of life and the meaning of old age. In T. R. Cole & S. Gadow (Eds.), *What does it mean to grow old?* (pp. 9–40). Durham, NC: Duke University Press.

Moody, H. R., & Carroll, D. (1997). *The five stages of the soul: Charting the spiritual passages that shape our lives*. New York: Doubleday.

Morris, J. N., Murphy, K., & Nonemaker, S. (1995). *Long Term Care Facility Resident Assessment Instrument (RAI) user's manual (for use with version 2.0 of the Health Care Financing Administration's Minimum Data Set)*. Washington, DC: Health Care Financing Administration (Government Printing Office 1995-404-792/43460).

Pargament, K., Tyler, F. B., & Steele, R. (1979). Is fit it? The relationship between church–synagogue fit and the psychosocial competence of the member. *Journal of Community Psychology, 1979*(7), 243–252.

Pargament, K. I. (1999a). Meaning. In Fetzer Institute (Ed.), *Multidimensional measurement of religiousness/spirituality for use in health research* (pp. 19–24). Kalamazoo, MI: John E. Fetzer Institute.

Pargament, K. I. (1999b). Religious/spiritual coping. In Fetzer Institute (Ed.), *Multidimensional measurement of religiousness/spirituality for use in health research* (pp. 43–55). Kalamazoo, MI: John E. Fetzer Institute.

Payne, B. P. (1982). Religiosity. In D. J. Mangen & W. A. Peterson (Eds.), *Research instruments in social gerontology: Social roles and social participation* (vol. 2, pp. 343–362). Minneapolis: University of Minnesota Press.

Picot, S. J., Debanne, S. M., Namazi, K. H., & Wykle, M. L. (1997). Religiosity and perceived rewards of black and white caregivers. *Gerontologist, 37*(1), 89–101.

Princeton Religious Research Center (1994). Importance of religion. *PRCC Emerging Trends, 16*, 4.

Rokeach, M. (1969). Religious values and social compassion. *Review of Religious Research, 11*, 3.

Rokeach, M. (1973). *The nature of human values*. New York: Free Press.

Sapp, S. (1996). Religious views on legacy and intergenerational transfers. *Generations, 20*(3), 31–36.

Sherril, K., Larson, D., & Greenwold, M. (1993). Is religion taboo in gerontology? *American Journal of Geriatric Psychology, 1*(2), 109–118.

Thibault, J. M., Ellor, J. W., & Netting, F. E. (1991). A conceptual framework for assessing the spiritual functioning and fulfillment of older adults in long-term care settings. *Journal of Religious Gerontology, 7*(4), 29–45.

Tobin, S. S., Ellor, J. W., & Anderson-Ray, S. M. (1986). *Enabling the elderly: Religious institutions within the community service system*. Albany: State University of New York Press.

Underwood, L. G. (1999). Daily spiritual experiences. In Fetzer Institute (Ed.), *Multidimensional measurement of religiousness/spirituality for use in health research* (pp. 11–17). Kalamazoo, MI: John E. Fetzer Institute.

Walton, C., Beck, C., Shultz, C., & Smith, R. (1990). *Development of a self-transcendence scale*. Little Rock: University of Arkansas College of Nursing.

Williams, D. R. (1999). Commitment. In Fetzer Institute (Ed.), *Multidimensional measurement of religiousness/spirituality for use in health research* (pp. 71–74). Kalamazoo, MI: John E. Fetzer Institute.

Williams, R. (1989). *The trusting heart: Great news about type A behavior*. New York: Times Books.

Zinnbauer, B. J., Pargament, K. I., Cowell, B., & Scott, A. (1996). *Region and spirituality: Unfuzzying the fuzzy*. Paper presented at the American Psychological Association Annual Conference, Toronto, Ontario, Canada, August 9–13.

Zuckerman, D. M., Kasl, S. V., & Ostfelt, A. (1984). Psychosocial predictors of mortality among the elderly poor. *American Journal of Epidemiology, 119*, 410–423.

# 11

# Assessment of Family Caregivers
# of Older Adults

JOSEPH E. GAUGLER, ROSALIE A. KANE, AND JOAN LANGLOIS

The forerunner of this book (Kane & Kane, 1981) was silent about tools for assessing family caregiving or family caregivers. Although sociologists have been interested in exploring intergenerational relationships within families for some time (Shanas, 1962; Shanas & Streib, 1965; Hill et al., 1970; Bengtson & Lovejoy, 1973; Sussman, 1976), the actual care provided to elderly family members was virtually ignored before 1980. Two decades later, an explosion has occurred in assessment tools and research findings related to family care. Gerontologists at the end of the twentieth century are keenly interested in studying family caregiving, and the literature is replete with related published work. Systematic measures of family care are part of the operational protocol of many programs that aim to assess and provide services to older people, and a wide choice of instruments is available to measure the consequences, or impact, of family caregiving. Such scales tend to emphasize the negative and are often summarized under the classification of *burden.*

## WHY ASSESS FAMILY CARE?

At least three considerations have fueled the interest in measuring aspects of family care:

1. Scholars, policy-makers, and practitioners are widely aware of the pivotal role that family members play in enabling frail older people to remain in the community. Simply put, long-term care programs *rely* on the family. The *formal care* provided by paid personnel (working either for themselves or for social and health agencies) is distinct from *informal care,* that is, the uncompensated care that is given by family and friends. With awareness of family care came a need for tools to characterize its magnitude, nature, and adequacy in order to determine what formal services, if any, a debilitated older person might need.

2. Family care is now widely understood to be potentially stressful, so much so, in fact, that family caregivers themselves have become the object of assessment. Most clinical efforts to assess caregiver burden are motivated by a desire to ease or eliminate negative caregiving experiences as much as possible, and most research efforts are directed at determining what increases or mitigates burden. Measures are needed to conduct research that eventually leads to the design and evalua-

tion of beneficial programs for family caregivers. Caregiving instruments should also guide program operations during phases of implementation.

3. The increases in prevalence and awareness of Alzheimer's disease and other forms of dementia have led to specialized efforts to measure both the inputs and the effects of family care in this particularly challenging context. With dementia, the need for care and oversight may be continuous, while positive feedback to the family caregiver may be spotty, minimal, or nonexistent. Many family caregiver measures have been developed specifically for dementia care with items gleaned from focus groups, research interviews, and clinical experience that identify aspects of dementia care that family members find stressful. The Alzheimer's Association, which has become a formidable political force in the last few decades, adds to this emphasis because its leadership tends to be composed of spouses and adult children of people with dementia. Many of the programs it advocates or sponsors, such as support groups, day services, and respite care, are meant to relieve the burden of family caregivers. Appropriate measures are needed to test the efficacy of such programs.

Most chapters in this book focus on measures that are applied directly to older people. Caregiver measures, in contrast, are applicable to adults of all ages who provide care to elderly family members. Certainly, heterogeneity is the watchword for family caregivers; they come in all ages, ethnic and cultural backgrounds, incomes, life situations, and kin relationship. Most family members (i.e., spouses, children, siblings, and other relatives) who bear major responsibility for the care of elderly relatives are themselves, however, over the age of 60 years (Kane & Penrod, 1995).

## DEFINING FAMILY CAREGIVING

Markedly different estimates exist regarding the prevalence of family caregiving, partly because studies adopt different conventions for what should count as family care (Stone, 1991). Some studies count caregiving as the activities reported by relatives of frail older people without reference to the actual needs of the older person. Other studies require that the older person meet some threshold of need before family caregiving can be said to occur. Some studies count only hands-on help with specific tasks (e.g., household help, personal care, nursing assistance, and transportation), whereas others count the arrangement and oversight of care or even affective care (such as worrying about an older relative or lending emotional support). In the least restrictive approaches, family caregivers are simply those who define themselves as occupying that role. In the most restrictive approaches, family caregivers are people who have major responsibility for an older relative or friend and who devote at least a specified amount of time (e.g., 4 hours a week) to providing that care. An astonishing number of books and articles on family caregivers simply avoid the matter of definition.

For the purposes of this review, we adopt a rather inclusive definition: *Family caregivers are relatives or friends of an older person who provide, arrange, or oversee services that the older person needs because of functional disabilities or health needs.*

The tasks performed by family caregivers are as varied as the needs of the older person. Family caregivers may be called on to bathe, dress, and feed the older person, help him or her ambulate or use the toilet, cook, clean, and do laundry. Caregivers may assist with medications, health procedures, or therapies, and be present to ensure the older person's safety. Caregivers may help with transportation, arrange medical appointments, and provide care management; they also may perform errands for the older person or accompany him or her on errands such as shopping or banking. Considering the nature of the work, family caregiving is hard to quantify. The following problems plague efforts to pinpoint and quantify family care.

### Distinguishing Family Care from Ordinary Family Life

Various kinds of assistance are performed within families that are independent of functional disability among family members. For example, if a wife *always* prepared meals for her husband, how should the meal preparation be counted after his stroke prevents him from doing it himself? How does the extra laundry, due to a relative's incontinence, get noted? Once an elderly mother living alone becomes functionally impaired, how does one distinguish between the visits from her adult daughter that are part of oversight and those that are a continuation of the mother–daughter relationship?

### Live-In Caregivers

When a family caregiver lives in a different household from the impaired elderly relative, it is somewhat more straightforward to quantify the time spent in providing care (although, as mentioned above, this is complex when differentiating care provided from time visiting). When the caregiver lives in the same household as the care recipient, however, the durations of tasks are difficult to determine; typically, care tasks are integrated into the life of the household.

### Supervision for Safety

The problem of quantifying the time expended in supervision for safety is an extension of quantifying live-in family care. Such supervision may be continuous, yet the family caregiver may well be engaging in other activities, even sleeping, at the same time as "supervising" the relative. Either the time spent providing care is overestimated (because every waking and possibly sleeping minute of the caregiver's time is counted), or it is underestimated.

### Focus on Caregiver–Care Recipient Dyads

Family caregiving is typically examined with reference to the care that *one* family caregiver provides to *one* care recipient. Often, but not always, one person bears the lion's share of family caregiving responsibility, gets dubbed the *primary caregiver,* and is the informant on family care for a given individual. If we count only the care from this primary caregiver, however, we are likely to undercount care given to a particular person by his or her other family members. This problem arises in reverse if we are interested in determining, from the perspective of the caregiver, how different inputs in family care affect perceived burden. Some family members simultaneously undertake care responsibilities for more than one relative, and, without direct inquiry, we may overstate the provision of assistance to the care recipient of interest.

### Recognizing and Measuring Family Care for Relatives in Institutions

Family members provide tangible hands-on care to nursing home residents and, increasingly, assisted living residents. Caregivers may literally feed residents and help them ambulate. They may bring food or take laundry home to be washed. Caregivers may also be responsible for transportation and arrangements for medical care. No consensus has emerged about whether and how to count this as family care. If we were counting assistance in terms of societal costs borne by family caregivers, we might not want to count activities that fail to result in less expense for formal caregivers. If we are counting help to examine correlates of family burden, we surely would want to include such care.

## CONCEPTUALIZING CAREGIVING IMPACT

There have been numerous attempts to develop conceptual frameworks that describe the family caregiving process. Early efforts were spent documenting the various effects of care provision on individuals who provided intensive assistance to disabled elderly relatives (Deimling & Bass, 1986; Greene et al., 1982; Rabins, Mace, & Lucas, 1982; Zarit, Reever, & Bach-Peterson, 1980). These initial studies provided researchers with the first measurable constructs that assessed the overall impact of the caregiving experience. As the literature grew more refined, comprehensive theoretical models were developed that emphasized the complex and multidimensional interplay of caregiving over time (Aneshensel et al., 1995; Pearlin et al., 1990; Zarit, 1990). The development of theoretical frameworks has raised a number of important issues pertaining to assessment; as various dimensions of caregiving impact were identified, it became necessary to refine and review the measurement tools used to assess the phenomenon.

## Caregiver Burden

For the most part, early research referred to the impact of caregiving as *burden*. Although the term carries various connotations throughout the literature, burden generally represents the emotional, psychological, physical, and financial "load" assumed by caregivers, as well as their subjective appraisals of how task performance affects their lives (George & Gwyther, 1986; Poulshock & Deimling, 1984; Zarit, 1990; Zarit, Todd, & Zarit, 1986). The earliest conceptualizations of the caregiving process often attempted to correlate contextual variables (e.g., duration of care, relationship of caregiver to care recipient), and care demands (e.g., severity of behavior problems, intensity of cognitive impairment, extent of activities of daily living [ADL] dependencies) with unidimensional constructs representing burden. Measures that treated burden as a unidimensional construct often focused on the "subjective" aspects of burden, that is, the negative emotional reactions related to the intensive provision of family care

(Morycz, 1985; Robinson, 1983; Zarit et al., 1980).

Critical evaluations of caregiving research soon revealed that the construct of burden suffered from several limitations (George & Gwyther, 1986; Moritz, Kasl, & Berkman, 1989). Criticisms focused on both the definition of burden and its scope as a measurable construct. For example, George and Gwyther (1986) questioned the desirability of burden measures that are specifically designed to measure caregiving experiences because comparisons with people who are not family caregivers are impossible. Also, measures of burden often require caregivers to relate care demands to potential impacts (generally categories such as emotional, social, or financial implications), thus confounding "stressors" (i.e., burden) with more global assessments of well-being, such as depression. Third, unidimensional conceptualizations of burden obscure the presence of multiple dimensions.

These concerns led to a refinement in the conceptualization and assessment of burden. Research comparing the effects of caregiving with other life events found that people providing care scored significantly worse on measures of well-being than noncaregiving controls (Anthony-Bergstone, Zarit, & Gatz, 1988). In addition, use of specific burden measures allow researchers to determine how caregivers perceive that a certain stressor is affecting their lives (Zarit, 1990), which is impossible if more global measures of well-being and psychological distress (e.g., depression) are applied. For example, a caregiver may not suffer from depression or deficits in physical health, but that caregiver may still feel unable to provide the necessary amount of care to the elderly care recipient and choose to institutionalize the relative. Recent research has emphasized the importance that burden (in the form of negative appraisals of caregiving) has in predicting the care recipient's early admission to a nursing home (Aneshensel, Pearlin, & Schuler, 1993; Montgomery & Kosloski, 1994).

One limitation in early caregiving research was the reliance on single summary scores as indicators of burden. Specifically, the use of summary scores may obscure a domain of the construct that is likely to have differential impacts on care-related outcomes (Zarit, 1990). For example, a factor analysis of one popular measure of burden found that two dimensions (anger and perception of a patient's care demands as excessive) predicted one particular outcome, institutionalization, as effectively as the total summary score (Hassinger, 1986).

Other approaches separate measures of caregiver burden into "objective" and "subjective" dimensions (Montgomery, Gonyea, & Hooyman, 1985; Thompson & Doll, 1982). Objective indices of burden reflect the disruptions and degree of changes caregivers experience in various life domains (e.g., family relationships, employment, and social/recreational activities). Subjective burden refers to caregivers' emotional reactions to care demands (e.g., exhaustion, feelings of being trapped in the caregiving role). Studies that incorporate this conceptualization of burden have found variability in what predicts objective and subjective burden, underscoring the theoretical usefulness in approaching the consequences of caregiving as a multifaceted construct (Lawton et al., 1989; Montgomery et al., 1985; Poulshock & Deimling, 1984).

## Stress Process Models of Caregiving

As research proliferated, studies began to emphasize the multidimensional and longitudinal nature of caregiving. The complexity of the caregiving process motivated investigators to develop comprehensive theoretical frameworks that organized some of the interrelationships among constructs, thus providing a useful heuristic to explain how caregiving becomes troublesome for certain individuals. In addition, well-developed theoretical models provide some insight as to what constructs should be assessed when determining the impact of caregiving.

Theoretical conceptualizations of caregiving are largely grounded in sociological perspectives of stress (i.e., Lazarus, 1966; Lazarus & Folkman, 1984). Specifically, this approach suggests that the occurrence of some environmental demand that is potentially harmful (the stressor) is appraised by the individual in terms of whether or not the demand is threatening (primary appraisal) (Lawton et al., 1989). If the demand is appraised as threatening and there is a lack of resources available to stem that threat, the likelihood of poor adaptation increases (e.g., negative mental or physical health outcomes).

In the past decade, a number of researchers have significantly contributed to the literature by developing and testing various conceptual models of the caregiving process (Aneshensel et al., 1995; Lawton et al., 1989); Pearlin et al., 1990; Zarit, 1990). Figure 11.1 presents one of the most comprehensive caregiving models to date, the Stress Process Model. There are several important components to the model, including contextual factors, primary stressors, appraisals of primary stress, secondary stressors, outcomes, and various mediators/buffers of stress. Although this model was developed specifically for caregivers of patients with Alzheimer's disease, its grounding in general sociological theory makes it potentially applicable to caregivers of older adults with other kinds of disabilities and impairments.

Several contextual factors have a potential impact on the stress process. A key element is the family context of care. For example, a frequently studied variable is the relationship of the caregiver to care recipient. Feelings of obligation, commitment, and burden often vary by kin relationship, such as adult child, spouse, or sibling (Anthony-Bergstone et al., 1988; Cohler et al., 1989; Deimling et al., 1989; Gaugler et al., 1999). Additional family-level indices, however, such as quality and size of family support networks, are often ignored in descriptive analyses of caregiving (Zarit,

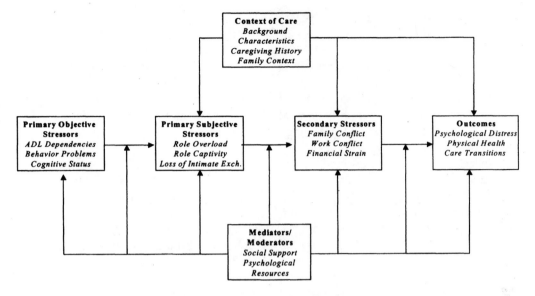

**Figure 11.1.** The Stress Process Model.

1990). Other important contextual variables include the type and nature of living arrangements (e.g., variations in the caregiving experience among separate and shared households), culture and ethnicity, social and economic characteristics of the caregiving household, and caregiving history (e.g., duration of care).

Although context provides a general picture of the caregiving experience, the heart of the Stress Process Model is its identification of multiple components of stress and how these various components interact over time. In particular, the Stress Process Model is guided by the concept of "proliferation," or the spread of stress, strain, and conflict from the actual provision of care to other life domains (e.g., family, work, social). As caregiving stress proliferates, global indicators of functioning are likely to be affected, such as psychological well-being (e.g., depression, anger, guilt) and physical health (Aneshensel et al., 1995; Pearlin et al., 1990; Zarit, 1994).

The Stress Process Model first identifies *primary stressors*. Primary stressors are those challenges or problems that are embedded in the caregiving situation and are a direct result of the care recipient's illness or disability. Primary stressors have "ob-

jective" and "subjective" components. Primary objective stressors refer to the occurrence of care demands, which include the care recipient's need for help with ADLs or instrumental activities of daily living (IADLs) (Lawton & Brody, 1969), intensity of the care recipient's behavior problems, severity of his or her memory impairment, and the care recipient's resistance to the assistance offered. Caregivers' emotional reactions to the occurrence of care demands represent primary subjective stressors (or "appraisals of primary stress"). Similar to subjective dimensions of burden, primary subjective stressors represent the degree to which caregivers *perceive* care demands as exhausting, confining, distressing, or, conversely, uplifting. Primary subjective stress also includes the loss of intimacy and emotional contact with the care recipient, presumably due to the care recipient's illness (Aneshensel et al., 1995; Pearlin et al., 1990; Zarit, 1990).

Primary stressors are embedded in the caregiving situation; however, the strain and stress that results from intensive care provision may spread to other life domains. This outgrowth of primary stress is termed *secondary stress*. Although the term *secondary* is used to describe these various forms of stress, they are potentially powerful predictors of negative outcomes (Aneshensel et al., 1995; Pearlin et al., 1990; Zarit, 1990). Secondary stress can include family tension and conflict (disagreements between the caregiver and other family members over a variety of care issues), work conflict (caregiving's impact on the quality and frequency of employment), and financial strain (e.g., reduction in income and increased expenditures due to caregiving responsibilities). In some respects, secondary stress is similar to the "objective" dimensions of burden highlighted above. In terms of assessment, some measures combine different areas of secondary stress into one scale, thus obscuring the effects of family conflict, work conflict, and financial strain (Zarit, 1990). As illustrated below, however, there have been a few attempts to measure and empirically determine the implications of various secondary stressors independently (Aneshensel et al., 1995; Gaugler et al., 1999; Semple, 1992).

In addition to stressors, several components of the Stress Process Model potentially stem the proliferation of stress. These *mediators/moderators* include social support and psychological resources (e.g., mastery). Social support is either instrumental or emotional. Indices of social support may also encompass objective indicators (e.g., the amount of support received) or subjective indicators (e.g., the caregiver's perception of adequate support; Gaugler et al., 1999; Zarit, 1994).

The final component of the Stress Process Model includes global outcomes. *Outcomes* refer to indicators of negative mental health (e.g., depression, anger, anxiety, guilt) and physical health (e.g., blood pressure, reduced immune system response) (Anthony-Bergstone, 1988; Kiecolt-Glaser et al., 1987; Zarit, 1990). In addition, certain transitions in the caregiving process are conceptualized as outcomes, such as the institutionalization of an elderly care recipient (Kowloski & Montgomery, 1995; Pruchno, Michaels, & Potashnik, 1990).

Documenting the different components of the Stress Process Model provides insight into those constructs that best represent the impact of caregiving. Several sources (including chapters in this volume) address the assessment issues surrounding indices of everyday functioning (e.g., ADLs) and well-being (e.g., depression, subjective health) among older adults. Little attention has, however, been given to the assessment of caregiving impact. For the purpose of this review, *impact* refers to measures of burden and appraisals of primary stress and secondary stress. These measures of impact are specific to the caregiving experience and assess the various emotional, social, and financial implications of care provision. Because of their importance, a review of the measures utilized to assess impact is warranted.

## MEASUREMENT CHALLENGES

The theoretical discussion above translates directly into practical quandaries of measurement.

### Dimensionality of Constructs

As emphasized earlier, the impact of caregiving is likely multifaceted, and the complexity of the care process should be reflected in measures of burden and appraisals of primary stress and secondary stress. Early studies utilizing various scales of burden simply summed item responses to represent aggregate feelings of burden (Horowitz & Dobrof, 1982; Robinson, 1983; Zarit et al., 1980); however, later analyses began to differentiate between objective and subjective dimensions of burden (Montgomery et al., 1985; Vitaliano, Young, & Russo, 1991b). Greater refinement occurred when comprehensive theoretical models were developed to conceptualize the caregiving process (Aneshensel et al., 1995; Pearlin et al., 1990; Zarit, 1990). A major issue in reviewing measures of caregiving impact is determining their usefulness as multidimensional constructs. Is there evidence that multidimensional measures of burden and stress have greater utility in explaining the impact of caregiving (George & Gwyther, 1986; Zarit, 1990; Vitaliano et al., 1991a)?

## Subjective versus Objective Dimensions of Burden

A specific issue related to the dimensionality of burden is the distinction between objective and subjective components (Montgomery et al., 1985; Vitaliano et al., 1991a). *Objective burden* refers to disruptions in finances, family life, and social relations, while *subjective burden* represents feelings of embarrassment, overload, confinement in the caregiving role, resentment, and exclusion (Thompson & Doll, 1982). Although the two dimensions of burden are conceptually distinct, the potential confounding of objective and subjective burden is problematic (Stephens & Kinney, 1989). In addition, items included in measures of objective and subjective burden often overlap with indices of global physical and psychological well-being, thereby producing spurious associations between burden and outcomes. As Stephens and Kinney emphasize (1989), there is a need to establish conceptual independence between predictor and criterion variables, particularly if stress process models are utilized (i.e., the occurrence of care demands → caregiver stress → caregiver outcomes). Zarit (1990), however, provides a competing argument. Although the separation of burden and outcome is important on an abstract level, caregivers evaluate their experiences in terms of how care demands actually affect their lives. By assessing the meaning and significance of the caregiving situation through measures of burden/stress appraisal, we can better understand how caregivers make crucial decisions.

## Specificity of Burden to the Caregiving Situation

Another important issue is the specificity of burden measures' to the caregiving situation. Because some of these measures are embedded in the caregiving process, they cannot be administered to non-caregiving populations. Therefore, it is difficult to assess the relative burden of care provision or whether or not family caregivers are worse off than other groups in similar life situations (George and Gwyther, 1986). Past research has provided estimates of stress impact among caregivers and other populations (Anthony-Bergstone et al., 1988). Comparisons among caregivers of disabled older adults and other populations are few, however, and there is a need to demonstrate the variability of stress and burden across heterogeneous populations.

## Tapping Positive Dimensions of Caregiving

Measures that describe the caregiving process often frame care as an overwhelmingly negative and adverse life experience. Most analyses provide limited or no attention to the potentially positive effects of caregiving. Several researchers have developed measures of caregiving uplift and satisfaction, including Lawton and coworkers (1989), Kinney and Stephens (1989a), and Picot, Youngblut, and Zeller (1997). One of the major issues in the measurement of caregiving is to understand the sense of fulfillment and mastery that may result from the provision of assistance and to place such constructs into an overall theoretical model of the caregiving process. A related issue pertains to the reliance on quantitative measures of caregiving impact. Reinardy and colleagues (1999) compared results from the Montgomery Burden Scale (see below) with open-ended items that assess how caregiving affects the respondent's life (i.e., "positively" or "negatively"). The open-ended questionnaire was administered to caregivers a few weeks after the Montgomery Burden Scale. Although the general findings were comparable, in the open-ended approach caregivers did not always mention the burdens they had checked affirmatively on the closed-ended scale, and they did indicate various positive effects.

## Cross-Cultural Assessment of Caregiving Impact

Few studies have examined caregiving among diverse ethnic groups. The overwhelming majority of caregiving research deals largely with white families. Early research stressed the kinship network of African-American families, and caregiving within this context was hypothesized to extend beyond the nuclear family and into other families and non-kin relations (Morycz, 1993; Gelfand, 1982; Mindel, 1983). Findings of burden among white and African-American caregivers of patients with Alzheimer's disease seem to suggest some differences in perceived strain and stress among the two groups (i.e., whites indicate greater strain and stress than their African-American counterparts; Morycz et al., 1987; Stueve, Vine, & Struening, 1997). Much more work needs to be done, however, before any conclusions can be drawn with regard to these results; unfortunately, there is a dearth of data exploring the differential impact of caregiving among individuals of heterogeneous ethnic backgrounds. Meanwhile, measures of caregiving impact are open to charges of being culturally insensitive because their analyses are often conducted with mainstream samples.

## REVIEW OF MEASURES

The following sections review common measures of caregiving impact. A general description of the measure is provided, as well as its method of administration. Then, the psychometric properties of each measure are considered, including reliability and validity (if assessed). Table 11.1 provides an overview of the measures discussed. Some scales were developed with small samples, and some appear to have been used only within the confines of a single research study. Even so, this long table presents tools selectively; many more have been reported. We highlight those tools that play a seminal role in extending

our understanding of family caregiving and represent a departure from preceding instruments.

## Measures of Burden

### The Burden Interview

The 29 item Burden Interview (Zarit et al., 1980) and a 22 item modified version (Zarit & Zarit, 1983) were developed to measure caregivers' perceptions of burden. The Burden Interview was originally designed to assess perceived stressors among caregivers of individuals with dementia in a small study (n = 29). Its specific items were generated from clinical experience as well as early research that examined care provision for mentally disabled older adults (Lowenthal & Berkman, 1967). Respondents are asked to appraise several different "problem areas" that may affect caregiving, including health, psychological well-being, social life, relationship between the caregiver and care recipient, and finances. The Burden Interview was originally conceptualized as a unidimensional measure, although factor analyses have identified specific dimensions of the scale (Hassinger, 1986).

The Burden Interview can be completed by the caregiver either as part of a questionnaire or by in-person or phone interview (Table 11.2). The caregiver responds to the 22 statements about the impact of the care recipient's disabilities on his or her life by indicating how often he or she has felt that way. Item responses range from "never" (0) to "nearly always" (4), with a possible total point score of 88; higher scores indicate greater burden. Population norms for the Burden Interview have not been calculated, but the preliminary classification by Zarit and Zarit (1987) used the following categories: 0–20 total points, little or no burden; 21–40 points, mild to moderate burden; 41–60 points, moderate to severe burden; and 61–88 points, severe burden. Internal reliability for the Burden Interview is generally high; reliability coefficients of 0.88 are not uncommon (e.g., Hassinger, 1986).

There have been several efforts to explore the validity of the Burden Interview. Construct validity was determined with a single global rating of burden and the Brief Symptom Inventory (Derogatis et al., 1971). Additional evidence of construct validity was found when burden scores were correlated with psychiatric symptoms, morale, and the quality of the caregiver-care recipient relationship (Scharlach, 1987; Winogrond et al., 1987; Zarit, Anthony, & Boutselis, 1987).

## Revised Memory and Behavior Problems Checklist (RMBPC)

The care demands of the impaired care recipient and the caregiver's emotional reactions to these demands can be measured with the Revised Memory and Behavior Problems Checklist (RMBPC) (Teri et al., 1992). The RMBPC includes 24 items derived from Zarit and Zarit's original Memory and Behavior Problems Checklist (1983). The RMBPC was administered to 201 caregivers of elderly patients in a geriatric assessment clinic. The RMBPC rates three domains of patient problems: behavior, memory, and depression. Each behavior is rated on two scales: frequency (i.e., "never occurs" [0]; "occurs infrequently and not in the last week" [1]; "occurred 1–2 times in the last week" [2]; "occurred 3–6 times in the last week" [3]; and "occurs daily or more often" [4]) and reaction, which represents the degree to which the caregiver finds the particular problem upsetting ("not at all" [0]; "a little" [1]; "moderately" [2]; "very much" [3]; and "extremely" [4]). Examples include "asking the same question over and over," "losing or misplacing things," "destroying property," "doing things that embarrass you," "waking you or other family members at night," "crying and tearfulness," and "comments about feeling worthless or being a burden to others." Internal consistency was high for both frequency of problems and caregivers' reactions to problems ($\alpha = 0.75$; $\alpha = 0.87$, respectively). Validity was established by conducting correlations between the RMBPC dimensions and several established measures: the Hamilton Depression Rating Scale (HDRS; Hamilton, 1967); the Center for Epidemiological Studies Depression Scale (CES-D; Radloff, 1977); the Caregiver Stress Scale (Deimling & Bass, 1984); and the Mini-Mental Status Examination (MMSE; Folstein, Folstein, & McHugh, 1975). Teri and coworkers (1992) found that (1) the frequency of depression subscale was significantly associated with the HDRS and the CES-D (concurrent validity), (2) the frequency of memory problems was reliably correlated with the MMSE and dementia diagnosis (concurrent validity), and (3) the frequency of behavior problems was significantly related to the HDRS (construct validity). Finally, the reaction subscales were correlated with the CES-D and the Caregiver Stress Scale, providing further evidence of the construct validity of the RMBPC.

The comprehensive nature of the Burden Interview and the RMBPC and their widespread use have made these instruments "gold standards" for assessing burden among caregivers of older adults suffering from dementia. There are, however, several limitations to the measures. Although the Burden Interview and RMBPC provide a broad overview of care recipient problems and caregivers' emotional reactions to these problems, there is no assessment of caregiver-centered problems that may contribute to feelings of burden and distress. Nevertheless, the Burden Interview and RMBPC remain two of the most widely used measures of caregiving impact. Moreover, although the symptoms and behaviors that comprise the items in the RMBPC were designed as dementia specific, only 7 of the 24 items refer directly to forgetfulness and difficulty in concentrating. It is possible that the RMBPC, either as is or with modification,

**Table 11.1.**
Summary of Measures of the Impact of Family Caregiving

| Instrument | Domains assessed | Administration | Item responses | Reliability | Validity |
|---|---|---|---|---|---|
| Burden Interview (BI) (Zarit, 1980) | Negative feelings about caregiving | Self-report or interview; primary caregivers of older adults with senile dementia (n = 29) | 22 items; responses range from "never" (0) to "nearly always" (4) | α = 0.88 | Construct validity: BI was correlated with single rating of burden, the Brief Symptom Inventory, psychiatric symptoms, morale, and quality of the caregiver–care recipient relationship |
| Revised Memory and Behavior Problems Checklist (RMBPC) (Teri et al., 1992; Zarit & Zarit, 1983) | Various "problem areas" of the care recipient (behavior, memory, and depression) and caregivers' perceptions of those demands | Interview; caregivers of elderly patients attending a geriatric clinic (n = 201) | 24 items; frequency of problems rated in past week ("never occurs" [0] to "occurs daily" [4]); degree of upset ranges from "not at all" (0) to "extremely" (4) | α = 0.75 for frequency; α = 0.87 for perception | Construct and concurrent validity: Correlations between the RMBPC and the Hamilton Depression Rating Scale, the CES-D, the Caregiver Stress Scale, and the MMSE |
| Objective and Subjective Burden Inventory (Montgomery et al., 1985) | Changes and disruptions in life (objective burden); emotional responses (subjective burden) | Interview; family caregivers of elderly relatives with a variety of health needs (n = 81) | 9 item objective inventory with 5 point response (from "a lot more better" to "a lot less worse"); 13 item subjective inventory with 5 point response ("rarely or never" to "most of the time") | α = 0.85 for objective burden; α = 0.86 for subjective burden | Construct validity: Empirical associations between burden inventories and background variables and caregiving tasks |
| Caregiver Strain Index (CSI) (Robinson, 1983) | Series of "strains" related to care provision (e.g., physical, personal, family, financial) | Interview; caregivers who provided assistance to recently hospitalized older adults (n = 85) | 13 items; caregivers respond "yes" or "no" | α = 0.86 | Construct validity: CSI scores were correlated with care recipient characteristics, caregiver's subjective perceptions, and caregiver's emotional well-being |

| Instrument | Measures | Method/Sample | Items and responses | Reliability | Validity |
|---|---|---|---|---|---|
| Poulshock and Deimling Model (Poulshock & Deimling, 1984) | Measures burden in direct relation to care recipient impairments and impact on caregiving life | Interview; 614 caregivers and the elderly care recipients with whom they lived | Mental impairment: Caregivers rate degree of upset for each memory problem as "tiring," "difficult," "upsetting" (range 0–3) ADL dependencies: Caregivers rate degree of upset for each ADL with responses ranging from "not at all" (1) to "a great deal" (3) | α = 0.88 and 0.80 for "impact on life" subscales (negative changes in family relations, restrictions in activity, respectively) | Construct validity: Burden subscales were correlated with care recipients' ADLs, cognitive functioning, Zung Depression Scale, and impact on life subscales |
| Family Strain Scale (Morycz, 1985) | Caregivers' subjective burden (emotional/psychological affect, changes in living patterns, changes in relationships/health | Interview; family caregivers of patients with Alzheimer's disease (N = 80) | 14 items; responses range from "not experienced at all" (0) to "experienced a great deal" (4) | α = 0.77 | Construct validity: The Family Strain Scale was correlated with the Zung Depression Scale |
| Relatives' Stress Scale (RSS) (Greene et al., 1982) | Severity of caregivers' emotional response and disruptions in family/social life | Interview; 38 primary caregivers of day hospital patients suffering from dementia | 15 items; responses ranged from "not at all" (0) to "considerably" (4) | α = 0.85 | Construct validity: The RSS was associated with the Behavior and Mood Disturbance Scale (see Greene et al., 1982), caregiver distress, and care recipient disruption |
| The Caregiver Burden Inventory (CBI) (Novak & Guest, 1989; Caserta, Lund, & Wright, 1996) | Restrictions on time, chronic fatigue, adverse effects on health, role conflict, negative feelings toward care recipients | Interview or self-report; originally administered to 171 caregivers of dementia patients (Novak & Guest, 1989) | 24 items (with 5 subscales of burden: time dependence, developmental, physical, social, and emotional); responses range from "not at all descriptive" (0) to "very descriptive" (4) | α = .85 for time dependence; α = 0.87 for developmental; α = 0.86 for physical; α = 0.69 for social; α = 0.81 for emotional | Construct validity: The CBI was correlated with the CES-D and the Memory and Behavior Problems Checklist |

(continued)

**Table 11.1.** Summary of Measures of the Impact of Family Caregiving—Continued

| Instrument | Domains assessed | Administration | Item responses | Reliability | Validity |
|---|---|---|---|---|---|
| Screen for Caregiver Burden (SCB) (Vitaliano et al., 1991a) | The occurrence of care demands (objective burden) and distress associated with them (subjective burden) | Interview; 191 spousal caregivers of patients with Alzheimer's disease | 25 items; responses range from "no occurrence" (0) to "occurrence with severe distress" (4); objective burden subscore sums whether event occurred; anchor points, range from "no occurrence/ occurrence but no distress" (1) to "severe distress" (4) | $\alpha = 0.85$ for objective burden; $\alpha = 0.88$ for subjective burden | Construct validity: The burden subscales were correlated with measures of behavioral and cognitive functioning, caregiver distress, and caregiver personality Criterion validity: Burden scores were compared with age- and sex-matched controls |
| Caregiver Hassles Scale (CHS) (Kinney & Stephens, 1989b) | Hassles in dealing with ADLs, memory problems, behavior problems, and support network | Interview; 60 primary caregivers of patients with Alzheimer's disease | 42 items; responses range from "not at all a hassle/event did not occur" (0) to "a great deal of hassle" (4) | $\alpha = 0.91$ for total scale; $\alpha = 0.79$ for basic ADLs; $\alpha = 0.75$ for IADLs; $\alpha = 0.82$ for cognitive; $\alpha = 0.89$; for behavior; $\alpha = 0.74$ for support network | Construct validity: The CHS was correlated with caregiver reports of care recipient functioning as well as various measures of caregiver well-being |
| Perceived Burden Measure (Macera et al., 1993) | The amount of support caregivers provide and associated levels of stress | Interview; 82 caregivers of family members with a diagnosis of dementia | 15 items; sum of the stressful assistance caregiver provided (range = 0–15) | $\alpha = 0.87$ | Construct validity: The Perceived Burden Measure was correlated with the CES-D |
| Caregiver Burden Scale (Gerritsen & van der Ende, 1994) | The quality of the caregiver–care recipient relationship (i.e., "negative relationship") and limitations in the personal life of the caregiver (i.e., "personal consequences") | Interview; 89 caregivers of psychogeriatric patients suffering from some form of senile dementia | 20 items; responses to statements recoded as dichotomies (0 = "disagree," 1 = "agree") | $\alpha = 0.84$ for total scale; $\alpha = 0.77$ for both personal consequences and negative relationship subscales | Face validity: Established with the consultation of academics, caregivers, and students Construct validity: Depression was correlated with the total Caregiver Burden Scale as well as the subscales; deviant behavior was correlated with the total scale and the personal consequences subscale |

| Measure | Construct/Dimensions | Sample/Method | Items/Responses | Reliability | Validity |
| --- | --- | --- | --- | --- | --- |
| Novel Caregiver Burden Scale (NCB) (Elmståhl, Malmberg, & Annerstedt, 1996) | Various dimensions of subjective burden, including general strain, isolation, disappointment, emotional involvement, and environment | Interview; 150 family caregivers of dementia and stroke patients (for factor and reliability analysis); 35 caregivers of stroke patients (for validity analyses) | 20 items; responses include "not at all" (1), "seldom" (2), "sometimes" (3), and "often" (4) | $\alpha = 0.87$ for strain; $\alpha = 0.70$ for isolation; $\alpha = 0.76$ for disappointment; $\alpha = 0.70$ for emotional involvement; $\alpha = 0.53$ for environment | Construct validity: The total NCB score was correlated with patient's extroversion and quality of life (see Eysenck & Eysenck, 1964; Jadbäck et al., 1993) |
| Caregiver Appraisal Measure (Lawton et al., 1989) | Caregiving satisfaction, perceived caregiving impact, caregiving mastery, caregiving ideology, and subjective caregiving burden | Interview; based on study of 632 caregivers of older adults with dementia and study of 123 family caregivers of older adults screened for nursing home admission | 47 items with each response on two 5 item scales; responses range from "never" to "nearly always" and "strongly agree" to "strongly disagree" | $\alpha = 0.85$ for subjective burden; $\alpha = 0.67$ for caregiving satisfaction; $\alpha = 0.70$ for caregiving impact | Construct validity: Significant associations were found among three subscales (subjective burden, caregiving satisfaction, and caregiving impact) and measures of affective states, quality of the caregiver–care recipient relationship, and emotional burden |
| Caregiving Uplifts (Kinney & Stephens, 1989a) | The "uplifts" associated with care in 4 domains: ADLs, care recipient's cognitive status, care recipient's behavior, and items involving the practical aspects of care | Interview; 60 caregivers of family members with Alzheimer's disease | 110 items; caregivers asked whether or not a care-related event occurred; caregivers rated each event for degree of uplift associated with it; responses ranged from "not at all" to "a great deal" (4 point scale) | Test–retest reliability was estimated at 0.89; internal reliability for the 4 subscales ranged from 0.71 to 0.90 | Construct validity: The ADL and Behavior Subscales were associated with caregiver depression; however, caregivers with greater uplift scored higher on depression measures |
| The Picot Caregiver Rewards Scale (PCRS) (Picot et al., 1997) | External and internal rewards associated with the provision of care | Interview; 83 African-American female caregivers (nonrandom) and random sample of 256 African-American and white caregivers | 16 items; caregivers rated items in terms of their reward; responses ranged from "not at all" (0) to "a great deal" (4) | $\alpha = 0.88$ for the entire measure | Content validity: Experts reviewed the content of the PCRS. Construct validity: PCRS was correlated with CES-D and the Burden Interview |

*(continued)*

Table 11.1. Summary of Measures of the Impact of Family Caregiving—Continued

| Instrument | Domains assessed | Administration | Item responses | Reliability | Validity |
|---|---|---|---|---|---|
| Caregiver Reaction Assessment (CRA) (Given et al., 1992) | Caregivers' reactions to the various impacts of care provision such as impacts on schedule, esteem/self-worth, family support, physical health, finances | Interview/questionnaire; 276 caregivers of cancer patients and 101 older adults suffering from dementia | 24 items; item responses range from "strongly agree" (1) to "strongly disagree" (5) | $\alpha$ = 0.82 for schedule; $\alpha$ = 0.90 for esteem; $\alpha$ = 0.85 for lack of family support; $\alpha$ = 0.80 for health; $\alpha$ = 0.81 for finance | Construct validity: The CRA subscales were correlated with the CES-D (Radloff, 1977) and a checklist of ADL dependencies |
| Aspects of the Caregiving Role (Schofield et al., 1997) | A variety of domains, including life satisfaction, positive and negative affect, physical health, social support, overload, family environment, and the caring role | Phone interview; 976 caregivers of family members suffering from a chronic disability; 219 noncaregivers. Sixty-seven caregiver–care recipient dyads were also included for validity analyses | Life satisfaction (6 items, 5 point scale ranging from "very dissatisfied" to "very satisfied"); positive and negative affect (20 items); health (1 item, 4 point scale ranging from "excellent" to "poor"); social support (7 items, 5 point scale ranging from "strongly disagree" to "strongly agree"); overload (3 items, 5 point scale ranging from "strongly disagree" to "strongly agree"); family environment (6 items, responses include "more," "the same," and "less") and caring role (15 items) | Internal reliability ranged from $\alpha$ = 0.60 to $\alpha$ = 0.88 | Construct validity: Clinical assessments used to validate caregivers' assessments of ADL dependency, severity of care recipient disability, and problematic behavior |
| Role Overload (Aneshensel et al., 1995; Pearlin et al., 1990) | Feelings of exhaustion and fatigue related to care responsibilities | Interview; 555 family caregivers of elderly relatives suffering from dementia | 3 items; responses range from "not at all" (1) to "completely" (4) | $\alpha$ = 0.78 | Construct validity: It was associated with ADLs and problematic behavior over 1 yr; role overload was also predictive of depression over a 1 and 3 yr period |

| Measure | Description | Sample | Items and responses | Reliability | Validity |
|---|---|---|---|---|---|
| Role Captivity (Aneshensel et al., 1995; Pearlin et al., 1990) | Feelings of being "trapped" in the caregiving role | Interview; 555 family caregivers of elderly relatives suffering from dementia | 3 items; responses range from "not at all" (1) to "very much" (4) | α = 0.83 | Construct validity: It was associated with problematic behavior over a 1 and 3 year period; role captivity was also predictive of depression over a 3 year period |
| Loss of Intimate Exchange (Aneshensel et al., 1995; Pearlin et al., 1990) | Decrements in caregiver's personal relationship with the care recipient | Interview; 555 family caregivers of elderly relatives with dementia | 3 items; responses range from "completely" (1) to "not at all" (4) | α = 0.76 | Construct validity: Related to cognitive impairment and indirectly related to depression over 1 year period |
| Family Conflict (Pearlin et al., 1990; Semple, 1992) | Disagreements and tension experienced with family members outside of the caregiving situation | Interview; 555 family caregivers of elderly relatives suffering from dementia | 12 items; responses range from "no disagreement" (1) to "quite a bit" (4) | α = 0.90 | Construct validity: Family conflict was related to role captivity and depression over a 1 year period |
| Work Conflict (Aneshensel et al., 1995; Pearlin et al., 1990) | Degree of job–caregiving conflict due to care responsibilities | Interview; 555 family caregivers of elderly relatives suffering from dementia | 5 items; responses range from "strongly disagree" (1) to "strongly agree" (4) | α = 0.75 | Construct validity: Work conflict was related to role captivity and depression over a 1 year period |
| Financial Strain (Aneshensel et al., 1995; Pearlin et al., 1990) | Pressure on family finances due to the increased expenditures of caregiving | Interview; 555 family caregivers of elderly relatives suffering from dementia | 3 distinct items; (1) expenditures due to care ("much less now" [5] to "much more now" [1]); (2) able to make ends meet on a monthly basis ("not enough" [3] to "some money left" [1]); (3) reductions in income over time | N/A | Construct validity: One item (reductions in income) was associated with role overload over a 1 year period |

**Table 11.2.**

**The Zarit Burden Interview\***

*Do you feel:*

1.   That your relative asks for more help than he/she needs?
2.   That because of the time you spend with your relative you don't have enough time for yourself?
3.   Stressed between caring for your relative and trying to meet other responsibilities for your family or work?
4.   Embarrassed over your relative's behavior?
5.   Angry when you are around your relative?
6.   That your relative currently affects your relationship with other family members in a negative way?
7.   Afraid of what the future holds for your relative?
8.   Your relative is dependent on you?
9.   Strained when you are around your relative?
10.  Your health has suffered because of your involvement with your relative?
11.  That you don't have as much privacy as you would like because of your relative?
12.  That your social life has suffered because you are caring for your relative?
13.  Uncomfortable having friends over because of your relative?
14.  That your relative seems to expect you to take care of him/her as if you were the only one he/she could depend on?
15.  That you don't have enough money to care for your relative in addition to the rest of your expenses?
16.  That you will be unable to take care of your relative much longer?
17.  You have lost control of your life since your relative's illness?
18.  You wish you could just leave the care of your relative to someone else?
19.  Uncertain about what to do about your relative?
20.  You should be doing something more for your relative?
21.  You could be doing a better job in caring for your relative?

Overall, how burdened do you feel in caring for your relative (not at all, a little, moderately, quite a bit, extremely)?

\*Items 1–21 measured as never, rarely, sometimes, quite frequently, nearly always.

Source: Zarit (1980).

could be administered to a wide variety of caregivers.

### Montgomery Burden Inventories

Montgomery and associates (1985) conducted structured interviews in the homes of 81 caregivers who assisted elderly family members with a variety of health needs. They identified two dimensions of burden: objective (or changes and disruptions in life) and subjective (i.e., attitudes and emotional responses of caregivers; Table 11.3). On the 9 item objective inventory, caregivers indicate the degree to which the provision of care has affected several areas of life, including finances, privacy, social activity, health, and interpersonal relationships (Vitaliano et al., 1991b). Response categories on the objective burden inventory range from "a lot more (better)," "a little more (better)," "the same," "a little less (worse)," and "a lot less (worse)." Subjective burden was assessed on a 13

item inventory that asked caregivers the frequency with which they have experienced particular feelings. The 13 items were adapted from the Burden Interview (see earlier), but appropriate for use with caregivers whose relatives have a variety of disabilities. Item responses were rated on a five-point scale of "rarely or never," "a little of the time," "sometimes," "often," and "most of the time." Using Cronbach's alpha coefficients, Montgomery and colleagues (1985) found that both inventories exhibited high internal consistency (i.e., 0.85 for objective burden, 0.86 for subjective burden).

To determine the viability of the two dimensions, Montgomery and associates (1985) performed a series of correlational and regression analyses that included a number of care-related variables (age, gender, employment status and household income of caregiver, functional status of care recipient, living arrangement, relationship of caregiver to care recipient, number of

**Table 11.3.**

Montgomery Burden Inventories

*Objective Burden**

*As a result of giving care, how would you rate*
1. The amount of time you have to yourself
2. The amount of privacy you have
3. The amount of money you have to meet expenses
4. The amount of personal freedom that you have
5. The amount of energy that you have
6. The amount of time you spend in recreational and/or social activities
7. The amount of vacation activities and trips you take
8. Your relationship with other family members
9. Your health

*Subjective Burden*

*Rating: rarely/never, a little of the time, sometimes, often, most of the time*
1. I feel it is painful to watch my _____ age
2. I feel useful in my relationship with my _____
3. I feel afraid for what the future holds for my _____
4. I feel strained in my relationship with my _____
5. I feel that I am contributing to the well-being of my _____†
6. I feel that my _____ tries to manipulate me
7. I feel pleased with my relationship with my _____†
8. I feel that my _____ does not appreciate what I do for him/her as I would like
9. I feel nervous and depressed about my relationship with my _____
10. I feel that my _____ makes requests that are over and above what he/she needs
11. I feel that I don't do as much for my _____ as I could or should
12. I feel that my _____ seems to expect me to take care of him/her as if I was the only one he/she could depend on
13. I feel guilty over my relationship with my _____

*1–7 are rated as a lot more, a little more, the same, a little less, a lot less; 8 and 9 are rated as a lot better, a little better, the same, a little worse, a lot worse.*

† Reverse scoring.

Source: Montgomery et al. (1985).

additional family members providing care, type and number of tasks, and total hours spent in caregiving) as well as the two dimensions. Initial analyses found that the objective and subjective burden dimensions were significantly correlated. The dimensions shared only 12% of common variance, however, suggesting that the factors associated with each type of burden were likely different (e.g., see Thompson & Doll, 1982). Subsequent regression analyses supported this assertion; certain caregiver tasks (i.e., nursing care, bathing, dressing, walking, transportation, and errands) and the number of family members assisting with care responsibilities were significant predictors of objective burden. Two variables were predictive of subjective burden (caregiver's income and age of caregiver). Additional analyses of validity

for the objective and subjective burden inventory are not available. Other concerns include the lack of conceptual correspondence between the items on each scale and the difficulty in assessing specific demands that are actually distressing to the caregiver (Vitaliano et al., 1991b).

### Caregiver Strain Index (CSI)

Some research views strain (those enduring problems that potentially harm the individual; see Pearlin & Schooler, 1978) as interchangeable with the concept of burden, and the simple presence of a problem is seen as a likely precursor to general distress. The Caregiver Strain Index (CSI) assumes this approach (Robinson, 1983). It was developed with a sample of caregivers (in this case, family members or friends/neighbors; n = 85) who provided assistance to recently hospitalized older adults (e.g., for hip surgery or arteriosclerotic heart disease).

The CSI is a relatively brief and easily administered instrument that asks caregivers to respond "yes" (1) or "no" (0) to 13 items representing various domains of strain related to care provision (e.g., physical, personal, family, financial). Examples are given for each item to clarify meaning (Table 11.4). Total scale scores range from 0 to 13. The internal consistency of the CSI was high ($\alpha$ = 0.86). Construct validity of the measure was also supported by correlating total CSI scores with care recipient characteristics, caregivers' subjective views of the caregiving situation, and the emotional well-being of caregivers (see Bradburn & Caplovitz, 1965; McNair, Lorr, & Droppleman, 1971).

A potential limitation of the CSI is its conceptualization of burden: Does the presence of certain strains actually demonstrate caregiver burden? In addition, the dichotomous scaling of the items, although easily administered and scored, may lack the refinement of other measures that assess the degree of strain/burden for different responsibilities.

### Poulshock and Deimling Model

In their research on dementia care, Poulshock and Deimling (1984) proposed a model that attempted to identify the complex dynamics of caregiving impact by measuring the construct of "burden" in direct relation to actual caregiving problems (e.g., elder complains or criticizes things, elder interferes with caregiver and other household members, elder fails to respect privacy, elder disrupts meals or makes them unpleasant), care recipient impairments (e.g., elder is confused, elder hears or sees things that are not there, elder wanders inside the house), and positive characteristics (e.g., elder is interesting to talk to, elder is enjoyable to be with, elder is cooperative, elder is appreciative or grateful).

In the Poulshock and Deimling (1984)

---

Table 11.4.
Caregiver Strain Index

*I am going to read a list of things that other people have found to be difficult after somebody comes home from the hospital. Would you tell me if any of these apply to you (respond yes or no):*

1. Sleep is disturbed (e.g., because _____ is in and out of bed or wanders around at night)
2. It is inconvenient (e.g., because helping takes so much time or it's a long drive over to help)
3. It is a physical strain (e.g., because of lifting in and out of a chair or the effort or concentration required)
4. It is confining (e.g., helping restricts free time or I cannot go visiting)
5. There have been family adjustments (e.g., because helping has disrupted routines or there has been no privacy)?
6. There have been changes in personal plans (e.g., I had to turn down a job or could not go on a vacation)
7. There have been other demands on my time (e.g., from other family members)
8. There have been emotional adjustments (e.g., because of severe arguments)
9. Some behavior is upsetting to me (e.g., incontinence, _____ has trouble remembering, or _____ accuses people of taking things)
10. It is upsetting to find _____ has changed so much for his/her former self (e.g., he/she is a different person than he/she used to be)
11. There have been work adjustments (e.g., because of having to take time off)
12. It is a financial strain
13. I am feeling completely overwhelmed (e.g., because of worry about _____; concerns about how I will manage)

Source: Robinson (1983).

model, functional and behavioral impairments serve as the independent variables, impact on life is the dependent variable, and burden (or caregivers' emotional responses) is the mediator. Impairment was a multidimensional construct consisting of two factors: ADL dependency and three measures of mental impairment derived from a factor analysis (i.e., sociability, disruptive behavior, and cognitive incapacity).

Two dimensions of impact were derived from a factor analysis: an 11 item scale of Negative Impact on Elder–Caregiver Family Relationships and an 8 item Caregiver Social Activity Restriction Scale (Table 11.5). Poulshock and Deimling's initial analysis included 614 elderly relatives who

**Table 11.5.** Two Impacts of Caregiving Scales Derived from Factor Analysis

*Negative Impact on Elder–Caregiver Relationships*

Caregiver feels angry toward elder

Caregiver's relationship with elder makes caregiver depressed

Caregiver relationship with elder is strained

Caregiver feels resentful toward elder

Elder has negatively affected relationship with family members

Caregiver feels elder tries to manipulate caregiver

Caregiver wishes elder and caregiver had better relationship

Caregiver relationship with elder gives pleasure

Caregiver feels elder makes more requests than necessary

Caregiver feels pressured between giving care to elders and others in family

Caregiver feels that elder can only depend on caregiver

*Caregiver Social Restriction*

Caregiver takes part in group and organized activities less

Caregiver takes part in theater, concerts, and shows less

Caregiver visits family and friends less

Caregiver takes part in volunteer activities less

Caregiver feels social life has suffered because of elder

Caregiver doesn't have enough time for self

Caregiver takes part in church-related activities less

Caregiver takes part in other social activities less

Source: Poulshock and Deimling (1984).

received personal care assistance from a co-residing family caregiver. Interviews were administered in the homes of caregivers.

Two burden measures were administered that corresponded with the ADL and mental impairment dimensions. For each ADL dependency, caregivers rate whether or not help with that ADL is "tiring," "difficult," or "upsetting." Items are given one point for each rating, with a total item response range of 0–3. For the three mental impairment scales, caregivers indicate how much a particular impairment upsets them or creates a problem. Item responses include "not at all" (1), "somewhat" (2), and "a great deal" (3).

Subsequent analyses reported that reduced versions of the "impact on life" subscales (negative changes in the family relationship and restrictions in caregivers' activities) had high internal reliability ($\alpha = 0.88$ and $\alpha = 0.80$, respectively). Construct validity of the burden measures was demonstrated in several studies; the burden measures were significantly correlated with care recipients' cognitive and ADL functioning, negative change in the caregiver–care recipient relationship, restrictions in caregivers' activities, caregiver mental health as measured with the Zung Depression Scale, and institutionalization decisions (Deimling & Poulshock, 1985; Poulshock & Deimling, 1984).

It does not appear that the Deimling and Poulshock impact measures have been used widely outside the studies for which they were designed. The conceptualization of burden as a mediating process, however, influenced the development of subsequent caregiving models (e.g., Pearlin et al., 1990). Another strength of this approach is that burden is measured as a construct in direct relation to care recipient impairments. Vitaliano and colleagues (1991b), however, note several limitations, such as the exclusion of family disruptions as indicators of "life impact." In addition, global depression in the Poulshock and Deimling model is conceptualized as an antecedent to burden, whereas subsequent models tended to conceptualize global indicators of well-being and distress as outcomes of the caregiving process. More research in needed on possible "feedback" loops among these constructs. Also, the noncontinuous scaling of some burden items makes the determination of psychometric properties difficult.

### Family Strain Scale

The Family Strain Scale (Morycz, 1985) was designed to measure caregivers' subjective burden. The scale was utilized in a large study that analyzed the role of caregiver characteristics in the institutionalization process. The Family Strain Scale was administered through in-person interviews to 80 family caregivers of persons with Alzheimer's disease. The 14 items represent specific measures of strain and are viewed as outcomes of the subjective experience of caregiving. Items include information related to caregivers' emotional and psychological affect, perceived changes in living patterns, perceptions of change in relationships, and health. Items are rated on a four-point scale and responses include "not experienced at all" (1), "not experienced too much" (2), "somewhat experienced" (3), and "experienced a great deal" (4). Total point scores range from 14 to 56, with higher scores signifying greater family strain.

The Family Strain Scale has shown good internal reliability ($\alpha = 0.77$). There is also some evidence for construct validity; the Family Strain Scale was correlated with the Zung Depression Scale. Several limitations regarding the content of the Family Strain Scale have, however, been noted. Stephens and Kinney (1989) emphasize that the Family Strain Scale is more representative of general well-being than caregiver stress because the items do not use actual caregiving responsibilities as a referent. Therefore, the Family Strain Scale is not conceptually distinct from measures of global psychological distress such as depression.

### Relatives' Stress Scale (RSS)

The 15 item Relatives' Stress Scale (RSS) was developed to assess the amount of stress and upset experienced by family caregivers of elderly relatives (Greene et al., 1982). In particular, the RSS measures severity of emotional response and disruptions in family and social life. Items were worded for nonprofessionals and were drawn from the literature as well as the authors' experiences. The measure can be administered through in-person interview, phone, or survey.

The RSS was originally administered with the Behavior and Mood Disturbance Scale (BMDS) to 38 primary caregivers of day hospital patients suffering from dementia (Greene et al., 1982). The BMDS provides a frequency count of 34 common behavioral problems. Response categories for the BMDS range from "never" (0) to "always" (4), whereas item responses for the RSS include "not at all" (0), "a little" (1), "moderately" (2), "quite a lot" (3), and "considerably" (4). Construct validity was established through empirical associations with the BMDS as well as measures of caregiver distress and care recipient disruption. A factor analysis was also conducted and three subscales were identified, although the small sample size validating these dimensions makes any conclusions tenuous (Vitaliano et al., 1991b). Internal consistency for the entire scale was high ($\alpha = 0.85$). In their review of burden scales for cognitively impaired populations, Vitaliano and colleagues (1991b) emphasize the strength of including measures of problem frequency and caregiver distress (see The Revised Memory and Behavior Problems Checklist, earlier). The BMDS and the RSS, however, tap distinct content domains, with little or no correspondence between the occurrence of behavior disruptions and the stress associated with the actual problems.

### The Caregiver Burden Inventory (CBI)

The Caregiver Burden Inventory (CBI) is a multidimensional instrument designed for caregivers of older adults suffering from dementia (Novak & Guest, 1989). Items were drawn from the experiences of caregivers as well as from previously developed burden measures (Table 11.6). The CBI was originally administered to 171

**Table 11.6.**
Caregiver Burden Inventory

*How descriptive is this statement of your situation (from 0, not at all descriptive; to 4, very descriptive)?*

*Factor 1: Time Dependence*

1. My care-receiver needs my help to perform many daily tasks
2. My care-receiver is dependent on me
3. I have to watch my care-receiver constantly
4. I have to help my care-receiver with many basic functions
5. I don't have a minute's break from my caregiving chores

*Factor 2: Developmental Burden*

1. I feel that I am missing out on life
2. I wish I could escape from this situation
3. My social life has suffered
4. I feel emotionally drained due to caring for my care-receiver
5. I expected that things would be different at this point in my life

*Factor 3: Physical Burden*

1. I'm not getting enough sleep
2. My health has suffered
3. Caregiving has made me physically sick
4. I am physically tired

*Factor 4: Social Burden*

1. I don't get along with other family members as well as I used to
2. My caregiving efforts aren't appreciated by others in my family
3. I've had problems with my marriage
4. I don't do as good a job at work as I used to
5. I feel resentful of other relatives who could but do not help

*Factor 5: Emotional Burden*

1. I feel embarrassed by my care-receiver's behavior
2. I feel ashamed of my care-receiver
3. I resent my care-receiver
4. I feel uncomfortable when I have friends over
5. I feel angry about my interactions with my care-receiver

Source: Novak and Guest (1989).

caregivers of dementia patients (Novak & Guest, 1989). The method of administration of the CBI is flexible.

To confirm the presence of multiple dimensions, Novak and Guest (1989) performed a factor analysis on the 24 item measure, which produced five interpretable factors: time-dependence burden (burden associated with restrictions on caregivers' time; 5 items), developmental burden (caregivers feeling "out of sync" in development relative to their peers; 5 items), physical burden (feelings of chronic fatigue and adverse effects to the caregiver's health; 4 items), social burden (feelings of role conflict; 5 items), and emotional burden (negative feelings of caregivers toward care recipients; 5 items). Item responses range from "not at all descriptive" (0) to "very descriptive" (4). The maximum subscale score for all of the dimensions (except physical burden) is 20; for the physical burden subscale, the maximum score is 16.

Recent research has explored the psychometric properties of the CBI further (Caserta, Lund, & Wright, 1996). Caserta and colleagues administered the CBI and other measures (e.g., CES-D, the MBPC) to 160 primary caregivers of older adults suffering from Alzheimer's disease or related disorders. The five dimensions of the CBI all demonstrated sufficient internal consistency ($\alpha = 0.85$ for time dependence; $\alpha = 0.87$ for development; $\alpha = 0.86$ for physical; $\alpha = 0.69$ for social; $\alpha = 0.81$ for emotional). There was also some evidence of construct validity, as all of the subscales were found to significantly correlate with the CES-D. In addition, three of the subscales (time dependence, developmental, physical) were associated with the Memory and Behavior Problems Checklist.

Although short, the CBI takes a comprehensive approach to assessing burden, making it a useful measure. The identification of multiple dimensions is another noteworthy contribution of the CBI; as mentioned above, one of the early detractions of burden measures was their unidimensional orientation. Whether the CBI is appropriate for different types of caregivers is unknown, although most items do not pertain specifically to dementia.

### Screen for Caregiver Burden (SCB)

The Screen for Caregiver Burden (SCB) is a 25 item measure that assesses the objective and subjective burdens of caregivers (Vitaliano et al., 1991a). The measure was administered to 191 caregivers of spouses with Alzheimer's disease via in-person interviews. The items of the SCB include a series of potentially troublesome experiences that are presented to the caregiver, who responds on the following 5 point scale: "no occurrence of the experience" (0); "occurrence of the experience, but no distress" (1); "occurrence with mild distress" (2); "occurrence with moderate distress" (3); and "occurrence with severe distress" (4). The total objective burden score simply sums whether an event has occurred or not (i.e., 0 = did not occur, 1 = occur), while the total subjective burden score measures the distress associated with caregiving experiences. The anchor points for each subjective burden item are 1 (no occurrence/occurrence but no distress), 2 (mild distress), 3 (moderate distress), and 4 (severe distress). The range of scores for objective burden is 0–25, while the range for subjective burden is 25–100.

Vitaliano and colleagues (1991a) have demonstrated the psychometric properties of the SCB among several independent samples. Reliability coefficients were 0.85 for the objective burden subscale and 0.88 for the subjective burden subscale, respectively. Construct validity was established by analyzing the relationships of the objective burden subscale with measures of behavioral and cognitive functioning among care recipients. Similarly, the subjective burden subscale was associated with caregiver distress and personality variables (Vitaliano et al., 1991a). Criterion validity was demonstrated by comparing burden scores with age- and sex-matched controls.

There are several limitations to the SCB.

The SCB was solely administered to spousal caregivers in early demonstrations of the measure's psychometric properties. An additional concern that Vitaliano and coworkers (1991b) express is the inclusion of subjective statements in the objective burden subscale; some of the items included in the objective burden score are actually appraisals. Demonstrations of validity, however, offer some evidence for the conceptual and empirical distinction between the two dimensions.

### Caregiving Hassles Scale

The Caregiving Hassles Scale (CHS) is a 42 item scale designed to assess the daily hassles associated with caring for an elderly relative with dementia. In contrast to caregiving responsibilities that occur over a long period of time, the CHS focuses on the daily events of caregiving and uses a short time reference (e.g., last week). The concept of hassles was derived from a transactional framework in which stress is characterized as a minor irritation of daily life that the individual perceives as threatening to his or her well-being (Lazarus & Folkman, 1984). Although hassles are weak threats individually, the accumulation of the daily stressors over time can have a negative impact on an individual's well-being (e.g., social roles and relationships, emotional states, and physical health).

The CHS consists of 42 items with five subscales: hassles in assisting with basic ADLs (9 items), hassles in assisting with IADLs (7 items), hassles with the care recipient's cognitive status (9 items), hassles with the care recipient's behavior (12 items), and hassles with the caregiver's support network (5 items; Table 11.7). Caregivers report which events occurred during the previous week, whether they are appraised as a "hassle," and if so, to what degree. Each item that occurred is rated on a four-point scale, with responses ranging from "not at all, a hassle/event did not occur" (0) to "a great deal of hassle" (4). Summing the item responses creates a total score, while subscale scores are calcu-

**Table 11.7.**

Caregiving Hassles Scale

*How much was this a hassle in the last week (from 0, not at all/doesn't occur; to 4, a great deal of hassle)?*

1. Care recipient criticizing/complaining
2. Care recipient declining mentally
3. Assisting care recipient with walking
4. Extra expenses due to caregiving
5. Friends not showing understanding about caregiving
6. Care recipient losing things
7. Undesirable changes in care recipient's personality
8. Assisting with care recipient's toileting
9. Transporting care recipient to doctor/other places
10. Conflict between care recipient and family
11. Care recipient not showing an interest in things
12. Bathing care recipient
13. Family not showing understanding about caregiving
14. Care recipient yelling/swearing
15. Care recipient not cooperating
16. Care recipient's forgetfulness
17. Assisting care recipient with exercises/therapy
18. Doing care recipient's laundry
19. Care recipient leaving tasks undone
20. Care recipient being confused/not making sense
21. Lifting or transferring care recipient
22. Not receiving caregiving help from friends
23. Care recipient frowning/scowling
24. Care recipient living in past
25. Helping care recipient eat
26. Picking up after care recipient
27. Care recipient verbally inconsiderate/not respecting feelings
28. Being in care recipient's presence
29. Care recipient talking about/seeing things that aren't real
30. Dressing care recipient
31. Not receiving caregiving help from family
32. Care recipient asking repetitive questions
33. Care recipient not recognizing familiar people
34. Giving medications to care recipient
35. Preparing meals for care recipient
36. Care recipient wandering off
37. Care recipient's agitation
38. Assisting care recipient with health aids (e.g., dentures/braces)
39. Care recipient requiring day supervision
40. Leaving care recipient with others at home
41. Care recipient hiding things
42. Care recipient requiring night supervision

Source: Kinney and Stephens (1989b).

lated by summing ratings across the items that comprise that subscale.

Psychometric properties were determined among a group of primary caregivers of patients with Alzheimer's disease (n = 60). Alpha and test–retest reliabilities for the total scale were high (0.91 and 0.83, respectively); however, these values were calculated with the same sample that was used to construct the CHS. An independent sample is needed to test the psychometric properties of the CHS further. Reliability coefficients were also high for each of the subscales (basic ADLs = 0.79; instrumental ADLs = 0.75; cognitive = 0.82; behavior = 0.89; support network = 0.74). Construct validity was supported by correlating total and subscale scores of the CHS with caregiver reports of care recipients' functioning (i.e., physical limitations, behavior, and cognitive impairment) as well as various measures of caregiver well-being (London Psy-

chogeriatric Rating Scale, Hersch, Kral, & Palmer, 1978; Caregiver Social Impact Scale, Poulshock & Deimling, 1984; and SCL-90-R Derogatis, 1983).

As noted by Vitaliano and colleagues (1991b), a conceptual concern is whether hassles are indicative of burden. For example, some responsibilities may be perceived as a hassle, but whether such tasks are reflective of actual burden is not assessed by the CHS. The time frame of the CHS is another issue; Vitaliano and colleagues (1991b) note that limiting the time frame of the CHS to a weekly basis may obscure the fact that some responsibilities or demands may not have occurred in the past week but are still a source of significant worry to the caregiver. Stephens and Kinney emphasize (1989), however, that restricting the time frame of the measure enhances precision. In sum, the CHS can potentially serve as an effective compliment to general measures of burden.

## Perceived Burden Measure

The Perceived Burden Measure assesses the amount of support the caregiver provides and the associated levels of stress for 15 care responsibilities (Macera et al., 1993). Areas of assistance range from walking to yard work. The Perceived Burden Measure was administered as an in-home interview to 82 caregivers of family members with a diagnosis of dementia.

"The number of patient needs" was the sum of items for which the patient required assistance in the previous month. "The number of caregiver tasks" was the sum of items for which the patient required assistance and the caregiver provided help. The range of both of these subscales is 0–15. "Perceived burden" was defined as the sum of items for which the caregiver provided assistance that was deemed stressful. The range of the perceived burden subscale (or the Perceived Burden Measure) is 0–15, and the alpha coefficient was 0.87 in the original analysis. Construct validity was also determined, and the Perceived Burden Measure was significantly correlated with the CES-D (Radloff, 1977).

The Perceived Burden Measure has several strengths, including its practical format and ease of administration. It is also focused on specific care tasks, as opposed to more general measures of burden. The small sample size, however, makes it difficult to confirm findings of reliability or validity. In addition, the dichotomous coding schemes do not allow for an assessment of how stressful each individual care responsibility is to the caregiver.

## Caregiving Burden Scale

Although caregiving research emphasizes the need for assessment tools that are generalizable and multifaceted, there have been several efforts to develop more specific measures of burden. Gerritsen and van der Ende (1994) note that the conceptual diversity present in the literature makes it difficult to determine the impact of caregiving burden on care recipients' functioning and caregivers' psychological well-being. Therefore, Gerritsen and van der Ende developed a measure that highlighted two dimensions of burden: the quality of the caregiver–care recipient relationship and the limitations in the personal life of the caregiver.

The sample used to test the Caregiving Burden Scale consisted of 89 caregivers of psychogeriatric patients. All care recipients suffered from some form of senile dementia. Items in the Caregiving Burden Scale were derived from previously developed measures (Vernooij-Dassen, 1993; Zarit et al., 1980). The face validity of the items were assessed with the consultation of academics, caregivers, and students ($n = 39$). Additional factor analyses identified two major components of the scale: "personal consequences" (or the subjective impact of care provision on the caregiver [6 items]) and "relationship" (which represented negative evaluations of the caregiver–care recipient relationship [7 items]). Item responses include "disagree very much" (1), "disagree" (2), "agree on the one hand, disagree on the other" (3), "agree" (4), and "agree very much" (5). These responses are then re-coded as dichotomies ($1 - 2 = 0$; $3 - 5 = 1$).

Internal reliability was strong for the entire measure ($\alpha = 0.84$) and for the subscales (relationship = 0.77; personal consequences = 0.77, respectively). Construct validity was also established, with correlations present among the Caregiving Burden Scale, depression, and deviant behavior problems. Activities of daily living dependencies were not significantly associated with the Caregiving Burden Scale. Depression was significantly related to both subscales, and deviant behavior was most strongly associated with personal consequences.

Although Gerritsen and van der Ende (1994) note that the correlation between the subscales was low enough to conclude that the two dimensions were distinct (i.e., $r = 0.58$), the degree of association warrants some concern when characterizing the Caregiving Burden Scale as "multidimensional." In addition, the reliance on dichotomous scoring, although not necessary, does reduce the measure's ability to assess the severity of burden. Also, larger samples are needed to demonstrate the validity, reliability, and factor structure of the Caregiving Burden Scale.

### Novel Caregiver Burden Scale (NCB)

Although Sweden has an extensive and well-integrated formal care system, the family is still the major provider of assistance to the elderly. Elmståhl, Malmberg, and Annerstedt (1996) developed a Novel Caregiver Burden (NCB) scale to assess burden among family caregivers of patients who suffered stroke in Malmö, Sweden. Reliability and factor analyses were studied using 150 family caregivers of dementia or stroke patients. Various aspects of validity were examined among a group of 35 family caregivers of stroke patients.

The 20 item NCB was largely based on a previous measure developed by Oremark (1988) that assessed subjective burden among caregivers of chronically ill older persons. Item responses include "not at all" (1), "seldom" (2), "sometimes" (3), and "often" (4). Factor analyses revealed five dimensions of burden: general strain (8 items), isolation (3 items), disappointment (5 items), emotional involvement (3 items), and environment (3 items). The reliability for general strain, isolation, disappointment, and emotional involvement were high ($\alpha = 0.87$, $\alpha = 0.70$; $\alpha = 0.76$; $\alpha = 0.70$, respectively). Reliability for the environment subscale was low ($\alpha = 0.53$). Limited construct validity was also found; the total score of the NCB was significantly correlated with the patient's degree of extroversion and quality of life (see Eysenck & Eysenck, 1964; Jadbäck, Nordbeck, Hagberg, & Johansson, 1993).

Although there is some evidence that the NCB is useful for different types of caregivers, there are several limitations. First, some of the dimensions specified in the analysis by Elmståhl and associates (1996) show little conceptual distinction from more global measures of well-being (e.g., isolation). In addition, there is a need to better demonstrate the psychometric properties of the measure; it is unknown if the dimensions of the NCB exhibit construct validity with measures of care recipient functioning or caregiver well-being.

### Caregiving Appraisals

As is evident from the earlier review of measures, caregiving burden has attracted a great deal of attention in the literature. Early analyses of burden served as the foundation for later efforts that sought to conceptualize caregiving as a complex process characterized by multiple components. In many instances, these models developed new, more specific instruments designed to assess caregiving impact, although their relation to general measures of burden are readily apparent.

Several studies have focused on caregivers' subjective appraisals (emotional reactions) of care demands and tasks. In many ways, subjective appraisals are similar to subjective dimensions of burden. Appraisals are, however, more directly associated with the responsibilities of caregiving. In addition, subjective appraisals are not necessarily negative; several studies have attempted to document the positive nature of care provision to disabled older adults. Some measures that assess caregivers' subjective appraisals are reviewed below.

### Caregiver Appraisal Measure

Several conceptual contributions have adopted a diversified approach when determining the stress of a particular care demand. The occurrence of a care demand is not necessarily indicative of stress; rather, stress is determined by subjective appraisal (Lazarus & Folkman, 1984). For the most part, research has emphasized the negative aspects of care provision, but subjective appraisal is not inherently negative or positive.

Lawton and coworkers (1989) proposed a multifaceted model of caregiving appraisal that entailed several dimensions. Data from two studies of caregiving were analyzed to empirically confirm this conceptual approach. The first analysis was based on data from a respite evaluation that included 632 caregivers of older adults with dementia. The second analysis included 123 family caregivers of impaired older adults who had either applied or were screened for nursing home admission.

The 47 items of the Caregiver Appraisal Measure augment standard measures of burden with items that potentially tap positive dimensions of the caregiving experience. Each item is scored with two 5 point scales that ask the extent to which the statement is true ("never" to "nearly always") and the extent to which the caregiver agrees ("strongly agree" to "strongly disagree"). A factor analysis was conducted in both studies that confirmed the presence of five factors: *(1)* subjective caregiver burden, represented by poor health, isolation, loss of control, and depression; *(2)* caregiving impact, or the effect of care provision on one's social life (e.g., negative family relations, lack of privacy, restriction on socialization); *(3)* caregiving mastery; *(4)* caregiving satisfaction; and *(5)* caregiving ideology (e.g., family tradition, religious tradition). For subsequent analyses, Lawton and associates (1989) excluded the caregiving ideology factor because it was most heavily correlated with lower education (as opposed to other factors in the model). In addition, caregiving mastery was dropped because its factor structure was not as consistent as the other three dimensions. (Table 11.8 lists the 18 items that comprise the three factors.)

Internal consistencies were similar across the respite and institutionalization samples (subjective burden = 0.85 and

**Table 11.8.**
Caregiver Appraisal Measure

*Measured on five-point scales with responses either from "never" to "nearly always" or from "strongly agree" to "strongly disagree."*

*Subjective Burden*

You can fit in most of the things you need to do in spite of the time taken by caring for _____
It's hard to plan things ahead when _____'s needs are so unpredictable
Taking care of _____ gives you a trapped feeling
Because of the time you spend with _____, you don't have enough time for yourself
Your health has suffered because you are caring for _____
Your social life has suffered because you are caring for _____
You are very tired as a result of caring for _____
You will be unable to care for _____ much longer
You have lost control of your life since _____'s illness

*Caregiving Satisfaction*

You really enjoy being with _____
Taking responsibility for _____ gives your self-esteem a boost
Helping _____ has made you feel closer to him/her
_____ shows real appreciation of what you do for him/her
_____'s pleasure over some little things gives you pleasure

*Caregiving Impact*

_____ currently affects your relationships with other family members in a negative way
Caring for _____ doesn't allow you as much privacy as you would like
You are uncomfortable having friends over because of _____
Caring for _____ has interfered with your use of space in your home

Source: Lawton et al. (1989).

0.76, respectively; caregiving satisfaction = 0.67 and 0.68, respectively; caregiving impact = 0.70 and 0.65, respectively). There was also some evidence of construct validity; significant associations among the three subscales and measures of affective states, quality of the caregiver–care recipient relationship, and emotional burden were found (Vitaliano et al., 1991b).

By taking a more comprehensive approach to assessing caregiving impact, the Caregiver Appraisal Measure represents a major step forward. The incorporation of an appraisal model provides a framework to explore the complex interrelationships among positive and negative dimensions of stress. Lawton and associates (1989) caution the use of the Caregiver Appraisal Measure subscales, however, because their confirmation via factor analyses was not conclusive. In addition, it is necessary to further explore the psychometric properties of burden, satisfaction, and impact.

### Caregiving Uplifts

In addition to assessing daily hassles, Kinney and Stephens (1989a) analyzed the potential "uplifts" of family caregiving. Using a 110 item Caregiver Hassles and Uplifts Scale (the CHUS, which was later pared down to focus only on caregiver hassles; see earlier), 60 caregivers of family members with Alzheimer's disease were asked whether a certain event was a hassle, an uplift, or neither. The four categories in the CHUS are ADL limitations (12 items), care recipients' cognitive status (20 items), care recipients' behavior (53 items), and items involving the practical and logistical aspects of care provision (25 items). In the CHUS, caregivers indicate whether or not an event has occurred in the past week and, for each occurring item, rate how much of a hassle or uplift the event was on a 4 item scale. Response categories range from "not at all" to "a great deal." A total uplift score is created by summing across all of the items, and the CHUS also provides subscale uplift scores.

Sixteen items reported hassles only, and 1 item reported an uplift only. Most items could be seen as both. The items most frequently endorsed as uplifts, all of which were endorsed by half or more of the sample, were seeing the recipient calm, pleasant interactions between care recipient and family, seeing care recipient responsive, care recipient showing affection, friends showing understanding about caregiving, family showing understanding about caregiving, care recipient recognizing familiar people, care recipient being cooperative, leaving care recipient with others at home, care recipient smiling/winking, being in the care recipient's presence, and receiving caregiving help from family.

Intercorrelations within each subscale were analyzed to provide evidence for multiple dimensions of uplift. The test–retest reliability of the total uplift score was 0.89 at a 1 day interval, and the internal reliability of the uplift subscales ranged from 0.71 to 0.90. In terms of construct validity, total uplift scores were not related to indicators of well-being (i.e., SCL-90-R, Caregiver Social Impact Scale; see Derogatis, 1983; Poulshock & Deimling, 1984). The ADL and Behavior Uplift Subscales were significantly associated with depression; however, caregivers who reported greater uplift on these subscales were more likely to experience depression.

The length of the CHUS makes it a difficult measure to include or administer in a comprehensive analysis of caregiving. Moreover, the fact that most caregiving events could be interpreted by some as hassles and some as uplifts renders it difficult to derive a short "uplifts" scale. In addition, the "uplifts" approach should not be considered a measure of caregiving satisfaction because its items are derived narrowly in reaction to daily caregiving tasks. Other research suggests that satisfactions found in caregiving are related to more general phenomena such as fulfilling duty, demonstrating competence, reciprocating love of the care recipient, feeling close to the care recipient, and enjoying the care recipient's company (Reinardy et al., 1999; Kane & Penrod, 1995). In sum, the findings of Kinney and Stephens (1989a) raise some interesting implications for the role of uplifts in the caregiving situation; for example, uplifts may not necessarily serve to "buffer" stress and alleviate negative mental health. Instead, uplifts may be a result of caregivers attempting to find meaning in a situation fraught with chronic stress.

### The Picot Caregiver Rewards Scale (PCRS)

The Picot Caregiver Rewards Scale (PCRS) includes general positive feelings that are not tapped in the Uplifts Scale just discussed. The 16 item PCRS (Table 11.9) was derived from the choice and social exchange theory (Nye, 1978), caregiver interviews, and a review of the literature (Picot et al., 1997). The PCRS is administered via an in-person interview and was tested on a nonrandom sample of 83 African-American female caregivers and a random sample of 256 African-American and white caregivers who provided assistance to an elderly relative.

The PCRS was hypothesized to contain two subscales: (1) external rewards, which consist of verbal and/or nonverbal praise from God, health care professionals, and the care receiver; and (2) internal rewards, which represent caregivers' feelings of personal achievement and growth. Caregivers were asked to rate items that assessed the pleasant feelings, positive consequences, and satisfaction associated with care. Item

**Table 11.9.**

Picot Caregiver Reward Scale

*Now I'd like to ask you about some of the ways people feel about caring for another person. Please tell me how you feel now about caring for your _____. Choose only one answer for each statement from the following (responses: 5 point scale ranging from "a great deal" [4] to "not at all" [0]):*

1. I feel God will bless me
2. I feel better about myself
3. I feel I have become a stronger, tolerant, and/or patient person around persons with sickness or handicaps
4. I feel having others say that taking care of my relative is the right thing to do is important
5. I feel that my relative will remember me in his/her will for my care
6. I feel someone will take care of me when I need it
7. I feel nurses, doctors, and social workers work hard to care for my _____ too
8. I feel that placing my _____ in a nursing home will be avoided
9. I feel that doctors, nurses, and social workers do not know everything about my _____'s chances for getting better
10. I feel receiving a smile, touch, or eye contact from my _____ is important
11. I feel I have a closer relationship with my _____
12. I feel I have an opportunity to repay my _____ for a past debt
13. I feel receiving a "Thank you" from my _____ is important
14. I feel I have become a better person by learning new information
15. I feel I have become a better person by learning new ways to care for the elderly
16. I feel that I have made many new friends
17. I feel more important
18. I feel I have the freedom to make decisions that matter
19. I feel I do not need to hold a job
20. I feel receiving praise and admiration for my efforts from doctors, nurses, and social workers is important
21. I feel I can now plan my own schedule each day
22. I feel happier now than I did before I started caring for my _____
23. I feel that caring for my _____ has made our family grow and work closer together
24. I feel my family members now look up to me because of my efforts under difficult circumstances
25. [If caregiver lives with respondent/elder care recipient] I feel having my relative live with me means added money coming into the house

responses were on a 5 point scale, ranging from "not at all" (0) to "a great deal" (4). A confirmatory factor analysis provided empirical support for a unidimensional approach in scoring the PCRS. The internal consistency of the PCRS was high (α = 0.88). Picot and colleagues (1997) performed several additional psychometric analyses of the measure, which generally provided good evidence for content and construct validity. Several measurement experts were consulted to confirm the content validity of the PCRS. In addition, the PCRS was reliably associated with constructs such as depression (CES-D) and caregiver burden (the Burden Interview). In contrast to other assessments of caregiver rewards and uplifts (e.g., Kinney & Stephens, 1989a), high scores on the PCRS (which reflect greater rewards) were predictive of lower depression and burden.

The PCRS represents one of the latest attempts to assess the rewards associated with caregiving, and initial psychometric results suggest that the PCRS is a reliable and valid instrument. There is a need, however, for further psychometric testing. Given that a significant portion of the sample included in the psychometric analyses was also involved in the initial generation of items, it is necessary to conduct reliability and validity analyses on independent samples. There may also be a need to distinguish between objective and subjective rewards of caregiving (Picot et al., 1997). Before using it to claim racial differences, white samples must also be tested.

### The Caregiver Reaction Assessment (CRA)

More recent analyses of caregiving impact have stressed the need for *(1)* multidimensional assessment and *(2)* the applicability of measures for older adults with a wide variety of impairments. This led to the Caregiver Reaction Assessment (CRA) of Given and coworkers (1992). Their objective was to develop a multidimensional instrument that assesses the reactions of

family caregivers of elderly relatives with chronic impairments (i.e., Alzheimer's disease, cancer, and physical debilitation; Table 11.10). After a comprehensive review of the literature as well as in-depth interviews with caregivers, Given and colleagues (1992) identified 40 items that assessed various dimensions of caregiving impact, including health, daily schedule, finances, negative impact on life, self-worth, and family support. Initially, Given and colleagues (1992) conducted an exploratory factor analysis on these 40 items with

**Table 11.10.**
Caregiver Reaction Assessment

*Responses: 5 point scale from strongly agree to strongly disagree.*

*Impact on Schedule*

I stopped work to give care
I eliminated activities from my schedule
My activities are centered on care
I visit family and friends less
I have interruptions because of care

*Caregiver's Esteem*

It is a privilege for me to give care
I want to give care
I enjoy caring
Caring makes me feel good
Caring is important to me
I can never do enough to repay
I resent having to care†

*Lack of Family Support*

It is difficult to get help
I feel abandoned
My family left me alone
Our family works together†
Others dump caring on me

*Impact on Health*

I have the physical strength to care†
I am healthy enough to care†
My health has gotten worse
I am tired all the time

*Impact on Finances*

It is difficult to pay for care
Finances are adequate†
There is a financial strain on the family

†Reverse scoring.

Source: Given et al. (1992). The scale was constructed from the article. For exact wording and ordering of items, contact author.

a sample of 377 caregivers of elderly patients who suffered from physical impairments, dementia, or a combination of both. The exploratory factor analysis led to the retention of 24 items for a subsequent confirmatory factor analysis that determined the multidimensionality of the scale. For the confirmatory analyses, an independent sample was drawn consisting of caregivers of both cancer patients (n = 276) and older adults suffering from dementia (n = 101).

The method of administration of the CRA is flexible, although items were developed in a questionnaire format. Item responses are on a 5 point scale, ranging from "strongly agree" (1) to "strongly disagree" (5). Confirmatory factor analyses identified five factors that assessed caregivers' reactions to the provision of assistance: *(1)* impact on schedule (5 items), *(2)* caregiver's esteem/self-worth (7 items), *(3)* lack of family support (5 items), *(4)* impact on physical health (4 items), and *(5)* impact on finances (3 items). The alpha coefficient within each subscale was high (schedule = 0.82; esteem = 0.90; lack of family support = 0.85; health = 0.80; finance = 0.81). To establish construct validity, the various subscales of the CRA were correlated with the CES-D depression scale (Radloff, 1977) and a checklist of ADL dependencies. All of the subscales were moderately (albeit significantly) correlated with ADL dependencies and strongly associated with depression.

The strength of the CRA is its comprehensive approach. It is a well-developed scale that has undergone rigorous psychometric testing. In addition, it is generalizable to caregivers of older adults with a variety of impairments, thereby enhancing the opportunity of comparisons across heterogeneous samples. Although Given and colleagues (1992) do not offer a theoretical model that helps to explain how the occurrence of care demands, caregiver reactions, and outcomes are interrelated, the CRA itself is a strong measurement tool.

## Aspects of the Caregiving Role

Similar to Given and colleagues (1992), Schofield and colleagues (1997) attempted to develop a "generic" measure of caregiving impact that would be applicable to different types of caregivers as well as noncaregivers. Their instrument assesses experiences directly pertinent to caregiving as well as socioemotional well-being in general. The development of the measure took place in three steps: First, the research literature was reviewed to identify relevant measures and items; second, appropriate items were incorporated into their measure; and third, exploratory interviews were conducted with various caregivers to generate additional items. A representative sample of caregivers from Victoria, Australia, were identified and initially contacted. Caregivers were defined as someone who provided assistance to an older adult or an individual suffering from a long-term illness or disability. A random sample of those who did not meet the criteria of "caregiver" were selected as noncaregivers. In all, 976 caregivers and 219 non-caregivers were identified and interviewed over the phone. An independent sample of 67 caregiver–care recipient dyads were also included for the purposes of external validation via clinical assessments.

A variety of measures were administered, most of which had been previously developed in other studies. These instruments included life satisfaction (6 items, responses are on a 5 point scale ranging from "very dissatisfied" to "very satisfied"; based on work from Headey & Wearing [1992]), positive and negative affect/psychological well-being (20 items; Watson, Clark, & Tellegen, 1988), health (single item subjective rating of health; responses include "excellent," "good," "fair," and "poor"), social support (7 items assess perceived support from family members and friends on a 5 point scale with responses ranging from "strongly disagree" to "strongly agree"; derived from the Provision of Social Relations Scale — see Turner, Frankel, & Levin, 1983), and overload (3 item measure assessing caregiver's feelings of exhaustion and fatigue on a 5 point scale ranging from "strongly disagree" to "strongly agree" — see Pearlin et al., 1990). Two additional measures were administered solely to caregivers: family environment (consisting of two 3 item measures that assess closeness and conflict in family relations; item responses include "more," "the same," or "less") and the caring role. The caring role includes three dimensions. Caregiver satisfaction is tapped by 7 items on a five-point response scale (ranging from "agree" to "disagree") that measure positive emotional reactions toward the care recipient and caregiving role (i.e., I get satisfaction seeing _____ accomplish things; caring for _____ has made me more confident dealing with others; I get a great deal of satisfaction from caring, I would really feel at a loss if _____ were not around; I worry about what would happen to _____ if something happened to me; I feel reassured knowing that as long as I am helping _____, he/she is getting the proper care; I grieve for opportunities _____ does not have). Caregiver resentment it tapped by 5 items on the same scale (i.e., I have lost control of my life since caring for _____; I regret the opportunities I don't have; my friends don't visit us as often because I am caring for _____; I care for _____ because no one else can; caring for _____ takes up most of my time and I neglect the rest of the family). Caregiver anger is tapped through 4 items on the same response scale (I am angry when I am around _____; nothing I can do seems to please _____; I am embarrassed over _____'s behavior; I feel guilty about _____). Finally, caregivers were asked to determine care recipients' ADL dependencies, severity of disability, and the extent of problematic behavior. For the final three measures,

clinician assessments were used to determine construct validity. The internal reliabilities for all of the measures ranged from $\alpha = 0.60$ to $\alpha = 0.88$.

A major strength of the approach of Schofield and coworkers (1997) is that their assessment instruments are applicable to caregivers across various disabilities. In addition, the positive aspects of caregiving are considered. For these reasons, the analysis by Schofield and colleagues represents a major progression in the assessment of caregiving. It must be noted that the validity of the measures used to assess caregivers' reactions was not determined, and it is not clear how different constructs are related to each other in a theoretical sense. The instruments developed by Schofield and colleagues, however, show great potential across a wide range of settings.

### The Stress Process Model

Earlier in this chapter, we highlighted the noteworthy contributions made by Pearlin and associates (see Aneshensel et al., 1995; Pearlin et al., 1990). Here we describe the actual measures this research group developed for primary and secondary stressors unique to their model: role overload, role captivity, loss of intimate exchange, family conflict, work conflict, and financial strain. All have the advantage of being brief measures, and all have been carefully studied. Table 11.11 lists these measures' specific items.

Appraisals of primary stress are divided into three related dimensions: *role overload, role captivity,* and *loss of intimate exchange.* Role overload refers to feelings of exhaustion and fatigue due to the occurrence of care demands and is assessed by three items that reflect the "energy level and time it takes to do things." Item responses are on a 4 point scale ranging from "not at all" (1) to "completely" (4). Similarly, role captivity represents the involuntary aspects of caregiving; caregivers feel trapped and have no choice in their

## Table 11.11.
Measures Specifying the Caregiver Stress Process

*Role Captivity*

*How much does each statement describe your thoughts about your caregiving (very much, somewhat, just a little, not at all)? How much do you*
1. Wish you were free to lead a life of your own
2. Feel trapped by your relative's illness
3. Wish you could just run away

*Role Overload*

*How much does each statement describe you (completely, quite a bit, somewhat, not at all)?*
1. You are exhausted when you go to bed at night
2. You have more to do than you can handle
3. You don't have time just for yourself
4. You work hard as a caregiver but never seem to make any progress

*Loss of Intimate Exchange*

*How much have you personally lost the following (completely, quite a bit, somewhat, not at all)?*
1. Being able to confide in your relative
2. The person whom you used to know
3. Having someone who really knew you well

*Family Conflict*

*How much disagreement have you had with anyone in your family concerning any of the following issues (quite a bit of disagreement, some disagreement, just a little disagreement, no disagreement)?*
1. The seriousness of your relative's memory problem
2. The need to watch out for your relative's safety
3. What things your relative is able to do for himself/herself
4. Whether your relative should be placed in a nursing home
*How much disagreement have you had with people in your family because they*
1. Don't spend enough time with your relative
2. Don't do their share in caring for your relative
3. Don't show enough respect for your relative
4. Lack patience with your relative
5. Don't visit or telephone you enough
6. Don't give you enough help
7. Don't show enough appreciation for your work as a caregiver
8. Give you unwanted advice

*Work Conflict*

*Do you strongly agree, agree, disagree, or strongly disagree with these statements about your present work situation?*
1. You have less energy for your work
2. You have missed too many days
3. You have been dissatisfied with the quality of your work
4. You worry about your relative while you're at work
5. Phone calls about or from your relative interrupt your work

*Financial Strain*

*Compared with just before you began to take care of your relative (responses: much less than now, somewhat less than now, about the same, somewhat more than now, much more than now):*
1. How would you describe your total household income from all sources?
2. How would you describe your monthly expenses?
3. In general, how do your family finances work out at the end of the month? *(response: not enough to make ends meet, just enough to make ends meet, some money left over)*

Source: Pearlin et al. (1990).

role responsibilities. Role captivity is assessed on a 3 item measure that asks respondents to describe their thoughts and feelings as caregivers. Item-responses are on a four-point scale ranging from "not at all" (1) to "very much" (4). Loss of intimate exchange represents decrements in the caregiver's personal relationship with the care recipient due to the progression of illness. Three items measure the extent to which the caregiver has lost affective aspects of his or her relationship with the care recipient. Item responses range from "completely" (1) to "not at all" (4).

Secondary stressors include *family conflict, work strain,* and *financial strain.* Family conflict is assessed on a 12 item measure that asks caregivers to determine the degree of interpersonal tension they have experienced with other family members due to *(1)* the severity of the patient's condition, *(2)* the involvement of other family members with the care recipient, and *(3)* family members' treatment of the caregiver. Response categories range from "no disagreement" (1) to "quite a bit" (4). Individuals are also provided with several statements representing the degree of job–caregiving conflict experienced due to care responsibilities. Work strain was measured on a 5 item scale, with item responses ranging from "strongly disagree" (1) to "strongly agree" (4). Financial strain represents the pressure on family finances due to expenditures of care and decreased earnings. Financial strain is assessed by three indicators that determine the following: *(1)* expenditures due to care (one item on a five-point scale, with responses ranging from "much less now" [5] to "much more now" [1]); *(2)* whether there is enough money to make ends meet on a month-to-month basis (one item on a 3 point scale with responses ranging from "not enough to make ends meet" [3] to "some money left over" [1]), and; *(3)* reductions in total household income over time.

The various dimensions of subjective and secondary stress have been included in a number of empirical analyses (e.g., Aneshensel et al., 1993, 1995; Gaugler et al., 1999; Semple, 1992; Zarit et al., 1998). The primary evaluation of these components, however, took place in the Caregiver Stress and Coping Study, a longitudinal analysis of 555 family caregivers of elderly relatives suffering from Alzheimer's disease or related forms of dementia (Aneshensel et al., 1995). Respondents were interviewed at year-long intervals to determine their caregiving experiences and the status of the care recipient (e.g., at home, institutionalized, or passed away).

All of the appraisals of primary stress showed good reliability at baseline (role overload = 0.78; role captivity = 0.83, loss of intimate exchange = 0.76). In addition, the measures demonstrated good construct validity with other indicators of the stress process. Over a 1 year period, ADL dependencies were significantly predictive of role overload, severity of the care recipient's cognitive impairment was associated with loss of intimate exchange, and problematic behavior was predictive of role captivity. In addition, problematic behavior was reliably predictive of role overload and role captivity over a 3 year period. The longitudinal analysis by Aneshensel and associates also found that role overload was significantly associated with depression (as measured by the HSCL; see Derogatis et al., 1971) over a 1 year period, with loss of intimate exchange and role captivity indirectly impacting depression. Finally, over a 3 year period, both role overload and role captivity were directly related to depression. Additional analyses have found that appraisals of primary stress (role captivity in particular) play an important role in the institutionalization process (Aneshensel et al., 1993).

As with appraisals of primary stress, secondary stressors showed good internal reliability (family conflict = 0.90; work conflict = 0.75). Because of the heterogeneous items included in the financial strain measure, it was not possible to determine internal consistency. Although several studies have conducted factor analyses on the family conflict measure to determine the presence of multiple dimensions (Gaugler et al., 1999; Semple, 1992), the high intercorrelations between subscales warrant the use of a unidimensional approach. Secondary stressors showed good construct validity over a 1 year period. Both family conflict and work conflict were related to role captivity, while a single indicator of financial strain (changes in income) was significantly associated with role overload. Both family conflict and work conflict were predictive of depression, as well. Secondary stress did not, however, appear to play an important role in depressive symptomatology over a 3 year period.

In sum, the various measures developed by Pearlin and colleagues represent a multidimensional, theoretically guided approach to understanding the caregiving process. There are, however, some limitations. For example, the small number of items used to measure appraisals of primary stress may not capture the actual extent of overload, captivity, or loss of intimate exchange. For this reason, recent analyses have added new items to these measures (see Zarit et al., 1998). In addition, more research must be conducted to determine the role of secondary stress in the caregiving process, and the positive impact of caregiving does not receive adequate attention in the Stress Process Model. Even with these limitations, the Stress Process Model remains a comprehensive theoretical framework that has significantly added to our understanding of the caregiving experience.

## CONCLUSIONS AND FUTURE ISSUES

There is certainly no shortage of instruments to draw on when measuring family caregiving. Many have been developed in a research context with careful attention to their psychometric properties, but are also sufficiently brief to be helpful in clinical situations. Some of the instruments described in this chapter are most appropri-

ate for caregivers of people with dementia, whereas others are more generic. Nonetheless, the assessment of caregiving impact needs further development in terms of instrumentation, and much work is needed to advance practical applications.

### Better Measures of Caregiving Inputs

Most measures focus on caregiving impact (often the dependent variable of interest), but better measures of caregiving inputs are needed. The usual approach is to ask about the performance of caregiving tasks within a specified time period. Each type of task (e.g., ADL assistance, housekeeping assistance) can be classified in a variety of ways: dichotomously as present or not present, on a rating scale to tap intensity of care, or, if the time period is recent and short enough, an accounting of actual hours or minutes spent on a particular task. Unless the time period is quite recent, caregivers' recall is unlikely to be accurate, but when certain events are relatively rare (e.g., bringing a relative to the doctor, helping with exercises), a 1 or 2 week time window might be insufficient to capture them for many people who actually perform these tasks. Also, because so many tasks are accomplished together, research that seeks actual time estimates might be better served to make clear the types of help that will count and then determining the time spent on *all* types of care. Although some promising work with diaries and other assessment tools has been performed recently, there is a need to test and compare these methods with more traditional measures of caregiving inputs (e.g., Davis et al., 1997; Jones, 1994). Also of interest for clinicians would be some way to assess the capability and adequacy of family caregivers. Such a measure could be used to help target caregiver instruction and also to determine when formal care may be necessary.

### Item-Weighting and Refinement of Measures

The refinement of caregiving measures also deserves attention in future research. Even in measurements that adopt a multidimensional approach, all items are assumed to impact caregivers to the same degree. It may be, however, that certain care demands within the same construct/dimension may exert a greater influence on adaptation than others (e.g., incontinence during the night time hours vs. hallucinations). Statistical procedures such as weighting, however, have not been consistently applied among measures of caregiving impact. Doing so may better reflect the severity of certain care demands.

## Dementia Focus

Many caregiver measures were developed as dementia specific. Although they may readily be extended to people with diseases that are also accompanied by cognitive loss (Parkinson's, stroke), it would be useful to generate items that are specific to other chronic illnesses and disabilities. More generic instruments should be developed and refined, as well. Many items on the scales presented here are pertinent to a variety of conditions requiring care (e.g., time demands, anxieties about safety, sense of isolation), but more work is needed to develop and test generic tools.

## Positive Dimensions of Caregiving

Several instruments include positive aspects of family caregiving, and a few tap positive dimensions exclusively. This is an important area of work to continue. Emphasizing the negative in our measures tends to "pathologize" caregiving and may inadvertently socialize family caregivers to expect burden.

## Natural History of Caregiving Not Well Measured

Although family caregiving is a dynamic process, little is known about support patterns in early stages of need. It is difficult to characterize the onset of family care because, until it takes on rather large proportions, it seems to be part of everyday life. The lack of tools available to describe the onset of care provision precludes a thorough critique of the concept of "primary caregiver" or an examination of caregiving dynamics.

## Care Recipient's Perspective Is Lacking

Because so much focus has been directed at nurturing, supporting, and minimizing the negative implications of caregiving, almost nothing is known about how the care recipient reacts to family care. Similarly, we know little about the features of family caregiving that are most associated with satisfaction among care recipients. It would be useful to have some common way of asking the older person about family caregiving.

## Incorporating Measures into Practice

Professionals such as hospital discharge planners, community-based care managers, or home care providers make judgments about family care. They use these judgments to determine whether the older person is safe at home (is there enough family care of adequate quality?) and whether formal care is needed (how is the family caregiver adapting?). Increasingly, some standardized questions on family care have been inserted into comprehensive assessments of older people, and the assessor is enjoined to speak to the family member who fills out that portion of the instrument. In practice, however, there seems to be a somewhat haphazard approach to assessing family care, which is surprising when one considers how far the field has advanced in the research context. Often, insufficient attention is given to who is assessed: Convenience and accessibility appear to govern the selection of the research informant rather than actual care responsibility. In addition, there is no provision for talking to multiple family caregivers when their inputs are equal. Similarly, there is no conventional wisdom about the degree of privacy needed to interview an individual about the care of a relative. Often, both the caregiver and care recipient are present when an interview is administered.

Assessing caregiving is a challenge because of the difficulties in distinguishing family care from ordinary exchanges of support and disentangling the effects of care provision from general reactions to life's challenges. Furthermore, a new development, that of using public funds to pay family members for providing care, has added another complexity in the systematic assessment of family caregiving. Despite these inherent difficulties, the last two decades have fostered remarkable progress in the development of relevant assessment tools (from almost none to a great abundance). Those instruments that have been successfully applied in research contexts should surely be used to inform and improve clinical practice and long-term care.

## REFERENCES

Aneshensel, C. S., Pearlin, L. I., Mullan, J. T., Zarit, S. H., & Whitlatch, C. J. (1995). *Profiles in caregiving: The unexpected career*. San Diego: Academic Press.

Aneshensel, C. S., Pearlin, L. I., & Schuler, R. H. (1993). Stress, role captivity, and the cessation of caregiving. *Journal of Health and Social Behavior, 34,* 54–70.

Anthony-Bergstone, C., Zarit, S. H., & Gatz, M. (1988). Symptoms of psychological distress among caregivers of dementia patients. *Psychology and Aging, 3,* 245–248.

Bengtson, V. L., & Lovejoy, M. C. (1973). Values, personality, and social structure: An intergenerational analysis. *American Behavioral Scientist, 16,* 880–912.

Bradburn, N. M., & Caplovitz, D. (1965). *Reports on happiness*. Chicago, IL: Aldine.

Caserta, M. S., Lund, D. A., & Wright, S. D. (1996). Exploring the Caregiver Burden Inventory (CBI): Further evidence for a multidimensional view of burden. *International Journal of Aging and Human Development, 43*(1), 21–34.

Cohler, B., Groves, L., Borden, W., & Lazarus, L. (1989). Caring for family members with Alzheimer's disease. In E. Light & B. Lebowitz (Eds.), *Alzheimer's disease, treatment and family stress: Directions for research* (pp. 50–105). Washington, DC: U. S. Printing Office.

Davis, K. L., Marin, D. B., Kane, R., Patrick, D., Peskind, E. R., Raskind, M. A., & Puder, K. L. (1997). The Caregiver Activity Survey (CAS): Development and validation of a new measure for caregivers of persons with Alzheimer's disease. *International Journal of Geriatric Psychiatry, 12,* 978–988.

Deimling, G. T., & Bass, D. M. (1984). *The strengths and resources of families caring for impaired elders: A report to the retirement research foundation*. Cleveland, OH: The Benjamin Rose Institute.

Deimling, G. T., & Bass, D. (1986). Symptoms of mental impairment among elderly adults and their effects on family caregivers. *Journal of Gerontology, 41,* 778–794.

Deimling, G. T., Bass, D. M., Townsend, A. L., & Noelker, L. S. (1989). Care-related stress: A comparison of spouse and adult-child caregivers in shared and separate households. *Journal of Aging and Health, 1*(1), 67–82.

Deimling, G. T., & Poulshock, S. W. (1985). The transition from family-in-home care to institutional care. *Research on Aging, 7,* 563–576.

Derogatis, L. R. (1983). *SCL-90-R administration, scoring, and procedures manual* (vol. 2). Baltimore, MD: Clinical Psychometric Research.

Derogatis, L. R., Lipman, R. S., Covi, L., & Rickels, K. (1971). Neurotic symptom dimensions. *Archives of General Psychiatry, 24,* 454–464.

Elmståhl, S., Malmberg, B., & Annerstedt , L. (1996). Caregiver's burden of patients 3 years after stroke assessed by a Novel Caregiver Burden Scale. *Archives of Physical Medicine and Rehabilitation, 77,* 177–182.

Eysenck, H. J., & Eysenck, S. (1964). *Manual of the Eysenck Personality Inventory*. London: Brown Knight & Truscott Ltd.

Folstein, M. F., Folstein, S., & McHugh, P. R. (1975). Mini-mental state: A practical method for grading the cognitive state of patients for the clinician. *Journal of Psychiatric Research, 12,* 189–198.

Gaugler, J. E., Zarit, S. H., & Pearlin, L. I. (1999). Caregiving and institutionalization: Perceptions of family conflict and socioemotional support. *International Journal of Aging and Human Development, 49*(1), 15–38.

Gelfand, D. E. (1982). *Aging: The ethnic factor*. Boston: Little, Brown.

George, L. E., & Gwyther, L. P. (1986). Caregiver well-being: A multidimensional examination of family caregivers of demented adults. *Gerontologist, 26*(3), 253–259.

Gerritsen, J. C., & van der Ende, P. C. (1994). The development of a care-giving burden scale. *Age and Ageing, 23,* 483–491.

Given, C. W., Given, B., Stommel, M., Collins, C., King, S., & Franklin, S. (1992). The Caregiver Reaction Assessment (CRA) for caregivers to persons with chronic physical and mental impairments. *Research in Nursing and Health, 15,* 271–283.

Greene, J. G., Smith, R., Gardiner, M., & Timbury, G. C. (1982). Measuring behavioural disturbance of elderly demented patients in the community and its effects on relatives: A factor analytic study. *Age and Ageing, 11,* 121–126.

Hamilton, M. (1967). Development of a rating scale for primary depressive illness. *British Journal of Social and Clinical Psychology, 6,* 278–296.

Hassinger, J. M. (1986). *Community-dwelling dementia patients whose relatives sought counseling services regarding patient care: Predictors of institutionalization over a one-year follow-up.* Unpublished Ph.D. thesis, University of Southern California, Los Angeles.

Headey, B., & Wearing, A. J. (1992). *Understanding happiness: A theory of subjective well-being.* Melbourne: London Cheshire.

Hersch, E. L., Kral, V. A., & Palmer, B. (1978). Clinical value of the London Psychogeriatric Rating Scale. *Journal of the American Geriatrics Society, 26,* 348–354.

Hill, R., Foote, N., Aldous, J., Carlson, R., & MacDonald, R. (1970). *Family development in three generations.* Cambridge, MA: Schenkman.

Horowitz, A., & Dobrof, R. (1982). *The role of families in providing long-term care to the frail and chronically ill elderly living in the community.* New York: Hunter College, Brookdale Center on Aging.

Jadbäck, G., Nordbeck, B., Hagberg, B., & Johansson, B. (1993). Livskvalitet efter stroke. *Sjuksköterstidningen, 7,* 216–219.

Jones, C. J. (1994). Household activities performed by caregiving women: Results of a daily diary study. *Journal of Gerontological Social Work, 23*(1/2), 109–134.

Kane, R. A., & Kane, R. L. (1981). *Assessing the Elderly: A Practical Guide to Measurement.* New York: Springer.

Kane, R. A., & Penrod, J. D. (Eds.) (1995). *Family caregiving in an aging society: Policy perspectives.* Thousand Oaks, CA: Sage.

Kiecolt-Glaser, J. K., Dura, J. R., Speicher, C. E., Trask, O. J., & Glaser, R. (1987). Chronic stress and immunity in family caregivers of Alzheimer's disease patients. *Psychosomatic Medicine, 3,* 523–535.

Kinney, J., & Stephens, M. (1989a). Hassles and uplifts of giving care to a family member with dementia. *Psychology and Aging, 4*(4), 402–408.

Kinney, J., & Stephens, M. A. P. (1989b). Caregiver Hassles Scale: Assessing the daily hassles of caring for a family member with dementia. *Gerontologist, 28,* 328–332.

Kowloski, F., & Montgomery, R. J. V. (1995). The impact of respite use on nursing home placement. *Gerontologist, 35,* 67–74.

Lawton, M. P., & Brody, E. M. (1969). Assessment of older people: Self-maintaining and instrumental activities of daily living. *Gerontologist, 9,* 179–186.

Lawton, M. P., Kleban, M. H., Moss, M., Rovine, M., & Glicksman, A. (1989). Measuring caregiving appraisal. *Journal of Gerontology, 44*(3), P61–P71.

Lazarus, R., & Folkman, S. (1984). *Stress, appraisal, and coping.* New York: Springer.

Lazarus, R. S. (1966). *Psychological stress and the coping process.* New York: McGraw-Hill.

Lowenthal, M. F., & Berkman, P. (1967). *Aging and mental disorder in San Francisco.* San Francisco: Jossey-Bass.

Macera, C. A., Eaker, E. D., Jannarone, R. J., Davis, D. R., & Stoskopf, C. H. (1993). A measure of perceived burden among caregivers. *Evaluation and the Health Professions, 16*(2), 204–211.

McNair, D. M., Lorr, M., & Droppleman, L. F. (1971). *Profile of mood states.* San Diego: Educational and Testing Service.

Mindel, C. H. (1983). The elderly in minority families. In T. H. Brubaker (Ed.), *Family relationships in late life* (pp. 193–208). Beverly Hills: Sage.

Montgomery, R. J. V., Gonyea, J., & Hooyman, N. (1985). Caregiving and the experience of subjective and objective burden. *Family Relations, 34,* 19–25.

Montgomery, R. J. V., & Kosloski, K. (1994). A longitudinal analysis of nursing home placement for dependent elders cared for by spouses vs. adult children. *Journal of Gerontology Social Sciences, 49*(2), S62–S74.

Moritz, D. J., Kasl, S. V., & Berkman, L. F. (1989). The health impact of living with a cognitively impaired elderly spouse: Depressive symptoms and social functioning. *Journal of Gerontology, 44,* S17–S27.

Morycz, R. (1993). Caregiving families and cross-cultural perspectives. In S. H. Zarit, L. I. Pearlin, & K. W. Schaie (Eds.), *Caregiving systems: Formal and informal helpers* (pp. 67–73). Hillsdale, NJ: Lawrence Erlbaum Associates.

Morycz, R. K. (1985). Caregiving strain and

the desire to institutionalize family members with Alzheimer's disease: Possible predictors and model development. *Research on Aging, 7*(3), 329–261.

Morycz, R. K., Malloy, J., Bozich, M., & Martz, P. (1987). Racial differences in family burden: Clinical implications for social work. *Journal of Gerontological Social Work, 10,* 133–154.

Novak, M., & Guest, C. I. (1989). Application for a multidimensional Caregiver Burden Inventory. *Gerontologist, 29,* 798–803.

Nye, F. I. (1978). Is choice and exchange theory the key? *Journal of Marriage and the Family, 40,* 219–233.

Oremark, I. (1988). *ABS-eb abhörigbelastningsskala.* Paper presented at the IXth Nordic Congress of Gerontology, Bergen.

Pearlin, L. I., Mullan, J. T., Semple, S. J., & Skaff, M. M. (1990). Caregiving and the stress process: An overview of concepts and their measures. *Gerontologist, 30*(5), 583–594.

Pearlin, L. I., & Schooler, C. (1978). The structure of coping. *Journal of Health and Social Behavior, 19,* 2–21.

Picot, S. J. F., Youngblut, J., & Zeller, R. (1997). Development and testing of a measure of perceived rewards in adults. *Journal of Nursing Measurement, 5*(1), 33–52.

Poulshock, W., & Deimling, G. (1984). Families caring for elders in residence: Issues in measurement of burden. *Journal of Gerontology, 39,* 230–239.

Pruchno, R. A., Michaels, J. E., & Potashnik, S. L. (1990). Predictors of institutionalization among Alzheimer's disease victims with caregiving spouses. *Journal of Gerontology, 45,* S259–S266.

Rabins, P. V., Mace, N. L., & Lucas, M. J. (1982). The impact of dementia on the family. *Journal of the American Medical Association, 248,* 333–335.

Radloff, L. S. (1977). The Center for Epidemiologic Studies—Depression Scale: A self-report depression scale for research in the general population. *Applied Psychological Measurements, 3,* 385–401.

Reinardy, J. R., Kane, R. A., Call, K. T., & Shen, C.-T. (1999). Beyond burden: Two ways of looking at caregiving burden. *Research on Aging, 21*(1), 106–127.

Robinson, B. C. (1983). Validation of a caregiver strain index. *Journal of Gerontology, 38*(3), 344–348.

Scharlach, A. E. (1987). Relieving feelings of strain among women with elderly mothers. *Psychology and Aging, 2*(1), 9–13.

Schofield, H. L., Murphy, B., Herrman, H. E., Bloch, S., & Singh, B. (1997). Family care-giving: Measurement of emotional well-being and various aspects of the caregiving role. *Psychological Medicine, 27,* 647–657.

Semple, S. J. (1992). Conflict in Alzheimer's caregiving families: Its dimensions and consequences. *Gerontologist, 19,* 438–447.

Shanas, E. (1962). *The health of older people: A social survey.* Cambridge, MA: Harvard University Press.

Shanas, E., & Streib, G. (Eds.) (1965). *Social structure and the family: Generational relations.* Englewood Cliffs, NJ: Prentice-Hall.

Stephens, M. A. P., & Kinney, J. M. (1989). Caregiving stress instruments: Assessment of content and measurement quality. *Gerontology Review, 2*(1), 41–54.

Stone, R. (1991). Defining family caregivers of the elderly: Implications for research and public policy. *Gerontologist, 31*(6), 724–725.

Stueve, A., Vine, P., & Struening, E. L. (1997). Perceived burden among caregivers of adults with serious mental illness: Comparison of black, hispanic, and white families. *American Journal of Orthopsychiatry, 67*(2), 199–209.

Sussman, M. B. (1976). The family life of old people. In R. H. Binstock & E. Shanas (Eds.), *Handbook of aging and the social sciences.* First Edition, (pp. 218–243). New York: Van Nostrand Reinhold.

Teri, L., Truax, P., Logsdon, R., Uomoto, J., Zarit, S., & Vitaliano, P. P. (1992). Assessment of behavioral problems in dementia: The revised memory and behavior problems checklist. *Psychology and Aging, 7*(4), 622–631.

Thompson, E. H., & Doll, W. (1982). The burden of families coping with the mentally ill: An invisible crisis. *Family Relations, 31,* 379–388.

Turner, J. R., Frankel, B. G., & Levin, D. M. (1983). Social support: Conceptualization, measurement and implications for mental health. *Community and Mental Health, 3,* 67–111.

Vernooij-Dassen, M. (1993). *Dementie en thuiszorg.* Amsterdam: Swets & Zeitlinger.

Vitaliano, P. P., Russo, J., Young, H. M., Becker, J., & Maiuro, R. D. (1991a). The screen for caregiver burden. *Gerontologist, 31*(1), 76–83.

Vitaliano, P. P., Young, H. M., & Russo, J. (1991b). Burden: A review of measures used among caregivers of individuals with dementia. *Gerontologist, 31*(1), 67–75.

Watson, D., Clark, L. A., & Tellegen, A.

(1988). Development and validation of brief measures of positive and negative affect: The PANAS Scales. *Journal of Personality of Social Psychology, 54*(6), 1063–1070.

Winogrond, I. R., Fisk, A. A., Kirsling, R. A., & Keyes, B. (1987). The relationship of caregiver burden and morale to Alzheimer's disease patient function in therapeutic setting. *Gerontologist, 27*(3), 336–339.

Zarit, S. H. (1990). Interventions with frail elders and their families: Are they effective and why? In M. A. P. Stephens, J. H. Crowther, S. E. Hobfoll, & D. L. Tennenbaum (Eds.), *Stress and coping in later life families* (pp. 241–265). New York: Hemisphere Publishing Co.

Zarit, S. H. (1994). Research perspectives on family caregiving. In M. H. Cantor (Ed.), *Family Caregiving: Agenda for the Future* (pp. 9–24). San Francisco: American Society on Aging.

Zarit, S. H., Anthony, C. R., & Boutselis, M. (1987). Interventions with caregivers of dementia patients: Comparison of two approaches. *Psychology and Aging, 2*(3), 225–232.

Zarit, S. H., Reever, K. E., & Bach-Peterson, J. (1980). Relatives of the impaired elderly: Correlates of feelings of burden. *Gerontologist, 20*(6), 649–655.

Zarit, S. H., Stephens, M. A. P., Townsend, A., & Greene, R. (1998). Stress reduction for family caregivers: Effect of adult day care use. *Journal of Gerontology, 5*, S267–S278.

Zarit, S. H., Todd, P. A., & Zarit, J. (1986). Subjective burden of husbands and wives as caregivers: A longitudinal study. *Gerontologist, 26*, 260–266.

Zarit, S. H., & Zarit, J. M. (1983). Cognitive impairment. In P. M. Lewinsohn & L. Teri (Eds.), *Clinical Geropsychology* (pp. 38–81). Elmsford, NY: Pergamon Press.

Zarit, S. H., & Zarit, J. M. (1987). Molar aging: The physiology and psychology of normal aging. In L. L. Carstensen & B. A. Edelstein (Eds.), *Handbook of clinical gerontology* (pp. 18–32). Elmsford, NY: Pergamon Press.

# 12

# Assessment of Physical Environments of Older Adults

## LOIS J. CUTLER

Environmental conditions affect the growth and development of a person. This chapter defines the environment on the basis of four categories—the physical, social, psychological, and cultural—each composed of characteristics that individually or collectively affect the physical, social, and cognitive functioning of the older person. The physical environment is composed of objective, measurable characteristics such as stairs, noise, corridors, windows, and door width and is but one supporting component of the total environment. Characteristics of the psychological environment include preferences, memories, reactions, images, and sensory stimuli, and they are individual and difficult to measure. The social environment refers to the interaction of people in the older person's environment. Privacy is a measurable attribute of the social environment. Social isolation results from too much privacy, while crowding offers too little privacy. The cultural environment refers to traditions, values, norms, and symbols. The current emphasis on residential-like settings for the elderly provides a good example of the cultural environment. The combination of these four categories creates a setting. The level of characteristics present

in a setting is determined by the purpose of the setting. An environmental assessment measures the characteristics of the environment, the interaction between the users and the characteristics of their environment, and the outcome of that interaction.

Assessments are carried out in settings that range from independent living residences in the community to institutions that provide complete geriatric care. All environments can be measured against the principles of universal design, wherein a residential setting should be adaptable, supportive, accessible, and safe. Adaptability is the key element of universal design, as the needs of users change over time. A person who currently walks with a cane may someday need a wheelchair, necessitating modifications to the environment to accommodate the change. The foundation of universal design includes concepts of the diversity of people and the changes in functioning across the life span.

A variety of professionals perform environmental assessments, most often for research, management, or health care purposes. The practicality of an environmental assessment suggests that families, too, can benefit from assessing their current living conditions. By creating an awareness of deficiencies in the environment, a proactive approach toward finding solutions can be taken rather than reacting to a crisis situation when time is often at a premium. Along with identifying goals of assessing different settings, this chapter describes environmental measures currently available and provides suggestions for determining if an environment can not only sustain normal aging but also compensate for losses in cognitive and physical functioning.

## WHY IS ASSESSING THE ENVIRONMENT IMPORTANT?

As the aging process continues and the gap between the demands of the environment and the older person's competence widens, a loss of mastery over necessary environmental characteristics can lead to older persons living limited lives in their environments or prematurely giving up their homes. Unfortunately, research in this area has been limited, but there is evidence that peoples' behavior in their environment is directly related to the design of the space and that an optimal environment is designed to meet the specific needs and preferences of an individual (Kahana, 1975; Christenson, 1990). The theoretical basis for this research is Lawton and Nahemow's Ecological Model (1973). This model theorizes that behaviors are a function of the interaction of personal factors with the physical, psychological, and social dimensions of the environment. Behavior and affect are defined as outcomes of a person's level of competence (functioning ability in the areas of biologic health, sensorimotor capacity, and cognition) interacting with an environment's level of press, or challenge.

An environment's level of press is defined as the demands placed on people by their environment. Thus, highly competent persons can function in environments that are not very supportive of their limitations, whereas less competent people func-

tion at a diminished capacity. The physical environment makes certain functions impossible while encouraging others. To perform successfully and adapt to changes in functioning, a person must match ability levels to demands of the environment. The adaptation level is the point where the person is functioning at a comfortable level relative to external demands. For example, a three-level home with multiple steps will place more demands on the person who has recently suffered a hip fracture than a single level home would. The environment can also place too little demand on the person, as in a nursing home where boredom and anxiety can result from sensory deprivation. A challenging environment raises competence by requiring problem solving. Excessive environmental demand, in relation to competence, leads to negative outcomes while inadequate demand leads to disuse. The environmental docility hypothesis, an outcome of this theory, suggests that the lower the level of competence, the greater the influence of the environment on behavior. This is not a static relationship but is dynamic as changing levels of functioning lead to changing environmental demands.

## GOALS OF ASSESSMENT

Housing the older person is a major concern that ultimately affects all of us. People of all ages want safe and comfortable housing. Although consumers, managers, policy-makers, and researchers have different reasons for assessing the environment, the goal of an environmental assessment remains the same: to determine the level of environmental characteristics present, the interaction effect between the users and the characteristics of their environment, and the outcome of that interaction.

The evolving needs of the elderly consumer, changing discretionary resources, combined with the desire to be independent and age-in-place has necessitated consumers to become involved in issues concerning their living arrangement. Losses in vision, mobility, coordination, strength, hearing, and mental functioning can cause a previously well-matched environment to become less supportive, necessitating that changes be made. An assessment can assist by determining if the present environment is detrimental to optimal functioning or, on the other hand, compensates for a loss in functioning. Does the environment compensate for a disability as well as provide a challenge? An assessment can determine the adaptability of the environment to wheelchair accessibility. An increasingly important function of an assessment is to determine if the environment hinders or facilitates caregiving. Finally, an assessment can identify if modifications to the home are possible or help determine if it is time to relocate. Whether an older person relocates to a more supportive environment or completes home modifications, other behavior and affective domains will also improve even though the underlying disease and impairment may remain the same (Connell, 1996).

Managers of congregate housing and long-term care facilities need to determine periodically how well their facility is achieving its purpose. An assessment provides quantitative measurements of resident and family satisfaction. It can indicate if expectations and preferences are being met. An assessment can also identify areas that need improvement, evaluate programs, determine resource and staff allocation, identify code compliance and staff efficiency, and assist with long-range planning.

Architects and designers acknowledge past failures when developing theories. They have had difficulty predicting the outcomes of interventions and have not been trained to work with professionals in disciplines other than design (Preiser, Rabinowitz, & White, 1988). An assessment can provide them with improved design criteria, ideas about the type of intervention to utilize and ways to test the efficacy of an intervention, as well as updated standards and guidance literature. Environ-mental research can provide design directives to architects and policy-makers with the expectation that they will not repeat past errors in future senior housing programs.

## WHAT IS BEING ASSESSED? HOW DOES AN ENVIRONMENTAL ASSESSMENT DIFFER FOR AN AGING POPULATION?

The variety of living arrangements available to older persons ranges from community independent living to settings that provide full geriatric care with an assortment of semi-independent alternatives in between. Each has a unique combination of physical characteristics. These living arrangements can be categorized by type of housing, characteristics present in the environment, and programs/services provided. Unfortunately, there is little consensus on either terminology or a systematic approach for classifying different options, but in general nursing homes focus on disabilities and other types of senior purpose–built housing focus on abilities.

Even though the type, level of characteristics, and programs/services offered in these settings differ, a basic level of physical characteristics is present in each, and these can be measured using the four standardized categories of universal design. Residential settings must adhere to the principles of being supportive, adaptable for changes in functioning, accessible, and safe. The foundation of universal design includes the concepts of the diversity of people and the dynamics of functioning across the life span. The objective of universal design is as an extension of the Americans with Disabilities Act (ADA). When the principles are followed, functioning becomes easier for all persons throughout their life spans. For example, a cut-out curb is easier for both the person pushing a baby stroller and the person using a wheelchair (Schwartz, Brent, & Hennigh, 1995; Osterberg, Davis, & Danielson, 1995). The goal of the design field is to take a proactive approach, where universal design is incorporated into all new construction. This will ensure the next generation's ability to age in place without the environment requiring major modifications.

Four characteristics define the salient issues of a successful universal environment:

- Supportive: An environment that is both therapeutic and prosthetic supports autonomy by providing a substitute for a loss in functioning and attributes that challenge the resident. The focus is on the older person's active participation rather than on passive support of disabilities as occurs in nursing homes.
- Accessible: An environment is accessible when it can be entered by a person using a wheelchair, crutches, or other mobility aids.
- Adaptable: An environment is adaptable if it can be modified or added to so as to accommodate the needs of persons with different degrees of disability and is able to respond to future changes in functioning.
- Safe: A safe environment, including the neighborhood and the physical setting, protects against hazards but is not restrictive to the point of preventing autonomy.

In addition to the characteristics that are measured by universal design, other attributes of the environment need to be addressed when assessing for an aging population. Included are private and shared spaces in purpose-built housing, prosthetic and therapeutic characteristics, location, stimulation/challenge, sensory compensatory elements, familiarity/residential appearance, personalization, territoriality, privacy, and symbolism. It is not enough that the characteristics be present; what is important is understanding the interaction of the user and his or her environment. For example, a dementia special care unit must not only be accessible to disabled persons but also include wandering paths, exit control, sensory considerations, and

orientation cues that provide a supportive environment for the residents. These features distinguish a special care unit from other settings (Zeisel, Hyde, & Levkoff, 1994).

The level at which an assessment is conducted is determined by the setting. For example, older persons who live independently but have a changed mobility status and now require a wheelchair can assess their environment for accessibility using a simple checklist. This type of assessment assists the homeowner in identifying potential modifications that can accommodate the change in functioning. For the consumer checklist to be useful, it must also include recommended design solutions and a list of product resources. An assisted living facility or special care unit requires a more elaborate assessment by which interaction effects between the physical, social, and psychological environments are measured and the absence or presence of characteristics specific to the setting are identified. Descriptions of senior housing based on a continuum from independent to purpose built, along with a sample assessment for each type, are presented in Tables 12.1 through 12.3, starting with community independent living.

In 1990, about 80% of Americans aged 55 years and over were homeowners and lived independently in their homes. Most of them preferred to age-in-place (American Association of Retired Persons, 1996). Those not living in single family houses lived independently in mobile homes, apartments, town houses, condominiums, or boarding houses. Many senior apartments are a result of a federal housing program created in the early 1960s to alleviate a shortage of housing opportunities for low-income seniors. This program created new design opportunities for senior housing, but, unfortunately, no research-based design solutions were available at the time. No services are provided in independent living situations, although services (the level depending on the adaptability of the environment) are routinely brought in. Ta-

**Table 12.1.**
Wheelchair Accessibility Checklist for the Home

| Entrance | Flooring | Living room | Kitchen | Bedroom | Bathroom |
|---|---|---|---|---|---|
| Curb cutout | Carpet pile no higher than half inch | Sturdy armchairs provide support for rising out of a chair | 60 Inch turning radius in center of room | Fitted bedspread is easier to transfer onto | 17 inch toilet or raised toilet seat facilitates transferring |
| Ramp, 1:20 pitch | No scatter rugs | Outlet 27 inches from floor | Side/side refrigerator for easy access | Higher bed to facilitate transferring | Toilet arm support |
| Door width at least 36 inches | No loop carpet | Casters on furniture allow easy passage | No over-the-counter storage | Closet rods 36–48 inches and adjustable are optimal | Transfer bath bench |
| Remove screen door | Floor sill inserts available to lower threshold | Chair raising aids are available | Roll-out shelves are very convenient | Bed rails offer security and support | Tub lift |
| Threshold no higher than one-half inch | Remove inside doors and door frames to provide additional width | | Counter height 28–36 inches is optimal | Motion sensor light offers security and convenience | Swing out door with swing clear hinges |
| Mailbox located 45 inches high | Lever door handles are easier to use | | Table 27–30 inches high with space underneath | | Horizontal and vertical grab bars 1.5 inch diameter |
| Shelf by door | | | Angled mirror over range assists with viewing | | Side wall medicine cabinet 44 inches high |
| Possible stair glides, elevator or lift | | | Range controls in front are safer and more accessible | | Walk-in shower with seat, hand-held control, and elevated drain control |
| | | | | | Lever-type faucet |
| | | | | | Angle mirror |

ble 12.1 presents an independent living accessibility checklist that focuses on wheelchair accessibility in the home. This checklist is useful for homeowners in determining if their present homes can be modified to accommodate a wheelchair user.

Falls resulting from failing senses, degenerative bone conditions, reduced muscular strength, coordination problems, and slower reaction time are the most frequent types of accident that older people have. Assessing the home for the possibilities and prevention of falls is a priority because fewer than 25% of the survivors of hip fractures will regain their prior mobility (Connell, 1996).

Semi-independent living is available in purpose-built congregate housing that provides limited support services such as at least one meal a day, transportation, activities, and often an alarm system. Assisted living facilities are a recent addition to this category of housing and include a higher level of services. The concept emerged out of a desire to provide services in a residential setting. The size, scale, and configuration of a building define a residential setting, not the cosmetic features present. Regnier (1994) noted that assisted living needs to be more than a decorated nursing home to be a viable alternative. Some of the efficiency and convenience of the nursing home comes at the cost of losses of privacy, autonomy, and independence of the residents.

Regnier (1994, p. 1) defined assisted living as "a long-term care alternative which involves the delivery of professionally managed personal and health care services in a group setting that is residential in character and appearance in ways that optimize the physical and psychological independence of residents." Kane and Wilson (1993, p. 1) define assisted living as "any group residential program that is not licensed as a nursing home, that provides personal care to persons with need for assistance in the activities of daily living (ADL), and that can respond to un-

scheduled needs for assistance that might arise." This definition focuses on services, whereas Regnier's definition focuses on the physical environment. There has been tremendous growth in the number of residential care facilities, but differences in terminology have created confusion for long-term care consumers. Table 12.2 presents examples of the four characteristics that define the salient issues of universal design. It illustrates that, when combined, the four categories create a comprehensive assessment guide.

Long-term care is defined as a set of health, personal care, and social services delivered over a sustained period of time to persons who have lost some degree of functional capacity. It is equated with a nursing home setting and uniform management of all residents (Kane & Kane, 1987). A nursing home stresses societal values of safety and physical health over a normal life style that emphasizes psychological and social well-being. Special care units are located in nursing home settings, and they typically offer geographic segregation, services tailored to dementia, specially designed environments, and special programs. Table 12.3 presents characteristics that one would expect to find in a dementia special care unit.

## WHO SHOULD PERFORM THE ASSESSMENT?

Who should assess is directly related to the purpose of the assessment. Organizations such as the American Occupational Therapy Association provide checklists that professional health care workers and social service providers can use for discharge and care plans. County extension offices and insurance companies are becoming involved by offering checklists, videos, and other informative literature to assist the consumer with performing a home assessment or when assessing facilities for relocation purposes. Facility managers often hire a marketing firm to assess their residents' satisfaction or a specific environ-

**Table 12.2.**

Categories of Universal Design that Apply to an Assisted Living Facility

| | Supportive | Accessible | Adaptable | Safe |
|---|---|---|---|---|
| | | Shared Spaces | | |
| Site attributes | Community resources within one-fourth mile Patio area with garden | Curb cuts, reserved parking, automatic door | Increased exit control for higher levels of dementia | Neighborhood low crime Security system |
| Lobby | Furniture can be rearranged for small groups Daily newspapers Resident council | Reception counter 30–34 inches Shelf by mailboxes Furniture spaced to accommodate wheelchair Signage 54–56 inches with light on dark contrast | Table lamps with adjustable intensity Different methods of communicating activities Arrangement encourages interaction but allows privacy Elevator or stairs | Visible waiting area Front door visible from reception desk |
| Dining area | Choice of tables Minimal background noise to facilitate conversation Age-appropriate music | Tables 27–30 inches high | Furniture and utensils ergonomically designed | Chairs are sturdy and have arm rests |
| Residential services | Exercise room, laundry facility | Laundry machines front loading | Laundry-adjustable shelves Instructions communicated in several ways | Windows in laundry room open to corridor |
| Corridors | Functional length Indented entry Decorations | Wide enough for passage of wheelchairs No pile carpet | Resting places along corridor Increased cueing features | Nonglare flooring Increased light levels Handrails on both sides of corridor and around corners |
| | | Private Spaces | | |
| Entry way | Personalized entry Bench to sit on to remove boots | Threshold not to exceed 0.5 inch Door width 5 feet minimum | Lighted Audible doorbell Lever handle, rocker light switches | Ability to lock door and preview guest Large type thermostat |
| Kitchen | Cooking opportunities | Counter microwave | Adjustable storage Removable cabinet under sink | Control knobs in front No garbage disposal |
| Bathroom | Lighting considerations Magnifying mirrors Toilet 18.5 inches high | Turn around and transfer space 5 feet diameter | Reinforced walls for additional bars | Door opens out, alarm system, medicine cabinet preferably in kitchen |
| Bedroom | Furnishings stable enough to provide support | Ample space to accommodate wheelchair | Low window to the world | Night light or motion sensor |

**Table 12.3.** Environmental Characteristics Found in Nursing Home Dementia Special Care Units

Exit control designed so that residents are unaware of exits, locks, and security devices
Increased surveillance
Wandering paths that are continuous with visual cues
Optical barriers
Residential scale furnished with residents' belongings
Shared spaces differentiated by function and supportive of individual use
Sensory considerations
   Cueing features
   Muted color choices
   Low lighting levels
   Low noise levels
   Low visuals
Orientation and wayfinding
Individual away spaces
Immediate access to secure outdoor area
Choice of music available in room
Support autonomy through choices

mental concern. Government inspectors are responsible for code compliance even though many are poorly trained. Academic researchers are becoming more involved in assessments, often designing instruments for a specific project that are never used again.

## CHOOSING A MEASURE

If sufficient instruments were available for assessing the environment, the task would be much easier and the outcomes more reliable. Unfortunately, past instruments have often resulted in subjective, descriptive, and global data rather than data that are objective, evaluative, and discrete. This is the result of a lack of a standardized framework or purpose for assessing the environment. In recognition of this lack of instruments, Lawton, Weisman, and Calkins (1997, p. 96) suggest that "the goal of the ideal environmental assessment battery might thus be to represent with user- and context-specific content limited ranges in each generic dimension." The book *Beautiful Barrier-Free: A Visual Guide to Accessibility* is a valuable tool for identifying

the generic dimensions that Lawton and coworkers emphasize (Leibrock, 1993).

## SOURCES OF DATA

An abundance of methods for assessing the environment are available, but unfortunately there is an over-reliance on the standard methods of interviews, observation at one point in time, or questionnaires, often completed by a proxy. The problem with these methods is that they can result in a lack of understanding of how the residents interrelate with their environment on an individual and continuing basis. It is pertinent to be aware of the ecological fallacy that patterns found at a group level will translate to an individual level. A residential satisfaction survey can be a useful assessment tool if the instrument includes questions relevant to both the resident and the family's use of the facility. Once again, however, the ecological fallacy must be avoided. Focus groups are an underused source of information in environmental assessments. A focus group offers an opportunity to observe behavior, gain individual perspectives on how well the environment works for the resident, and provides a time for socialization. A checklist for evaluation at the basic level of the presence, frequency, and location of environmental characteristics, based on code or ADA requirements, is useful for social workers and health care providers. More sophisticated methods are also available to gain a comprehensive understanding of the interaction between residents and their environment.

Observing behaviors means systematically watching how people use their environment over a period of time. "Behavioral measures, based on observation of the client's actual functioning, are particularly useful because they typically are the most direct expression of the problem and therefore tend to have a great deal of validity. Also, because behavior can be counted and defined fairly specifically, this form of measurement can add a good deal to the precision and reliability of one's assessment" (Corcoran & Fischer, 1987, p. 28). Having floor plans that detail each room by size, configuration, furnishings, and design features together with schedules of activities facilitates behavioral mapping. Observing physical traces by recording them with photographs or notations can be an unobtrusive measuring tool for the researcher studying patterns of use. Visual impressions can identify unusual patterns of wear or indicate the success or failure of furniture groupings in shared spaces. Observation, when performed reliably by trained observers over a sustained period of time, can provide an objective assessment of staff and resident behaviors. Data can be gathered through direct assessment or videotaping followed by coding by trained raters. The process is time consuming and expensive but effective if strict standardization procedures are followed. Item definitions, rater training, data collection times, and techniques all must be standardized. Use of several methods will increase the reliability of an assessment.

## METHODOLOGICAL ISSUES

Assessing an environment is not as simple as measuring blood pressure. A good assessment must take into account the setting, the users, and the interactions between the two to fully understand the person–environment fit. Bias is always a concern when assessing older persons because they assess their environments in a more positive light than experts do, and they tend to understate housing dissatisfaction. These characteristics reflect a resistance to changes, including relocation, home modification, and, to a lesser extent, support services except when linked to hospitalization. This perspective can be labeled "psychological adaptation." Elderly persons adapt psychologically and socially to their environment but not always physically. Attachment to home, resistance to change, self-reliance, and denial can all be attributed to the subjective assessment of

their home versus the objective view of the researcher. Past research has been criticized for being preoccupied with the physical side of the environment at the expense of behavioral aspects (Goland, 1991; Filion, Wister, & Coblentz, 1992). It has been found that multidimensional intervention strategies that focus on physiological, psychological, and social needs are more successful in preventing falls than are those that concentrate solely on environmental factors (Connell, 1996).

A problem with the use of proxies to obtain information is the potential of systematic errors. A multilevel, multimethod weighted approach to data collection— collection of data independently from several sources and on more than one occasion—enhances the validity of a measurement. An environment may be congruent in some respects but incongruent in others. Different aspects of the residential setting should not necessarily be assigned equal weight or salience in a consideration of their impact. Using direct observations by different raters can put reliability at risk; however, inter-rater agreement can be increased with rater training and precise measurement domains (Goland, 1991). Experience with and an understanding of the interactions of the physical, social, and psychological environment are necessary for assessing an environment. One problem with past environmental research is that standardized questionnaires with explicit instructions for coding responses have not been utilized. The policy has been to create a new instrument for each assessment, resulting in a divergent assortment of results but no central base on which to build future design solutions.

## COMMONLY USED
## ENVIRONMENT MEASURES

### Multiphasic Environmental Assessment Procedure (MEAP)

The most comprehensive environment evaluation instrument is the Multiphasic Environmental Assessment Procedure (MEAP) developed by Moos and Lemke (1996). As shown in Table 12.4, it is a five part measurement designed to evaluate the physical and social environments in nursing homes, residential care facilities, and congregate apartments, not including independent community dwellings. It was not originally designed to be used with frail elderly but is salient for this group. The MEAP is intended to analyze the relationship between the objective characteristics of a program (aggregate resident and staff characteristics, physical and policy factors), personal factors, social climate, residents' coping responses, and resident adaptation. The MEAP's Physical and Architectural Feature, Policy and Program Information Form, and Sheltered Care Environment Scale each has a Form I available to assess individual preferences or what the respondent would consider an ideal facility.

The MEAP is designed for flexibility. The scales can be administered either singly or in combination for a given facility. Moos and Lemke (1996) have included the five MEAP instruments along with a discussion of their previous use in the book *Evaluating Residential Facilities*. This book provides a comprehensive collection of checklists and scales. Lawton and coworkers (1997) consider the MEAP the most extensive and best-developed battery of environmental assessment instruments currently available.

## Satisfaction Assessment Questionnaire for Assisted Living Residents (SAQ)

The Satisfaction Assessment Questionnaire for Assisted Living Residents (SAQ) was developed by the American Health Care Association (1996) to assist facilities in measuring customer satisfaction. Factors of quality, as defined by long-term care customer groups, are measured through in-person and telephone interview with this easy-to-use instrument. Table 12.5 describes the SAQ briefly. This chapter is only concerned with the facility setting and the security and safety components of this measure. Chapter 9 provides a more

comprehensive description of satisfaction measures.

## Elderly Resident Housing Assessment Program (ERHAP)

The Elderly Resident Housing Assessment Program (ERHAP) is a computer program that assesses the housing needs of older persons living independently (Brent & Brent, 1987). As summarized in Table 12.6, this evaluation tool uses 300 design rules to identify present and potential housing inadequacies specific to the resident's health and constraints. The ERHAP is geared primarily toward social service professionals assessing the suitability of the home. The assessment takes about 75 minutes and is conducted by interview and direct observation. Photographs document problems for further analysis. Participants receive a follow-up that identifies environmental risks and modification recommendations. Minimal training of raters is necessary. A commercial version "Home Safe Home" is available (Brent & Brent, 1993).

## LivAbility

LivAbility is an easy-to-use environmental measurement tool designed for the older person living independently (Christenson, 1997). This consumer-oriented tool includes a descriptive video along with a questionnaire that focuses on the person's home environment as well as the respondent's physical characteristics, health, and fitness. The questionnaire is self-explanatory and does not need to be used in conjunction with the video, although the video could be very useful for group viewing and discussion as it provides specific tips for minimizing risks in the home environment. The core of the program is the personalized LivAbility report that is prepared from the questionnaire responses. It provides ideas and solutions specific to the respondent as well as valuable information geared toward aging-in-place. Table 12.7 summarizes the LivAbility instrument.

**Table 12.4.**

Multiphasic Environmental Assessment Procedure

| Description | Components | Data collection | Time estimate |
|---|---|---|---|
| Physical & Architectural Feature Checklist (PAF)<br><br>153 items measure location, physical features inside and outside of facility, and space allowances with a focus on availability of these resources—not their use<br><br>Form I is available to assess resident's preferences for physical resources in a facility. | Section I: Neighborhood context<br><br>Section II: Exterior of building<br><br>Section III: Interior of building<br><br>1. Community accessibility<br>2. Physical features for comfort and involvement, physical amenities<br>3. Social–recreational aids<br>4. Supportive physical features and prosthetic aids<br>5. Orientation aids<br>6. Safety features<br>7. Staff facilities<br>8. Space availability | Data collection is by direct observation and floor measurements performed by raters with additional information from staff. Most of the components are measured "yes" or "no," with values of 0 and 1 totaled for a percentage score<br><br>Individual unit scores are either on a square foot basis or a 3 part scale<br><br>Form 1 data can be collected in three ways: self-administered, group administered, or interview. Responses are "not important," "desirable," "very important," or "essential" | 2 h needed to complete checklist; additional time required if facility is large<br><br>Form I requires approximately 1 h to complete |
| Resident and Staff Information Form (RSIF)<br><br>104 scored items that measure characteristics and behaviors of residents and staff in senior congregate housing<br><br>6 subscales | 1. Resident and staff information<br>2. Resident heterogeneity<br>3. Resident functional abilities<br>4. Resident activity level<br>5. Resident activities in the community<br>6. Staff resources | Administrator and satff interviews, observation of residents and staff by rater, facility records, and optional resident questionnaires.<br><br>Scoring is either on a percentage basis or "yes/no" for resident heterogeneity and staff resource sections | 3 h to locate and tabulate data for 100 residents |
| Policy and Program Information Form (POLIF)<br><br>130 scored items that measure policies, room | 1. Expectations for functioning<br>2. Acceptance of problem behavior | Interviews with administrators and staff<br><br>Scoring is either on a "yes/no" basis or a 0/1 | 1 h. Form I also requires 1 h |

*(continued)*

## MEASURES FOR DEMENTIA SPECIAL CARE UNITS

### Professional Environmental Assessment Protocol (PEAP)

The Professional Environmental Assessment Protocol (PEAP) was developed to provide a standardized method for assessing special care units (Teresi et al., 1994). The comprehensive measure, summarized in Table 12.8, focuses on the therapeutic environment, including the physical settings, the philosophy of care, level of resi-dent capability, constraints of regulations and budget, and other organizational policy and social contexts. The assessment is at the facility level rather than on the individual resident and includes fixed, semi-fixed, and nonfixed features of the environment.

### Nursing Unit Rating Scale (NURS)

The Nursing Unit Rating Scale (NURS) measures policy and program features in dementia special care units in nursing

## Table 12.4.
### Multiphasic Environmental Assessment Procedure—Continued

| | | | |
|---|---|---|---|
| types, organization, and services.<br><br>9 subscales in 3 groups<br><br>Form I is available to measure preferences about facility polices and services | 3. Policy choice<br>4. Resident control<br>5. Policy clarity<br>6. Provision for privacy<br>7. Availability of health services<br>8. Availability of daily living assistance<br>9. Availability of social recreational activities | basis with allowed/tolerated scored as 1 and discourage/intolerable scored as 0. Individual sections are totaled for a percentage score<br><br>Form 1 is scored on a 4 point scale of "definitely not," "preferably not," "preferably yes," or "definitely yes" | |
| Sheltered Care Environment Scale (SCES)<br><br>63 yes/no items that measure the social climate of residential setting. This scale is equally useful for measuring individual levels or aggregating the scores to assess the social climate of the residents as a group<br><br>7 subscales in 3 groups<br><br>Form I assesses preferences about residential setting | 1. Relationship dimensions<br>  Cohesion<br>  Conflict<br>2. Personal growth dimensions<br>  Independence<br>  Self-disclosure<br>3. System maintenance and change dimensions<br>  Organization<br>  Resident influence<br>  Physical comfort | Scale-administered either individually by interview or in a group setting<br><br>Responses are coded yes/no and averaged for the facility | 30 min in a group or 15–30 min per resident if interviewing individual resident<br><br>Form 1 requires 15–30 min |
| Rating Scale<br><br>24 items that measure observers' impressions of physical environment and staff and resident functioning. Intended to rate subjective aspects of settings such as attractiveness, resident activity, and interactions | 1. Physical environment<br>  Physical attractiveness<br>2. Environmental diversity<br>3. Resident functioning<br>4. Staff functioning | Direct observation by trained rater<br><br>Scoring is on a 0–3 point scale that requires a subjective assessment of the facility | 15 min if completed with PAF |

Source: Moos and Lemke (1996).


## Table 12.5.
### Satisfaction Assessment Questionnaire for Assisted Living Residents

| Description | Components | Data collection | Time estimate |
|---|---|---|---|
| A three section satisfaction survey for measuring customer satisfaction. Ten themes are addressed along with an annual survey section that provides general trend data and demographic data on residents | 1. Facility setting survey<br>2. Staff survey<br>3. Management survey<br>4. Owners survey<br>5. Health and services<br>6. Transition aids<br>7. Safety and security<br>8. Family, friends, and community<br>9. Programs<br>10. Meals and dining | Resident or family in-person and/or telephone interview. This easy to use form is scored on a 5 point scale | 30 min per resident |

Source: American Health Care Association (1996).

**Table 12.6.**
Elderly Resident Housing Assessment Program

| Description | Components | Data collection | Time estimate |
| --- | --- | --- | --- |
| A 300 design rule computer program that identifies present and potential housing inadequacies in three domains and at four levels | *Domains*<br>1. Safety<br>2. Functioning<br>3. Comfort<br>*Levels*<br>1. Lighting, fire safety, electrical<br>2. Health, safety, security<br>3. Gross motor safety<br>4. Fine motor safety | Interview homeowner, direct observation, and photographs by rater | Approximately 75 min per house |

Source: Brent and Brent (1993).

facilities (Grant, 1996). This measure addresses important domains (shown in Table 12.9) at the unit level but does not consider individual levels or the interactions effect between the residents and their environment, and it is limited by staff self-report.

### The Therapeutic Environment Screening Scales (TESS)

The Therapeutic Environment Screening Scale (TESS) measures five therapeutic functions of the physical environment based on a 12 item observational scale that assess physical features of a special care unit (Table 12.10) (Sloane & Mathew, 1990). The TESS-2+ (Sloane et al., 1995), a modified version of the TESS-2, is a unit observation checklist that provides information on the physical environment of a dementia special care unit (Table 12.11). The checklist is organized in eight parts containing, collectively, 49 questions. The instrument provides a comprehensive index for quantitatively assessing the physical environment through observation but does not measure the interaction effect between the resident and the physical features of the environment. Standardized observation methods such as clear definitions of variables, careful training of raters, and standardization of data collection times and techniques attempt to minimize observer bias and increase validity. The TESS-2+ is a useful tool that could be adapted to assess a variety of purpose-built senior housing.

**Table 12.7.**
LivAbility, Choices for Better Living

| Description | Components | Data collection | Time estimate |
| --- | --- | --- | --- |
| A consumer-oriented program for assessing the independent living environment. A computer-scored questionnaire, based on individual responses, provides the basis for a personalized LivAbility report. Optional video that describes evaluation process is available | *Housing*<br>1. Living arrangement<br>2. Exterior features<br>3. Interior features<br>4. Kitchen<br>5. Laundry<br>6. Bathroom<br>7. Bedroom<br>*Physical characteristics, health, and fitness* | Consumer self-administered questionnaire formatted for computer scoring. The instructions are easy to understand, and excellent use of color assists the respondent in deciphering the different sections | Approximately 30 min to complete questionnaire Personalized LivAbility report mailed to home in about 1–2 weeks |

Source: Christenson (1997).

**Table 12.8.**

Professional Environmental Assessment Protocol

| Description | Components | Data collection | Time estimate |
|---|---|---|---|
| 8 dimension instrument for measuring a dementia special care unit. Focus on physical setting with an understanding of context of social, organizational, and policy environment | 1. Maximizes safety and security<br>2. Maximizes awareness and orientation<br>3. Supports functional abilities<br>4. Facilitates social contact<br>5. Provides privacy<br>6. Personal control opportunities<br>7. Quality and regulation of stimulation<br>8. Allows for continuity of self | Interview and direct observation by rater used to prepare narrative description and evaluation of environmental quality<br><br>Each section is scored on a 5 point scale. An example of scoring for section 3 on "supports functional abilities": a score of 5 indicates extraordinarily high support, 4 = high level of support, 3 = moderate support for competent behavior, 2 = low level of support, and 1 = support absent | Specific time not available. Expect a time-consuming process considering how comprehensive the instrument is |

Source: Teresi et al. (1994).

## Environment–Behavior Model

The Environment-Behavior Model (E-B Model) for special care units measures the relationship between environmental influences and behavioral effects, including behavior, perception, and attitudes (Zeisel et al., 1994). Each of the eight design criteria has two dimensions that represent a link between a design feature and performance criterion. The dimensions are scored along different axes on a chart with four cells that represent the most positive to the least desirable resident outcomes. Each cell of the table represents a performance-based therapeutic outcome statement. Although the scoring technique involves additional training, it is worth the effort because the instrument does predict outcomes likely to occur given the design features and the performance criteria of the setting being measured. The model assists the researcher in understanding the relationships between the purpose of a setting, the performance criteria, design decisions, and therapeutic outcomes. Even though the instrument

**Table 12.9.**

Nursing Unit Rating Scale

| Description | Components | Data collection | Time estimate |
|---|---|---|---|
| The Nursing Unit Rating Scale is a 6 domain rating scale that assesses policy and program features in SCUs that are not easily observable. The domains assess how people with dementia adapt to the institutional environment of an SCU | 1. Separation<br>2. Stimulation<br>3. Stability<br>4. Complexity<br>5. Control/tolerance<br>6. Continuity | Face-to-face or telephone interviews with supervisory nurse<br>Some questions are scored on a 5 point scale and some on a 4 point scale, and others are open-ended questions | 45 min to 1 h + |

SCU, special care unit.

Source: Grant (1996).

**Table 12.10.**

Therapeutic Environment Screening Scale — TESS-2

| Description | Components | Data collection | Time estimate |
|---|---|---|---|
| The Therapeutic Environment Screen Scale (TESS-2) is a 12 item observation scale of SCU physical features based on five therapeutic functions | *Therapeutic functions*<br>1. Noxious stimuli<br>2. Mood enhancement and self-image<br>3. Safety<br>4. Social activities<br>5. Outdoor access<br>*Physical features*<br>1. Absence of shiny or slippery floor surfaces<br>2. Absence of glare<br>3. Absence of odor or cleaning solutions<br>4. Absence of odor of bodily excretions<br>5. Absence of distracting noise<br>6. Adequate light level<br>7. Presence of personal items<br>8. Presence of home-like decor<br>9. Presence of protected accessible outdoor area<br>10. Availability of separate room for family or friends<br>11. Absence of TV use in shared space<br>12. Kitchen available for supervised resident use | Direct observation by rater to complete this 12 question checklist<br>Score ranges from 0 (worst) to 24 (best). Questions scored either no/yes or on a yes/moderate/no scale | 1 h |

SCU, Special care unit.

Source: Sloane and Mathew (1990).

**Table 12.11.**

Therapeutic Environment Screening Scale — TESS-2 + )

| Description | Components | Data collection | Time estimate |
|---|---|---|---|
| The TESS-2 +, a modified version of the Therapeutic Environment Screening Scale (TESS-2), is a unit observation checklist of the physical environment of a dementia SCU<br>The instrument is organized in 8 parts containing 49 questions | 1. General design (nursing station, resident rooms, security at exits, views to exterior and overall floor plan)<br>2. Maintenance (cleanliness, odors, and obstacles)<br>3. Space/seating (specialized areas and overall character)<br>4. Lighting<br>5. Noises (presence and control)<br>6. Residents' rooms (orientation cues, privacy, personalization, furnishings, and storage)<br>7. Programming orientation (stimulation and appearance)<br>8. Overall ratings (subjective rating of interaction involvement) | Standardized observation using standardized item definitions, raters training, data collection times, and techniques<br>This is a useful instrument, but the scoring ranges from 0/1 to 1 through 4 to a measurement of square feet and counting of environmental attributes<br>The overall rating scale is a subjective 10 point scale | 1.5 to 3 hs, depending on experience of rater |

SCU, Special care unit.

Source: Sloane et al., 1995)

**Table 12.12.**
Environment-Behavior Model for Special Care Units

| Description | Components | Data collection | Time estimate |
|---|---|---|---|
| The Environment–Behavior model (E-B Model) is composed of 8 environmental–behavior concepts along with two related dimensions that link a design feature to performance criteria | *Exit control*<br>1. Immediacy of control<br>2. Unobtrusiveness<br>*Wandering paths*<br>1. Continuousness<br>2. Wayfinding<br>*Individual away places*<br>1. Privacy<br>2. Personalization<br>*Common space*<br>1. Quantity<br>2. Variability<br>*Outdoor freedom*<br>1. Availability<br>2. Supportiveness<br>*Residential scale*<br>1. Size<br>2. Familiarity<br>*Autonomy support*<br>1. Safe<br>2. Prosthetic<br>*Sensory comprehend*<br>1. Noise management<br>2. Meaningfulness to residents | Direct observation by trained rater<br>Each dimension is rated high or low, generating four-cell tables where each cell represents a condition correlated with therapeutic outcomes, along with a performance-based therapeutic outcome statement | Approximately 1.5 h, depending on size of facility and experience of rater |

Source: Zeisel et al. (1994).

was designed for special care units, it could be adapted for assessments of other types of senior purpose–built housing. Zeisel and colleagues (1994) suggest that the concepts and elements of this model can be tested, refined, and developed employing established methods for systematic Post-Occupancy Evaluations, which is a systematic collection of data on the physical environment of a setting, the people who use the setting, and the interaction between the two. The E-B Model is summarized in Table 12.12. Table 12.13 contrasts the various environmental measures discussed in this chapter.

## CONCLUSIONS

The lack of standardized instruments is partially due to the lack of consistency and uniformity in defining industry-wide standards for senior housing. The infinite ways to describe a residential setting, combined with varying state regulations and building codes, has created a situation in which it is difficult to create a standardized tool. Universal design is the first step toward standardization and is slowly but firmly gaining in acceptance by design professionals. Universal design is a start, but it cannot be used as an isolated concept.

Time and again, environmental assessments are conducted with a single measure of observation (users or characteristics), a residential satisfaction survey, or, worse yet, an interview with a proxy as the only source of data. Interaction effects are not assessed sufficiently. An environmental assessment needs to be a process, not a single procedure. The process must take into account the goals of the setting, the management, the demographics of the occupants (needs, disabilities, preferences, and so forth), overall resident satisfaction and dissatisfaction, building performance, and occupants' use of the space. Data must come from several sources, including observation, behavioral mapping, traces,

**Table 12.13.**
Summary of Environment Measures

| Measure | Description | Psychometric | Application |
|---|---|---|---|
| MEAP (Multiphasic Environmental Assessment Procedure) (Moos & Lemke, 1996) | Five instruments: PAF, physical and architectural; POLIF, policy and programs; RESIF, resident and staff; SCES, perceived social climate; and RS, evaluates facility using direct observation, interviews, records and questionnaires | Cronbach's alpha for PAF items: community accessibility, 0.84; physical amenities, 0.71; social recreational aids, 0.73; prosthetic aids, 0.82; orientation aids, 0.62; safety features, 0.71; staff facilities, 0.81; space availability, 0.66<br><br>Confounds unit and facility level effects; requires a degree of subjective interpretation | This comprehensive measure assesses nondementia senior purpose built housing at the facility level but unfortunately has limited use at the unit level. This measure allows for a systematic comparison with other facilities<br><br>An assessment of a 200 unit congregate housing facility built in 1975 found that compared with a normative sample of other similar facilities it rated high on social-recreational aids and low on physical amenities and staff facilities |
| ERHAP (Elderly Resident Housing Assessment Program) (Brent & Brent, 1987) | 300 rule computer program organized for room by room walk through assessment utilizing universal design considerations. An interview with the homeowner, observation of the environment, and photographs are utilized in this consumer-specific measure | Total validation score, 96%. Overlap between categories; same question not asked in each room | A comparative analysis (n = 44 and 46) of independent living identified housing inadequacies common to senior housing<br><br>Bathroom and kitchen were the most environmentally challenging, possibly because they incorporate the largest number of activities. This hierarchical model serves as a useful tool in prioritizing needs. Safety inadequacies contributed to functioning and as a result contributed to overall comfort<br><br>Assessment provides resident with results and design suggestions specific to their needs |
| LivAbility (Christenson, 1997) | A self-administered questionnaire for the healthy independent living older person that measures housing and physical characteristics as they relate to functioning in the environment. A customized report is generated for the respondent | A pilot study conducted approximately 4 months after the evaluation found 54% of the respondents acted on the individualized suggestions | This consumer-oriented tool is useful and easy to use but is limited by its application only to the healthy independent living senior<br><br>The video could be useful in group settings such as senior centers and church gatherings to create an awareness of the role the environment plays in well-being |
| NURS (Nursing Unit Rating Scale) (Grant, 1996) | Six dimensions (separation, stimulation, stability, complexity, control/tolerance, and continuity) are rated by staff interviews | Cronbach's alpha: separation, 0.94; stability, 0.83; stimulation, 0.70; complexity, 0.86; control/tolerance, 0.95; continuity, 0.76 | This study found the NURS to be a useful tool for assessing policy and program features of SCUs<br><br>The domains of continuity and stimulation resulted in low total item correlations. Perceptions held by nurse supervisors were reflected, but the question remains if other staff members feel |

*(continued)*

**Table 12.13.** — Continued

| | | Study of 400 nursing units in 124 Minnesota facilities. Correlational analysis examined relationships between scales with ANOVA used to compare SCUs and non-SCUs | the same way. The lack of clear distinctions between units is problematic in attempting to compare SCUs with non-SCUs<br><br>This tool measures a person's adaptation to his or her environment, but does not assess the physical environment as well as the TESS-2+ does |
|---|---|---|---|
| TESS (Therapeutic Environment Screening Scale) (Sloane & Mathew, 1990) | 12 item observation scale of SCU physical features based on 5 therapeutic functions (noxious stimuli, mood enhancement and self image, safety, activities, and outdoor access) are assessed by direct observation | Comparative analysis of 31 SCUs and 32 traditional units in five states<br><br>Scores on the aggregate scale ranged from 3 to 24, with a mean score of 12 and a standard deviation of 3.77<br><br>Study showed dementia units scored significantly better on supportive characteristics than traditional nursing home units | This is a comprehensive instrument designed for assessing skilled care facilities. Attention has been given to standardization of data collection times and techniques |
| TESS 2+ (Therapeutic Environment Screening Scale) (Sloane et al., 1995) | This modified version of the TESS-2 assesses 8 domains (general design features, maintenance, inventory of spatial amenities and seating capacity, lighting, noise, amenities, programming, and global environment) in dementia SCUs | Cronbach's alpha = 0.825<br><br>Validity not tested | This modified version is useful for descriptive purposes that focus on physical features common to a dementia unit<br><br>A subjective rating scale of the overall atmosphere of the unit is problematic because of the possibility of rater's bias |
| PEAP (Professional Environmental Assessment Protocol) (Teresi et al., 1994) | This 8 dimension SCU-specific instrument focuses on the physical setting and the extent to which it supports the needs of people with dementia | Kappas ranged from 0.69 for facilitation of social contact to 0.85 for continuity of self in study of 20 SCUs in Kansas<br><br>Number of residents ranged from 8 to 64, with facilities divided between rural and urban | This instrument differentiates three levels of the physical setting (the fixed or structural features, the semifixed features, and the nonfixed features) as they relate to the social, organizational, and policy environment |

*(continued)*

377

**Table 12.13.**
Summary of Environment Measures—Continued

| Measure | Description | Psychometric | Application |
|---|---|---|---|
| E-B Model (Environment-Behavior model for SCUs) (Zeisel et al., 1994) | 8 environment–behavior concepts, along with dimensions that link a design feature to a performance criteria, measure the relationship between environmental influences and behavioral effects | No psychometric measurements | This instrument requires additional training for the raters, but the effort is worth it. It has the potential to predict therapeutic outcomes by indirectly measuring interaction effects between the residents and their environment |
| | | | The authors note that no environmental instrument should be used in isolation but should involve a systematic collection of data on the physical setting, the people who use the setting, and their interactions |

SCU, special care unit.

floor plans, questionnaires, interviews, and focus groups. All of these steps are necessary to understand the congruence between the older person and his or her environment.

Environmental measures to date have been developed on a "felt need" basis. Occupational therapists have evolved numerous checklists to examine the safety and adaptability of the home environment, as have various programs in home modifications for low-income seniors. Measures have also followed the interests of the research community, with tools developed to study hypothesized relationships. The interest in Lawton's theories about the need to create optimal levels of environmental press required test measures of person–environmental fit. One approach to assessing environments is for seniors and others to report on the environment; another is direct observation. Observation works particularly well for the physical environment, including furnishings, fixtures, and equipment, but less well for use made of the environment. Moos and Lemke (1996) have contributed major theoretical work, and their efforts in measurement development have been extensive. They view all those who live and work in an environment as part of that environment and gather input from all to characterize environmental cultures. Their MEAP, however, is much too extensive to use in its entirety except with major research funding.

Direct observations of nursing home special care units were a direct result of the National Institute on Aging's funding on that topic. The TESS, MEAP, and PEAP are examples of largely observational approaches to the special care unit, whereas Grant's NURS (1996) is an example of an interview format in which the unit coordinator answers questions about practices and that allows scoring the degree of separation or integration of the person with dementia, the amount of stimulation in the environment, and so on. In the 1990s, trade associations for assisted living have also taken a keen interest in assessing the state of physical environments in the industry and relating these to price and occupancy.

The result of all this activity is, in part, long questionnaires to administrators that have not yet been validated or shown to be reliable, multiple marketing tools to prospective customers that certainly do not rise to the level of research tools, and observation tools, notably for Alzheimer's disease special care units, that have proved reliable in the hands of trained raters but that have a great deal of subjectivity. Two lines of work need to be developed in the future: brief generic self-reported tools that tap the older person's experience and satisfaction with various types of living environments that could be used to compare *across* environments; and detailed observational tools that are as objective as possible to capture detail about the built environment where the older person resides. As researchers learn which aspects of physical environments and which practices in the use of the environment are associated with better outcomes for the older person, the short self-report tools will be better designed to address these issues.

## REFERENCES

American Association of Retired Persons (1996). *Understanding senior housing: Into the next century.* Washington, DC: American Association of Retired Persons.

American Health Care Association. (1996). *Satisfaction assessment questionnaire for assisted living residents.* Washington, DC: American Health Care Association.

Brent, E., & Brent, R. (1987). EFHAP: An artificial intelligence expert system for assessing the housing of elderly residents. *Housing and Society, 14,* 215–230.

Brent, E., & Brent, R. (1993). *Home Safe Home.* Columbia, MO: Idea Works.

Christenson, M. (1990). *Aging in the design environment.* Binghamton, NY: Haworth Press.

Christenson, M. (1997). *LivAbility, choices for better living.* New Brighton, MN: Lifease.

Connell, B. R. (1996). Role of the environment in falls prevention. *Clinics in Geriatric Medicine, 12*(4), 859–880.

Corcoran, K., & Fischer, J. (1987). *Measures for clinical practice: A sourcebook.* New York: Free Press.

Filion, P., Wister, A., & Coblentz, E. J. (1992). Subjective dimensions of environmental adaptation among the elderly: A challenge to models of housing policy. *Journal of Housing for the Elderly, 10,* 3–32.

Goland, S. M. (1991). Matching congregate housing settings with a diverse elderly population: Research and theoretical considerations. *Journal of Housing for the Elderly, 9,* 21–38.

Grant, L. A. (1996). Assessing environments in Alzheimer special care units. *Research on Aging, 18*(3), 275–291.

Kahana, E. (1975). A congruence model of person environment interaction. In P. G. Windley, T. Byherts, & E. G. Ernst (Eds.), *Theoretical Development in Environments and Aging.* Washington, DC: Gerontological Society.

Kane, R. A., & Kane, R. L. (1987). *Long-Term Care: Principles, Programs, and Policies.* New York: Springer.

Kane, R. A., & Wilson, K. B. (1993). *Assisted living in the United States: A new paradigm for residential care for frail older persons?* Washington, DC: American Association of Retired Persons.

Lawton, M. P., & Nahemow, L. (1973). Ecology and the aging process. In C. Eisdorfer & M. P. Lawton (Eds.), *Psychology of adult development and aging.* Washington, DC: American Psychological Association.

Lawton, M. P., Weisman, G. S. P., & Calkins, M. (1997). Assessing environments of older people with chronic illness. *Journal of Mental Health and Aging, 3,* 83–100.

Leibrock, C. (1993). *Beautiful barrier-free: A visual guide to accessibility.* New York: Van Nostrand Reinhold.

Moos, R. L., & Lemke, S. (1996). *Evaluating Residential Facilities.* Thousand Oaks, CA: Sage.

Osterberg, A. E., Davis, A. M., & Danielson, L. D. (1995). Universal design: the users' perspective. *Housing and Society, 22,* 1–2.

Preiser, W., Rabinowitz, H., & White, E. (1988). *Post-occupancy evaluation.* New York: Van Nostrand Reinhold.

Regnier, V. (1994). *Assisted living housing for the elderly.* New York: Van Nostrand Reinhold.

Schwartz, B., Brent, R., & Hennigh, G. (1995). Internalizing values: Universal design in the design studio. *Housing and Society, 21,* 91–96.

Sloane, P. D., & Mathew, L. J. (1990). Therapeutic environment screen scale. *American Journal of Alzheimer's Disease and Associated Disorder, 5,* 22–26.

Sloane, P. D., Mitchell, C. M., Long, K., & Lynn, M. (1995). *TESS+ Instrument B: Unit Observation Checklist—Physical Environment. A report on the psychometric properties of individual items and initial recommendations on scaling.* Chapel Hill, NC: Unpublished.

Teresi, J., Lawton, M. P., Ory, M., & Holmes, D. (1994). Measurement issues in chronic care populations: Dementia special care. *Journal of Alzheimer Disease and Associated Disorder, 8*(Suppl 1), S144–S183.

Zeisel, J., Hyde, J., & Levkoff, S. (1994). Best practices: An environment–behavior (E-B) model for Alzheimer special care units. *American Journal of Alzheimer's Care and Related Disorders and Research, March/April,* 4–21.

# II

# Applications of Assessment

# 13

# Comprehensive Geriatric Assessment and Management

CRISTINA F. URDANGARIN

Comprehensive Geriatric Assessment (CGA), the multidisciplinary evaluation and care planning of older adults by more than one health professional, has become a cornerstone of geriatric care systems. The principle behind CGA is that the simultaneous presence of many problems (physical, psychological, and social) and the unmet health care needs facing the older patient require an assessment more complex than can realistically be provided by a routine diagnostic examination.

Comprehensive evaluation of an elderly individual's health status requires an assessment of four principal domains: functional ability, physical health, cognitive and mental health, and socioenvironmental factors. This assessment constitutes the basis of the older person's treatment and rehabilitation plan designed to prevent or delay the onset of disability and to reduce expensive hospital care and poor quality of life. By taking all of the patient's needs into consideration simultaneously, CGA offers a health care model that integrates medical care with social support.

The concept of a comprehensive assessment of the elderly person dates back to the 1930s. It is a part of good geriatric medicine, something that has been infor-

mally done in many cultures for centuries but that has become a more formal contemporary challenge. Comprehensive Geriatric Assessment is usually too complex, too time consuming, and too poorly reimbursed to be provided routinely by most practitioners. It requires skills in the medical, social, and psychological aspects of care and familiarity with providers of various types of services for the elderly and with the complicated systems used by third-party payers. To compensate for some of the problems that limit the use of CGA, standard geriatric assessment protocols and technology have been developed for use by primary care physicians and by nonphysician staff, and techniques for enhancing the cooperation between geriatrically trained teams and primary care physicians have been developed.

Comprehensive Geriatric Assessment has played a central role in the evolution of the geriatric care system toward an integrated community program of social and medical services for older persons with complex problems. It has been shown to reduce health care costs (Tulloch & Moore, 1979; Williams et al., 1987; Rubin, 1993; Engelhardt et al., 1996) while improving patient satisfaction (Engelhardt et al., 1996) by providing early detection of and timely intervention for problems (Tulloch & Moore, 1979; Silverman et al., 1995) and a better match of services to patient. At the same time, CGA could increase costs if used with people who are too healthy to derive much benefit, if the evaluation and the recommendations are not carefully focused on those conditions that are most responsive to treatment, or if it leads to unnecessary or duplicative services.

Studies have, however, shown that the strategy of assessing problems and making recommendations is not effective by itself (Solomon, 1988), because only 50%–70% of the recommendations are followed (Cefalu et al., 1995; Epstein et al., 1990; Shah et al., 1997; Barker et al., 1985; Katz, Dube, & Calkins, 1985). It is now believed that in order to be effective, assessment must be linked closely with direct prevention and treatment services (Silverman et al., 1995; Solomon, 1988; Applegate & Burns, 1996; McVey et al., 1989). The expanded process, which includes a management or treatment component as well as an assessment component, is called *Geriatric Evaluation and Management* (GEM). Because many CGA recommendations address iatrogenic problems, simply returning the older patient to his or her prior care situation may not suffice even when recommendations are offered to the primary care physician.

Geriatric assessment and management should therefore be viewed as a three-stage process, and each component must be adequately addressed.

1. Identification or targeting of an appropriate patient: a frail elder
2. Assessment of the patient and development of recommendations
3. Implementation of the recommendations by physician and patient

Programs can be unsuccessful when screening is inappropriate, the most appropriate recipients remain unidentified, or recommendations are not implemented.

## HISTORY OF GERIATRIC ASSESSMENT

Geriatric assessment originated in England in the 1930s before the British National Health Service was founded. The successful work of the early pioneers (Marjory Warren, Lionel Cosin, and Sir Ferguson Anderson) helped forge the principles of special, comprehensive, and interdisciplinary assessment of elderly patients. These principles were later successfully incorporated into the British National Health Service, resulting in the establishment of geriatric assessment units as a point of entry into the health system and of universal coverage of geriatric assessment for all elders. In this system, elderly patients requiring hospital admission or admission to another institution are first admitted to a geriatric assessment/evaluation unit, where each patient receives a comprehensive assessment of medical, functional, and psychosocial problems and where care plans are developed, usually by an interdisciplinary team. Less intensive assessments are also provided to elderly patients through programs such as consultation clinics, home visits, and day hospitals. Since the 1930s, many countries (e.g., Israel, Finland, Norway, Australia, the Netherlands, Italy, and Canada) have followed the British model (Rubenstein, 1987).

In the United States, CGA has steadily grown in importance since the pioneering work of T. F. Williams in the 1970s, with a rapid proliferation of local programs but no large-scale and consistent provision of geriatric assessment to all elderly patients. In the late 1980s, the Department of Veterans Affairs, which had previously provided extensive support for research, education, and clinical work in geriatrics with the formation of the geriatric research and education clinical centers, fostered the development of geriatric evaluation units at VA medical centers. With increasing recognition of the need to include management along with evaluation, the GEM approach to care was adopted and is now a fundamental component of geriatric clinical care.

A variety of models for implementing CGA have been developed and tested. These programs vary in their purpose, comprehensiveness, staffing, site, targeting, structural, and functional components. Table 13.1 summarizes types of geriatric assessment programs by site (Rubenstein, 1987).

Goals are different for each type of CGA, depending on where the program is implemented, the complexity of the medical problems encountered, and the intensity of the assessment. Programs usually have several goals. It is of particular importance for the goals of the programs to be defined clearly and for assessment and treatment to be directed toward those goals. For example, a program with community residence as a major goal should direct its efforts toward improving patients' functional status or strengthening their social supports. Table 13.2 summarizes the variety of goals a CGA may have.

Early reports on the efficacy of CGA and GEM interventions were positive but were based largely on uncontrolled case studies or on controlled but nonrandomized designs. In the 1990s, more methodologically rigorous studies have been conducted in a variety of clinical settings, and the outcomes of patients treated in various programs have been published. Most of these studies have reported at least one positive outcome. The design of the trials, the implementation of the pro-

**Table 13.1.** Types of Geriatric Assessment Programs by Site

Acute hospital inpatient units
  Geriatric assessment/evaluation units
  Geropsychiatric assessment units
  Geriatric rehabilitation units
Chronic hospital inpatient assessment units
Inpatient geriatric consultation services
Hospital outpatient departments
Home visit assessment
Nursing home assessment
Office setting or free-standing units

**Table 13.2.** Summary of Potential Goals of Comprehensive Geriatric Assessment Programs

Improve diagnostic accuracy
Determine optimal placement
Plan therapy
Facilitate primary care and case management
Maintain or recover functional ability
Maintain or recover independence or discharge to the community
Increase quality of life
Facilitate hospital discharge
Increase cost effectiveness and coordination of care
Reduce medical costs
Reduce hospital utilization
Increase patient's and provider's satisfaction
Decrease mortality

grams, and the outcome measures (and the tools used to evaluate them) have, however, been very variable and incompletely described in the literature. Whereas some studies report good outcomes, several trials show poor results. For these reasons it is difficult to draw firm conclusions about the programs' efficacies, and one should be cautious when reviewing and comparing results from different studies and pay attention to the study design, type of intervention being studied, alternatives to which the intervention is compared, target population, control group, outcome measures being assessed, assessment techniques being used, and negative outcomes observed (Reuben et al., 1996; Burns, 1994).

A specific component of the design or analysis of a study may be partly responsible for its overwhelming number of positive results. Sometimes CGA is compared with very poorly defined forms of usual care; other times the control group receives a high standard medical care and findings underestimate the benefits that may occur if compared with usual medical care (Williams et al., 1987; Reuben et al., 1996). In other studies, poor results could be partially explained by lack of adequate sample size and therefore lack of statistical power to detect differences between the study groups (Williams et al., 1987; Rubin, 1993; Reuben et al., 1992, 1996) by contamination bias—when all study subjects receive care from the same medical staff and potential differences between groups are minimized (McVey et al., 1989); or by selection bias—when only a small percentage of the potential population elects to participate in the study (Stuck et al., 1995). In other studies, only a few of the components of the intervention are being compared, nonvalidated assessment tools are used (Vetter, Jones, & Victor, 1984), and, in general, very little information about the actual assessment technique is given.

## RANDOMIZED CLINICAL TRIALS

Because of the limitations of nonrandomized study designs, this chapter focuses on randomized clinical trials of CGA and GEM in different settings. In general, studies of CGA/GEM have been done in three settings: inpatient units, outpatient clinics, and specialized types of home care.

Some of the most successful results have been observed in GEM programs in inpatient settings. The inpatient hospital Geriatric Evaluation and Management Unit is a specialized unit in an acute care or rehabilitation hospital designed to provide assessment and treatment services to a target population (Applegate & Burns, 1996; Rubenstein et al., 1984; Reuben et al., 1995). The cost of such interventions is high, however, which encourages experimentation with less expensive outpatient settings (Boult et al., 1998). The results of inpatient geriatric consultation programs, in contrast, have yielded conflicting results, and no firm conclusions can be drawn from these studies (McVey et al., 1989; Becker, McVey, & Saltz, 1987; Allen et al., 1986; Fretwell, 1992; Siu, Morishita, & Blaustein, 1994). Geriatric Evaluation and Management Unit programs provide an assessment of the elderly patient by an interdisciplinary team with expertise in evaluating and managing older patients. Table 13.3 summarizes the results of inpatient geriatric assessment randomized clinical trials (CGA and GEM).

Outpatient geriatric evaluation and management programs are ambulatory-based, interdisciplinary GEM programs performed in targeted, functionally impaired elderly persons who are community dwelling. The results of outpatient GEM programs have been inconsistent as well, but individual programs have reported a number of benefits compared to usual care: greater diagnostic accuracy, improved functional ability, greater satisfaction with health care, increased use of home services, and decreased mortality, anxiety, depression, stress for caregivers, use of emergency rooms, use of hospital services, and health care costs (Williams et al., 1987; Rubin, 1993; Engelhardt et al., 1996; Silverman et al., 1995; Cefalu et al., 1995; Epstein et al., 1990; Rubin et al., 1992; Siu et al., 1994; Teasdale et al., 1983; Bernabei et al., 1998; Yeo et al., 1987; Burns et al., 1995; O'Donnell & Toseland, 1997). Results from a randomized clinical trial of an outpatient GEM program that provided 6 months of targeted intensive care versus usual care to community dwelling Medicare beneficiaries 70 years of age and older in Minnesota are expected to be published soon. Preliminary analysis of the data shows high satisfaction ratings of patients and their primary physicians and less decline in function and affect in the GEM group participants than the usual care group (Boult, 1998; Morishita et al., 1998). Table 13.4 summarizes the results of outpatient CGA/GEM.

Attention has also been placed on less medically intensive untargeted home-based CGA programs. Despite earlier emphasis on targeting, three randomized studies (Stuck et al., 1995; Vetter et al., 1984; Hendriksen, Lund, & Stromgard, 1984) have demonstrated that continued in-home assessment of elderly persons and referral for the care of any problems uncovered may have substantial benefits, although neither intervention is technically a CGA because only one discipline is involved. Hendriksen and coworkers (1984) randomly selected 600 nontargeted community dwelling persons over 75 years old

**Table 13.3.**
Outcomes of Inpatient Geriatric Randomized Clinical Trials

| Author | Intervention | Target (age group) | Duration | Functional ability | Cognitive ability | Affect | Mortality | Satisfaction | Use of services |
|---|---|---|---|---|---|---|---|---|---|
| Rubenstein et al. (1984) | GEM VA | 65+ frail | 1 year | IG* | IG | IG* | IG* | NE | IG* |
| Allen et al. (1986), Becker et al. (1987), McVey et al. (1989) | CGA VA | 75+ | Discharge | EQ | NE | NE | NE | NE | EQ |
| Applegate et al. (1990) | GEM | 65+ functionally impaired | 1 year | IG* | EQ | EQ | NE | EQ | CG |
| Fretwell et al. (1990) | CGA | 75+ | 2 months after discharge | EQ | EQ | EQ | EQ | NE | EQ |
| Reuben et al. (1995) | CGA HMO | 65+ screened | 12 months | EQ | EQ | NE | EQ | NE | NE |
| Siu et al. (1996) | CGA | 65+ screened | 60 days | EQ | EQ | EQ | EQ | CG | EQ |

CG, outcome more favorable for control group; CGA, Comprehensive Geriatric Assessment; EQ, outcome equal for GEM and control groups; GEM, Geriatric Evaluation and Management; HMO, health maintenance organization; IG, outcome more favorable for intervention group; NE, not evaluated; VA, Veterans Administration.

*$p < 0.05$.

# Table 13.4.
Summary of Randomized Clinical Trials on Outpatient Geriatric Assessment

| Author | Intervention | Target | Follow-up | Mortality | Functional ability | Cognitive ability | Affect | Use of services | Costs | Satisfaction |
|---|---|---|---|---|---|---|---|---|---|---|
| Tulloch & Moore (1979), UK | CGA | 70+ | 2 yr | NE | EQ | NE | NE | Hospital admission, CG; hospital days, IG* | IG | |
| Williams et al. (1987), US | CGA | 65+ frail | 1 yr | EQ | IG | IG | NE | Hospital days, IG; home service, CG; nursing home, CG | Hospital, IG; nursing home, IG | EQ |
| Yeo et al. (1987), US | GEM VA | 65+ | 18 mo | CG | IG* | EQ | EQ | Primary care, CG*; home services, CG; dental, eye, ear, CG* | NE | NE |
| Epstein et al. (1990), US | CGA HMO | 70+ | 1 yr | EQ | EQ | EQ | EQ | Primary care visit, CG* | NE | NE |
| Rubin et al., (1992), Rubin (1993), US | GEM | 70+ hospitalized frail | 1 yr | EQ | ADL, EQ; IADL, IG* | EQ | NE | Home service, IG* | Hospital, IG* | EQ |
| Burns et al. (1995), US | GEM VA | 65+ hospitalized frail | 1 yr | IG* | IG | IG | IG* | Hospital use, EQ | NE | IG |
| Silverman et al. (1995), US | CGA Multisite | 65+ frail | 1 yr | EQ | EQ | EQ | Anxiety, IG* | EQ | NE | IG |
| Engelhardt et al. (1996), US | GEM VAMC | 55+ frail VA | 16 mo | EQ | EQ | NE | EQ | Primary care, CG*; emergency room, IG* | Outpatient, CG* | IG* |
| Boult et al. (1998), US | GEM | 70+ | 18 mo | EQ | IG* | NE | IG* | EQ | EQ | IG* |
| Reuben et al. (1999), US | CGA + adherence intervention | 65+ frail | 15 mo | IG | IG* | NE | NE | NE | NE | EQ |

ADL, activity of daily living; CG, outcome more favorable for control group; CGA, Comprehensive Geriatric Assessment; EQ, outcome equal for GEM and control groups; GEM, Geriatric Evaluation and Management; HMO, health maintenance organization; IADL, instrumental ADL; IG, outcome more favorable for intervention group; NE, not evaluated; VAMC, Veterans Administration Medical Center.

*p < 0.05.

and randomized them to receive quarterly home assessment visits by a trained nurse or usual care. The nurses assessed the patients in a comprehensive manner and then arranged for appropriate medical or social services. The intervention group utilized significantly more in-home social services and experienced a significant reduction in mortality, lower repeated hospitalizations, and a trend toward lower nursing home use. The impact of functional status was not assessed. Vetter and colleagues (1984) randomized a sample of persons over age 70 years registered in two general practices (one urban and one rural) to receive one extra visit per year from a home visitor (more if problems were found). In the urban practice, the intervention group experienced a lower mortality rate over 2 years and greater use of in-home nursing visits and home health. There were no differences in utilization or mortality in the rural practice.

In an intervention offering in-home CGA by a geriatric nurse practitioner, Stuck and associates (1995) reported results from a 3 year randomized clinical trial in which an annual in-home CGA and follow-up resulted in a lower prevalence of disability as measured by ADL scales and less use of long-term nursing home care at a savings of $6,000 per disability-free year. Table 13.5 summarizes the results of these three randomized clinical trials of in-home assessment.

Recently, a randomized clinical trial that evaluated the impact of a 1 year, senior center–based chronic illness self-management and disability prevention program on health, functioning, and health care utilization in frail older adults demonstrated an improvement in function and reduction in inpatient utilization by participants assigned to the intervention group compared with a control group (Leveille et al., 1998). This study provides evidence of the effectiveness of a new model of preventive care, which uses a prevention-oriented assessment and self-management program led by a geriatric nurse practitioner in collaboration with primary care providers. More recently, a randomized clinical trial of outpatient CGA coupled with an intervention to increase adherence to recommendations showed a reduction in functional and health-related quality of life decline among community dwelling older persons (Reuben et al., 1999). This study demonstrates that a relatively inexpensive CGA program that incorporates features of successful but more intensive programs can confer many of the same benefits.

**Table 13.5.**
Randomized Clinical Trials of Home-Based Assessment

| Author | Intervention | Significant results* |
|---|---|---|
| Hendriksen et al. (1984), Denmark | Quarterly home visits and coordination of care by a nurse | Fewer emergency calls, fewer hospital admissions, fewer hospital days, lower mortality. Increased number of in-home services |
| Vetter et al. (1984), UK | Annual home visits and coordination of care by a nurse | Urban patients: More services at home, lower mortality<br>Rural patients: no significant differences |
| Stuck et al. (1995), US | Annual home visits and coordination of care by gerontological nurse practitioners | Reduction in the number of persons who required assistance in performing the basic activities of daily living and reduction in the number of permanent nursing home admissions. Increased use of services promoting socialization |

*Associated with the intervention ($p < 0.05$).

In 1993, Stuck et al. (1993) published a meta-analysis of 28 international controlled trials comprising 4912 controls and 4959 subjects allocated to five comprehensive geriatric assessment types: inpatient geriatric evaluation and management units, inpatient consultation services (provided on a consultative basis to hospitalized patients in nondesignated units), home assessment service (in-home CGA for community dwelling elderly persons), hospital–home assessment services (in-home CGA for frail patients discharged from acute care), and outpatient assessment services (Stuck et al., 1993). Although the meta-analysis on selected reports may be biased to some degree (Ioannidis, Cappelleri, & Lau, 1998; Cappelleri et al., 1996), the results provide important information about the clinical value of CGA. The reduction of mortality found in early studies of institutional CGA units and home assessment was essentially confirmed: The odds ratio for combined mortality for all CGA programs was 0.86. Institutional programs and outpatient and home assessments had a favorable effect on likelihood of living at home at 12 months as well. Hospital geriatric evaluation and management units had a favorable effect on cognitive and physical functioning at follow-up. Finally, CGA programs taken together reduced the likelihood of hospitalization during follow-up.

The meta-analysis also identified several factors of the programs associated with successful outcomes: Services with strict targeting criteria seemed to be more effective and were often associated with decreased total costs. All studies on preventive home visits were, however, untargeted. Programs that delivered an intervention that combined assessment and strong sustained treatment (GEM) with long-term extensive outpatient follow-up improved the results even further. Benefit was more likely among patients with treatable chronic conditions that wear down the quality of life and require expensive medical institutional care.

Overall, the success of most American geriatric assessment programs has been limited. Some explanations could be the lack of a national health service that facilitates the comprehensive geriatric assessment systems, the limited supply of geriatricians and primary care doctors trained in geriatrics, the declines in length of hospital stay that interfere with programs aimed at hospitalized patients, difficulties with reimbursement of programs that feature extended post-acute assessment and rehabilitation after acute hospitalization (e.g., of ambulatory programs), and the separate funding sources (Medicare and Medicaid) for different programs for the elderly.

## LEVELS OF COMPREHENSIVE GERIATRIC ASSESSMENT

Forms of comprehensive assessment comprise a continuum of care from superficial periodic screening of all members of a population to comprehensive geriatric evaluation and management of frail elderly patients.

### Comprehensive Screening and Untargeted Preventive Assessment of Older Populations

Different approaches to comprehensive screening, including these performed periodically by mailed questionnaire or face-to-face interview in the community, have been tested. Some health maintenance organizations (HMOs) mail multidimensional, self-administered health risk appraisals to their older clients. Responses are scored according to defined algorithms, and reports of high-risk conditions and behaviors are sent to the clients and their primary physicians in order to stimulate follow-up diagnoses, treatment, and changes in behavior. Some HMOs also use brief questionnaires to identify enrollees at high risk of using hospitals exclusively (Boult et al., 1993; Boult, Boult, Pirie, & Pacala, 1994; Boult, Pacala, & Boult, 1995). This sort of activity is not, however, considered CGA.

Other organizations collect multidimensional screening information through questionnaires or interviews of older persons at their homes or at meeting places (e.g., meal sites, senior centers, churches, and community education sites). Randomized trials have reported some positive results—improvements in functional ability and immunization rates and reductions in mortality, falls, and use of hospitals, nursing homes, and emergency rooms—derived from periodic untargeted home visits by nurses (Stuck et al., 1995; Vetter et al., 1984; Hendriksen et al., 1984). In contrast, a one-time screening and referral by trained lay volunteers at community gathering sites did not produce positive outcomes (Reuben et al., 1993).

## Preventive Assessment of Community Dwelling Elderly People in Primary Care Without Access to a Multidisciplinary Team: Case Finding

Case finding refers to the independent geriatric assessment performed by an experienced health professional and incorporated into the primary care services of the elderly patient. This assessment can be performed by the primary care physician and/or a nurse practitioner or case manager trained in geriatrics during regular outpatient or home visits. The same professional who initiates the assessment usually implements part or all of the recommendations stemming from the assessment or arranges the provision of health services, or both. This model introduces the concept of continuity of care in which patients could be assessed at baseline and periodically reassessed at subsequent visits. Such assessment provides a health and functional baseline for each patient or community dwelling older person, helps detect changes in health or function at subsequent visits, picks out the frail elder and those at risk of becoming frail (screening), and institutes measures to prevent or ameliorate decreasing health or function. It may also improve health or function by appropriate referral, case management, and education

of the elders and may help the robust elder remain that way by improving self-efficacy, health, and safety behaviors.

The practice of repeated CGA in older people in the community is not easy to implement in private practice because of time and cost. A strategy to accomplish this model requires some changes in our system of care delivery such as changes in the reimbursement policy, use of nonphysician staff to perform part of the assessment, and the development of simpler and standardized tools for CGA. A study of the use of CGA techniques by community physicians found that the average family physician saw more than 166 patients per week and had only 12 minutes per encounter (Tryon, Mayfield, & Bross, 1992). According to these results, it would be very difficult to perform a 45–60 minute CGA as recommended (Fretwell, 1992). A model that calls for performing the assessment over several visits may be more realistic (Hamm, 1986).

## Preventive Assessment of Community Dwelling Elderly People by a Community Geriatric Unit

Assessment in a geriatric unit is similar to the previous type of assessment in that it targets elderly people living in the community. The difference resides in the subjects receiving case management and care planning by a nonmedical unit in coordination and close collaboration with general practitioners. In addition to the general practitioners, the community geriatric unit may include a geriatrician, social worker, and several nurses. Case managers perform the initial assessment, complement the information with a medical history obtained from general practitioners, and report the results to the geriatric evaluation unit. This unit determines the services that the patients need and are eligible for and design and implement individualized care plans in agreement with the general practitioners. All services considered necessary are then provided in an integrated fashion. In this model the community geriatric evaluation unit represents the gatekeeper to health services. It supports and integrates the activity of the general practitioner, but ultimately the general practitioner retains full responsibility of the patient. Such an integrated community care program implemented by an interdisciplinary team including a general practitioner and a intensively trained case manager reduced the risk of hospital admission and length of hospital and nursing home stay (Bernabei et al., 1998).

## Comprehensive Geriatric Assessment

Because geriatric assessment in various clinicl settings and long-term facilities comprises an evaluation of the patient in several areas, in practice it is probably better performed by an interdisciplinary or multidisciplinary team of health care professionals. This is particularly true for elders with complex needs that require more in-depth evaluation before effective plans of actions can be established.

The geriatric team performs the assessment in accordance with the patient's needs and caregiver expectations, but, because the team does not include the direct participation of the primary care provider, it has no control over the implementation of the recommendations and treatment plan, which are usually initiated by the primary care provider. It follows that this type of CGA is helpful in making diagnoses, but it will not improve patient outcomes if the recommendations are not followed and a treatment plan implemented. Primary care physicians must first implement recommendations, and patients must then adhere to them.

The most common problems associated with these models are the various degrees of noncompliance with the recommendations arising from the assessment process (Cefalu et al., 1995; Shah et al., 1997; Maly, Abrahamse, Hirsch, Frank, & Reuben, 1996; Saltz, McVey, Becker, Feussner, & Cohen, 1988; Reuben et al., 1999). Compliance with recommendations may be affected by the nature and characteris-

tics of the recommendations, the direct care providers, and the patient (Allen et al., 1986).

## Geriatric Evaluation and Management

In the Geriatric Evaluation and Management (GEM) programs, the interdisciplinary team that performs the assessment maintains responsibility for managing the patients beyond the initial comprehensive assessment period and ensures that the treatment regimen is followed and is effective. This treatment may later be continued by others either within institutional settings or on an outpatient basis in primary health care. Some of the most successful programs have assumed temporary control over the patient's care, but at the cost of interrupting a patient's tie to a primary care physician, which is not always desired by primary care physicians, patients, or family members. Efforts should be made to involve the primary physician, patient, and family members in the decision-making process.

## WHO PROVIDES COMPREHENSIVE GERIATRIC ASSESSMENT?

There appears to be no consensus about the best number or composition of the assessment team, which varies from a single individual to an array of specialists. In the context of screening, case finding, and community geriatric units, an experienced primary health provider (geriatrician, primary care physician, nurse, nurse practitioner, case manager) can effectively conduct a comprehensive and systematic assessment of the elderly patient. A nurse practitioner is recommended because he or she has the medical background to perform the medical aspects of the assessment. Usually, however, the assessment is conducted by a geriatric team. A core team generally consists of a social worker, nurse, and physician, but it may differ depending on the problem and conditions of the patients. Other professionals participating in the assessment may include one or more from psychiatry, audiology, clinical psychology, pharmacology, physical therapy, nutrition, occupational therapy, dentistry, and ophthalmology.

Each member of the team should have—but usually does not have—well-defined tasks. The geriatrician or physician generally supervises the CGA; the nurse usually performs most of the evaluation tests and interviews to assess impairments, resources, and demands; and the social worker performs the psychosocial assessment. In the interdisciplinary teams, members meet individually with the patient and assesses according to their area of expertise. All of the professional staff meet to review the findings and develop a collective care plan. In the multidisciplinary teams, each professional prepares an evaluation and a set of recommendations that one of the team members then integrates into a plan of care.

These geriatric teams are usually established on specialized assessment units, but, as previously stated, they may also be organized within the primary care system. The responsibility for implementing the recommendations varies according to the model of care.

## WHO RECEIVES COMPREHENSIVE GERIATRIC ASSESSMENT?

There are conflicting recommendations regarding who should receive CGA. Research shows that the highly specialized and more expensive unit programs of CGA and GEM are usually more cost-effective when provided to persons at high risk of functional decline or who rely heavily on health services (Stuck et al., 1993), but the results are not consistent. In some less specialized unit programs, CGA has been efficiently provided to all elders (Stuck et al., 1995).

The process of selecting the most appropriate patient for a given program is termed *triage* or *targeting* (Rubenstein et al., 1991). Currently three targeting strategies are used to identify recipients of CGA and GEM: periodic screening, referrals,

and analysis of administrative records. These approaches are not mutually exclusive; ideally, a combination of the three should be used to identify elders who would benefit from GEM.

### Periodic Screening of the Population

Screening is designed to identify those elders who are most likely to benefit from a CGA/GEM program. It is the process by which a CGA program uses targeting criteria to select potential recipients of CGA. Different methods of screening have been used in the past, but the ability of such instruments to predict clinical outcomes in the general elderly population has not been conclusively proved (Maly et al., 1996). Age, functional impairment, the presence of physical illness or common geriatric clinical syndromes (e.g., falls, confusion, polypharmacy, or incontinence), the use of health services (e.g., home health care or adult day care), psychosocial conditions and perceived need for services, and the occurrence of sentinel events (e.g., recent hospital admission, new incontinence, or the death of a spouse) are the most common criteria, used individually or in combination (Maly et al., 1996; Winograd, 1991). The targeting approaches of the different CGA/GEM programs will differ with the needs and goals of each.

The case finding models used in the primary care physician's office or the emergency room can also be used as a means of identifying frail elders in need of a more in-depth comprehensive assessment. Furthermore, a short questionnaire has proved to be a sensitive, reliable, inexpensive, and acceptable screening test to systematically identify elders in the community at high risk of future hospitalization (Boult et al., 1993, 1994, 1995; Pacala, Boult, & Boult, 1995a). This questionnaire, the probability of repeated admission (Pra) questionnaire, has been validated in different populations. Periodic screening of the elderly population by mail with this questionnaire will help to identify those older adults who might be appropriate recipients of interventions such as GEM designed to reduce their need for hospital care.

## Referrals

Comprehensive Geriatric Assessment and GEM recipients can also be identified by referrals. Most frequently referrals come from family members, caregivers, social service workers, or self-referral, but they can also come from primary health care providers, hospital personnel, and emergency services personnel. Events that can trigger CGA include applications for admission to a nursing home, a health or life crisis, or a change in the patient's usual status.

## Information Systems

An analysis of administrative records by diagnosis or by clinical characteristics can be used to identify high-risk persons. In HMOs, the organization's electronic management information systems can be used to identify appropriate enrollees. International Classification of Disease codes recorded at office visits can be flagged by the management information system as triggers for further evaluation and management. Information comparable with that described earlier for the probability of repeated admission questionnaire may be generated from administrative data (Coleman et al., 1998).

## COMPREHENSIVE GERIATRIC ASSESSMENT: INSTRUMENTS AND DOMAINS

Comprehensive Geriatric Assessment may be initiated independently of the site, provided that competence and adequate tools are available. Instruments used for efficient screening or case finding assessment are different from instruments needed for indepth CGA/GEM programs of frail elders. In the first case, assessment of each domain is less complex than in CGA programs and can even be completed (partially or totally) at home by the older patient and his or her family or caregivers. The use of standardized instruments in these programs is not essential, although they are preferred to make the process reliable and efficient. The assessment should include evaluation of the four principal domains (function, physical health, mental and cognitive health, and socioenvironmental factors) and the evaluation of common geriatric problems such as vision, hearing, nutrition, medication, falls, and vaccines.

Table 13.6 outlines a set of items designed to help primary care physicians, nurses, and other health care workers to perform screening or case finding assessment of older patients. It includes elements from a tool recommended by the American College of Physicians and parts of instruments that have been validated and field-tested for a specific randomized clinical trial (Boult, in press).

In a more specialized assessment unit (inpatient CGA, CGA consultative unit, and GEM), the assessment of the four domains mentioned earlier should be more extensive and should be performed on those accepted into the program by an interdisciplinary/multidisciplinary team according to a well-defined protocol. Examination of common geriatric problems, special senses, motivation for rehabilitation, wishes for the future, and laboratory tests such as finger stick hematocrit and glucose, dipstick urinalysis, and fecal occult blood testing are usually included in the assessment as well. Follow-up assessments to determine adherence to recommendations and to identify new problems that develop over time could then be performed periodically.

The use of valid, reliable, and standardized assessment instruments and specially adapted and standardized data collection forms will ensure that evaluation is efficient, consistent, and reproducible as different social workers, nurse practitioners, physicians, and so forth. rotate onto the team. It will also facilitate communication among the health care providers.

**Table 13.6.**
Example of an Assessment Instrument Designed for Use by Primary Care Physicians

| Domain | Items |
| --- | --- |
| Daily functioning | How much difficulty do you have in bathing, dressing, using the toilet, moving between bed and chair, feeding yourself, controlling your urine and bowels? |
| | How much difficulty do you have with preparing meals, cleaning lightly, using a telephone, using transportation, shopping, taking medicine, handling finances? |
| Affect | Do you often feel sad or depressed? |
| Cognition | Ability to remember three objects after 1 min |
| Nutrition | Height, weight |
| | Have you lost 10 pounds in the past 6 months without trying? |
| Gait, balance | How many times have you fallen in the past 6 months? |
| | Time required to raise from a chair, walk 20 feet, turn around, return, and sit down |
| | Extent of maximal standing forward reach with upper extremity |
| Sensory ability | Ability to report three numbers whispered 2 feet behind head |
| | Ability to read Snellen chart at 20/40 or better (with lenses, if used) |
| Upper extremity | Ability to clasp hands behind head and back |
| Medications | Prescription and nonprescription |
| Human assistance | Use of paid caregivers (e.g., nurses, aides) |
| | Use of unpaid caregivers (e.g., family, friends, volunteers) |
| Assistive devices | Personal (e.g., cane, walker, wheelchair, oxygen) |
| | Environmental (e.g., grab bars, shower bench, hospital bed) |
| Prevention | Women: Pap smear, mammogram, thyroid-stimulating hormone, calcium/vitamin D intake |
| | Men and women: Blood pressure, stool hemoccult, colonoscopy, immunizations (influenza, pneumococcal, tetanus), dental care, exercise, smoke detectors |
| Advance directives | Living will |
| | Durable power of attorney for health care |
| Substance abuse | Have you ever felt that you should cut down the amount of alcohol you drink? |
| | Have people ever annoyed you by criticizing your use of alcohol? |
| | Have you ever felt guilty about your drinking? |
| | Have you ever had an "eye-opener" drink in the morning? |
| | Do you smoke cigarettes? |

The quality of the geriatric assessment depends on the competence of the assessor and the tools used for the assessment. Numerous assessment tools have been introduced for use with elderly patients, but in routine clinical settings usage is considered to be low. For example, most family physicians employ some selected age-related assessment techniques, but less than 25% perform functional assessment techniques considered unique to the geriatric patient, such as mental status or activities of daily living (ADLs) (Tryon et al., 1992).

Some scales are comprehensive and therefore time consuming, making them infeasible for clinicians. Some are not accepted by the patient or the physician, and some are difficult to use or interpret. It is important to emphasize that assessment tools should not replace the routine clinical evaluation, but complement it. In reviewing the quality of any assessment tool, a number of characteristics should be reviewed. All tools should be valid, reliable, acceptable to the patient, responsive to change, presented in an appropriate format, and easy to administer. It is also important that the assessment tool does not demand an extensive course of training and that it is easily understood by the patient, the family members or caregivers, and the assessor or geriatric team. Efforts should be made to use assessment tools that minimize respondent burden and maximize the collection of objective and valid information from individuals and proxies. The collection of the most critical measures (e.g., physical function) should be done at the beginning of the assessment before the respondent becomes fatigued,

**Table 13.7.**
Domains and Assessment Tools in Different Studies

| Domain | Assessment tool | Study |
|---|---|---|
| Functional ability | Katz ADL scale | Rubin (1993), Keller and Potter (1994), Boult et al. (1998) |
| | Barthel ADL Index | Rubenstein et al. (1984), McVey et al. (1989) |
| | Lawton IADL Scale | Burns et al. (1995), Stuck et al. (1995) |
| | IADL OARS Scale | Rubin (1993), Silverman et al. (1995), Boult et al. (1998) |
| | Personal Self-Maintenance Scale | Rubenstein et al. (1984) |
| | Functional Independence Measure | Engelhardt et al. (1996) |
| | Functional Status Questionnaire (FSQ) | Reuben et al. (1993) |
| | Timed "Up and Go" | |
| | Medical Outcomes Short Form-36 | Boult et al. (1998) |
| | Restricted Activity Days | Siu et al. (1994) |
| | | Leveille et al. (1998), Boult et al. (1998) |
| | Bed Disability Days | Leveille et al. (1998), Boult et al. (1998) |
| Physical health | Tinetti Balance and Gait Evaluation | Engelhardt et al. (1996) |
| | Cumulative Illness Rating Scale (CIRS) | Keller & Potter (1994) |
| | Sickness Impact Profile (SIP) | Boult et al. (1998), Epstein et al. (1990) |
| Cognitive function | Mini-Mental State Examination | Keller and Potter (1994); Cefalu et al. (1995) |
| | Kahn-Goldfarb Mental Status Questionnaire | Rubenstein et al. (1984) |
| | Short Portable Mental Status Questionnaire | Rubin (1993); Engelhardt et al. (1996) |
| | Clinical Dementia Rating Scale (CDR) | Silverman et al. (1995) |
| | Rand Mental Index | Reuben et al. (1993) |
| | Mental Status Questionnaire | Alessi et al. (1997) |
| Mood disorders: Depression, anxiety | Yesavage Geriatric Depression Scale | Cefalu et al. (1995), Engelhardt et al. (1996), Boult et al. (1998) |
| | Center for Epidemiological Studies Depression test (CES-D) | Burns et al. (1995), McVey et al. (1989) |
| | Diagnostic Interview Schedule (DIS) | Silverman et al. (1995) |
| | Zung Self-Rating Depression Scale | Yeo et al. (1987), Fretwell et al. (1990) |

(continued)

which could bias the results. It is important to define adequate outcome measures according to program objectives and to use tools appropriate to evaluate them.

Table 13.7 lists use CGA/GEM program assessment tools that have been used in different studies. (These tools are described in more detail in other chapters.)

The team or person who carries out the assessment develops a *problem list* for each patient, specifies *goals and priorities of care* (outcomes that need to be maximized), and finalizes a *treatment plan* or set of recommendations for each individual according to the best services available. If the patient is a referral, a follow-up appointment with the primary physician is made. The primary physician is informed of the treatment plan, reviews the recommendations, and implements them at his or her discretion. If the patient is assessed in a GEM unit, the GEM team provides most of the care.

**Table 13.7.** — Continued

| | | |
|---|---|---|
| | Bradburn's Affect Balance Scale | Yeo et al. (1987) |
| | Philadelphia Geriatric Center Morale Scale — Revised | Engelhardt et al. (1996) |
| | Lawton Morale Scale | Rubenstein et al. (1984) |
| Self-perception of health | Medical Outcomes Study Short-Form Health Survey (SF-20) | Engelhardt et al. (1996) |
| | Self-Rated Health | Yeo et al. (1987), Boult et al. (1998) |
| Medical disorders | Computerized Severity Index (CSI) | Engelhardt et al. (1996) |
| | Review of medical charts | Silverman et al. (1995) |
| | Brief Symptom Inventory | Toseland et al. (1996) |
| Polypharmacy and drug use | CAGE questionnaire of alcohol abuse | Reuben et al. (1993) |
| | Veteran Alcoholism screening test | McVey et al. (1989) |
| Family and social support | Lubben Social Network Scale (LSNS) | Engelhardt et al. (1996) |
| | Satisfaction with Support Scale | Toseland et al. (1996) |
| | Support Services Questionnaire | Toseland et al. (1996), Engelhardt et al. (1996) |
| Visual impairment | Ability to read Snellen chart at 20/40 or better | |
| Hearing impairment | Audiometry | |
| | Welch Allyn Audioscope | |
| Nutrition | Nutrition Screening Initiative (NSI) | Cefalu et al. (1995), Boult et al. (1998) |
| | BMI | Alessi et al. (1997), Boult et al. (1998) |
| Dental problems | Self-reported | |
| Immobility and pressure sores | Physical examination | |
| Falls and fractures | Review of medical charts | Silverman et al. (1995) |
| | Self-reported | |
| Urinary incontinence | Review of medical charts | |
| Caregiver burden | Caregiver Burden Scale | Silverman et al. (1995), Boult et al. (1998) |
| | Morycz Family Strain Scale | |
| Economics | Financial Benefits Questionnaire | Toseland et al. (1996) |
| Satisfaction with care | One overall question | Silverman et al. (1995) |
| | Pressing Problem Index | Toseland et al. (1996) |
| | Patient Satisfaction Questionnaire | Engelhardt et al. (1996) |
| Life satisfaction | Life Satisfaction Index | Yeo et al. (1987), Rubin (1993) |
| Social activity | Social Activity Scale | Epstein et al. (1990) |
| | Lubben Social Network Scale | Engelhardt et al. (1996) |
| Quality of Life | Quality of Well-being Scale | Siu et al. (1996) |

ADL, activity of daily living; IADLS, instrumental activities of daily living; OARS, Older Americans Resources and Services; BMI, basal metabilic index.

## CARE PLANNING AND IMPLEMENTATION

A beneficial outcome of CGA requires a prompt implementation of the treatment plan. Comprehensive Geriatric Assessment has proved to be ineffective in some studies because only 50%–70% of the recommendations in the treatment plan are usually followed, and adherence to those recommendation is variable (Cefalu et al., 1995; Shah et al., 1997; Allen et al., 1986).

In a preventive CGA model without access to a multidisciplinary team (screening or case finding), the person implementing the assessment is often a nurse practitioner. As a result of the evaluations performed in the CGA, he or she identifies specific problems, specifies goals and priorities of care, and recommends a multidisciplinary treatment plan for each individual. The recommendations are then reviewed with the patient or caregiver. Some recommendations can be implemented directly by the nurse practitioner without physician approval (case management, counseling, education); some are implemented directly by the physician, patient, or caregiver; and some need the approval of the primary care physician for before implementation (e.g., arrangements for occupational therapy, rehabilitation, physical therapy). If the person implementing the assessment in this model of CGA is the primary care physician, he or she implements recommendations accordingly.

In the model of preventive assessment by a community geriatric unit, the case managers and primary care physicians design and implement individualized care plans. This integration of medical and social services with case management programs, if cost effective, could become a model for better delivery of health services to the healthy elderly population.

In most consultative programs, the patient goes back to his or her own primary care physician for implementation of the treatment plan that stemmed from the assessment. A successful outcome requires that both primary care physicians and patients believe that the recommendations suggested by the CGA will be effective.

Recommendations in the treatment plan may include self-care activities, diagnostic testing, treatment of medical problems and referral to a specialist, referral to a case manager (case managers arrange and coordinate social, health, and community services), referral to a nonphysician professional or community service for rehabilitation, adjustment of medications, education, counseling, mental health services, family conferences, community services, caregiver services, home health services, advance directives, prevention activities, aids and devices, and so forth. In some situations the primary physician may arrange for a member of the assessment team to remain involved with the patient for re-evaluation and advice from the CGA team whenever needed or for the interdisciplinary team to take charge of the patient.

The degree of physician implementation of CGA recommendations varies according to target condition and type and number of recommendations, with higher rates for those related to falls, medication adjustment, and rehabilitation and lower for those related to depression, mental disorders, and physical impairment, speech, and occupational therapy (Cefalu et al., 1995; Shah et al., 1997; Allen et al., 1986). The relatively low physician implementation rate for some recommendations (e.g., physical impairment, mental disorders, urinary incontinence) may reflect physicians' beliefs that such geriatric conditions or impairments are a "normal" part of aging (Shah et al., 1997). Physician implementation rates could be increased through education of the primary care physician regarding the need for aggressive evaluation and management of geriatric problems, generalist/specialist interaction, and so forth (Reuben et al., 1999).

Patient adherence to physician-initiated recommendations is usually higher than to self-care recommendations (exercise, counseling, and joining support groups). Lifestyle changes are the most difficult to follow. To help patients make such lifestyle changes it may be necessary to educate them regarding the benefits of such changes and use strategies to help alter those lifestyles. An intervention that gave patients information and skills and encouraged them to discuss important questions and concerns with their physicians increased patient involvement and improved disease outcomes (Greenfield, Kaplan, & Ware, 1985; Reuben et al., 1999).

In GEM programs, patients receive most of their care from the GEM team: The geriatrician or physician generally supervises follow-up treatment and provides some direct medical care. The nurse provides some medical treatment and educates the patient and caregiver (if available) about treatments and medications, the use of home health equipment, and the appropriate use of emergency services. The social worker's primary functions are psychosocial counseling of the patient and caregiver, referral to appropriate financial, social, and psychological services, and in the event of hospitalization, the coordination of discharge planning. Referrals to medical specialists or to support groups and community services are also made when necessary. Communication is a key factor in the success of a GEM program. It requires the physician and the other health professionals to work as a team and also to inform the primary provider, the patient, and the family of the decisions made. In the GEM program patient progress and treatment plans are closely monitored, ongoing reassessments are performed, and review and adjustment of treatment plans are made at periodic team meetings. Family members are encouraged to be present at visits and are informed about the treatment plan. The geriatric nurse practitioner or physician updates the patient's primary care physician on a regular basis.

Discharge from the GEM program occurs when the patient no longer requires or benefits from the GEM program. This may happen because the therapeutic goals have been accomplished or a stable condition has been reached and there is nothing else the team can do for the patient. For some patients this may never happen, and they should continue to receive care in the geriatric unit and never be discharged from the program. The social worker usually works with the patient and family to make the arrangements necessary to achieve permanency in the community and maintain continuity of care in the geriatric unit after discharge. It is very important to periodically monitor the post-discharge status of the patients through a series of phone calls or mailed questionnaires

## EVALUATION OF THE COMPREHENSIVE GERIATRIC ASSESSMENT OR GEM PROGRAM

Program-specific and appropriate outcome measures should be used to assess the effectiveness of the CGA/GEM program. Some health status measures used in the process of geriatric assessment are adequate to measure patient health, but they may not be sensitive to the measurement of change. These measurements utilize a relatively gross categorization of conditions and may be unable to detect the small and specific changes that may result from geriatric assessment (Silverman et al., 1995). To document changes in different domains, standardized, reliable, valid, and sensitive-to-change measurement instruments have to be used. Engelhardt and coworkers (1996) examined the sensitivities of some instruments used to measure change in each domain and concluded that functional status measures such as ADLs did not detect any decline in functioning for patients over a period of 16 months, although one would expect at least some decline in frail older outpatients. Measures focused on instrumental activities of daily living (IADLs) may detect more subtle effects of the intervention not captured by measures that focus on ADL scales alone (Toseland et al., 1996). It may be even more difficult to measure change in health status when recipients of CGA/GEM are not extremely frail (Epstein et al., 1990). Another methodological issue is the appropriate timing for the measurement of change (when does the change occur? how long does it last?) and the appropriate ascertainment of the outcomes. Assessment of outcomes should optimally be blinded (Feussner, 1991). Table 13.8 offers some examples of different types of information that have been used to measure the outcomes of CGA.

## ECONOMICS

The potential of CGA for enhancing the health status of older persons while containing the costs is very appealing. But CGA is not free. The assessment itself costs money, and whether it saves money in the long run or produces better outcomes is not yet clear.

To date there are no complete results on the cost effectiveness of CGA/GEM programs. The negative cost-effective results

**Table 13.8.** Examples of Information Sources for Outcomes in CGA/GEM Programs by Domain

| Type of information | Source |
|---|---|
| Mortality | Death certificates |
| Morbidity | Review of medical charts |
| Utilization measures | Length of hospital stay |
| | Admission/readmission rates |
| | Outpatient visits |
| | Nursing home admissions |
| Functional status | Change in scores on the scale used |
| Quality of life | Change in scores on the scale used |
| Patient/caregiver satisfaction | Answer to an overall satisfaction question or questionnaire |
| Cost | Total inpatient cost |
| | Total outpatient cost |
| | Total nursing home cost |
| | Total health care cost |
| | Total cost of the CGA/GEM program |

CGA/GEM, Comprehensive Geriatric Assessment/Geriatric Evaluation and Management.

described in some studies should, however, be interpreted with caution. Costs of CGA/GEM programs include the initial costs of setting up the program, developing standardized questionnaires and protocols, training of staff, and so forth. They also include the costs of comprehensive assessment and follow-up visits to address conditions revealed by the assessment that usually leads to higher use of immediate short-term inpatient and outpatient services to treat them. The rates of reimbursement allowed by Medicare (about $275) do not come close to covering even the costs of targeting, laboratory testing, and personnel (about $1,700) (Boult et al., 1998). Such an investment is thus premised on expected improvements in quality of life and reduction in subsequent use of expensive medical care as well. The reduction of heath care costs reported in some studies results almost exclusively from a reduction in the number of days of hospitalization of CGA/GEM patients (Williams et al., 1987). Because hospitalization generates an enormous expense, any reduction in this area produces substantial savings.

One of the goals of most CGA/GEM is to maintain or recover the function and independence of the patient and to facilitate sustained residence in the community. As a result, higher rates of utilization of home health care services to assist in monitoring and treating the patients have already been seen in some studies, and a shift in care and resource utilization from the inpatient setting to the outpatient setting may occur with time. Investment in health promotion and prevention for older persons has rarely translated into immediate cost reductions. The emphasis on health promotion and more attempts to diagnose and treat health problems before they become exacerbated may translate into future lower hospitalization rates and hence a lower cost of health care.

Separate funding sources of health care programs and inadequate CGA reimbursement by Medicare interfere with optimal provision and coordination of services. If convinced of the value of CGA/GEM care, large practices might find it worthwhile to designate a geriatric evaluation team; smaller practices could arrange for a team meeting about to review outpatient cases, once a month perhaps in conjunction with nursing home rounds, hospital discharge planning rounds, or another regularly scheduled meeting that assembles the team members from social work, nursing, pharmacy, and psychology. Coordinating the care delivery to elderly patients will also improve the cost effectiveness of programs like CGA and GEM. These programs will probably be more cost effective as part of other programs for seniors at risk existing in the community. Transitional care units, case management, home care, and geriatric hospital units offer good locales for GEM.

## FUTURE DIRECTIONS

Managed care experience with older adults is relatively new. The number of HMOs contracting with the Health Care Financing Administration (HCFA) for provision of Medicare services grew rapidly during the 1980s. Wagner's survey (1996) of 75% of all HMOs with Medicare contracts in 1991 found that most did not have a formally trained geriatrician or generalist with a Certificate of Added Qualifications in Geriatrics on staff, and most were not systematically assessing functional status and other important social or health characteristics. Systematic approaches to major geriatrics syndromes like polypharmacy or inactivity and deconditioning were rare (Friedman & Kane, 1993).

Within the actual capitated system, group/staff model HMOs have the potential and the incentives to provide the most effective care for older adults at reasonable cost without the constraints of Medicare reimbursement guidelines. They are generally nonprofit, integrated delivery systems with their own staff, their own facilities, and long-term involvement in their own communities. Physicians are salaried, full-time employees of the organization or of a medical group that provides the health-related services (Wagner, 1996). These traditional HMOs have structural characteristics that could enhance the care of older people through the implementation of preventive programs like CGA and GEM. They serve a clearly defined population, each member of which has an accountable health care provider. They also have the full complement of professionals and services needed to care for older people with various needs and integrated data systems that facilitate planning and evaluation of care.

These managed care organizations can deliver low-intensity CGA programs to a large number of seniors for a relatively low per capita cost. To be cost-effective, the more intensive programs will have to focus selectively on those most likely to benefit and with more in-depth needs. Until recently, however, HMOs had neither the motivation nor the knowledge to renovate their delivery systems to better meet the needs of older chronically ill patients. Market pressures and high costs have provided the motivation (Wagner, 1996). The full potential of managed care to address chronic care has not, however, been realized (Kane, 1998). Some HMOs have begun to develop case management programs to manage the care and costs of older adults under the incentives of capitation. Social HMOs are experimenting with adding coordinated psychosocial and long-term care to the acute care package of services offered by traditional HMOs (Pacala et al., 1995b).

The implementation of preventive CGA and GEM programs in the fee-for-service model of care is a bigger challenge. Accomplishing continuity of care, in which patients are continuously reassessed and treated, requires some changes in the system of delivery of care. Some of these steps include establishing a computerized population-based medical information system, changing the current payment approach in Medicare, providing financial incentives, using nonphysician staff—nurses and social workers—and a proper integration of the currently fragmented acute and long-term care delivery systems. A population-based computerized medical information system is recommended to support health providers in the care of their elderly patients by systematically identifying high-risk elderly, tracking the care delivered, tracking the outcomes associated with the care, and sharing the data with members of the clinical team (Kane, 1998).

A change in the payment method used in Medicare-managed care models would remove some of the current disincentives to enroll the chronically ill in managed care. At present, Medicare pays a set amount per patient (average amount spent for a Medicare beneficiary) independently of his or her actual health status and hospitalization risk. This payment formula encourages HMOs to enroll healthy clients and avoid the sickest. A new formula based on better risk adjustments that properly recognize the costs associated with caring for people with different conditions and lower payments for healthy would be more appropriate. Public policy efforts to change fee-for-service reimbursement policies to increase reimbursement for geriatric care (especially outpatient visits) are necessary. Practicing physicians are well aware of the extra time that it takes to provide adequate care for frail elderly patients (time is needed for longer histories, discussion with family and other caregivers, and assessment of cognitive, functional, and affective status) (Goldstein, 1995). In most cases, geriatric assessment teams will have to work in partnership with primary care physicians who provide the majority of the care for the elderly population; in other settings, nurses working in teams with physicians could be trained to periodically implement the assessments of elders.

Integration of the existing health delivery systems would also improve the efficiency and quality of care. The fragmentation of services increases the cost of health, duplicates services, and increases the load of paperwork and confusion in the health care milieu. Additional attempts to develop realistic and cost-effective methods of CGA delivery are needed. Such approaches must use costly inputs (interdisciplinary team, home care etc) efficiently, fit in with the prevailing organizational practice framework that includes managed care, and work effectively in partnership with the primary care physician when appropriate. Comprehensive Geriatric Assessment ultimately should assist physicians in managing frail and complicated older patients. If the cost effectiveness of outpatient CGA/GEM programs is finally established, they will become more attractive to managed care, where guidelines for targeting and conducting the assessment and management of patients can be implemented and monitored.

There is also room for improvement in other areas of the health care of elderly patients. Additional research is needed to prevent and treat the health problems associated with aging. More efforts should be made to identify which components of the assessment process are strongly associated with improved outcomes and lower hospitalization rates. Standardized data gathering procedures and classification would ensure that each patient receives comprehensive evaluation and would facilitate comparisons among different programs.

## REFERENCES

Alessi, C. A., Stuck, A. E., Aronow, H. U., Yuhas, K. E., Bula, C. J., Madison, R., Gold, M., Segal-Gidan, F., Fanello, R., Rubenstein, L. Z., & Beck, J. C. (1997). The process of care in preventive in-home comprehensive geriatric assessment. *Journal of the American Geriatrics Society, 45,* 1044–1050.

Allen, C. M., Becker, P. M., McVey, L. J., et al. (1986). A randomized controlled clinical trial of a geriatric consultation team: Compliance with recommendations. *JAMA, 255,* 2617–2621.

Applegate, W., & Burns, R. (1996). Geriatric medicine. *JAMA, 275,* 1812–1813.

Applegate, W. B., Blass, J. P., & Williams, T. F. (1990). Instruments for the functional assessment of older patients. *New England Journal of Medicine, 322*(17), 1207–1214.

Barker, W. H., Williams, T. F., Zimmer, J. G., Van Buren, C., Vincent, S. J., & Pickrel, S. G. (1985). Geriatric consultation teams in acute hospitals: Impact on back-up of elderly patients. *Journal of The American Geriatrics Society, 33*(6), 422–428.

Becker, P. M., McVey, L. J., & Saltz, C. C. (1987). Hospital-acquired complications in a randomized controlled clinical trial of a geriatric consultation team. *JAMA, 257*(17), 2313–2317.

Bernabei, R., Landi, F., Gambassi, G., Sgardari, A., Zuccala, G., Mor, V., Rubenstein,

L. Z., & Carbonin, P. (1998). Randomised trial of impact of model of integrated care and case management for older people living in the community. *BMJ, 316,* 1348–1351.

Boult, C. (in press). Comprehensive geriatric assessment, *Merck Manual of Geriatrics (3rd edition).*

Boult, C., Boult, L., Morishita, L., Smith, S. L., & Kane, R. L. (1998). Outpatient geriatric evaluation and management. *Journal of the American Geriatrics Society, 46*(3), 296–302.

Boult, C., Dowd, B., McCaffrey, D., Boult, L., Hernandez, R., & Krulewitch, H. (1993). Screening elders for risk of hospital admission. *Journal of the American Geriatrics Society, 41,* 811–817.

Boult, C., Pacala, J. T., & Boult, L. (1995). Targeting elders for geriatric evaluation and management: Reliability, predictive validity and practicality of a questionnaire. *Aging Clinical and Experimental Research, 7*(3), 159–164.

Boult, L., Boult, C., Pirie, P., & Pacala, J. T. (1994). Test–retest reliability of a questionnaire that identifies elders at risk for hospital admission. *Journal of the American Geriatrics Society, 42*(7), 707–711.

Burns, R. (1994). Beyond the black box of comprehensive geriatric assessment. *Journal of the American Geriatrics Society, 43,* 1130.

Burns, R., Nichols, L. O., Graney, M. J., & Cloar, F. T. (1995). Impact of continued geriatric outpatient management on health outcomes of older veterans. *Archives of Internal Medicine, 155,* 1313–1318.

Cappelleri, J. C., Ioannidis, J. P., Schmid, C. H., deFerranti, S. D., Aubert, M., Chalmers, T. C., & Lau, J. (1996). Large trials vs meta-analysis of smaller trials: How do their results compare? *JAMA, 276,* 1332–1338.

Cefalu, C. A., Kaslow, L. D., Mims, B., & Simpson, S. (1995). Follow-up of comprehensive geriatric assessment in a family medicine residency clinic. *Journal of the American Board of Family Practice, 8,* 263–269.

Coleman, E. A., Wagner, E. H., Grothaus, L. C., Hecht, J., Savarino, J., & Buchner, D. M. (1998). Predicting hospitalization and functional decline in older health plan enrollees: Are administrative data as accurate as self-report? *Journal of the American Geriatrics Society, 46,* 419–425.

Engelhardt, J. B., Toseland, R. W., O'Donnell, J. C., Richie, J. T., Jue, D., & Banks, S. (1996). The effectiveness and efficiency of outpatient geriatric evaluation and management. *Journal of the American Geriatrics Society, 44,* 847–856.

Epstein, A. M., Hall, J. A., Fretwell, M., Feldstein, M., DeClantis, M. L., Tognetti, J., Cutler, C., Constantine, M., Besdine, R., Rowe, J., & McNeil, B. J. (1990). Consultative geriatric assessment for ambulatory patients. *Journal of the American Medical Association, 263*(4), 538–544.

Feussner, J. R. (1991). Geriatric evaluation and management units: Experimental methods for evaluating efficacy. *Journal of the American Geriatrics Society, 19,* 19S–24S.

Fretwell, M. D. (1992). Comprehensive functional assessment: An overview. *Family Medicine, 24,* 453–456.

Fretwell, M. D., Raymond, P. M., McGarvey, S. T., Owens, N., Traines, M., Silliman, R. A., & Mor, V. (1990). The Senior Care Study: A controlled trial of a consultative/unit-based geriatric assessment program in acute care. *Journal of the American Geriatrics Society, 38*(10), 1973–1081.

Friedman, B., & Kane, R. L. (1993). HMO medical directors' perceptions of geriatric practice in Medicare HMOs. *Journal of the American Geriatrics Society, 41,* 1144–1149.

Goldstein, M. K. (1995). Comprehensive geriatric assessment: Is it too comprehensive for compliance and cost-effectiveness? *Journal of the American Board of Family Practice, 8*(4), 337–340.

Greenfield, S., Kaplan, S. H., & Ware, J. J. (1985). Expanding patient involvement in care: Effects on patient outcomes. *Annals of Internal Medicine, 102*(4), 520–528.

Hamm, R. J. (1986). Assessment, *Geriatric Medicine Annual* (pp. 223–254). Oradell, NJ: Medical Economic Books.

Hendriksen, C., Lund, E., & Stromgard, E. (1984). Consequences of assessment and intervention among elderly people: A three-year randomized controlled trial. *BMJ, 289,* 1522–1524.

Ioannidis, J. P. A., Cappelleri, J. C., & Lau, J. (1998). Issues in comparisons between meta-analysis and large trials. *JAMA, 279,* 1089–1093.

Kane, R. L. (1998). Managed care as a vehicle for delivering more effective chronic care for older persons. *Journal of the American Geriatrics Society, 46,* 1034–1039.

Katz, P. R., Dube, D. H., & Calkins, E. (1985). The use of a structured functional assessment format in a geriatric consultative service. *Journal of the American Geriatrics Society, 33,* 681–686.

Keller, B., & Potter, J. (1994). Predictors of

mortality in outpatient geriatric evaluation and management of clinic patients. *Journal of Gerontology, 49*(6), m246–m251.

Leveille, S. G., Wagner, E. H., Davis, C., Grothaus, L., Wallace, J., LoGerfo, M., & Kent, D. (1998). Preventing disability and managing chronic illness in frail older adults: A randomized trial of a community-based partnership with primary care. *Journal of the American Geriatrics Society, 46*(10), 1191–1198.

Maly, R. C., Abrahamse, A. F., Hirsch, S. H., Frank, J. C., & Reubens, D. B. (1996). What influences physician practice behavior? An interview study of physicians who received consultative geriatric assessment recommendations. *Archives of Family Medicine, 5,* 448–454.

McVey, L. J., Becker, P. M., Saltz, C. C., Feussner, J. R., & Cohen, H. J. (1989). Effect of a geriatric consultation team on functional status of elderly hospitalized patients. A randomized, controlled clinical trial. *Annals of Internal Medicine, 110,* 79–84.

Morishita, L., Boult, C., Boult, L., Smith, S., & Pacala, J. T. (1998). Satisfaction with outpatient geriatric evaluation and management. *Gerontologist, 38,* 303–308.

O'Donnell, J. C., & Toseland, R. W. (1997). Does geriatric evaluation and management improve health behavior of older veterans in psychological distress? *Journal of Aging and Health, 9*(4), 473–497.

Pacala, J. T., Boult, C., & Boult, L. (1995a). Predictive validity of a questionnaire that identifies older persons at risk for hospital admission. *Journal of the American Geriatrics Society, 43,* 374–377.

Pacala, J. T., Boult, C., Hepburn, K. W., Kane, R. A., Kane, R. L., Malone, J. K., Morishita, L., & Reed, R. L. (1995b). Case management of older adults in health maintenance organizations. *Journal of the American Geriatrics Society, 43*(5), 538–542.

Reuben, D. B., Borok, G. M., Wolde-Tsadik, G., Ershoff, D. H., Fishman, L. K., Ambrosini, V. L., Liu, Y., Rubenstein, L. Z., & Beck, J. C. (1995). A randomized trial of comprehensive geriatric assessment in the care of hospital patients. *New England Journal of Medicine, 332*(20), 1345–1350.

Reuben, D. B., Fishman, L. K., McNabney, M., & Wolde-Tsadik, G. (1996). Looking inside the black box of comprehensive geriatric assessment: A classification system for problems, recommendations and implementation strategies. *Journal of the American Geriatrics Society, 44,* 835–838.

Reuben, D. B., Frank, J. C., Hirsch, S. H., McGuigan, K. A., & Maly, R. C. (1999). A randomized clinical trial of outpatient comprehensive geriatric assessment coupled with an intervention to increase adherence to recommendations. *Journal of the American Geriatrics Society, 47,* 269–276.

Reuben, D. B., Hirsch, S. H., Chernoff, J. C., Cheska, Y., Drezner, M., Engelman, B., Frank, J. C., Schlesinger, M., & Siegler, C. F. (1993). Project safety net: A health screening outreach and assessment program. *Gerontologist, 33,* 557–560.

Rubenstein, L. Z. (1987). Geriatric assessment: An overview of its impacts. In L. Z. Rubenstein, L. J. Campbell, & R. L. Kane (Eds.), *Clinics in Geriatric Medicine.* Philadelphia: W. B. Saunders.

Rubenstein, L. Z., Goodwin, M., Hadley, E., Patten, S. K., Rempusheski, V. F., Reuben, D., & Winograd, C. H. (1991). Working group recommendations: Targeting criteria for geriatric evaluation and management research. *Journal of the American Geriatric Society, 39,* 37S–41S.

Rubenstein, L. Z., Josephson, K. R., Wieland, G. D., English, P. A., Sayre, J. A., & Kane, R. A. (1984). Effectiveness of a geriatric evaluation unit: A randomized clinical trial. *New England Journal of Medicine, 311*(26), 1664–1670.

Rubin, C. D. (1993). A randomized controlled trial of outpatient geriatric evaluation and management in a large public hospital. *Journal of the American Geriatrics Society, 41,* 1023–1028.

Rubin, C. D., Sizemore, M. T., Loftis, P. A., Adams-Huet, B., & Anderson, R. J. (1992). The effect of geriatric evaluation and management on Medicare reimbursement in a large public hospital: A randomized clinical trial. *Journal of the American Geriatrics Society, 40,* 989–995.

Saltz, C., McVey, L. J., Becker, P. M., Feussner, J. R., & Cohen, H. J. (1988). Impact of a geriatric consultation team on discharge placement and repeat hospitalization. *Gerontologist, 28*(3), 344–350.

Shah, P. N., Maly, R. C., Frank, J. C., Hirsch, S. H., & Reuben, D. B. (1997). Managing geriatric syndromes: What geriatric assessment teams recommend, what primary care physicians implement, what patients adhere to. *Journal of the American Geriatrics Society, 45,* 413–419.

Silverman, M., Musa, D., Martin, D. C., Lave, J. R., Adams, J., & Ricci, E. M. (1995). Evaluation of outpatient geriatric assessment: A randomized multi-site trial. *Jour-*

nal of the American Geriatrics Society, 43, 733–740.

Siu, A. L., Kravitz, R. L., Keeler, E., Hemmerling, K., Kington, R., Davis, J. W., Mitchell, A., Burton, T. M., Morgensten, H., Beers, M. H., & Reuben, D. B. (1996). Postdischarge geriatric assessment of hospitalized frail elderly patients. Archives of Internal Medicine, 156, 76–81.

Siu, A. L., Morishita, L., & Blaustein, J. (1994). Comprehensive geriatric assessment in a day hospital. Journal of the American Geriatrics Society, 42, 1094–1099.

Solomon, D. H. (1988). Geriatric assessment: Methods for clinical decision making. Journal of the American Medical Association, 259, 2450–2452.

Stuck, A. E., Aronow, H. U., Steiner, A., Alessi, C. A., Bula, C. J., Gold, M. N., Yuhas, K. E., Nisenbaum, R., Rubenstein, L. Z., & Beck, J. C. (1995). A trial of annual in-home comprehensive geriatric assessments for elderly people living in the community. New England Journal of Medicine, 333(18), 1184–1189.

Stuck, A. E., Siu, A. L., Wieland, G. D., Adams, J., & Rubenstein, L. Z. (1993). Comprehensive geriatric assessment: a meta-analysis of controlled trials. Lancet, 342, 1032–1036.

Teasdale, T. A., Shuman, L., Snow, E., & Luchi, R. J. (1983). A comparison of placement outcomes of geriatric cohorts receiving care in a geriatric assessment unit and on general medicine floors. Journal of the American Geriatrics Society, 31(9), 529–534.

Toseland, R. W., O'Donnell, J. C., Engelhardt, J. B., Hendler, S. A., Richie, J. T., & Jue, D. (1996). Outpatient geriatric evaluation and management: Results of a randomized trial. Medical Care, 34, 624–640.

Tryon, A. F., Mayfield, G. K., & Bross, M. H. (1992). Use of comprehensive geriatric assessment techniques by community physicians. Family Medicine, 24, 453–456.

Tulloch, A. J., & Moore, V. (1979). A randomized controlled trial of geriatric screening and surveillance in general practice. J R Coll Gen Pract, 29, 733–742.

Vetter, N., Jones, D. A., & Victor, C. R. (1984). Effect of health visitors working with elderly patients in general practice: A randomized controlled trial. BMJ, 288, 369–372.

Wagner, E. H. (1996). The promise and performance of HMOs in improving outcomes in older adults. Journal of the American Geriatrics Society, 44(10), 1251–1257.

Williams, M. E., Williams, T. F., Zimmer, J. G., Jackson, Hall, W., & Podgorski, C. A. (1987). How does the team approach to outpatient geriatric evaluation compare with traditional care: A report of a randomized controlled trial. Journal of American Geriatrics Society, 35, 1071–1078.

Winograd, C. H. (1991). Targeting strategies: An overview of criteria and outcomes. Journal of the American Geriatrics Society, 39S, 25S–35S.

Yeo, G., Ingram, L., Skurnick, J., & Crapo, L. (1987). Effects of a geriatric clinic on functional health and well being of elders. Journal of Gerontology, 42, 252–258.

# 14

## Care Planning for Older Adults in Health Care Settings

### PATRICIA FINCH-GUTHRIE

Clinical assessments of elderly individuals' health and functional abilities are directly valuable for older adults only if they are actually used to make decisions about their care. To be useful in a clinical situation, assessment information must be analyzed and synthesized in a way that serves to direct, define, or evaluate care. Clinicians take action based on clinical assessments in order to provide appropriate care. To move beyond the assessment phase of care, diagnoses and problems must first be identified from the collected data. These are then prioritized so that interventions can be designed, implemented, and evaluated. The documentation of a planned process of assessment, problem identification, intervention, and evaluation is the patient's plan for care. Without a specified plan, the care given to an individual can be directionless, lacking coordination and continuity. A well-constructed care plan is especially important for older patients due to co-morbidities and complex health care needs. Care plans are part of standard practice in acute hospital care, subacute and nursing home care, rehabilitation settings, and home care. Wide variation exists, however, as to how care plans are developed and utilized.

This chapter defines and describes the care-planning process, provides a conceptual framework for care planning, identifies key differences in planning care for older adults as compared with other populations, and identifies and discusses care planning methods currently used for elderly patients. It details the types of assessments used in care planning and describes how those assessments are utilized in different care-planning methods. Problems that occur with different planning approaches are addressed and recommendations offered for improving care planning for older adults.

## WHAT IS CARE PLANNING?

Specifically, care planning is a dynamic decision-making process based on assessment. Assessment is a continuous, systematic process for collecting, validating, analyzing, and interpreting health information that becomes more complete and thorough as knowledge of the patient increases (Alfaro-LeFevere, 1998). Assessment is an integral part of the care planning process; the effectiveness of the care plan depends on the breadth, depth, and accuracy of assessments. The clinical product of the assessment process is development of an individualized care plan document that outlines necessary actions essential for achieving prioritized outcomes. Assessments have to be conducted systematically to produce information needed for decision making. Haphazard assessments lead to inappropriate, ineffective, and possibly harmful care.

Initial clinical assessments provide baseline information about an elderly individual's current health status, functional capabilities, health concerns, and personal health goals. Baseline information provides clinicians with a reference point for an assessment database and helps clinicians focus on the patient's individual needs. This database is useful for evaluating the patient's progress toward meeting health outcomes, as well as for identifying subsequent status changes. Focused assessments explore in more depth health concerns uncovered in baseline assessments. They provide additional, detailed information about a specific area of concern, such as mobility problems, incontinence issues, chronic pain, and nutritional needs.

Through data classification and synthesis of information from baseline and focused assessments, needs and diagnoses are identified and then prioritized based on several criteria, such as problem severity, importance to the individual, and effect on functional independence. After priorities for care are determined, actions or interventions are identified and designed by the professional caregiver and patient to achieve specific outcomes. Throughout the care-planning process, ongoing assessments are used to validate collected information, to monitor health status, and to evaluate the patient's progress in meeting outcomes. Based on continuous assessment, the care plan may then be maintained, modified, or terminated.

## WHY IS CARE PLANNING IMPORTANT?

Care planning is important for several reasons. First, care plans can facilitate the diagnosis and treatment of disease. Signs and symptoms are assessed, a diagnosis is determined, and treatment is prescribed that eliminates or manages the condition. The care plan for this purpose outlines assessments, such as laboratory tests and diagnostic procedures needed to determine etiology. Once the cause or causes are isolated, the plan of care can then be used to outline necessary treatment.

Second, care plans facilitate management of predictable or preventable health problems, with goals being to restore, maintain, or improve health. In the presence of known care problems, the most likely complications are identified and strategies put in place that prevent them from occurring or serve to manage outcomes if prevention is not possible. For example, a patient with diabetes is at risk for poor wound healing. Thus, a plan of routine foot care should be implemented in order to avoid ulcers and wound infections that often develop in the feet of individuals with diabetes. Additionally, risk factors for potential problems are identified and interventions implemented that eliminate, reduce, or control the effects of risk factors. Clinicians also need to assess for more general risk factors that could negatively affect health and initiate preventative strategies. For example, immunization against influenza and pneumoccal pneumonia is standard care for most older adults, especially the frail older adult, because of their decreased resistance to infection and the increased risk of significant morbidity and mortality.

Third, a written care plan provides a basis for establishing continuity of care. The care plan serves as a communication tool that facilitates coordination of care between disciplines, care sites, and agencies involved in the patient's care. A written plan helps to ensure that everyone is working toward the same goals and promotes consistent monitoring and evaluation. The transfer of care information becomes more important with increasing care complexity and when recovery involves several care locations. Many institutions have created interagency referral forms to ensure the transfer of information deemed necessary by the receiving agency for the continuation of care. For example, when a patient is transferred from acute hospital care to a long-term care facility, the discharge summary, interagency transfer form, assessment data such as laboratory test results, the plan of care, and physician orders generally accompany the individual. This transfer of information helps to ensure continued care and facilitates the patient's recovery, regardless of the care site.

## CONCEPTUAL FRAMEWORK

Care planning should be patient centered. Unfortunately, care planning often becomes a routine task completed more to satisfy federal and state regulatory requirements than to address patient needs. If a given diagnosis automatically triggers a standard approach, one care plan may look like another with little or no attention to the unique care needs of the individual. Thus, the framework most appropriate for planning care for older adults is a patient-centered approach that ensures individualized care. A patient-centered approach supports the older adult's values, preferences, and decisions, which enhances autonomy (see Chapter 8). A patient-centered approach empowers the patient and can improve health care outcomes, such as the reduction of stress levels, fatigue, and depression (Coulton, Dunkle, Chow, Haug, & Vielhaber, 1989; Brandreit, Lyons, & Benley, 1994; McWilliam et al., 1994). There are two key components to patient-centered care. First, patients are active participants in their care, and, second, the patient's family and support system are important parts of assessment, decision making, and care (Gage, 1994).

The term *patient centered* was first used in association with Rogers' approach to psychotherapy (1951). His methodology emphasized an active patient role in therapy. Today, the term *patient-centered* or *client-focused care* refers to a care process that emphasizes responding to patient needs first instead of what is convenient or more important for the institution or health care professional (Lathrop et al., 1991; Weber, 1991; Bernd, 1992; Gage, 1994). A patient-centered approach means that individuals and their needs or care priorities drive the care-planning process.

Resident rights, outlined by the 1987 Omnibus Budget Reconciliation Act, reinforce patient involvement in care planning in nursing homes (Table 14.1). Even though these rights were developed to apply to nursing homes, they are applicable to any care situation. Every older adult has the right to expect preventive, rehabilitative, and restorative care that improves function and respects the individual's opinions, desires, and decisions (Burger et al., 1996).

Ensuring patient participation in care and decision making is not a simple matter, and determining the number of older adults participating may not be the best measure for involvement for an institution. In one study, 40% of nursing home residents reported not being involved in their health care decisions (Wetle et al., 1988). However, 79.3% of those patients reported that the level of their participation was the right amount. This finding suggests a varying degree of preferences with regard to care involvement and ability to participate. Some individuals wanted family members or physicians to make most of the decisions. This variation in involve-

**Table 14.1.  Resident Rights Related to Care Planning**

To have access to adequate or appropriate health care
To be informed of your medical condition
To participate in planning your own treatment
To refuse medication and treatment
To participate in the discharge planning process
To review your medical record

ment may be related to whether patients expect to have personal control or whether they expect the situation to be out of their control (Coulton et al., 1988; Coulton et al., 1989). Thus, older adults need to be asked about the level of involvement they want in planning their own care and then given control of the decisions identified as important. Proxy decision-makers need to be specified if the older adult wants this kind of support. Older adults need to be given opportunities to be involved and make their own decisions, even if this means selecting others to make decisions for them.

Numerous barriers exist for patient involvement in care. The need to balance patient safety and autonomy, institutional convenience and patient preferences, and patient and family preferences along with lack of staff knowledge and understanding for the care needed by older adults and presence of cognitive impairment all com-

plicate care. Many professional caregivers and institutions have a paternalistic attitude toward older adults. An underlying belief that health care professionals "know what is best" and that older people are "child-like" prevails. Many care providers assess older adults as incapable of making informed, voluntary care choices (Avorn & Langer, 1982).

How is a patient-centered approach operationalized? The patient and/or family actively participates in all phases of the care-planning process, which is a circular process with the patient at the center (Fig. 14.1). Needs identification and assessment, diagnosis, priority setting, decision making and planning, plan implementation, and evaluation revolve around the patient's interests.

Assessments are made to clarify patient needs, health care concerns, and goals. Once data are classified as to areas of wellness, illness, disease, and social needs, the

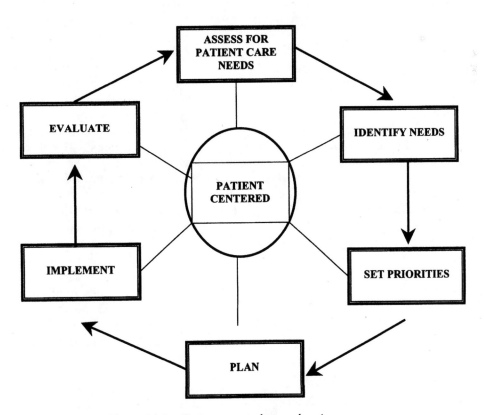

**Figure 14.1.** Patient-centered care planning process.

needs are prioritized with the patient. Priority setting determines which diagnoses or needs are addressed, the order in which they are addressed, the assessments needed on an ongoing basis, and frequency of reassessments. Criteria for determining priorities are listed in Table 14.2.

From a health perspective, conditions or needs that threaten life, safety, and security, are more severe and require immediate attention and action. A patient suffering from shortness of breath needs immediate intervention to improve oxygenation before they receive care for incontinence. In addition, core needs are dealt with first. Core needs are problems that, when not dealt with, cause other problems such as functional impairment. If a patient has mobility needs as a result of hip pain, the hip pain is dealt with before the mobility issues. The patient's priorities are also incorporated into the plan before issues that the older adult views as less important. It may seem that severity of care needs should always be the major criterion for determining care priorities. There is no strict hierarchical criteria, however, as decisions cannot be made outside the clinical context. Modifying factors, such as advanced age and frailty, have to be considered. A 90-year-old woman may view the removal of cataracts so that she can read a greater priority than treating her breast cancer. Often there is tension between the professional caregiver and family when dealing with patient safety versus satisfying the patient's preferences (see Chapter 8).

Once care priorities have been established, achievable outcomes must be determined. Outcomes serve two purposes: They help determine appropriate interven-

Table 14.2.
Criteria for Setting Priorities

Severity of the illness/need or disease prognosis
Presence of modifying factors
Core needs versus problems that are effects or
   consequences of unmet needs
Effect on functional independence
Safety needs
Patient priorities and care preferences

Table 14.3.
Criteria for Outcomes

Derived from the patient's prioritized care needs
Patient instead of discipline focused
Attainable given the patient's capabilities
Formulated with the patient
Realistic in relation to available resources
Documented in measurable terms

tions, and they are essential for evaluating the patient's progress. Outcomes need to meet several criteria to be useful for planning care (Table 14.3).

Generally, several outcomes can be selected for each priority problem. Including the patient in the decision making increases the likelihood that the outcome meets the needs of the patient. For example, if chronic pain is a priority problem, the patient outcome might be to achieve absence of pain, a specific number of hours of pain relief between treatments, or a decrease in pain severity. The patient may choose to have some pain versus taking stronger pain medication that causes drowsiness. The need to function normally may be a higher priority than total pain relief. If the clinician chooses the outcome of total pain relief without consulting the patient, the patient's need to function normally would be sacrificed.

After determining outcomes, the professional caregiver and patient identify appropriate interventions. Decisions are made as to which interventions will achieve specified outcomes by considering the risks and benefits associated with each intervention. The clinician's role is to support decision making by providing the information needed for the older adult to make informed choices based on what is right or desirable for himself or herself (Castellucci, 1998). Patients with cognitive deficits are included in the planning process to the fullest extent possible by providing opportunities for decision making within their cognitive limitations and by including the family. Involving the patient and/or family in risk/benefit discussions is extremely important. Some older individuals may choose a conservative approach to care if the risks associated with alternative treatment options outweigh the benefits (Kasper, Mulley, & Wennberg, 1992). Other patients may choose a treatment that has greater risk if the possible outcome includes restoring health to previous levels or improving functional independence.

The choice of interventions is also based on established care standards, research, or evidence of the best practice approach. Clinicians have a responsibility to resolve or control health issues, to minimize the risks associated with treatment, and to promote optimum health and independence for the older adult by recommending appropriate care. Once interventions are chosen, the timing, frequency, and duration of interventions need to be determined. Often decisions concerning how to operationalize an intervention are based on professional standards associated with the specific intervention, along with the clinician's experience with the treatment approach. The level of care complexity and skill required to implement actions determines who implements selected actions. Finally, practical constraints or limitations affect which actions are implemented. The cost of care, the clinical and social resources that are needed, the technology required, and the available locations for provision of care play significant roles in the implementation phase of the care plan.

The availability of financial resources is an important area to assess before a specific plan is implemented. Without a clear understanding of covered services, the best plan of care will be irrelevant if the insurance is inadequate to cover the care costs. It is better to know the financial limitations before a plan is developed so that services can be negotiated than to have to completely abandon the entire plan. Insurance plans often dictate the type of services that are covered, along with who can provide the services and where they can be provided. For example, Medicare will only cover intermittent intravenous antibiotic therapy in a hospital or extended care facility. The cost of administering this treatment in the home, however, is not covered (Health Care Financing Administration, 1994).

Technology impacts the plan of care substantially and is a double-edged sword. Although advanced interventions can improve the quality of care, they also create care complications that result in negative outcomes. For example, although mechanical ventilators have been successfully used to treat patients with acute respiratory failure, they have also created ventilator-dependent patients when used to intervene in end-stage pulmonary disease. Successful weaning from a respirator cannot always be accomplished in this patient population, leaving patients who need continuous care in facilities that specialize in caring for ventilator-dependent patients.

Evaluation focuses on the patient's achievement of outcomes and is based on the patient's progress. Together with the patient and family, the clinician compares the care results with planned outcomes. Based on this comparison, the plan is continued if the individual has not achieved the outcomes and barriers to the plan's effectiveness are not present. Time in this instance may be the needed factor for improvement. The plan is modified if outcomes have not been accomplished and additional needs, risk factors, or more effective interventions are identified. In this case, the planning cycle starts again. Finally, the plan is terminated if the individual has achieved the outcomes, no new problems or risk factors have been identified, and the patient is able to resume self-care (Alfaro-LeFevere, 1998). Often the evaluation phase of the care planning process is given minimal attention and as such the plan is not updated appropriately, loosing its usefulness for guiding care.

## PLANNING CARE FOR ELDERLY PERSONS

Although the basic elements of the care planning process are essentially the same for all age groups and patient populations (assessment, diagnosis or problem identification, intervention, and evaluation), specific differences must be considered when planning care for older adults. First, planning care for older patients must include an assessment of age-related changes that may be present, as well as the individual's adjustment to aging. Assessments of how age-related changes and other health risk factors work together to contribute to negative or positive patient outcomes will help to identify necessary interventions. Assessing only health risk factors, without considering age-related changes, gives the clinician a limited picture of the needs of older patients. For example, when assessing the older patient's inability to sleep, one must recognize normal age-related changes that occur in the sleep cycle in addition to assessing other causal factors such as pain, discomfort, medications, lack of exercise, and environmental factors. If patients believe the only normal sleep cycle is the way they slept as a younger individual, they probably have not adapted well to a change in their sleep pattern. This lack of adaptation could lead to anxiety and possibly to sleep impairment. Thus, the required interventions may include only education concerning age-related changes in the sleep cycle and exploration of ways to adapt to the change in pattern. If additional factors are present, ways to eliminate, reduce, or manage their effect would also be initiated.

Second, the practitioner must be alert to subtleties of disease presentation in older adults. For example, acute confusion can be the first sign of severe illness in an older individual. An older patient experiencing a myocardial infarction may have a sudden onset of confusion rather than complain of chest pain. These variations in presentation add to the difficulty of assessment, diagnosis, and problem identification and thereby delaying appropriate treatment.

Third, because chronic disease patterns are more prevalent than acute illness, assessment should emphasize functional changes. Many elderly patients have more than one chronic condition or health problem, and each problem tends to have many contributing factors with multiple ramifications. Consequently, assessments need to be multidimensional, and interventions need to be aimed at maximizing function. For example, the development of sudden cognitive changes may be related to exacerbation of chronic illnesses such as diabetes, heart disease, or kidney failure; multiple medications; pain and discomfort; sensory and mobility impairments; or environmental factors. As a result, assessment, treatment, and care become very complex. Changes in cognition affect older persons' abilities to engage in self-care and increase dependency on informal and formal support structures. All aspects of their lives and the lives of their family are affected.

Finally, planning care for older adults often includes the management of multiple care transitions. Frail, older adults with chronic disease often have acute exacerbations of their illnesses that require hospitalization followed by home care or extended care in long-term care settings. Response to treatment can vary by patient age. Recovery patterns for older patients may be prolonged, requiring extensive monitoring and evaluation. Older adults may experience a gradual functional decline, requiring more and more community care, eventually leading to nursing home placement when it is no longer appropriate to remain at home. Proactive planning is key to providing quality care to older adults that includes management of transitions.

## TYPES OF ASSESSMENTS USED IN PLANNING CARE

Five different forms of assessments are generally used throughout the care planning process: screening, baseline, focused, validation and monitoring, and evaluation assessments.

### Screening

Screening in the traditional sense is usually applied to the examination of well or asymptomatic people in order to classify their likelihood of having the condition being screened (Morrison, 1985). In a broader context, screening is an assessment process that utilizes only a portion of the usual examining procedures to identify the need for more focused assessment and intervention. Screening instruments are generally brief and contain only the essential diagnostic criteria or salient domains of the construct being assessed. Often referrals to specific disciplines for continuing care are made after screening for specific key risk factors.

Screening can have a positive impact on the quality and length of an individual's life by identifying three major areas for intervention: early or asymptomatic disease, behaviors that could be modified to achieve a more healthy lifestyle, and functions that could be maximized in order to restore or maintain abilities. Three categories of intervention (primary, secondary, and tertiary prevention) are then utilized to address issues uncovered by screening processes or instruments (U.S. Preventive Services Task Force, 1996) (Table 14.4).

Primary prevention is targeted toward reversing or eliminating risks that predispose an individual to develop a future illness or condition. An example of a screening instrument that would lead to primary intervention in older adults includes the Level I screen of the Nutrition Screening Initiative, which identifies those individuals at risk for poor nutrition (Dwyer, 1991). Well-known primary preventive interventions in older adults include immunizations. Individuals over age 65 years are recommended to receive pneumoccal vaccine, immunization for influenza, and tetanus-diphtheria boosters (U.S. Preventive Services Task Force, 1996). Additional interventions include counseling, teaching, and support for changing behavior, which addresses issues such as smoking, diet, and exercise.

Secondary prevention is aimed at preventing morbidity from disease in a preclinical or asymptomatic phase. Sloane (1984) advocates this type of screening for medical conditions that have effective interventions for older adults as a way to promote and maintain health. The report of the U.S. Preventive Services Task Force (1996) recommends blood pressure screening, mammography, Papanicolau tests, vision and glaucoma checks, hearing tests, fecal occult blood tests and/or sigmoidoscopy, monitoring of height and weight, and assessment for problem drinking for all persons age 65 years and older. The goals of this type of screening, for example, are to prevent stroke that can occur from uncontrolled high blood pressure, mortality and morbidity from advanced cancer, and blindness from untreated glaucoma.

Tertiary prevention focuses on identifying symptomatic but untreated disease, dysfunction, or disability. An example of a tertiary screening tool for identifying cognitive dysfunction is the Mini-Mental State Examination. A low score indicates a need for further neurologic examination to determine the cause of the impairment and subsequent treatment. The primary goal for this type of prevention is to slow deterioration or to maintain or restore health.

Table 14.4.
Categories of Screening and Intervention

| Categories | Screening and intervention |
|---|---|
| Primary screening | Identifying risk factors that predispose a future illness |
| Intervention | Reversing or eliminating predisposing risk factors |
| Secondary screening | Identifying preclinical or asymptomatic illness or disease |
| Intervention | Preventing morbidity from undetected illness or disease |
| Tertiary screening | Identifying symptomatic untreated disease or disability |
| Intervention | Slowing deterioration, maintaining or restoring health |

Rehabilitative programs are generally included in tertiary prevention.

### Baseline Comprehensive Assessments

Baseline assessments include comprehensive information gathered on initial contact with persons to assess all aspects of their health status (Alfaro-LeFevere, 1998). Baseline assessments are usually obtained on admission to a particular care service. This form of assessment helps to establish an initial database for planning and evaluating care. Ongoing assessments are compared with those obtained at baseline to determine patient progress. The goals of the baseline assessment are to identify current care needs and problems requiring referral to other disciplines; to describe symptoms that may indicate presence of disease; to clarify established health regimens; to provide a summary of the patient's medical history; to concentrate on conditions that may have an impact on the patient's current health status; to assess functional status; and to identify patient strengths important for achieving outcomes.

Often the baseline or initial comprehensive assessment is based on a structured format, established by a particular agency. In long-term care settings, the Omnibus Budget Reconciliation Act of 1987 mandated the use of a standardized interdisciplinary assessment tool called the Resident Assessment Instrument (RAI; see Chapter 16). Thus, the care plan for each individual in long-term care should include identified problems from the RAI and the strategies or actions that will prevent problems from occurring or that will restore health. The success of the RAI in improving care planning varies and depends heavily on how it has been operationalized in a particular nursing home. If the RAI and the care plan sit in a book at the nursing desk and the direct care staff do not have access to them or utilize them in providing daily care, they are much less likely to affect care.

Physicians often complete a medical history and physical examination before or at admission to a hospital and a discharge summary on transfer to a long-term care facility or discharge home. Admitting nurses in both acute and long-term care conduct initial assessments, concentrating on the patients' responses to their health and illness. Other disciplines may also conduct initial assessments, depending on the nature of the service and care provided. For example, intake assessments to a rehabilitation facility may be conducted by a physical or occupational therapist because the main care focus is rehabilitation. In long-term care settings, the RAI may be filled out by nurses or in collaboration with other disciplines who focus on specific areas of functioning. The RAI was developed to facilitate communication and problem-solving among an interdisciplinary group of care givers by creating a common language and knowledge base about the resident (Hawes et al., 1997) The goal was to create an instrument that was not profession specific, but could be used by physicians, nurses, social workers, or rehabilitation and recreational specialists.

The initial baseline assessment for care planning should include both subjective and objective data. Table 14.5 presents a comprehensive list of potential assessments to be included; few real-world assessments are this complete. Subjective data reflect the patients' views and include their own observations, descriptions, complaints, and perspectives about their health and health care, as well as their affective and social functioning. Subjective assessments can include cultural factors, the patients' knowledge of health care requirements, and aspects of their lifestyle that may impact health. Objective data are often equated with findings based on physical examinations and laboratory data. A broader definition, however, includes information apparent to the external observer. Baseline objective assessments include measures of physical health as well as physical and cognitive functioning.

The primary purpose of a comprehensive assessment of an elderly patient is to identify functional patterns that differ

**Table 14.5.**

Baseline Comprehensive Assessments for Care Plan Development

| Subjective Data | Objective data-Presence of age-related changes and health risk factors |
|---|---|
| a. Individual's identification and description of own health concerns | a. Physical health |
| b. Self-rating of health | Admitting diagnosis |
| c. Pain and discomfort | Physical appearance |
| d. Patient/family preferences and expectations for care | Organ/system changes (respiratory, cardiovascular, nervous, integumentary system, gastrointestinal, musculoskeletal, and genitourinary system) |
| e. Spirituality, values, and beliefs | Presence of disease/past history |
| f. Self-care practices | Observable signs/symptoms |
| g. Patient motivation and readiness for self-care | Sensory changes |
| h. Patients' identification of their strengths | Oral/nutritional status |
| i. Adaptation to age-related changes | Sleep/rest patterns |
| j. Affective functioning | Elimination patterns |
| Self-concept | Medications |
| Presence of depression and anxiety | Immunizations |
| Emotional integrity | Allergies |
| Coping patterns/stress tolerance | Smoking/substance abuse |
| k. Social functioning | b. Physical functioning |
| Social support | ADLs |
| Roles/relationships | IADLs |
| Social networks | Presence of compensatory mechanisms/devices |
| Recreation | Activity/exercise pattern |
| Elder abuse/neglect | c. Cognitive functioning |
| Advance directives | Alertness |
| l. Life style | Attention |
| m. Living situation | Orientation |
| n. Cultural factors | Memory |
| o. Self-care abilities and knowledge of health care requirements | Judgment |
| p. Sexual function | Language |
| | d. Safety and security needs |

ADLs, activities of daily living; IADLs, instrumental activities of daily living.

from accepted norms. These serve as a basis for interventions and care activities to meet the older patient's needs, ultimately improving quality of life. Unidimensional instruments and scales for assessing functional domains have been described in previous chapters and should be used routinely in the initial, baseline assessment. Standardization of measures included in baseline assessments can improve clinical decision making and care planning. Important aspects of care are less likely to be missed and communication between disciplines can be enhanced through application of recognized and accepted measures.

**Focused Assessments**

Focused assessments are more in-depth and individualized assessments for determining the status of an older adult's specific problems or conditions. Frequently, these assessments are based on signs and symptoms of illness, focused on specific body systems or on areas of poor function. Only patients at high risk for problems or complications or who are experiencing specific problems receive focused assessments. Focused assessments are completed by the discipline with the most specialized knowledge in managing the identified problem. The nature of the assessment determines who completes the assessment. For example, if the patient is found to be at nutritional risk because the individual has lost more than 10 pounds in a month, is taking multiple medications, has poor dentition, eats sporadically, and lives alone, a referral to a dietitian would be appropriate for a more complete assessment and care planning focused on the nutritional needs of the patient.

### Validation and Monitoring

Two types of assessments occur throughout implementation of the care plan: validation of the baseline assessments and monitoring. Additional assessments are done to validate data to ensure that assessments and diagnoses are accurate, complete, and reflective of the patient's status. Validation can be done by checking new information with the clinical record, family members, and professional and/or informal caregivers. For example, if a professional caregiver has been informed by a visitor that a patient has a history of substance abuse but it has never been documented in the patient's record, further assessments need to be done to validate whether this information is correct and to determine the nature and severity of the problem if it exists. If there is a substance abuse problem, the care plan needs to include assessment and treatment of this condition.

Monitoring addresses the ongoing assessments for evaluating the patient's progress in relation to the outcomes specified in the care plan. The frequency and nature of ongoing assessments, along with which discipline should monitor each aspect of care are determined by the type of health problem, severity of condition, outcomes to be achieved, and skill needed. Given the previous example of the patient who needs a focused nutritional assessment for weight loss, an outcome in terms of weight gain and improved dietary intake can be monitored by weekly weight measurements and daily calorie counts. Even though data collection can be delegated to nursing assistants, the nutritionist, nurse, or physician should be responsible for synthesizing and analyzing the information.

### Evaluation

The final type of assessment is the evaluation of the outcomes the patient achieved, along with evaluation of the care plan itself. Evaluation assessments are completed by all of the disciplines involved in the patient's plan of care. Physicians, nurses, and case managers evaluate the effectiveness of the medical care, as well as the overall plan. Other disciplines conduct more focused evaluations, concentrating on the care referred to them. A major problem around the evaluation process, especially when multiple disciplines are involved, is establishing communication and consistent feedback processes between clinicians when changes in the plan of care need to be made. For example, a nutritionist may recommend tube feedings for a patient who is not meeting nutritional outcomes. Initiating tube feedings requires a physician order, but the physician may not be informed of the recommendation in a timely manner, thereby delaying treatment.

Evaluating the overall care plan includes determining whether the plan was implemented as designed and identifying factors that supported or hindered achievement of the outcomes. In acute care settings the plan of care is assessed more frequently, based on severity of illness (e.g., every 8–24 hours). In long-term care, care plans are reviewed, evaluated, and updated at least every 90 days. Those residents who qualify for skilled care, may have their care plans reviewed every 30 days (Ignatavicius, 1998). Under the new Medicare nursing home prospective payment system (PPS), assessments are done even more often. Through this ongoing evaluation, a decision is made whether to continue, modify, or terminate the existing plan. Often care plans are updated in a perfunctory manner just to satisfy organizational policies and procedures and regulatory requirements.

## CARE PLANNING METHODS

The types of care planning methods utilized for older patients include the traditional approach, collaborative planning, discharge planning, management through critical pathways, and case management.

**Table 14.6.** Comparison of Goals for Different Care Planning Methods

| Goals | Traditional | Collaborative/ team | Discharge planning | Clinical pathways | Case management |
|---|---|---|---|---|---|
| Facilitate diagnoses and treatment of disease in order to cure | + | + | − | − | + |
| Facilitate management of predictable and/or preventable problems in order to restore, maintain, or improve health | + | + | − | + | + |
| Provide individualized care with respect to age-specific needs | −* | + | −* | − | + |
| Reduce length of stay | − | + | + | + | + |
| Smooth transition between providers | − | + | + | + | + |
| Prevent avoidable readmissions | − | + | + | + | + |
| Use resources cost effectively | − | + | + | + | + |
| Facilitate interdisciplinary collaboration and continuity of care | − | + | −* | + | + |
| Incorporate existing standards, practice guidelines, and research findings | −* | −* | − | + | + |

+, Goal is present; −, goal not present.

*Goal may or may not be present.

The philosophy of care and goals behind these care planning methods differ, as do the assessments that are utilized (Tables 14.6 and 14.7). For example, screening in the traditional approach to care planning focuses on detection of disease, whereas screening methods for discharge planning are used to identify patients at risk for lengthy hospital stays. Each of these approaches has limitations for older adults. Each of the planning methods is discussed.

## Traditional Approach

### Description and Assessments

The traditional approach is based on the "medical model" and includes assessment of health risk factors, along with current and potential problems associated with disease. A plan is generated to address the individual's care needs, including interventions designed to restore, improve, or maintain health. In this model, the primary care physician takes major responsibility for care management decisions. Multidisciplinary involvement depends on referrals from the physician. Personnel from other disciplines, such as physical and occupational therapists, respiratory therapists, nutritionists, and social workers, operate primarily in parallel rather than in an integrated approach. Everyone performs their own work independently, but with little understanding of the roles, responsibilities, or contributions of other disciplines.

### Problems and Pitfalls

The most crucial issue for the traditional approach is fragmented care, which often occurs due to lack of collaboration and communication. For older patients, this arrangement is especially problematic because their complex needs generally require a more comprehensive care approach. Often the traditional plan of care is discipline specific; there may be separate medical, nursing, and therapy plans rather than one coordinated plan. Separate plans provide no guarantee that the disciplines involved will establish the same priorities, and one discipline may inadvertently thwart the interventions of other professional caregivers (Pike et al., 1993). Under this model, most of the different disciplines' plans of care are generally based on the medical diagnosis and tend to be prob-

**Table 14.7.**
Comparison of Assessments Utilized by Care Planning Methods

| Assessment | Screening | Baseline | Focus | Monitoring | Evaluation |
|---|---|---|---|---|---|
| Traditional | Uses multiple tests for detection of disease and risk factors | Initial assessment<br><br>Serves as a database for comparison and for identifying additional care problems | Done only as needed<br><br>Referrals to the most appropriate discipline with the most expertise | Not specified, based on clinical judgment and determined by severity of illness and the treatments initiated | Patient's progress<br><br>Problem focused |
| Collaborative/Team | Detection of disease and risk factors for health<br><br>Functional status | Same as traditional<br><br>Focus is more on identifying appropriate outcomes, strengths, and weaknesses of the patient | Team approach for assessing problems/concerns | May be same as the traditional approach<br><br>May use clinical pathways and interdisciplinary plans of care | Outcome oriented |
| Discharge Planning | [Initiated on Admission: Risk for prolonged recovery (Blaylock, 1992)] Risk Assessment CAAST (continence, age, ambulation, social background, and thought processes)<br><br>Organizational-specific criteria | Preadmission living arrangements<br><br>Previous community support<br><br>Patient preferences and expectations<br><br>Differences between patient and family expectations<br><br>Projected discharge date<br><br>Anticipated problems at discharge<br><br>Update database as patient progresses | Continuing care needs<br><br>Knowledge of care<br><br>Support needed<br><br>Ability to:<br>Learn, remember, and carry out instructions<br>Make own judgments and decisions about health and safety<br>Live in a less structured environment<br>Communicate needs and engage in self-care<br><br>Availability of social support<br><br>Adequacy of living arrangements<br><br>Financial concerns<br><br>Eligibility for resources | Monitoring the discharge plan to ensure relevance due to rapid status changes<br><br>Identifies:<br>Resolution of problems<br>Problems needing reassessment and replanning<br>New problems | Usually not evaluated once patients have left the facility<br><br>May have call back programs<br><br>May be evaluated for quality improvement<br><br>Feedback from Community services<br><br>Long-term care |

| | | | | |
|---|---|---|---|---|
| Critical Pathways | Some specific screens built into preoperative or preprocedural pathways<br><br>Also screen for the inclusion/exclusion criteria to see if use is appropriate | Baseline assessments are completed separate from the critical pathway, not usually part of the pathway | Specific assessments are identified in the pathway for assessing the patient's progress in meeting the specified outcomes<br><br>Prescribed by the pathway | Ongoing monitoring built into the pathway<br><br>Timing and frequency is specific and prescribed by the pathway | Variance data<br><br>Patient and systems data based on outcomes |
| Case Management | Case finding: those who incur high cost; have complex care needs, numerous admissions, numerous physician office visits; or require a team approach to their care. The case manager also applies additional screening as described in the traditional and collaborative approach<br><br>Health and wellness promotion | Same as the traditional method | Same as critical pathways if pathways are utilized as case management tools<br><br>May also be the same as the collaborative/team process | Directed by clinical pathways<br><br>Case management plans<br><br>Interdisciplinary action plans<br><br>Monitors service delivery:<br>Provided at the right time<br>By the appropriate caregiver<br>In the designated amounts<br>For the correct duration<br><br>Monitors changes in the client's status | Variance data<br><br>Patient and systems data based on outcomes<br><br>Evaluates the plan:<br>Is it realistic?<br>Obtainable?<br>Economical?<br>Flexible?<br>Effective?<br><br>Evaluates service delivery for meeting outcomes<br><br>Evaluations conducted at regular intervals |

lem rather than outcome oriented. Discharge planning is considered a separate care-planning process.

Coordination under this model becomes even more difficult when multiple physicians are involved and no physician has assumed the primary care role. There is no identifiable leader. For example, different specialists manage certain body systems. One physician may focus on the patient's heart problems, while another focuses on the patient's neurologic status, but no one coordinates the overall medical plan. The way nursing care is structured in many organizations also adds to this fragmentation. Nurses are often geographically assigned within institutions by nursing unit in which different levels of care or scope of practice defines the patient population. This differentiation impedes transferring of care responsibilities and maintaining continuity across units.

The traditional care-planning method usually has open time frames for assessments, interventions, and outcome achievement in which each individual clinician determines the goals and approaches to care. This variation in clinical practice depends to some degree on the individual clinician's education, experience or training, and practice location. Care is frequently based on routine and tradition. Physician practice patterns are known to vary substantially, and this variation continues throughout the care system, as physicians determine 80% of the care activities performed by other disciplines in a traditional care model (Eisenberg, 1986). In addition, the traditional approach has little fiscal accountability attached to the care planning process. Caregivers may or may not know the cost of services they are using or recommending to patients. Inappropriate utilization of scarce care resources occurs.

Ageism also exists, and ill health is sometimes equated with normal aging; as a result, medical problems are left untreated. For example, many clinicians interpret cognitive changes as the inevitable consequences of advanced age. If they assume that these changes result from dementia, the evaluation of sudden cognitive deterioration is delayed or averted, potentially retarding recovery.

## Collaborative Planning

Collaborative planning is a care planning method used by an interdisciplinary team for achieving shared patient outcomes. The term *interdisciplinary* is used instead of *multidisciplinary* to specifically describe the relationship among team members. Multidisciplinary teams include different disciplines but the members still primarily function independently. Limited integration and collaboration in planning and providing care occurs. Interdisciplinary team members, on the other hand, understand the roles and contributions of each discipline on the team. The team process includes methods for communication, collaborative care planning, and shared responsibility for client outcomes (Petrie, 1976; Clark, Spence, & Sheehan, 1987).

The collaborative planning method is intended as a patient-centered approach to reduce the fragmentation found in the traditional approach for care planning. The rationale behind interdisciplinary planning is that different disciplines working together provide more comprehensive assessments and intervention strategies. Each team member brings a different perspective, as well as assessment tools, interventions, and techniques, which broadens care that can be provided. Team members integrate their assessments and recommendations for intervention, which creates a comprehensive plan (Delfs, Stanley, & Yesner, 1995).

The patient-centered interdisciplinary care plan is based on four principles: *(1)* patient centered: the patient has an active role in the care process; *(2)* interdisciplinary involvement: disciplines, following their own patient assessments, meet to synthesize their findings; *(3)* setting of shared goals: the team reaches consensus for treating the patient; and *(4)* outcome measurement: the team utilizes feedback to evaluate the effectiveness of its clinical interventions (Gage, 1994). Team communication is fostered through team meetings, patient visits by various members on the team, and the generation of a written care plan that outlines the initial evaluation, care priorities, suggested interventions, and recommendations. This process leads to care continuity and comprehensive care. For a more complete discussion of the type of assessments that are utilized, along with the strengths and limitations of this model, refer to Chapter 13.

## Discharge Planning

Discharge planning is a special type of care planning focused on the transition between different care levels. For example, planning must occur to transfer care effectively and efficiently between agencies, such as from acute hospital care to nursing home care or subacute care to home care, to maintain uninterrupted care. Greater attention to discharge planning has occurred as a result of increasing numbers of older adults needing continuing care and lack of planning for this transition with traditional care planning methods. Also, there is a need to manage the finite resources available for continuing care in the community and to ensure appropriate levels of care (Volland, 1988; Proctor & Morrow-Howell, 1990; Naylor et al., 1994; Potthoff, Kane, & Franco, 1998).

The American Nurses Association describes discharge planning as "the part of the continuity of care process which is designed to prepare the patient for the next phase of care and to assist in making any necessary arrangements for that phase of care, whether it be self-care, care by family members, or care by an organized health care provider" (American Nurses Association, 1975, p. 10). To facilitate a timely discharge, discharge planning should start with the patient's admission. The feasibility of early discharge planning is, however, a major concern. Delayed discharge planning can increase length of stay and contribute to poor resource utilization.

Discharge planning is done by different disciplines, depending on the model adopted by the health care organization. In one approach, a designated discharge planner, either a nurse or a social worker, directs and implements the plan. In other models, the entire responsibility is shared by physicians and nursing staff. A third model has physicians and nurses sharing responsibility for identifying patients needing continuing care. After patient identification, a social worker assumes responsibility for developing the discharge plan, encompassing both physical and social care needs (Volland, 1988; Haddock, 1991). The key issues for discharge planning include (1) identifying patients needing discharge planning, (2) identifying patient and family goals and preferences for discharge, (3) defining the continuing care that needs to be provided, (4) determining timing of discharge, (5) identifying skill required to provide care, and (6) determining available financial resources for transitioning care (Zarle, 1987; Potthoff et al., 1998).

Four discharge dispositions are possible (Table 14.8) (Zarle, 1987). The primary discharge goal is for the patient to return home, which is the most appropriate destination for most patients. The patient's ability to engage in self-care is a major factor in determining the feasibility of discharge home. If going home is possible only if assistance is provided, the next goal is to discharge the individual with assistance from family and/or the community. The third discharge possibility is to transfer the individual to another facility that provides needed services for continuing care, either skilled or nonskilled support. Finally, some patients with terminal conditions need help to plan

**Table 14.8.**
Potential Discharge Dispositions

| |
|---|
| Return home |
| Return home with assistance from the family or community |
| Transfer to another facility for continued care |
| Preparation for death, transfer to hospice |

their death experience, including transfer to a hospice or other long-term care setting.

### Discharge Assessments

The patient assessments that are used in discharge planning are critical for ensuring continued quality of care. For example, a screening index for identifying patients needing discharge planning is considered important for the initiation of timely discharge planning, which reduces hospital costs and promotes efficient utilization of resources (Inui, Stevenson, Penda, & Murphy, 1981). The alternative to screening is to thoroughly assess the physiological, psychological, and social needs of every patient to plan the appropriate disposition. Assessing all patients would impose a huge burden on the case loads of social workers and nurses and would be prohibitively costly. Unfortunately, little work has been done to develop the needed screening measures. Available screening instruments include the Blaylock Discharge Planning Risk Assessment Screen (BRASS) and the CASST index. Another, the Uniform Needs Assessment Instrument (UNAI), is currently being tested for mandatory use with all Medicare patients.

The BRASS, developed by Blaylock and Cason (1992), is a tool designed to be administered as part of the hospital admission process in order to identify elderly patients at risk for prolonged hospitalization and who may need discharge planning services. The instrument identifies patients with more complex care needs and shows promise as an effective screening measure (Table 14.9).

The advantages of the BRASS instrument is that it is quick, simple, and "bedside friendly" (Blaylock & Cason, 1992). The tool takes an average of 15 minutes to complete by an admitting nurse. The instrument has a high degree of usability, but very little psychometric testing has been done; nor has the BRASS's accuracy in predicting which patient will need discharge planning been compared with other discharge planning measures. A relationship was found between BRASS scores and age ADLs, (activities of daily living); IADLs (instrumental activities of daily living).
and length of hospital stay. In a study of 206 patients, those with low BRASS scores had an average age of 48 years with an average length of stay of 8 days. Those with moderate BRASS scores had an average age of 58 years and a length of stay of 14 days. Those with the highest BRASS scores had an average age of 69 years and an average hospital stay of 19 days (Blaylock & Cason, 1992). Additional testing is needed to establish validity of the instrument before it can be recommended for routine clinical use. An evaluation of the instrument's sensitivity and specificity needs to be done to determine if BRASS scores effectively identify patients needing discharge planning.

Another objective clinical index for identifying patients needing discharge planning is Glass and Weiner's CAAST criteria (1976). The five parameters that correlate with difficulty in planning an appropriate disposition include whether the patient is continent, the patient's ability to ambulate, and the patient's age, social background, and thought or cognitive processes (see Table 14.9).

The scale was originally designed for physicians to assess their patients on hospital admission. Again, psychometric testing on this instrument is limited. The instrument was successful in identifying a population at risk for discharge planning (Glass & Weiner, 1976). The CAAST parameters were predictive of extended hospital stays when time was spent on planning a patient's disposition after medical care needs had been met. Problems with thought processes, social background, and age were each significantly associated with extended social stays.

Inui, Stevenson, and Plorde compared techniques of identifying hospital patients who needed early discharge (see Inui et al., 1981). They compared the CAAST with two interval scales developed specifically for the study. One scale rated projected dependency of a patient at discharge (11 point interval linear scale with scale end points labeled as totally independent and totally dependent), while the other scale rated probability of nursing home placement post-hospitalization (10 point interval scale with end points labeled 0% likelihood to 100% likelihood). (See Table 14.9 for correlations between the CAAST and the linear scales.) This study indicated that as many as 37% of patients requiring discharge planning were not identified by these screening instruments. These results are not clinically acceptable if the goal is to improve quality of discharge planning. Additional work is needed to improve the scale's sensitivity.

The Uniform Needs Assessment Inventory (UNAI) is a standardized assessment instrument designed by the Health Care Financing Administration that includes a screening process to identify hospitalized patients needing discharge planning and a focused assessment process to determine needs, goals, preferences, and support. The goal of this instrument is to decrease the variation in information that is assessed and utilized in discharge planning in hospitals (see Chapter 16). Most agencies do not use tested screens to determine which patients require discharge planning. Instead, organization-specific screens are used, which rely on the unique focus and experience of the particular organization to evaluate patient needs (Fitzig, 1988). The clinical judgments and expertise of the clinicians involved in the discharge planning are essential. For example, the discharge planner reviews the admission assessment and the physician's plan of care to identify high-risk patients. A hospital specializing in oncology may use a terminal prognosis or a new cancer diagnosis for triggering discharge planning. Additionally, most of the screening instruments for discharge planning have been designed for acute care settings. With the advent of

subacute care and short-term nursing home placement, instruments designed for these settings need to be developed and tested.

Discharge planning also includes focused assessments initiated to facilitate the transition of care once a patient has been identified at risk for a prolonged stay. These assessments help to determine the level of care and support needed by the patient in the community. Caregivers assess the patients' knowledge of their illness, treatment, and care as well as their ability to carry out instructions. The patients' ability to engage in self-care depends on their ability to make judgments and decisions about their own health and safety, to communicate needs to others, and to live in a less structured environment. The differences between patient and family expectations and preferences must also be determined.

Bull has developed a Discharge Planning Questionnaire (DPQ) to assist in identifying differences between the patients' perspectives and their family caregivers with regard to need for post-hospital care (Bull, 1994). The DPQ contains 51 items that ask hospitalized elderly patients questions concerning ADLs and IADLs, social support, environment, preferences with regards to disposition, and their family preferences for discharge. A parallel form has been developed to give to patients' family members. Disagreement between the patients' and family members' ratings for care expectations can be identified. For example, if the patient answers the question (listed in the social support section of the questionnaire) that he or she has a friend, relative, or neighbor that can be called on to do the laundry and the family answers the same question by stating that the patient does not have any one to complete this task, an obvious discrepancy exists that needs to be clarified.

The DPQ has undergone extensive psychometric testing (see Table 14.9) and shows promise for clinical use by those in-

Table 14.9.
Discharge Planning Instruments

| Instrument | Domains assessed | Scoring | Reliability/Validity | Usability |
|---|---|---|---|---|
| **BRASS** | | | | |
| Type of assessment: Screening instrument for discharge planning<br><br>Purpose: Identify elderly hospitalized patients at risk for prolonged hospitalization and needing discharge planning services | Age; living situation/social support; functional status—IADLs and ADLs; cognitive status; behavior pattern; mobility; sensory status—hearing and vision; number of previous admissions or emergency room visits; number of active medical problems; number of medications taken at home | Total score, 0–40; score < 10, anticipate self-care at discharge; score = 10, at risk for home care resources; score = 11–19, at risk for extended discharge planning; score > 20, at risk for placement other than home | Inter-rater reliability r = 0.84; intraclass correlation coefficient = 0.87;<br><br>Validity has not been tested | 15 min to complete; user friendly; can be completed on admission to the hospital; designed for nurses to complete |
| **CAAST** | | | | |
| Type of assessment: Screening instrument for discharge planning<br><br>Purpose: Identify patients with complex care needs that may require planning in order to arrange an appropriate disposition | Continence, ability to ambulate, age, social background, thought or cognitive processes | Total score, 0–10; higher score reflects complex care needs<br><br>Scores for each category range from 0 to 2, with 0 indicating no problem and 2 representing persistent problems<br><br>Age is scaled with 0 for patients below 65 years, 1 for those between the ages of 65 and 79, and 2 for those 80 years of age or greater | Reliability has not been determined<br><br>Validity parameters predictive of extended days<br><br>Correlated with the following scales: projected dependency scale, r = 0.74, p < 0.001; probability of nursing home placement scale, r = 0.74, p < 0.001 | Originally designed for physicians to assess and assign a CAAST score on hospital admission |

*DPQ*

| Type of assessment: Focused assessment instrument for discharge planning<br><br>Purpose: Identifying patient needs and preferences for discharge. Parallel form for identifying family perspectives for discharge | ADLs, IADLs, social support, environmental factors, preferences for disposition, family preferences | ADLs and IADLs scored 0–4, with 0 representing complete independence and 4 representing complete dependence. A score of 1.1 is given if respondent is unsure of abilities<br><br>For social support and environment, a score of 1 is given if there is support and a 2 if there are support or environmental issues. A score of 1.1 is given if the respondent is uncertain | Internal consistency: ADL subscale = 0.86; IADL subscale = 0.90; social support scale = 0.87; environment = 0.60<br><br>Validity ADL subscale compared with performance ADL scale by Kane et al. (1983), $r = 0.66$, $p < 0.001$; predictive validity ADL subscale correlated with number of community resources, $r = -0.65$, $p < 0.65$; support expected on DPQ correlated with that actually received, $r = 0.58$, $p = 0.003$ | Is self-administered by clients and families<br><br>Takes time to compare the client and family versions to identify discrepancies and areas of uncertainty |
| --- | --- | --- | --- | --- |

volved in discharge planning to better assess patient and family expectations and concerns. The tool's use is, however, dependent on a staff valuing the patient's perspective and willingness to take time to assess this area. A careful comparison of the patient's and family's responses is needed, with the ultimate goal being to incorporate information into the patient's discharge plan.

### Problems and Pitfalls

Discharge planning has not been entirely successful in improving the quality of care post-hospitalization. Risks exist with discharging patients from hospitals sicker and quicker (Anderson & Steinberg, 1984; McCorkle, 1987). This phenomenon is a legacy of prospective hospital reimbursement with Medicare payment based on diagnosis-related groups. The advent of managed care and capitation has served to further decrease length of hospital stays and has emphasized the need for quality post-hospital care (Department of Health and Human Services, 1987; Coulton, 1988; Stuen & Monk, 1990). Professional caregivers are pushed to develop plans rapidly to continue the patient's recovery in less costly settings as soon as medically possible. Unfortunately, hospitalized older patients are often more frail, do not recover as fast as younger patients, require more services and support post-discharge, and are at higher risk for poor outcomes post-discharge. Because of an increased need for care after acute care for older patients, a greater burden is placed on community services and informal caregivers. Several ethical dilemmas can occur with discharge planning: the competition between obligations to the patient, family, staff, and the organization; the need to choose between options equally unsatisfactory; the inability to determine risks or benefits of identified plans; and the need to divide time between current and future patients (Cummings & Cockerham, 1997).

Emphasis on resource utilization and cost has tended to usurp the patient from the center of the discharge planning process. Patients and families are often minimally included in discharge planning, and older patients can be stereotyped as being too infirm, frail, and senile to participate. The patients' desires and goals are often not explored. Many patients and family caregivers feel that discharge planning provided by institutions is coercive. They complain of automatic referral of high-risk patients for nursing home planning regardless of patient and family expectations, inadequate assessment of the patient's potential to be discharged home, rushed time frames for planning, and having to accept less then adequate or satisfactory solutions just so the hospital can discharge the patient within its time frame. Patients and family members believe that planners have more influence in post-hospital decision making than they actually do (Clemens, 1995).

Inadequate systems or organizational support for the discharge process is also an issue for many institutions, resulting in inadequate assessments, poor documentation, and fragmented implementation. Failure to establish who is in charge of discharge planning (physicians, nurses, or social workers) may lead to a system in which accountability and responsibility are poorly defined. A qualitative study aimed at identifying factors important in discharge planning reported negative outcomes that occurred with inadequate discharge planning (Bull & Kane, 1996). Two weeks after discharge, 91% of families interviewed (n = 253) had problems with managing their older relative's care. Similar results were found in a study of 75 nursing residents on a rehabilitation unit who were discharged home (Tappen, Hall, Stahura, & Blume, 1995).

To be effective, discharge planning needs to be initiated soon after admission whenever feasible, be patient focused, have interdisciplinary involvement, be continually assessed and updated through the length of stay, and include a coordinated follow-up evaluation program (Haddock, 1991,

1994; Naylor, 1990; Naylor et al., 1994). In many cases, however, discharge planning is not seen as a priority. It is delayed and left to just before the patient's actual discharge after the physician has written the discharge order. Many physicians are uncomfortable identifying projected discharge time frames because of the pressure that utilization management departments have exerted in the past to discharge a patient once a date has been identified, regardless of subsequent status changes. *Discharge planning* seems to be an outdated term and implies last minute planning. Many professional caregivers favor the idea of *continuity planning*, which is an ongoing process that includes participatory planning with the patient for the next level of care throughout all aspects of the care planning process (Haddock, 1991).

## Clinical Pathways

Another approach to improve and standardize care planning is the clinical pathway. A clinical pathway is a care planning tool that outlines important aspects of care necessary for meeting specific outcomes. Clinical pathways are aids for ensuring appropriate care and have been used in traditional care structures, collaborative team approaches, and case management models. The pathway is designed for the typical patient from a designated population, such as patients who have undergone hip replacement or coronary artery bypass graft surgery. Pathways work best when the expected recovery course is clear.

The pathway is a prewritten document that plots expected outcomes, interdisciplinary assessments, and interventions on a time line. Specific time frames are defined by hours, days, or phases of care (preoperative, perioperative, or postoperative; Zander, 1995). The time frame can form the headings for each column, while care categories are the row labels on the pathway document. Care categories may consist of outcomes, assessments, treatments, medications, diet, activities, patient education, and consultations. Lay versions of the pathway that mirror the clinician's document can be used by practitioners to promote patient participation and education.

Clinical pathways are based on systems theory, in which clinical and nonclinical processes directly relate to patient outcomes. Clinical pathways represent a way to operationalize continuous quality improvement in clinical practice (Hofmann, 1993; Kleinman, 1995; Zander, 1995; Gregor et al., 1996; Horne, 1996). The underlying premise is that standardizing work processes or inputs into the system decreases care variability and improves outcomes. Care variability is thought to be a major cause of poor outcomes. The care outlined on the pathway represents a research-based or best practice approach. The pathway is designed by the various disciplines routinely involved in the care of the designated patient population. Table 14.10 lists the potential benefits of using pathways. Many of the benefits that have been described are theoretical and have not been empirically demonstrated (Pearson, Goulart-Fisher, & Lee, 1995). The quality improvement literature, however, provides some evidence that clinical pathways do improve outcomes, specifically length of stay, cost, mortality, and morbidity (Strong & Sneed, 1991; Falconer et al., 1993; Hofmann, 1993; McGarvey &

**Table 14.10.** Theoretical Benefits of Clinical Pathways

Reduction in care variation that leads to poor outcomes

Improved clinical outcomes

Decreased length of stay

Reduction in cost

Structured process for evaluating population outcomes

Increased coordination of services

Improved interdisciplinary communication/ collaboration

Increased client/family involvement and satisfaction in care

Facilitation of discharge planning

Improved documentation of care

Harper, 1993; Gregor et al., 1996; Horne, 1996).

Clinicians (primarily nurses) frequently use clinical pathways in place of traditional care plans (Ignatavicius & Hausman, 1995; Zander, 1995; Horne, 1996). Physicians support the pathway through development of standardized orders that reflect the care outlined on the pathway. Pathways are used by case managers or collaborative care teams in order to structure and evaluate care for the individual and to evaluate care results for the population as a whole. For example, if the patient is not meeting specified outcomes for a particular day, additional interventions might be added to help the patient stay on track. The care manager or team is able to track population outcomes or care variances. Variances are defined as either positive or negative patient outcomes and care processes that deviate from those identified on the pathway (Potter, 1995). For example, if an elderly patient is not able to eat solid food by the second postoperative day as outlined on a pathway, a variance exists. The manager of the pathway must determine if this negative outcome was due to a clinical problem, such as nausea or vomiting, or whether the food was not advanced from a liquid to a solid diet as a result of a systems problem. This information is then used to further refine and develop care systems that support the pathway or to change the pathway itself. If nausea and vomiting were also found to be a consistent problem for many patients on this specific pathway, then the cause of the condition would need to be researched and additional interventions added routinely to the pathway to address the problem.

Clinical pathways originated in acute care settings and are now spreading to other settings. Pathways linking acute care with nursing homes or with home care are becoming a standard part of managing the care continuum. This type of expanded pathway helps caregivers in each setting know what care has been initiated, outcomes that have been met, and those left to achieve. A common example of these linkages is the total hip replacement pathways that includes a recovery phase in a subacute nursing unit (American Health Consultants, 1994).

A pathway used in subacute units differs from one used in an acute care setting because the subacute unit's patient population is in an advanced phase of recovery (Colucciello & Mangles, 1997). The pathway is designed to delineate the typical recovery pattern within a specified time frame. The essential elements are duration, functional health patterns, intensity or level of care, interdisciplinary team involvement, clinical treatment plan, tracking of variances, and expected outcomes. These elements are similar to the description of pathways in general except that the focus is on functional recovery. For example, duration is the time it takes the patient's condition to stabilize in order for the individual to transfer back to the community. Duration depends on severity or level of disability, amount of functional independence the patient exhibits and can achieve, resources needed to improve outcomes, and extent of interdisciplinary involvement. Functional health patterns include the patient's ability and desire to engage in self-care.

Pathways are also being developed for care delivered in home health. These pathways differ from those in acute care primarily with regard to time frame. Home care patients can be divided into those needing short-term versus long-term care. The outcome goals for long-term patients include the prevention of acute care and nursing home admissions. Long-term patients often require extended home care services to achieve these goals, and pathways are generally not used for this population (Corbett & Androwich, 1994). Relative short-term home care needs fit the pathway model better because care patterns are more easily defined and described. In this circumstance, the patient's degree of compliance with self-care regimens and amount of physician involvement required in care generally determines pathway duration. This loose determination of pathway duration is, however, starting to change. Third-party payers are gathering information to help establish specific numbers of home health visits needed per diagnosis (Freeman & Chamber, 1997).

### Clinical Pathway Assessments

Assessments outlined in the clinical pathway specify what is being assessed, along with the timing. The primary screening that occurs in clinical pathways is an assessment of inclusion/exclusion criteria to determine appropriate patients for the pathway. For example, in order for patients to be placed on a myocardial infarction clinical pathway, certain clinical parameters need to be present. The criteria may include elevated cardiac enzymes and/or presence of EKG changes. Exclusion criteria might include cardiogenic shock and inability to engage in cardiac rehabilitation. Other screening processes may also be built into the pathway, such as those that indicate need for interdisciplinary referrals, such as an assessment of ADLs or IADLs. Focused assessments and ongoing monitoring are also built into the pathway, in which timing and frequency of assessments are clearly defined. Evaluation is based on comparing outcomes outlined on the pathway with actual outcomes achieved by the patient.

### Problems and Pitfalls

Clinical pathways, while improving standardization, are criticized for not allowing enough individualization. Each patient has unique needs, but pathways generally do not allow time or include interventions necessary to meet these additional care requirements. Patients with complex care needs often are unable to meet the progressive pathway outcomes. Most of the successes reported for clinical pathways have been associated with procedural driven plans (Adler et al., 1995; Doran et al., 1997). It is more difficult to identify

care patterns for medical diagnoses and chronic illnesses, such as congestive heart failure, pneumonia, or diabetes, than for surgical procedures. Often these medical diagnoses do not occur in isolation, but occur with other conditions. In addition, clinical pathways are often based on care standards for a younger population and as such they do not meet the needs of elderly clients. Table 14.11, adapted from Gorbien (1995), identifies the special needs of older adults that confound the use of pathways.

Many disciplines, especially physicians, perceive pathways as cookbook medicine and another external source of control over clinical practice. Nursing, in contrast, has provided leadership in developing clinical pathways, which in some cases has threatened their acceptance by other disciplines. Some pathways have been too nursing focused and have not included enough interdisciplinary involvement to make them truly a collaborative patient care plan.

Obtaining reliable and valid information from pathways is a key part of the process and depends on the recorded assessments, operational outcome definitions, and consistency of documentation. Incomplete and inadequate documentation is a major issue in evaluating a pathway's effectiveness. Other problematic issues include difficulty in tracking outcome variances and managing multiple pathways. Many institutions have not created support systems to manage outcome data, such as personnel to ex-

**Table 14.11.** Needs of Older Adults that Confound Clinical Pathways

Impairments in physical functioning
Impairments in cognitive functioning
Presence of co-morbidities
Presence of mental illness
Atypical presentation of illnesses
Lack of resources necessary for discharge planning
Vulnerability for iatrogenic complications, such as adverse drug complications
Lack of "best practice" approaches for common syndromes that develop in older adults

tract data, computerized data bases, methods for data analysis, and standardized report generation. Additionally, as organizations add pathways for different diagnoses, patients may be on more than one pathway at the same time. Some third-party payers have also developed pathways, creating the possibility of patients with the same diagnosis in the same organization being on different pathways, depending on their insurance coverage. This variation makes it extremely difficult for staff to know the care requested on each pathway and to implement it accordingly. Loss of standardization lessens credibility.

The implementation of clinical pathways has raised many unanswered questions. It is often unclear when care should be individualized and under what circumstances pathways should be used for a given population. Also, the extent to which an institution's pathway design can be borrowed from other institutions and how much should reflect the institution's unique processes is not known. Some institutions have purchased prepared pathways created by consultants, without using interdisciplinary teams within their organization to identify their own clinical patterns and support systems. Generally, clinical pathways introduced in this manner have not succeeded in improving patient care. Clinicians must have some input into pathway development, and prepared pathways do not enhance staff ownership of the plan. Prepared pathways do not support a patient-centered approach because patient and family feedback is not incorporated into the continued development of the pathway. The criteria for discontinuing a pathway before completion of the plan are unclear. If the patient is not meeting outcomes or develops complications, should the pathway be continued? If the pathway is stopped prematurely, what plan of care should take its place?

## Care Coordination Through Case Management

Case management is a popular approach to care planning in health-oriented programs as a way to lessen service fragmentation. It is viewed as a valuable strategy across the continuum from ambulatory care to acute hospitalization to long-term care. It is a hallmark of managed care (Pacala, Boult, & Boult, 1995). There are considerable differences in the interpretation of the concept, however, and the way it is operationalized. There are many definitions: Case management has been referred to as a service, a process, and a care delivery model. White (1986) defines case management as a "service function directed at coordinating existing resources to assure appropriate and continuous care for individuals on a case-by-case basis." Henderson (1987) views case management as "a systematic approach to identifying high cost acutely ill patients, assessing potential opportunities in coordinating their care, developing treatment plans that improve quality and cost, and managing the patient's total care to ensure optimum outcome" (see Chapter 15). Case management in acute care has been viewed as a care delivery model that is nursing unit as well as population based in which the case manager either assists in directing care to a specific case load or provides care directly (Lulavage, 1991; Mahn, 1993; Hurt, 1995; Huggins & Lehman, 1997). These care delivery designs established in acute care have been extended to subacute, nursing home–sponsored units. Case management in health care settings focuses primarily on coordination of medical and nursing care and is different from social case management programs (see Chapter 15).

Regardless of the definition of case management, four major goals for case management in health care–oriented programs have been put forth: improve access to services, improve the health outcomes for patients, equitably distribute services, and contain costs (Kodner, 1993). Because of the variety of ways case management programs can be operationalized, several key elements should be examined in order to understand the approach being used (Table 14.12).

Coordination across the continuum of

**Table 14.12.**

Elements of a Case Management Program

Target population: Older adults versus younger clients

Risk groups: Seriously ill clients with multiple co-morbidities or those needing multiple services and extensive monitoring

Diagnostic categories: Range from frail elderly adults to clients with congestive heart failure

Duration and intensity: Time frame for service provision and the amount of involvement with the client and/or family

Control over resources: The extent of the "gatekeeping function" or management of funding for services

Field of the case manager: Social work, nursing, primary care physician,

Location of the case management program: HMO, hospital, nursing home, primary care organization, or insurance company

Source: Kodner (1993).

care means managing multiple transitions from one level of care to the next. Zander (1996) describes this process for acute care as management of crisis or entry to the hospital through stabilization and recovery. It includes following the patient to discharge and continuing care management in the community. In the community, the goal becomes management of health risks to prevent readmissions, accidents, abuse, and additional illnesses. Table 14.13 describes elements associated with various sites. Clinical case managers often follow a specific case type (diagnosis-related groups, procedure, or age group) using a

**Table 14.13.** Case Management/Care Coordination Across the Care Continuum

*Ambulatory Care*

Health promotion (education, counseling, and support)
Health maintenance (monitoring)
Illness prevention (primary and secondary screening)

*Acute Hospital Care*

Crisis management of acute illness
Stabilization
Health restoration

*Long-Term/Community Care*

Recovery
Convalescence/supportive care
Functional improvement (tertiary screening)
Prevention of hospital readmissions, abuse, and injuries
Management of health risk and chronic disease

service line approach such as cardiovascular, respiratory, or orthopedic services (Zander, 1995). These types of case managers tend to be advanced practice nurses.

In many models, a single case manager is assigned overall responsibility for care management functions, which include prevention, wellness, and disease management (Zander, 1995). The case manager assumes responsibility for assessing patient needs, planning and arranging service delivery, and monitoring provision of services and care outcomes. The case manager assists in communications and patient advocacy throughout the continuum of care. Additionally, services are negotiated and networks for maintaining continuity are established. Finally, effectiveness of planned interventions and use of resources are evaluated in relation to established goals. Outcome-based care is provided in case management systems within an appropriate length of time, in which health care services are integrated and coordinated. Collaboration between disciplines is at the basis of case management in which the patient is the center or focal point (Adler et al., 1995). The case manager creates an interdisciplinary process by serving as facilitator for interdisciplinary involvement.

## Case Management Assessments

Case management processes use screening assessments not only for detecting disease and care problems for individual patients but also for case finding. Case finding should identify patients in greatest need for case management. Various criteria have been used, including patients who incur the highest cost, have complex care needs requiring interdisciplinary involvement, have multiple admissions or numerous physician office visits, or are a high volume case type (Zander, 1995).

Some health maintenance organizations use simple, self-administered screening or case finding instruments to identify older clients at risk of hospitalization. Kaiser Permanente Northwest Region in Portland, Oregon, mails a standardized instrument (Health Status Form) annually to their older members to identify frail elderly individuals who could benefit from case management. Four items on the form have been determined to correctly classify 90%–95% of the Medicare Plus II members as frail or not frail. The four items included self-report of poor health, need for assistance with medication management, need for bathing assistance, and advanced age. Those individuals identified as frail and eligible for case management had hospitalization rates three time greater than those not identified as frail (American Health Consultants, 1996).

Seven factors that increase older adults' probability of readmission to the hospital include age over 75 years, male gender, diagnosis of diabetes, history of heart disease, an overnight hospital stay in the past 12 months, personal perception of poor health, and inability to name an individual who could take care of them for several days (Boult et al., 1994). Additionally, measures of patient acuity and case mix can alert the case manager to the need for extensive care planning (Bower, 1995).

Multidimensional, standardized functional assessments are incorporated into many of the case managers' standard approach for managing a case. Standardized assessments help to identify patient needs and facilitate monitoring and evaluation of provided services.

Monitoring for case management pri-marily focuses on ensuring that patients receive timely care services at the appropriate level and for the frequency and duration recommended. Monitoring also includes observations for detecting changes in the patient's condition or circumstances that may indicate need for changes in the care plan (Redford, 1992). Often the case manager utilizes standard care plans, such as clinical pathways, case management plans, or multidisciplinary action plans to monitor the patient's progress toward meeting established outcomes. Evaluation by case managers includes reassessments conducted at regular intervals. The goal is to ensure appropriateness and overall effectiveness of the service plan. Evaluation is outcome based at both patient and program level.

### Problems and Pitfalls

Some issues about case management have emerged. For example, although the basic elements of case management are similar across models, the manner in which these elements are implemented can differ widely. It is unclear who really should be called a case manager and what training or expertise is needed to implement the role effectively. There are inherent tensions between the roles of patient advocacy and the gatekeeping function. In some cases multiple case managers may be involved. (See Chapter 15 for a complete discussion of these issues.)

### Differences Among Care Planning Methods

The major differences between the traditional, collaborative planning, discharge planning, management through critical pathways, and case management strategies are related to the goals that they are designed to achieve (see Table 14.6). The traditional approach's primary goals include facilitation of diagnosis, treatment of disease, and management of predictable or preventable problems. The traditional approach is generally not patient centered. Although individual clinicians may practice using a patient-centered philosophy, the patient care system tends to be organizationally or disciplinarily focused. Care is designed for the convenience of the organization or the discipline providing care. Discharge planning's primary goals are to plan for transition between providers; reduction of length of stay in acute care, subacute care, and nursing homes; prevention of avoidable readmissions (especially to acute care facilities); and cost-effective utilization of resources. Discharge planning is generally a supplemental process used with the traditional approach to care planning. Discharge planning may or may not be patient centered, depending on the amount and type of involvement of the patient and family in the decision-making process.

Collaborative planning, clinical pathways, and case management have additional goals (see Table 6). Interdisciplinary collaboration and continuity planning are key for these approaches, but not for the traditional care planning method. According to Barnes (1997, p. 921) continuity means "persons are cared for whatever their location." Planning for care transitions occurs throughout the process rather than at the end of the recovery period. Interdisciplinary collaboration may or may not be present in discharge planning, depending on the discharge planning model utilized. Often discharge planning is delegated to specific staff, who develop and implement the plan in isolation.

Case management and collaborative planning by design incorporate the most objectives into the care planning process. These methods were developed to facilitate diagnoses and treatment of disease along with management of predictable or preventable problems. They are both interdisciplinary, patient-centered models that emphasize the provision of individualized care. Both were developed to improve patient care, reduce unnecessary utilization of services, assist in planning for care transitions, and prevent avoidable readmissions.

Clinical pathways differ from collaborative planning and case management because pathways are generally not designed to facilitate diagnosis. Pathways are usually implemented once the diagnosis has been established or a specific procedure initiated. Some exceptions, however, do exist. There are pathways in acute care for specific symptoms, such as chest pain in which ruling out a myocardial infarction is part of the pathway. In this case, diagnosis is one of the goals. Pathways are really tools for planning, structuring, monitoring, and evaluating care for a specific condition. Both the collaborative and case management models can include pathways as one of their care planning techniques. Collaborative team planning and case management, however, tend to address more aspects of care than are prescribed by a single pathway. When pathways are used in a traditional care model, they are primarily used by nurses with little involvement of other disciplines. Clinical pathways outline a standardized approach to care; individualized care is generally not the focus. Clinical pathways may, however, be indirectly patient focused if patient input is incorporated into the ongoing development of the patient care systems that support the pathway by mandating consistent measurement of patient satisfaction as one of the pathway outcomes.

## RECOMMENDATIONS FOR PLANNING CARE FOR ELDERLY PATIENTS

Because care planning depends on the accuracy and comprehensiveness of the conducted assessments, a consistent systematic approach needs to be adopted. Screening tools should be used that identify older adults at risk for health problems and care needs. Primary, secondary, and tertiary screening should be employed according to the recommendations made by the U.S. Preventive Services Task Force for the care of older adults. Methods are needed to obtain reliable and valid information for comprehensive and focused assessments, for measuring patient progress, and for identifying care concerns. Standardized instruments for recording comprehensive assessments offer a way to determine the patient's progress. A plan must be dynamic and change with the patient's changing needs. Moreover, innovative methods to incorporate standardized databases, such as the RAI, into the daily care routines must be encouraged so that assessments do not become just a paper exercise.

A patient-centered philosophy needs to be operationalized, which includes patient decision making, interdisciplinary involvement, and continuity of care planning. Continuity of care has been defined by some authors as synonymous with a patient-centered philosophy. For example, Zarle (1987) defines continuing care as "a decision-making process focusing on the patient, family, and significant others as the principal decision makers." The patient, in this model, is viewed as responsible for his or her own health care decisions. The role of the professional caregiver is to guide and facilitate decision making. Older adults need to have their autonomy respected and enhanced in order to prevent the cycle of dependency. Patient preferences, goals, values, and beliefs are incorporated into the plan of care to help the patient maintain, restore, or achieve health.

Continuity of care also refers to uninterrupted care that can be transferred from one level to the next level of care. Fragmented care is avoided by planned transitions in which discharge planning is incorporated into all phases of the care plan. Discharge planning must be given priority in order to improve patient outcomes. Table 14.14 lists the key elements of successful discharge planning.

Interdisciplinary involvement is important in care planning. The complex nature of the elderly patient's health care needs and the multitude of chronic health problems in the elderly population dictate the necessity for collaboration. An interdisciplinary team helps to improve the type, quantity, continuity, and comprehensiveness of services that can be offered. A team, working collaboratively, can complement each other's roles and expertise, resulting in improved patient outcomes. A collaborative planning model should help to strengthen interdisciplinary involvement.

A well-designed case management program can improve care planning by establishing accountability and consistent follow through to ensure positive patient outcomes and appropriate service delivery. Screening methods to identify patients who may benefit most from case management should be used. Clinical pathways also have a role in care planning for older adults, but should be designed for age-specific care and possibly limited to specific types of care, such as managing surgical or procedural care. They should be used as guides rather than as the only plan of care.

Table 14.14.
Key Elements for Successful Discharge Planning

Assigned responsibility and accountability for the coordination of discharge planning

Interdisciplinary involvement so that the medical, emotional, social, and financial needs of the patient are addressed

Early identification of the patient's post-discharge needs through utilization of preadmission and admission screening for determining discharge needs

Development of the plan with the patient and patient's family

Patient/family education

Use of a standardized documentation format to ensure completeness and communication

Post-discharge follow-up to ensure plan implementation

# REFERENCES

Adler, S. L., Bryk, E., Cesta, T. G., & McEachen, I. (1995). Collaboration: The solution to multidisciplinary care planning. *Orthopaedic Nursing, 14*(2), 21–29.

Alfaro-LeFevere, R. (1998). *Applying nursing process: A step-by-step Approach.* Philadelphia: Lippincott.

American Health Consultants (1994). Subacute geriatric path increases discharge home for hip patients. *Hospital Case Management, 2*(12), 207–211.

American Health Consultants (1996). Identifying at-risk seniors prevents costly admissions. *Case Management Advisor, 7*(2), 17–21.

American Nurses Association (1975). *Continuity of care and discharge planning programs.* Kansas City: American Nurses Association.

Anderson, C., & Steinberg, E. (1984). Hospital readmissions in the Medicare population. *New England Journal of Medicine, 311,* 1349–1353.

Avorn, J., & Langer, E. (1982). Induced disability in nursing home patients: A controlled trial. *Journal of the American Geriatrics Association, 30*(6), 397–400.

Barnes, S. J. (1997). Gerontological care in community care setting. In M. A. Matteson, E. S. McConnell, & A. D. Linton (Eds.), *Gerontological nursing* (2nd ed., pp. 897–929). Philadelphia: W. B. Saunders.

Bernd, D. (1992). Patient-focused care pays hospital-wide dividends. *Health Care Strategic Management, 10*(12), 9–12.

Blaylock, A., & Cason, C. L. (1992). Discharge planning: Predicting patients' needs. *Journal of Gerontological Nursing, 18*(7), 5–10.

Boult, L., Boult, C., Pirie, P., & Pacala, J. T. (1994). Test–retest reliability of a questionnaire that identifies elders at risk for hospital admission. *Journal of the American Geriatrics Society, 42*(7), 707–711.

Bower, K. (1995). Case management designed for the care continuum. In K. Zander (Ed.), *Managing outcomes through collaborative care: The application of care mapping and case management* (pp. 165–176). Chicago: American Hospital Publishing.

Brandreit, L. M., Lyons, M., & Benley, J. (1994). Perceived needs of post-stroke following termination. *Nursing and Health Care, 15,* 514–520.

Bull, M. J. (1994). A discharge planning questionnaire for clinical practice. *Applied Nursing Research, 7*(4), 193–207.

Bull, M. J., & Kane, R. L. (1996). Gaps in discharge planning. *Journal of Applied Gerontology, 15*(4), 486–500.

Burger, S. G., Fraser, V., Hunt, S., & Frank, B. (1996). *Nursing homes: Getting good care there (The National Citizens' Coalition for Nursing Home Reform).* San Luis Obispo, CA: Impact.

Castellucci, D. T. (1998). Issues for nurses regarding elder autonomy. *Nursing Clinics of North America, 33*(2), 265–273.

Clark, P. G., Spence, D. L., & Sheehan, J. L. (1987). A service/learning model for interdisciplinary teamwork in health and aging. *Gerontology and Geriatrics Education, 6*(4), 3–16.

Clemens, E. L. (1995). Multiple perceptions of discharge planning in one urban hospital. *Health and Social Work, 20*(4), 254–261.

Colucciello, M. L., & Mangles, L. M. (1997). Clinical pathways in subacute care settings. *Nursing Management, 28*(6), 52–54.

Corbett, C. F., & Androwich, I. M. (1994). Critical paths: Implications for improving practice. *Home Healthcare Nurse, 12*(6), 27–34.

Coulton, C. J. (1988). Prospective payment requires increased attention to quality of post hospital care. *Social Work in Health Care, 13*(4), 19–30.

Coulton, C. J., Dunkle, R. E., Chow, J. C., Haug, M., & Vielhaber, M. (1989). Locus of control and decision making for posthospital care. *Gerontologist, 29*(5), 627–632.

Coulton, C. J., Dunkle, R. E., Chun-Chun, J., Haug, M., & Vielhaber, D. (1988). Dimensions of post-hospital care decision-making: A factor analytic study. *Gerontologist, 28*(2), 218–223.

Cummings, S. M., & Cockerham, C. (1997). Ethical dilemmas in discharge planning for patients with Alzheimer's disease. *Health and Social Work, 22*(2), 101–108.

Delfs, J. R., Stanley, L., & Yesner, J. (1995). Geriatrics assessment programs: The Deaconess ElderCare Model. In J. J. Gallo, W. Reichel, & L. M. Anderson (Eds.), *Handbook of Geriatric Assessment* (2nd ed., pp. 219–234). Gaithersburg, MD: Aspen.

Department of Health and Human Services. (1987). *Posthospital care: Discharge planners report increasing difficulty in planning Medicare patients* (GAO/PMED-87-5BR). Washington, DC: US Government Printing Office.

Doran, K., Sampson, B., Staus, R., Ahern, A., & Schiro, D. (1997). Clinical pathway across tertiary and community care after an interventional cardiology procedure.

*Journal of Cardiovascular Nursing, 11*(2), 1–14.

Dwyer, J. (1991). *Nutrition screening initiative.* Washington, DC: Nutritional Screening Initiative.

Eisenberg, J. M. (1986). *Doctors' decisions and the cost of medical care.* Ann Arbor, MI: Health Administration Press Perspectives.

Falconer, J. A., Roth, E. J., Sutin, J. A., Strasser, D. C., & Chang, R. W. (1993). The critical path method in stroke rehabilitation: Lessons from an experiment in cost containment and outcome improvement. *Quality Review Bulletin, 19*(1), 8–16.

Fitzig, C. (1988). Discharge planning: Nursing focus. In P. J. Volland (Ed.), *Discharge planning: An interdisciplinary approach to continuity of care* (pp. 93–117). Owings Mills, MD: National Health Publishing.

Freeman, S. R., & Chamber, K. A. (1997). Home health care: Clinical pathways and quality integration. *Nursing Management, 28*(6), 45–48.

Gage, M. (1994). The patient-driven interdisciplinary care plan. *Journal of Nursing Administration, 24*(4), 26–35.

Glass, R. I., & Weiner, M. S. (1976). Seeking a social disposition for the medical patient: CAAST, a simple and objective clinical index. *Medical Care, XIC*(7), 637–641.

Gorbien, M. J. (1995). Clinical pathways: Too hard a course for complex patients? *Continuum: An Interdisciplinary Journal of Continuity of Care, 15*(5), 1–6.

Gregor, C., Pope, S., Werry, D., & Dodek, P. (1996). Reduced length of stay and improved appropriateness of care with a clinical path for total knee or hip arthroplasty. *Joint Commission Journal on Quality Improvement, 22*(9), 617–628.

Haddock, K. S. (1991). Characteristics of effective discharge planning programs for the frail elderly. *Journal of Gerontological Nursing, 17*(7), 10–14.

Haddock, K. S. (1994). Collaborative discharge planning: Nursing and social services. *Clinical Nurse Specialist, 8*(5), 248–252.

Hawes, C., Morris, J. N., Phillips, C. D., Fries, B. E., Murphy, K., & Mor, V. (1997). Development of the nursing home Resident Assessment Instrument in the USA. *Age and Ageing, 26*(Suppl 2), 19–25.

Health Care Financing Administration (1994). *The Medicare 1994 Handbook* (DHHS Publication No. HCFA 10050). Baltimore, MD: Health Care Financing Administration.

Henderson, M. (1987). *Case management defined.* Waltham, MA: Bigel Institute for Health Policy Studies, Brandeis University, Heller Graduate School.

Hofmann, P. A. (1993). Critical path method: An important tool for coordinating clinical care. *Joint Commission Journal on quality Improvement, 19*(7), 235–246.

Horne, M. (1996). Involving physicians in clinical pathways: An example for perioperative knee arthroplasty. *Joint Commission Journal on Quality Improvement, 22*(2), 115–124.

Huggins, D., & Lehman, K. (1997). Reducing costs through case management. *Nursing Management, 28*(12), 34–37.

Hurt, L. W. (1995). Care management: Providing a connecting link. *Nursing Management, 26*(11), 27–33.

Ignatavicius, D. D. (1998). *Introduction to long term care nursing: Principles and practice.* Philadelphia: F.A. Davis.

Ignatavicius, D. D., & Hausman, K. A. (1995). *Clinical Pathways for Collaborative Practice.* Philadelphia: W.B. Saunders.

Inui, T., Stevenson, K. M., Penda, D., & Murphy, I. (1981). Identifying hospital patients who need early discharge planning for special dispositions. *Medical Care, 19*(9), 922–929.

Kane, R. L., Bell, R., Riegler, S., Wilson, A., & Kane, R. A. (1983). Assessing the outcomes of nursing home patients. *Journal of Gerontology, 38,* 385–393.

Kasper, J. F., Mulley, A. G., & Wennberg, J. E. (1992). Developing shared decision-making programs to improve the quality of health care. *Quality Review Bulletin, 18*(6), 183–190.

Kleinman, J. (1995). The physician's new agenda. In K. Zander (Ed.), *Managing outcomes through collaborative care: The application of care mapping and case management* (pp. 39–57) Chicago: American Hospital Publishing.

Kodner, D. L. (1993). *Case management: Principles, practice, and performance.* New York: Institute for Applied Gerontology.

Lathrop, J., Suefert, G., MacDonald, R., & Martin, S. (1991). The patient-focused hospital: A patient care concept. *Journal of Social Health Systems 3,* 2.

Lulavage, A. (1991). RN–LPN teams: Toward unit nursing case management. *Nursing Management, 22*(3), 58–61.

Mahn, V. A. (1993). Clinical nurse case management: A service line approach. *Nursing Management, 24*(9), 48–50.

McCorkle, R. (1987). *The complications of early discharge from hospitals.* Paper presented at the Proceedings of the 5th National Conference: Human Values and Cancer, New York.

McGarvey, R. N., & Harper, J. J. (1993). Pneumonia mortality reduction and quality improvement in a community hospital. *Quality Review Bulletin, 19*(4), 124–130.

McWilliam, C., Brown, J., Carmichael, J., & Lehman, J. M. (1994). A new perspective on threatened autonomy in elderly persons: The disempowering process. *Social Science Medicine, 38*, 327–338.

Morrison, A. S. (1985). *Screening in Chronic Disease.* New York: Oxford University Press.

Naylor, M. (1990). Comprehensive discharge planning for hospitalized elderly: A pilot study. *Nursing Research, 39*(3), 156–161.

Naylor, M., Brooten, D., Jones, R., Lavizzo-Mourey, R., Mezey, M., & Pauly, M. (1994). Comprehensive discharge planning for the hospitalized elderly: A randomized clinical trial. *Annals of Internal Medicine, 120*(12), 999–1006.

Pacala, J. T., Boult, C., & Boult, L. (1995). Predictive validity of a questionnaire that identifies older persons at risk for hospital admission. *Journal of the American Geriatric Society, 43*, 374–377.

Pearson, S. D., Goulart-Fisher, D., & Lee, T. H. (1995). Critical pathways as a strategy for improving care: Problems and potential. *Annals of Internal Medicine, 123*(12), 941–948.

Petrie, H. G. (1976). Do you see what I see? The epistemology of interdisciplinary inquiry. *Journal of Aesthetic Education, 10*, 7–17.

Pike, A. W., McHugh, M., Cagney, K. C., Miller, N. E., Reiley, P., & Seibert, C. P. (1993). A new architecture for quality assurance: Nursing physician collaboration. *Journal of Nursing Quality Assurance, 3*(2), 11–18.

Potter, P. (1995). The uses of variance. In K. Zander (Ed.), *Managing outcomes through collaborative care: The application of care mapping and case management* (pp. 131–148). Chicago: American Hospital Publishing.

Potthoff, S., Kane, R. L., & Franco, S. J. (1998). Improving hospital discharge planning for elderly patients. *Health Care Financing Review, 19*(2), 47–72.

Proctor, E. K., & Morrow-Howell, N. (1990). Complications in discharge planning with Medicare patients. *Health and Social Work, 15*, 45–54.

Redford, L. J. (1992). Case management: The wave of the future. *Journal of Case Management, 1*(1), 5–8.

Rogers, C. (1951). *Client-centered therapy: Its current practice, implications, and theory.* Boston: Houghton Mifflin.

Sloane, P. D. (1984). How to maintain the health of independent elderly. *Journal of the American Geriatrics Society, 39*, 93–104.

Strong, A. G., & Sneed, N. V. (1991). Clinical evaluation of a critical path for coronary artery bypass surgery patients. *Progress in Cardiovascular Nursing, 6*(1), 29–37.

Stuen, C., & Monk, A. (1990). Discharge planning: Impact of Medicare's prospective payment on elderly patients. *Journal of Gerontological Social Work, 15*, 149–165.

Tappen, R. M., Hall, R. F., Stahura, P., & Blume, L. (1995). Adequacy of preparation for discharge from the rehabilitation units of a long-term care institution. *Rehabilitation Nursing Research, 4*(3), 98–103.

U.S. Preventive Services Task Force (1996). *Guide to clinical preventive services: Report of the U.S. Preventive Services Task Force (2nd ed.).* Baltimore, MD: Williams & Wilkins.

Volland, P. J. (Ed.). (1988). *Discharge planning: An interdisciplinary approach to continuity of care.* Owings Mills, MD: National Health Publishing.

Weber, D. O. (1991). Six months of patient-focused care. *Health-Care Forum Journal, 34*(4), 23–31.

Wetle, T., Levkoff, S., Cwikel, J., & Rosen, A. (1988). Nursing home resident participation in medical decisions: Perceptions and preferences. *Gerontologist, 28*(Suppl), 32–38.

White, M. (1986). Case management. In G. L. Maddox (Ed.), *The Encyclopedia of Aging* (pp. 92–96). New York: Springer Publishing.

Zander, K. (1995). Collaborative care: Two effective strategies for positive outcomes. In K. Zander (Ed.), *Managing outcomes through collaborative care: The application of care mapping and case management* (pp. 1–38). Chicago: American Hospital Publishing.

Zander, K. (1996). Evolving mapping and case management for capitation Part III: Getting control of value. *New Definition, 11*(2), 1–2.

Zarle, N. C. (1987). *Continuing care: The process and practice of discharge planning.* Rockville, MD: Aspen.

# 15

# Long-Term Case Management for Older Adults

## ROSALIE A. KANE

Since the early 1970s, case management has been steadily evolving as a feature of long-term care programs for elderly people. It is now the hallmark of home and community-based services (HCBS) programs designed to serve older people with disabilities outside nursing homes (Kane, Kane, & Ladd, 1998). These programs have a heavy state influence; long-term care and HCBS policy making are state prerogatives and account (albeit with federal matching) for a large portion of state budgets. The assessment tools used at the client level are vehicles for the implementation of these state policies.

Although HCBS case management programs vary widely, both between and within states, comprehensive assessment is their almost universal hallmark. This chapter discusses how measures for the various domains described in Part I of this book have been mixed and matched to ground HCBS case management. Ideally handled, this particular application of assessment technology can be a powerful force in helping older people. Unfortunately, the way to optimal case management is paved with problems, many of which have their root in the way that the assessment process is carried out and the results used.

## DESCRIPTIVE BACKGROUND

### What Is Case Management?

In language used by the Health Care Financing Administration in the 1981 legislation that enabled expanded HCBS programs under Medicaid waivers, *case management* refers to "coordinating and managing a group of services on behalf of a group of people" (Kane & Kane, 1997). As an advocate for each older person needing care, a case manager acts as a technical consultant and expert to identify and compensate for functional problems and marshal resources on behalf of people needing long-term care. As a gatekeeper to services and care, the case manager is expected to distribute societal resources in a fair and prudent manner. Obvious tensions exist between advocacy roles, which are said to have a "gate-opening" quality (Halter, 1999), and the resource allocation or gatekeeper roles. These tensions have made for exquisite ethical dilemmas (Kane & Caplan, 1993).

Despite the manifold variations in case management, widespread agreement has been achieved on general steps in the case management cycle (Applebaum & Austin, 1990; Austin, Roberts, & Low, 1985; White, 1995):

1. Case finding (or screening), which identifies people in a larger population who might benefit from case management
2. Comprehensive multidimensional assessment to determine the needs of the older person
3. Care planning, sometimes called *service planning*
4. Implementation of the plan, which sometimes is done through referrals but more usually involves authorization or purchase of services by the case manager
5. Monitoring the well-being of the consumer and the performance of service providers
6. Formal reassessment at prescribed intervals or as the situation may require

Steps 2 and 6 require the literal application of assessment approaches, but, less obviously, the case finding in Step 1 and the monitoring in Step 5 also apply assessment principles. Looking back to the opening chapter, the long-term care case management process often requires assessment as screening for both eligibility and case-finding purposes, assessment for clinical care management purposes, and assessment for monitoring and quality assurance purposes at both the individual and program level.

Case management in HCBS has an affinity to the care coordination and discharge planning activities described in Chapter 14. Indeed, the terms *care coordination* and *case management* are used almost interchangeably. Although the former is more commonly used in health-oriented programs and the latter in social service-oriented programs, the term itself does not signify which form of case management is in question.* Despite substantial overlap, case managers in health programs and case managers in socially oriented long-term care programs have markedly different

dominant tendencies and, at the extreme, are the proverbial ships in the night in terms of ability to communicate and collaborate. Consider the distinctions presented in Table 15.1.

## Who Performs Long-Term Care Case Management?

As stated before, case managers for HCBS are often social workers, sometimes because of formal training at the masters or bachelors level or sometimes because of job title. They may also be nurses. (Sometimes teams of social workers and nurses are involved, especially in the early phases of assessment.) Usually, case managers hold at least a college degree. Usually, too, however, they have had no specific education about case management before assuming the role, although some may be highly trained nurses, social workers, or others with advanced degrees. Typically, they have had little direct training or background in using their assessment tools.

Case managers are located at a wide range of employment sites. They may work in county health departments, county or regional social welfare departments, area agencies on aging, or voluntary heath and social services agencies (including home health and other home care programs, hospitals, and family service associations). Case managers for frail older people are also sometimes employed by financial institutions that manage care and finances for people with cognitive impairment. Some case managers work for themselves in solo or group practice and serve a privately paying clientele. In those situations, it is often the worried out-of-town relatives of the older person who arrange for the case management (and perhaps they also pay the bill).

States fulfill their responsibilities to provide long-term care for low-income people

---

*For convenience and to distinguish this content from that of the previous chapter, this chapter uses the unmodified term *case management* as distinguished from the care coordination and discharge planning activities discussed in Chapter 14. Also note

that some type of care coordination or case management is often incorporated into the more short-term and circumscribed activities of Geriatric Assessment and Management Units described in Chapter 13.

**Table 15.1.** Differences Between Case Management in Home and Community-Based Services (HCBS) and Care Coordination in Health Care

| Case management (care coordination) in HCBS | Care coordination (case management) in health programs |
|---|---|
| Usually done by social workers, sometimes with input of a nurse | Usually done by a nurse, sometimes with input of a social worker. Alternatively, done by "health care teams" with a nurse or other coordinator |
| Assessment concentrates on functional, cognitive, affective, and social domains with less attention to health-related items | Assessment concentrates on functional, cognitive, and health-related domains with less attention to broad psychological, social, and environmental domains |
| Care planning often, though not always, concentrates on meeting "unmet" needs of consumers and enhancing their general quality of life with less emphasis on improving functioning and health status | Care planning often, though not always, concentrates on improving, maintaining, or slowing decline in health and functional status and making the best use of a range of health and long-term care resources with less emphasis on quality of social life |
| Typically, though not always, the same case manager follows the consumer over time | Typically, though not always, the case manager is attached to the particular service the person receives (e.g., an outpatient clinic, a home care program, a nursing home) |
| High-risk individuals are typically identified on the basis of vulnerability and the risks to safety and well-being while living in the community. Those unable to manage their own plans because of complex needs, mental impairment, or physical health may be targeted | High-risk individuals are typically identified on the basis of their likelihood of using hospitals and other high-cost health services |
| Case managers are often, though not always, located outside the organizations providing services under the care plans | Case managers are often, though not always, located within complex service-providing organizations, including multilevel health care entities and managed care organizations at risk for the services provided |

and to oversee the general quality of long-term care for all people in a variety of ways. In financial terms, the Medicaid program is a major vehicle and one for which federal matching money can be claimed. Nursing home programs for low-income people are, of course, financed by Medicaid, as are limited home health programs. Many states have also opted to pay for HCBS services, particularly personal attendant services, through their state wide Medicaid programs. Since December 1981, HCBS Medicaid waiver money has also been available to states, permitting them to expand HCBS services to people who would otherwise be in nursing homes at Medicaid expense and to do so in a more gradual way, without the statewide requirements of the regular Medicaid program and to ease the financial eligibility as well.

The Medicaid waiver mechanism has accounted for the greatest growth in HCBS services in the United States over the last 20 years, but states also use funding from dedicated block grant funds (from the Older Americans Act), more open-ended social service block grant funds, and specially appropriated state funds (with no federal match) for long-term care, typically to fill in the cracks of the Medicaid and Medicaid waiver programs. In planning this care system, states have multiple goals: ending the predominant reliance on the nursing home (which is expensive for states and dreaded by consumers); avoiding a groundswell of new clientele for the more popular HCBS services (or at least ensuring that those served really *need* the care and help); and ensuring that those who receive HCBS services (such as homemaking, personal care at home, adult day care services, and HCBS services in new group residential settings licensed by the state) receive care of a quality that does not put their health at risk. Assessment at the consumer level is necessary to achieve all the goals just listed.

Inevitably, a state's HCBS case management program is structurally linked to its nursing home program, even if the state forgoes its right to perform aggressive case management once a person is in a nursing home under Medicaid (as most states do). States need to be reassured that nobody is served in those HCBS programs for which states are responsible if the client is deemed to "need" a nursing home and deemed unable to be served safely in the community. On the other hand (and this is somewhat of a Catch-22), to balance their ledgers, states also must target their services to those who "need" nursing homes. The paradox is reconciled somewhat by the shifting use of that term *need*.

The need for a nursing home in eligibility terms means that individuals are assessed as having the same functional limitations, disabilities, and needs that would (along with financial eligibility) render them eligible for nursing home care by state policy; if that need can be proved, they are eligible for HCBS funding under Medicaid waivers. In contrast, needing a nursing home in terms of being unsafe in the community requires assessment beyond the needs of the potential consumer. The case manager would need to assess that the circumstances in the community care are unsafe: typically, that requires assessing the adequacy of the person's physical environment, the adequacy of family assistance, and even the extent to which the older persons themselves cooperate with and contribute to the success of the HCBS plan. Professional judgments vary about whether an absolute need for a nursing home ever exists and the extent to which various long-term care programs can be interchangeable. This is obviously an area where value judgments flourish; some commentators envisage a perfect continuum with each individual slotted into the correct level of care based on an assessment, whereas others see much more potential overlap and suggest that a repertoire of services is a better metaphor than a continuum (Kane, 1993).

States also make their own structural decisions about the design of their HCBS case management programs. In some states, a great deal of centralization occurs; in the most centralized model, case managers are regional state employees; in a less centralized but still controlled model, the state devolves case management to local governmental or nonprofit agencies but maintains statewide consistency in procedures, including the use of a state-mandated assessment tool and state training for those who use it. Some programs have so much local autonomy that states can merely recommend a particular assessment tool.

## Variation in Long-Term Care Case Management

Case management varies substantially at the individual level, the level at which the case manager meets the client. The ways are numerous, and assessment must be tailored to the design of the particular program. Case management varies in scope, with some case management programs taking responsibility for a broader and some a narrower sphere of activity. Some case managers retain contact with their clients when they are hospitalized or temporarily placed in a nursing home, although most do not. A few case management programs work aggressively to relocate clients from nursing homes as well as to avert their admission in the first place. An early example of this emphasis occurred in Oregon, and Washington state is now moving in that direction (Kane et al., 1998). Case management also varies in intensity, from a minimal presence in the consumer's life to a highly involved relationship, with regard to the intervals of routine monitoring (weekly, monthly, or less frequently), the form of routine monitoring (by phone or in person), and the amount of systematic effort incorporated into determining the quality of service providers and the satisfaction of clients.

Related to all of the above, case management programs also vary in their relationships with service providers. In some programs, case managers refer most ongoing problem solving to the community agencies that provide care. The consumers may barely know that they have a case manager. In other programs, case managers maintain active relationships with their clientele. In some programs, case managers expect that service providers will bear the lion's share of quality assurance efforts, whereas in others the case managers themselves make conscious efforts at quality control (Kane & Degenholtz, 1997). In these latter programs, case managers may purchase or arrange services from self-employed workers as well as from formal organizations. In some case management programs, a single case manager handles all steps of the case management process, whereas in others the assessment process is separated from care planning and on-going case management. This separation can promote efficiency, but requires a special effort to generate meaningful assessments and to convey the information to the person following up on the case.

Case managers may be generalists or specialists working with a case load of consumers who share particular diagnoses or problems, and caseloads may vary from fewer than 20 to more than 200. All of these variations produce case management with widely varying costs. The striking cost discrepancies can be seen in both the average case management costs per consumer and the costs of case management as a percentage of the costs of all the services managed (Davidson et al., 1991).

A more subtle variation concerns the autonomy, individualization, and discretionary power of the case manager. In some programs, case managers are expected to follow fixed rules for their activities. Such rules determine the frequency of assessment and monitoring and the kind of services that are offered given the kinds of problems and needs observed. In other programs, case managers are encouraged

to reach their own decisions about the intensity of their involvement on a case by case basis and to creatively consider a wide range of ways to meet consumer needs, sometimes piecing together a program that goes well beyond arranging services from agencies with which the case management program has a formal contractual or collaborative arrangement.

## Goals of Case Managers

The effects long-term care case managers expect to accomplish can be addressed at the level of the individual consumers and their families and at the level of the system of care in the community. In both senses, the goals of case management are rarely monolithic or clearly expressed, and they are sometimes contradictory.

At the individual level, case management programs most frequently make some claim to keeping people out of nursing homes as an end in itself. More broadly, they may aspire to making sure that older consumers' needs can be met safely in the community, the tension already described. Almost as often, therefore, case management programs aim to "meet unmet needs" at some threshold of adequacy. But case management programs may also take as a goal a range of other outcomes, such as improved or sustained functional status, psychological well-being; and social well-being. Goals may also be related to the well-being of family members who may be providing much of the day-to-day care and safety supervision of the person needing assistance. Specific goals related to families could include improving the competence of family caregivers, relieving family anxiety over their relative's condition and their own abilities, keeping family efforts at a high level, or relieving family burden. Ideally, the assessment approaches developed would correspond to the program goals, although in practice things are rarely that well thought out.

At the individual level, some case management programs seek to maximize the choices and the personal autonomy of the consumers of care. This is a somewhat different type of goal than the others. If client autonomy and choice is a goal, then somehow the case managers need to become informed about client preferences and interests as part of the assessment and care-planning process. The kinds of assessment tools discussed in Chapter 8 would then be needed, and indeed some of those tools have been developed specifically so that state case management programs can be more responsive to consumer autonomy. For example, in the late 1990s, Ohio began a project to expand choice and control for HCBS consumers (Kane et al., 1998) and needed to incorporate an assessment of the extent to which the consumers wanted and could flourish with these greater amounts of control.

At the system level, case management may have any or all of the following goals: reduce the public and/or private costs of HCBS care in the community; improve access to services; allocate services equitably; assure quality of services; develop a broader range of services in the community; stimulate volunteer activities; and reduce unit price of services. These activities all suggest systematic approaches. The case management program uses its information systems and its purchasing power to bring about these kinds of system outcomes.

To illustrate how this may play out in a particular program, consider the Wisconsin Community Options Program (Kane et al., 1998). At the individual level, the goals for the consumers are particularly sweeping and ambitious and are embodied in the acronym RESPECT:

Relationships that are caring and respectful among consumers, care managers, and service providers with continuity over time

Empowerment of consumers to make choices

Services provided that are tailored to individual needs and unique circumstances

Physical and mental health, that is, services are intended to help consumers achieve optimum levels of functioning, including both physical and emotional health

Enhancement of participant reputations, that is, services are intended to maintain and enhance the consumer's sense of self-worth and community recognition for their value in every way

Community and family participation, that is, consumers are supported to maintain and develop friendships and participation in their families and communities

Tools for independence, which help consumers achieve maximum self-sufficiency

Because Wisconsin's case managers are held generally responsible for implementing the goals inherent in the RESPECT concept, their resident assessments should provide the information to do so and to evaluate success. For example, if they are to enhance social participation and self-esteem, they must have some way of assessing needs and accomplishments on those dimensions. Wisconsin is a state with strong county governments and a decentralized approach to actual case management and service delivery. Therefore, the state has needed to work indirectly through sensitization, training, and resource development, but its 1995 model long-term care assessment tool contains much more emphasis on social functioning and preferences than do those of most states, as well as many open-ended questions (Wisconsin Division of Community Service, 1995). Similarly, the state contracted with a consultant firm to develop a quality assurance assessment that case managers and others could use to monitor clients and see whether the aspirations of the RESPECT concept were fulfilled.

At the system level too, the Wisconsin program also has well-articulated goals. Program officials have stated that case management should achieve three general purposes: identifying those who meet the eligibility criteria established by the state; helping people make care plans and receive care that accords with their needs and individual preferences; and providing the state with information about the adequacy and effectiveness of long-term care programs within the state, including regional variation in quality, outcomes, and costs. These goals also have implications for assessments and how they are used.

## ASSESSMENT IN HCBS CASE MANAGEMENT

### Goals of Assessment

Linked to the goals of HCBS case management itself, the initial assessment and subsequent reassessments facilitate the case manager's need to

- Determine initial and continuing eligibility for the HCBS program itself and (if applicable) determine the levels of service and benefits to which the consumer will be entitled within the programs managed (sometimes, the case manager's assessment covers both financial and functional eligibility, but often the financial eligibility is a separate administrative function)
- Establish priorities for who should receive services if a waiting list is in effect or who should receive any particular service in short supply
- Develop and implement a care plan that accords with the consumer's needs and preferences and change the plan as needed
- Evaluate the effectiveness of the individual plan, including determining whether the consumer's needs are safely and adequately met in the community and recommending alternative living arrangements, if necessary
- Determine and improve the quality of services actually rendered
- Provide information that can be used to describe the clients, services, outcomes, and costs of the program, including local and regional variations in these elements

Some of these purposes are administrative (determining eligibility, managing waiting lists), and some of the administrative purposes relate less to a single program than to the use of assessment data as reported to a central body responsible for an overall program at a state or substate level. Other purposes are much more clinical in nature, meant to facilitate work with a particular client. Indeed, one of the challenges is to design an approach to assessment that is both specific and objective enough to be used to allocate services and clinically sensitive enough to guide the work of the case manager. If a newly assigned case manager picks up an assessment form for an ongoing client, it is unlikely that its completed check marks will convey a dynamic sense of the particular client in his or her family and community constellation and the unique nature of his or her needs. On the other hand, long narrative notes are insufficiently standardized, anchored, or user friendly to guide a case management program. Some assessment forms have adopted the convention of including items with fixed choices but leaving space after each dimension of the assessment (or sometimes with each item) for brief narrative notes that clarify ratings and additional information relevant to care planning. Such notes, however, are typically underutilized.

### Content of Assessment

The case manager's assessment typically covers a fairly wide range of content areas (see Table 15.2). At a minimum, the areas include functional status, a summary of health status, cognitive status, affective status, and social status (the latter incorporating information about social and economic resources and social support). The assessment may also include sections on the physical environment, behavior that puts the consumer at risk, and family-caregiver well-being. Some assessment protocols are modular with optional elements.

**Table 15.2.**

Typical Content Elements for Case Managers' Assessments

*Background Data*

✓ age, marital status, household composition, occupational status, gender, ethnicity, Medicaid status, insurance status
✓ driving instructions to person's home
✓ key contacts — family, doctor

*Presenting Problem*

(usually gathered through open-ended questions)

*Functional Abilities*

✓ ADL abilities
✓ IADL abilities
✓ mobility
✓ continence

*Health Status*

✓ active diseases and diagnoses
✓ recent use of hospitals & other health care
✓ medical coverage (name of primary care MD and active specialists)
✓ pain and discomfort
✓ vision and hearing
✓ prosthetic devices & medical equipment used
✓ nutritional status/eating habits
✓ fall risk and fall history

*Cognitive Functioning*

✓ memory (long-term and short-term)
✓ judgment
✓ disturbing or self-endangering behavior
  –wandering.
  –violent or aggressive behavior

*Emotional Functioning*

✓ history of or current psychiatric problems
✓ depression and anxiety

*Social Functioning*

✓ activities
✓ social network characteristics (size, proximity)
✓ social relationships

*Values and Preferences*

✓ for everyday routines and activities
✓ for place and type of care

*Expected and Actual Social Support*

✓ type of family help received
✓ amount of family help received
✓ number of family helpers
✓ expected permanence of family help
✓ use of paid helpers and caregivers
✓ income and assets
  –to purchase help
  –to determine eligibility for help

*Environment*

✓ safety of home and neighborhood
✓ adaptability of home to functional problems

*Alcohol and Substance Use*

*Family Assessment*

(done directly with identified primary family caregiver)
✓ care given — amount & type
✓ other obligations — labor force, children, other caregiving
✓ health status of family caregiver
✓ backup for primary caregiver
✓ effects of giving care
  –physical, emotional, social, financial
✓ willingness to continue caregiving

*Summary Judgments*

✓ unmet need
✓ safety in the community
✓ ability to manage care
✓ risk for abuse, neglect, victimization
✓ amount of help needed to say in community

ENTIRE ASSESSMENT

CARE PLAN

Some programs have further protocols for more intensive assessment should it be warranted by the initial exploration, for example, assessment of depression and suicide risk, assessment of alcohol and substance abuse.

The exact content of the assessment will depend on the populations whose care is being managed and on the extent of the case manager's responsibilities. As indicated below, some HCBS case managers also assess the appropriateness and necessity for all nursing home admissions, and the assessment must be tailored accordingly. Some case management programs also have responsibility for adult protective services for people who are abused, neglected, exploited, or self-neglecting or who are considered vulnerable for such conditions. If so, the case management program usually incorporates some measure of abuse into its assessment protocol, although typically a full abuse assessment would be triggered by some initial data that raise concern. Some case management programs, for example, in Illinois, offer "money management" as one of their services, and, therefore, the assessment examines in more depth how well money is being managed and the need for that kind of help. Typically, HCBS case managers act as feeders and links to mental health programs and other such programs in the state, and, when this is the case, it is reasonable to include a mental health screen to rationalize the referral process.

Case managers have a love–hate relationship with their assessment tools. Typically, they complain that the tools are too long. When groups of case managers meet to revise their assessments, however, typically they add rather than subtract components. Case management tools may incorporate alcohol and addiction assessments, nutritional assessments, smoking and other health practices assessments, and a variety of other batteries for which someone has lobbied.

## Relationship to Care Plan

The main purpose of the assessment is to generate a care plan. All the information that is illustrated in Table 15.2 is collected for the purpose of making a series of decisions: is help needed, what help is needed, is the person eligible for the help offered through the program, is the help needed available through the program at a cost that does not exceed nursing home care (a precondition for HCBS waiver funding), will the individual accept any of the help that the program can offer, and, finally, what services need to be in place.

The elements or content "building blocks" of the case manager's assessment echo the content discussed in the chapters in Section I of this book. Functional abilities, health status, emotional state, social functioning, environments, preferences, and caregiving were all discussed in earlier chapters, and all are relevant to this purpose. For the information to be useful for care planning, however, it needs to have a particular slant. For example, health status focuses on active and relevant health problems or conditions, not an entire health history. Similarly, other questions are pointed toward the kinds of help likely to be needed and the kinds problems for which the program offers help.

As indicated in Chapter 2, function can be measured in terms of capability to perform a particular function, whether a function is performed, the adequacy of the performance, and the difficulty of performing the function. One can also examine whether there is any unmet need in performing the activity. Functional status zeros in on tasks that must be done in the individual's environment that he or she cannot do and that nobody else can or will perform for the person. The last clause of the sentence is so important that many case managers' assessment tools blend the help received with the need for help into a single item. Case managers are interested in all of the above; indeed, they make judgments about the adequacy with which household tasks such as cleaning and cooking are performed. Their bottom line, however, is usually whether the individual has an unmet need. For that reason and because there is a desire to keep the questionnaires as short as possible, the items about performance ability are often combined and conflated with items about family help. For example, the choices about a given activity of daily living (ADL) activity might be no help needed, can perform task with equipment, receives some human help, receives complete help. The information generated will be much more useful, however, if separate columns are maintained for information about need for assistance, about capability, and about unmet needs.

Case management assessment tools are often quite practical in the way their items are defined and tailored. For example, the form may include an item about access to transportation or ability to read and speak English because the information gleaned will be pertinent to the kind of care plan developed. In one rural state, ability to chop and carry wood (or availability of help in doing so) was included among the functional topics; in wintry climates, snow removal is often included.

Typically, too, the case managers are expected to pay particular attention to risks, and the assessments are designed accordingly. These risks include nutritional risks, risks of being abused or victimized, and risks of falls. Special attention is paid to the individuals who live alone, especially those with cognitive impairment, and special attention is paid to the resilience and strength of family caregiving. Conflict in the family would, in particular, be noted.

## Style and Format for Assessment

The case management program's first contact with the client is through an initial referral or inquiry during which some information is collected about the presenting problem and brief parameters of functioning. This screening may be done on the telephone. The most effective screen is one that will help the care manager determine whether a full-fledged assessment is needed and, if so, whether it is needed on an urgent basis. If the screening indicates a specific delimited problem for which care can be arranged or that is of the magnitude and scope that the consumer can handle it, a referral may be made to a community resource. It is wasteful, for example, to respond with a full in-home assessment for someone who only needs help securing a ride in a van or a home-delivered meal. Unfortunately, little work has been done to examine the predictive value of screening tools (e.g., do they identify clients who really need help? Would the judgment that some people did not need an assessment and further care be borne out if they did receive a full assessment?).

Equally unfortunate, there is sometimes a tendency to use a full comprehensive assessment for everyone with no screening or triage whatsoever. There are a few exceptions. In the early 1990s, Florida went to enormous trouble to test its screening process for false negatives and false positives (Kane et al., 1991). During the same period, Ohio developed its triage concept, whereby a wide variety of community organizations had access to and training in the screening tool with the intent that they would refer for case management assessment only if indicated (Applebaum & Austin, 1990).

The comprehensive in-person assessment is usually done in the consumer's home, although some programs are also tied to hospital-based screening that offers consumers choices besides admission to nursing homes. An in-home assessment usually is about an hour or two in length, and, at the end of the assessment, at least a preliminary plan is typically reached. This may be important if the case manager needs to order services immediately. Family members are often present and indeed encouraged to be present so that they too can be assessed. If the consumer is cognitively impaired, a family member will serve as the observer (or proxy) who is asked to report on the consumer in terms of all the elements in the assessment. In addition, a family member may be interviewed with respect to his or her own caregiving and its effects on his or her life. The immediate involvement of family adds to the practicality of reaching a plan quickly, although family members' perceptions may affect the validity of the information gathered.

Most often the assessment protocols consist of rating scales for the interviewer to complete, interspersed with a few scales that require questions to be asked directly of the client or potential client. It is very unusual for the tool to be configured with items that are asked directly to the consumer. If questions are designed to be asked directly, these are usually for the cognitive and depression screens. Although some domains such as observed performance or physical environments may lend themselves quite well to rating scales, it seems ill-judged to use ratings for most items. It is unlikely that the case manager doing the initial assessment has had any previous encounter with the consumer; therefore, he or she will need to pose questions in order to conduct the assessment. In that case, an argument could be made for inclusion of actual items rather than characteristics to be rated on the basis of a less structured assessment. Some case managers' assessments provide more detail to guide the raters than do others. In some instances that detail is contained within bulky manuals, and in other examples the definitions may be contained on the page opposite the scales so that at least the case manager can consult what it is supposed to mean operationally to assert, for example, that the client "requires some help in dressing."

Case manager's assessment tools are predominately pencil-and-paper protocols. They may be prepared in duplicate or triplicate (often on no-carbon-required paper) so that copies can be kept locally, submitted to the state, and sent to care providers. Sometimes, the data from these "paper" assessments are entered into a computer file. In the last decade, however, some programs (notably, in Alabama, Indiana, and Connecticut) have made the investment in hardware, software, and training so that case managers enter their assessments on laptop computers that they bring to the client's home. This technology guides the case manager through the assessment, making skips and adding subsections as needed. It therefore improves the quality of the assessment by forcing the case manager through the instrument and guarding against error. It also, as is the case in Indiana, can be immediately incorporated into a database that provides an overview of clients, service providers, services, and outcomes to be used in both care planning and quality assurance (Kinney, Freedman, & Loveland-Cook, 1994).

## Tool Design

Many problems exist in the way comprehensive assessment tools are designed and formatted, which, in turn, affects the quality of the data and the potential usefulness of the tool clinically. Among the problems in design that we have noted in reviewing hundreds of case managers' assessment tools over the years are the following:

- There is no space for comments, elaborations, or summary judgments
- There is a lack of clarity about whether the notation is a case manager's judgment, question, or observation
- Most of the questions are in the form of rating rather than direct queries.
- Definitions are found in a telephone-book-size manual rather than on the form itself.
- No time dimensions are used.
- The case managers are instructed to change the assessment information by erasing or over-riding data in the computer if the condition changes, thus erasing the historical data from the record.

Table 15.3 illustrates an assessment tool that has dealt successfully with many of these issues: Idaho's Uniform Assessment Instrument developed in 1999. For example, a brief definition of each item is contained along with the item itself on the questionnaire, and on the back of each page (not shown in the example) the function is much more fully defined. Also note that the form distinguishes among the assistance needed (i.e., the disability level), the availability of family and others to provide that assistance, and unmet needs to be addressed by the case management program. Finally, note that the instrument is designed with ample room for written comments so that some individualization is possible for a case record. All these features are extremely positive. The questionnaire is stitched into a relatively thin booklet so that definitions on the back of the pages are readily visible to the assessor. On the less positive side, the items are phrased as ratings rather than as questions to be asked, and the terms *minimal, moderate, and extensive* are open to interpretation.

**Table 15.3.**

Example of Approach to Measuring Function

| SECTION TWO - Functional Abilities, Supports, and Related Information | | | |
|---|---|---|---|
| Assistance Required Column Directions:<br>Check one of the following codes in this column: N = None, MI = Minimal, MO = Moderate, E = Extensive, T = Total<br>Available Supports Column Directions:<br>Indicate the degree of existing supports received that are not paid by the Department of Health and Welfare or the Idaho Commission on Aging. Include supports received from family, friends, neighbors, volunteers, church, & paid caregivers, etc. Check N = None, MI = Minimal, MO = Moderate, E = Extensive, T = Total<br>Unmet Needs Column Directions:<br>Check the degree of unmet need to be met by the Department of Health and Welfare or the Idaho Commission on Aging. Check N = None, MI = Minimal, MO = Moderate, E = Extensive, T = Total | | | |
| | Assistance Required | Available Supports | Unmet Needs | COMMENTS: (If an AVAILABLE UNPAID or PAID SUPPORT exists, write the name in this section.) |
| 1. PREPARING MEALS: Identify the client's ability to prepare own food. Consider safety issues such as whether burners are left on. | ☐N ☐MI ☐MO ☐E ☐T | ☐N ☐MI ☐MO ☐E ☐T | ☐N ☐MI ☐MO ☐E ☐T | |
| 2. EATING MEALS: Identify the level of assistance needed to perform the activity of feeding and eating with special equipment if regularly used or special tray setup. | ☐N ☐MI ☐MO ☐E ☐T | ☐N ☐MI ☐MO ☐E ☐T | ☐N ☐MI ☐MO ☐E ☐T | |
| 3. TOILETING: Identify the client's ability to get to and from the toilet (including commode, bedpan, and urinal), manage colostomy or other devices, to cleanse after eliminating, and to adjust clothing. | ☐N ☐MI ☐MO ☐E ☐T | ☐N ☐MI ☐MO ☐E ☐T | ☐N ☐MI ☐MO ☐E ☐T | |
| 4. MOBILITY: Identify the client's physical ability to get around, both inside and outside, using mechanical aids if needed. | ☐N ☐MI ☐MO ☐E ☐T | ☐N ☐MI ☐MO ☐E ☐T | ☐N ☐MI ☐MO ☐E ☐T | |
| 5. TRANSFERRING: Identify the client's ability to transfer when in bed or wheelchair. | ☐N ☐MI ☐MO ☐E ☐T | ☐N ☐MI ☐MO ☐E ☐T | ☐N ☐MI ☐MO ☐E ☐T | |
| 6. PERSONAL HYGIENE: Identify the client's ability to shave, care for mouth, and comb hair. | ☐N ☐MI ☐MO ☐E ☐T | ☐N ☐MI ☐MO ☐E ☐T | ☐N ☐MI ☐MO ☐E ☐T | |
| 7. DRESSING: Identify the client's ability to dress and undress, including selection of clean clothing or appropriate seasonal clothing. | ☐N ☐MI ☐MO ☐E ☐T | ☐N ☐MI ☐MO ☐E ☐T | ☐N ☐MI ☐MO ☐E ☐T | |

Source: Uniform Assessment Instrument Idaho Department of Health & Welfare and Idaho Commission on Aging, Draft 1/01/99.

## Aggregation of Assessment Data

How do case managers summarize and make sense of the information they collect? How do case management programs use the data as a basis for fair allocation procedures? One approach is to generate cut-off scores — for example, a certain score needed to receive any service at all, a certain score that suggests the consumer's needs are too great for HCBS, and other scores to establish levels of care and benefits. Some programs have sought a way to score assessment data to identify those most at risk without services who, therefore, should get priority for service while others are on a waiting list.

There are advantages and disadvantages to scoring systems. From an administrative viewpoint, the scoring system offers at least the illusion of science and impartiality and seems to remove any question of partiality in the allocation of resources. As with Scholastic Achievement Tests or any established system for sorting people, there is refuge in "hiding behind the score." Moreover, scores are easily manipulated and may sometimes merely aggregate opinions of uncertain reliability and validity. Some programs adopt a middle course of decision-trees where certain key elements or combinations in the assessment plan will bump the client into a high need category—for example, having cognitive impairment and living alone; being unable to transfer.

If scoring systems are used, they can be developed somewhat arbitrarily or be empirically derived. To do the latter with a new instrument, one approach is to use it for a period of time and correlate the assessment items with actual needs and plans made by case managers regarded as clinically astute. Essentially, this is a process of backing into scores and weighting by making the implicit judgments of clinicians explicit. In truth, validation of these processes is extremely difficult. One is on safer ground if the score is used to signify high versus low need. When scores are used to signify "need for a nursing home" or some other plan designation, the worrisome suggestion seems to be that such life decisions can and should be made by protocol.

Aggregation of information is usually built around problems. Some would argue that the same information could be used to identify areas of client strength, resilience, resources, and resourcefulness (Kivnick, 1991) and that such summary information could be equally useful in guiding care plans. For the most part, however, information about strengths is simply not collected.

## Links to Preadmission Screening for Nursing Homes

Many of the assessment tools now in use are designed for Medicaid waiver programs, which, by definition, must be limited to clients who are "nursing home certifiable." Nursing home certifiability procedures and requirements differ from state to state (O'Keefe, 1996). Often a physician must attest to the "medical necessity" of a nursing home placement under Medicaid, which is arguably the least objective measure possible. HCBS waivers, constrained to serve only those eligible for nursing homes, typically design their statewide assessment forms to incorporate whatever the statutory and customary guidelines are for nursing home certifiability that the physician is expected to use. Reviews of these practices in all 50 states show remarkable variation from state to state and leave reason to doubt that the identical standards were being applied for nursing home eligibility and HCBS eligibility (Justice et al., 1991; O'Keefe, 1996).

Some states deploy their HCBS case managers as mandatory "preadmission screeners" for nursing home admission under Medicaid (or, in some states, for all nursing home admissions). Structurally, this requires a large and constant presence in hospitals, from which most nursing home admissions occur. Having HCBS case managers do preadmission screening should permit simultaneous determination of functional eligibility for HCBS services and offer a possibility of deflecting admissions. It also adds an enormous volume of work to the community program (some of which merely endorses an obvious need for a brief or long-term nursing home stay) and brings the HCBS case manager into potential conflict with the hospital discharge planners, whose coordinating role has been discussed in Chapter 14. The preadmission screening process in general offers a good example of how the best assessment tool cannot offset poor design and structure in its use. In some states, the task of doing preadmission screens was delegated to hospital personnel even though most rural hospitals themselves ran nursing homes (sometimes with many times more beds than the tiny hospital). Needless to say, when the hospitals were empowered to assess who needed nursing home care, every incentive favored filling those hospital-owned nursing home beds.

## Historical Evolution

Not all states mandate a single assessment form to guide their HCBS programs. As mentioned above, some states leave responsibility to counties or to contracted case managers to design their own protocols. The tendency, however, has been toward increased uniformity and the evolution of standardized assessment and information systems under state leadership. Indeed, by the 1980s many states had several statewide long-term care assessment tools in place with different forms to be used for case management under different funding programs. The recent trend has been to consolidate the multiple tools in use into a single tool. Sometimes, there is an effort to design a single assessment tool with branching modules for use across different populations with disabilities — older people, younger people with physical disabilities, people with developmental disabilities, people with aquired immunodeficiency syndrome. Failing that, at least the assessment tools for elderly people and people with physical disabilities lend themselves to consolidation even when separate tools are maintained for developmental disability, mental health, and children. Some states, such as Florida (Kane et al., 1991) and, to a lesser extent, Vermont (Reinardy, Kane, & Mollica, 1994), have undergone a rather elaborate process of consolidating assessment forms and procedures from different programs.

Some newer assessment tools, particularly the one developed in Florida, have the distinct advantage that they really are built around questions posed to the consumer or whoever is responding on the consumer's behalf rather than ratings based on the assessor reflection after an unstructured inquiry. Some states are deep into the process of developing their consolidated tool as this book goes to press. The task of combining assessment tools is difficult because it requires changes in the performances of both state and local agencies. Kansas, for example, went through a process that took many years to evolve a single assessment tool to replace one form used for older people served by the Department on Aging and another used for older people served by the Department of Social and Rehabilitation Services (Mollica et al., 1994). Its efforts were accelerated by state legislative action requiring that a preadmission assessment form be developed. In its misguided wisdom, the legislature mandated that the length of the form be no more than a single page, as though decisions about how to balance ease of completion and type size should be made at that political level.

Typically, when assessment tools are designed (either for the first time or in one of the frequent redesigns that occurs) one or more task forces are formed to consider the elements that need to be incorporated based on experience of clinicians and administrators, and consultants are hired to assist the state in crafting and testing an assessment that meets local needs. Usually this process is informed by competing desires to have the shortest assessment possible, yet to reflect a wide range of interests and issues (e.g., nutrition status, transportation needs, alcohol problems).

At this point, most states have at least one comprehensive assessment form in use for HCBS. Some states, for example, Massachusetts, Pennsylvania, Oregon, Florida, South Carolina, and Minnesota, have gone through numerous iterations of refining statewide HCBS assessment protocols that date back to the 1970s. In some instances, the state had an HCBS demonstration project in place that predated the HCBS waivers and used assessment tools developed for that purpose. In the early 1980s, the Long Term Care Channeling Project was conducted to determine whether

HCBS services were cost-effective alternatives to nursing homes; a common assessment tool was used for that controlled study, and many state HCBS assessments in place bear some resemblance to that instrument (Phillips, Kemper, & Applebaum, 1988). Indeed, the channeling demonstration and its precursor demonstrations did a great deal to define case management for the country (Christianson et al., 1988).

Undoubtedly, the development of assessment tools becomes a catalyst for community education and for refining HCBS systems and role relationships among providers and consumers. Yet it is fair to ask whether 50 or more HCBS assessment protocols are needed in the United States. Might not a single form suffice? Would not a single form provide a better basis for national comparisons? Chapter 16 discusses the nationally mandated assessment forms in use in nursing homes and in home health and the one under development for hospital discharge planning of older people. Certainly some authorities recommend that a version of the Minimum Data Set (MDS) protocol used in nursing homes under Medicaid also be used in HCBS programs. Also, some states perceive the advantages of being able to compare nursing home clientele with other long-term care populations. There is also reason to think that a federally mandated approach, however, rather than the current state-mandated approach would dilute the capability for rather sophisticated service planning developed by many state systems.

## CHALLENGES AND PROBLEMS

### Using the Assessment Properly

The best assessment forms with the most reliable individual scales deteriorate markedly if they are used haphazardly and incompletely or differently from case manager to case manager and from time to time by the same case managers. Too often this lack of precision occurs. HCBS case managers often come from a tradition of social work where less structured approaches to assessment were the norm. They sometimes believe that an assessment form, ordered in a particular way and, worse yet, with specifically worded questions, stifles the creativity of the assessor and ruins the relationship with the consumer. Sometimes, the assessment is perceived as dealing with the obvious, or forcing consumers to answer embarrassing questions when, after all, the case manager believes he or she knows the answer.

In fact, a great deal of training is needed to render case managers into reliable assessors. They need to understand the meaning and importance of each question, the extent to which clarifications are permitted, how to probe for clarity and additional information without leading the responder, and how to maintain a conversational approach while wielding specific questions. They need to practice these approaches and receive refresher courses. Such training can suggest ways to conduct the assessment with untalkative clients, anxious clients, angry or suspicious clients, and sad clients, relating to their concerns and feelings, yet keeping the integrity of the tool.

Too often line case managers perceive the assessment as something added to their work, something that must be done *in addition to* rather than *in the service of* getting to know the client and deciding what is needed. Of course, if the assessments are actually used as a basis for care planning at the individual level; discussion, and case conferencing, supervision, and training at the agency level; and program refinement at the state level, then case managers will take them more seriously. Insufficient attention has, however, been given to how case managers can make the assessment tool an organic part of their work, turning it into their stethoscopes, as it were.

Finally, just as one must guard against the case manager who does not ask the questions, makes guesses, fills out the assessment form later in the car and realizes he or she forget entire areas, the opposite problem needs to be headed off. Some case managers may be so intent on filling out boxes that they miss the cues around them, fail to listen to the information that the consumer is volunteering, or notice what the consumer wants to discuss. Using audiotaped encounters, Ann Dill (1990) vividly described how case managers, intent on finishing their forms, have subtly or not so subtly encouraged some responses and discouraged others and generally cut off communication.

## Using the Assessment Information

The observation that all care plans tend to look alike, or at least that they come in very few flavors is, by now, rather commonplace. In any given program, surprisingly little of the information gets translated into the care plans in observable ways. This calls into question whether too much information is being collected or, conversely, whether case managers have the skill, imagination, or administrative permission to enter into creative, individually tailored care plans. The assessment should guide but not dictate the care plan, which is a matter of negotiation, preference, creativity, and feasibility. The cookie-cutter approach where all care plans come in two or three forms is a problem. It is also a problem, however, if the care plan bears no relationship to the assessment data. When certain problems and issues are identified in the assessment, they should at least trigger some common approaches to identifying problems, further assessment, and consideration of a plan. The wheel need not be reinvented constantly.

A project in Philadelphia set out to provide case managers with tools to bridge the transition from the general comprehensive assessment to care planning around specific problems. The team identified key issues that plague case managers—for instance, people with cognitive impairment who live alone, people with alcohol problems, people who fall, people who are taking large numbers of medications, and people who are suspected of being victims of abuse. For 12 of these issues they devel-

oped general care plan templates that laid out further assessment strategies and possible plans to put in place. These care planning protocols come with training videos. Although the project was designed to be compatible with Pennsylvania assessment tools, program rules, and service environments, it is also a useful model for other states (Amerman, Schneider, & Frank, 1995).

There is doubt that assessment protocols have had much more attention than care planning protocols. This seems to reflect a naive belief that assessment could help anybody by itself. As early as the 1970s an early pioneer in studying long-term care case management, Raymond Steinberg, flagged the problem that many more resources and attention have gone to initial assessments than to planning the care and making the services available. He referred to people in such programs as "being all assessed with no place to go" (see Steinberg & Carter, 1982).

To guard against short-circuiting care planning and ending up with unimaginative plans, Schneider (1989), a nurse-researcher who helped develop case management tools for the national channeling demonstration, recommends the discipline of using extremely specific techniques in care planning. She recommends that a written care plan be based on a careful listing of all the problems identified in the assessment. Each specific action or plan element should be related to a problem, for example, "because the client's arthritis prohibits her from doing laundry, the homemaker will do laundry loads twice a week and linens will be sent out to a laundry." She cautions about expressing the problem generally—for example, "arthritis" instead of "difficulty doing laundry." Schneider also urges that a desired or expected outcome be assigned to each problem and plank in the care plan. She highlights as a common problem that the outcome is written as a restatement of the service rather than as a client status. For instance, a poorly constructed outcome would be "obtaining home delivered meals five days week"; a well constructed outcome would be "maintaining nutritional status" or "allowing the family member to work and therefore enabling the client to stay at home." Finally, the care plan, according to Schneider, should clearly specify who will be responsible for each service; it should calculate the anticipated costs of the publicly funded component of the plan; it should include services that are provided by family members and other sources; it should contain dates for review of each part of the plan; and it should be reviewed by, agreed to, and signed by client, family member, and case manager.

Although these ideas were promulgated more than a decade ago, one seldom finds care plans that meet these criteria for purposiveness and clarity. Furthermore, others have argued that clients and family members should be privy to information about the kinds of services that might be purchased under the plan; otherwise they are likely to think that the services that case managers order out of habit are the only ones available (Frankfather, Smith, & Caro, 1981). This strategy also is likely to lead to more creativity and variability in the plan. Finally, the plan should also specify how the case managers should behave toward and work with the client rather than simply iterate services that will be purchased (Kivnick, 1991).

### Incorporating Quality Assurance

The monitoring component of case management is also a mechanism for quality assurance. In essence, the client assessment at later points in time becomes a major vehicle for determining whether outcomes are achieved, especially if the assessment contains the kind of items that the plan would expect to influence. The previously mentioned computerized assessment tool developed in Indiana is a vehicle for care planning (because the screen suggests options to consider given various assessment combinations) and also for quality assurance (Kinney et al., 1994). The latter is

achieved because the client assessment data are linked to a database that includes care plans, services purchased, provider profiles, and client feedback about quality. This system facilitates reviewing the quality of services received by an individual, and it also enables the program at a local or state level to quickly generate overview tables relating to the quality of the program. For example, it is possible to assemble all the consumer feedback on a particular care provider or to examine the outcomes for all clients with particular characteristics.

Case management agencies for the HCBS service system in Massachusetts are currently working with researchers at the University of Massachusetts to explore the feasibility of incorporating Caro's Quality of Circumstance (COQ) protocol (Caro, 1999; Caro & Blank, 1988) into its case management work as a means to better be able to evaluate the effectiveness of their work. The QOC protocol was developed in the 1980s in New York City to enable objective appraisal of how well the needs of low-income older people were being met. In contrast to most of the Quality of Life Scales discussed Chapter 7, the areas assessed in the QOC endeavor to tap objective dimensions of daily living in behavioral terms. The original QOC had 11 "domains": shelter, privacy, safety, household provisions, meals and eating, choice, laundry, clothing, cleaning, quiet, and activity. The newer version created for Massachusetts has more. Each domain includes specific questions to be asked of the older person or proxy informant, perhaps observations to be made by the case manager, and a summary rating to be made by the case manager on the basis of the answers to the questions. In some cases the case manager makes multiple ratings. For example, after a somewhat longer set of items than in other domains on meals, the case manager rates both nutritional aspects and enjoyment aspects; telephone communication is rated in terms of receiving and sending messages. Table 15.4 illus-

**Table 15.4.**

An Illustration from the Quality of Circumstances Protocols*

**Financial Management**

1. Case manager observation
   With the permission of the client, check drawers and surfaces for financial documents. Check all of the following that apply.
   ____ unpaid bills
   ____ unopened bank statements
   ____ eviction notices
   ____ electricity shutoff notices
   ____ telephone shutoff notices

2. Ask the following questions directly of the client (or proxy).
   A. Do you pay your own bills or does someone else pay them for you?
      ____ pay own bills
      ____ someone else pays
      What is the relationship of that person to you? _____

   B. Are there any problems in the way your financial affairs are being handled. What are these problems?
      _____

   C. How often do your bills get paid?
      ___ more than once a month
      ___ once a month
      ___ less than once a month

   D. How many mistakes have been made in handling your bills in the past 3 months?
      ____ none      ____1-2 mistakes      ____ 3 or more mistakes

   E. How much difficulty have these mistakes created for you.
      ___ no difficulty      ___ minor difficulty      ____ major difficulty

*Comments.*

**Client Evaluation Page**

15. **Financial management**
    Which statement best describes how well the client's financial matters are being handled?
    ___ 1. All financial affairs are being handled **promptly and competently**.
    ___ 2. Financial affairs are being handled in a generally satisfactory way but there are **some delays and minor mistakes**.
    ___ 3. There are some mistakes and oversights that **could become serious**.
    ___ 4. There have been one or more **documented problems of a serious nature** in the handling of financial matters.
    ___ 5. Financial matters are regularly mishandled creating **continuing serious problems**.

*Note: This 65 page document follows the same template for 21 areas, including observations, direct questions, and one or more case manager ratings. The boldface makes it easy for case managers to identify the key concepts in the ratings. Ample room is provided for notes. To obtain a copy or more information about the document, contact Francis G. Caro, University of Massachusetts Boston, 617-287-7300 (Caro, 1999).

trates the approach with a short protocol on Financial Management. The QOC has not yet been applied outside a research and demonstration context. It is a long protocol, but its use would undoubtedly encourage case managers to follow up their assessments with more specific plans that themselves would be easily monitored.

Other approaches to quality assurance incorporate client satisfaction tools administered at intervals. In particular, Geron (1998) developed such tools specifically for monitoring HCBS case management practice. His satisfaction tool, which is reviewed in Chapter 9, is now being tested in case management programs in several states.

## CONCLUSION: GETTING THE EMPHASIS ON ASSESSMENT RIGHT

Multidimensional assessment is an integral and powerful tool to make HCBS case management work at the individual and program levels. It is also a powerful tool, which will become even more effective as we move away from paper and pencil tools to computerized forms and storage. Assessment presently occupies a strange, ambiguous role. It gets both too much attention and too little. It gets too much attention in that it is sometimes seen as an end in itself. Case management tends to be "front-loaded" with much more attention to bringing in the assessment, especially the first assessment, than to any of the subsequent activities. On the other hand, it does not get enough attention in the forms of assessors' training, continual refinement of the assessment tools, and information system design to manage the data. Striking the right balance is the next challenge.

## REFERENCES

Amerman, E., Schneider, B., & Frank, M. (1995). *Clinical protocol series in community based long-term care: Overview and trainers guide.* Philadelphia: Philadelphia Corporation for Aging.

Applebaum, R., & Austin, C. (1990). *Long-term care case management.* New York: Springer.

Austin, C. D., Roberts, L., & Low, J. (1985). *Case management: A critical review.* Seattle: University of Washington Institute on Aging.

Caro, F. C. (1999). *Quality of Circumstances Protocol: Massachusetts Performance-Based Home Care Project.* Boston: University of Massachusetts Boston, Conducted in collaboration with the Massachusetts Office of Elderly Affairs.

Caro, F. C., & Blank, A. S. (1988). *Quality impact of home care for the elderly.* New York: Haworth.

Christianson, J., Applebaum, R., Carcagno, G., & Phillips, B. (1988). Organizing and delivering case management services: Lessons from the national long-term care channeling demonstration. *Home Health Care Services Quarterly, 23,* 1–22.

Davidson, G., Penrod, J., Kane, R. A., Moscovice, I., & Rich, E. (1991). Modeling the costs of case management in long-term care. *Health Care Financing Review, 13*(1), 73–81.

Dill, A. (1990). Transformations of home: The formal and informal processes of home care planning. In J. Gubrium & A. Sankar (Eds.), *The home care experience: Ethnography and policy* (pp. 227–252). Newbury Park, CA: Sage.

Frankfather, D., Smith, M., & Caro, F. (1981). *Family care of the elderly: Public initiatives and private obligations.* Lexington, MA: DC Heath.

Geron, S. (1998). Assessing satisfaction of older adults with long-term care service. *Research on Social Work Practice, 8*(1), 103–119.

Halter, J. (1999). Physicians' roles in the geriatrics interdisciplinary team. In J. Campbell & N. Ikegami (Eds.), *Long-term care for frail older people: Reaching for the ideal system* (Vol. 4, Keio University Symposia for Life Science and Medicine, pp. 77–82). Tokyo, Japan: Springer-Verlag.

Justice, D., Folkemer, D., Donahoe, E., & Nelssen, H. (1991). *The integral role of case management in authorizing services under state community care programs.* Washington, DC: National Association of State United on Aging.

Kane, R. A. (1993). Dangers lurking in the "continuum of care." *Journal of Aging and Social Policy, 5*(4), 1–7.

Kane, R. A., & Caplan, R. (Eds.) (1993). *Ethical conflict in the management of home care: The case manager's dilemma.* New York: Springer.

Kane, R. A., & Degenholtz, H. (1997). Case management as a force for quality assurance and quality improvement in home care. *Journal of Aging and Social Policy, 9*(4), 5–28.

Kane, R. A., & Kane, R. L. (1997). *Long-term care: Principles, programs, and policies.* New York: Springer.

Kane, R. A., Kane, R. L., & Ladd, R. (1998). *Heart of long-term care.* New York: Oxford University Press.

Kane, R. L., Finch, M., Geron, S., Skay, C., Stoner, T., & McGuire, D. (1991). *Development and field testing of a uniform long-term client assessment instrument for Florida.* Minneapolis: Long-Term Care DECISIONS Resource Center, University of Minnesota School of Public Health. Report prepared for the Florida Department of Health and Rehabilitative Services.

Kinney, E., Freedman, J., & Loveland-Cook, C.

(1994). Quality improvement in community-based, long-term care: Theory and reality. *American Journal of Law and Medicine, 20*(1, 2), 59–97.

Kivnick, H. (1991). *Living with care, caring for life: The inventory of life strengths.* Minneapolis: Long-Term Care Decisions Resource Center, University of Minnesota School of Public Health.

Mollica, R., Reinardy, J., Kane, R., Fralich, J., Potthoff, S., Nyman, J., & Leone, A. (1994). *Preliminary findings and recommendation concerning Kansas long term care system.* Minneapolis: National Long Term Care Resource Center, University of Minnesota School of Public Health and National Academy for State Health Policy, Portland, ME.

O'Keefe, J. (1996). *Determining the need for long-term care services: An analysis of health and functional eligibility criteria in Medicaid home and community-based waiver programs* (No. 9617). Washington, DC: American Association of Retired Persons.

Phillips, B., Kemper, P., & Applebaum, R.

(1988). Case management under Channeling. *Health Services Research, 23,* 67–81.

Reinardy, J., Kane, R. A., & Mollica, R. (1994). *CAILS Assessment Project.* Minneapolis: National Long Term Care Resource Center, University of Minnesota School of Public Health (report prepared for Vermont Department on Aging and Disabilities).

Schneider, B. (1989). Care planning in the Aging Network. In R. A. Kane (Ed.), *Concepts in case management.* Minneapolis: National Long-Term Care Resource Center, University of Minnesota School of Public Health.

Steinberg, R., & Carter, G. (1982). *Case management and the elderly.* Lexington, MA: DC Health.

White, M. (1995). Case management. In G. Maddox (Ed.), *Encyclopedia of aging* (2nd ed., pp. 147–150). New York: Springer.

Wisconsin Division of Community Service (1995). *Model Long-Term Care Assessment.* Madison, WI: Division of Community Services, Wisconsin Department of Health and Social Services.

# 16

# Mandated Assessments

ROBERT L. KANE

The belief in the power of assessment has led to mandates for the use of formal assessments in several areas, including determining eligibility for public programs, improving quality of programs, and determining payment. Mandates come in several forms. Various programs and proposals for using specifically mandated structured assessment as a tool for quality improvement and as a basis for payment are reviewed in this chapter. Public programs, especially those at the federal level (like Medicare and Medicaid), rely increasingly on mandatory assessments as a source of data on which to build a regulatory structure. In some cases, the data derived are used to develop criteria for adequate performance. In others, there is a hope that collecting this information systematically and having it available will positively influence care by providing a structured information base for caregivers. The passage of the Nursing Home Reform Act in 1987 ushered in a major change in our approach to using information in long-term care. In the ensuing decade a national system of standardized information collection has been introduced into nursing homes, and a similar approach seems likely for other long-term care venues.

This chapter examines the implications of mandated assessments, especially the system universally used in nursing homes.

In the nursing home arena, a standardized approach to data collection, the Minimum Data Set (MDS), is required. Enthusiasm for such standardization has led to the development of comparable measures to be used in home care and other forms of post-hospital care. In several states, standardized assessments are mandated to establish eligibility for Medicaid-sponsored care. In many instances, potential clients must first be shown to be eligible for nursing home care in order to qualify for community long-term care.

In general, the content of the assessments for eligibility are quite distinct from those for quality. The components of assessments that determine payment may overlap with both. To the extent that payment is based on some measures of case mix (weighted on the basis of their implications for care needs), elements of both eligibility and quality may be involved. For example, functional dependency may be a components of all three. A certain level of dependency may be needed to become eligible for care. Changes in functioning may be a component of quality. Functional dependency, especially the need for human assistance, plays a major role in determining the costs of care. Nonetheless, the metric used in each case may be different. For example, functional improvement may be assessed by a change in the degree of difficulty experienced in performing a task or the extent of help required. The amount of help is important to the extent that it reflects the client's ability for self-care, but the actual number of persons providing the assistance has no bearing. For purposes of costing and care planning, however, help from two persons is much greater than from only one.

Structured assessment as the basis for determining eligibility has been used for some time in long-term care programs at both the state and federal levels. Although the algorithms for determining eligibility vary, many states use some form of standardized information collection to collect comparable information on clients to determine when their level of disability or dependency is sufficient to warrant public support (assuming that other requirements such as impoverishment) are also met. Some of these approaches employ the calculation of a specific point score with an arbitrary threshold for eligibility. Others rely on more categorical judgments that allow for professional input and synthesis. (This material is discussed in Chapter 15.)

Mandating the use of a specific assessment tool represents a means of ensuring that equivalent information is systematically collected across a jurisdiction. It is important, however, to distinguish possibilities from actualities. Specifying what is collected is not synonymous with specifying how it is collected. Variation can still occur in the thoroughness and unbiased nature of the data collection. The distinctions between the reliability of a tool and the reliability of its users (see Chapter 1) are especially apt here. Although one wants an assessment tool that is as reliable and valid as possible for such applications, there is still ample opportunity for variation due to the way it is applied in prac-

tice. Nonetheless, mandating the collection of the same data for all persons in a given program is an important step toward obtaining comparable information by which to compare case mix and outcomes.

## THE RESIDENT ASSESSMENT INSTRUMENT

In its 1986 report, the Institute of Medicine's Committee on the Quality of Nursing Home Care recommended that nursing homes be held accountable for accurate assessments of their residents' function as part of a new quality standard. This idea was translated into the implementation of a national program by which all residents of nursing homes supported by Medicare or Medicaid would be assessed regularly using a standard form. The Resident Assessment Inventory (RAI) mandated by the 1987 Nursing Home Reform Act (part of OBRA 1987) was the result. The RAI consists of two basic parts: the Minimum Data Set (MDS), a standard assessment to be completed on each resident at specified times, and the Resident Assessment Protocols (RAPs), a more detailed set of assessments for common problems among nursing home residents that are triggered by questions in the MDS.

### Minimum Data Set (MDS)

The goal of the MDS was to establish a standard set of information to be collected on every nursing home resident on admission and systematically thereafter every 3 months or when the resident's status changed (Hawes et al., 1997). This information was to be used for both care planning purposes and to serve as a basis for regulatory activity by providing a basis by which to judge the care delivered and the extent to which needs were met. Like most assessment instruments designed to serve several functions, the MDS became burdened with a variety of roles. It was initially intended to serve the dual purposes of improving care directly by serving as the basis for care planning and to facilitate accountability. The data derived, amplified by additional information collected through the RAPs, should flesh out the residents' problems and suggest the appropriate steps to deal with them. Quality could be judged by the adequacy of the care plans (in the context of the assessments) and the degree to which they were carried out. Another quality improvement role would be derived from using the data collected to identify specific outcomes. These could be judged on the basis of rates of events overall or for specific subgroups of residents at comparable risk for developing the problem. Alternatively, the outcomes could be assessed by comparing the change in status of subgroups over time.

The availability of comparable information for all nursing home residents led to other thoughts about how such information might be used. A natural extension was using the data as the basis for setting reimbursement rates. Substantial work had already been done to develop a Resource Utilization Groups (RUGs) program in New York, which translates information about residents' functional status and care needs into payments based on observed correlations between these variables and the time spent by various types of personnel in providing care.

As RAI information was used to establish care plans, each discipline involved in the care of nursing home residents was anxious that its concerns be reflected in the data collected so that their contributions would not be underestimated. The definition of the *minimum* data to be collected was thus challenged. The dominant profession in nursing home care (as the name suggests) is nursing. The MDS can thus be seen as largely reflecting elements that the discipline believes to be important. On the other hand, medicine has been conspicuously absent from nursing homes; this absence is reflected in the MDS, which contains little information needed to provide (or assess) the medical aspects of care (beyond checklists of diagnoses, health conditions, and psychoactive

and diuretic medications and an assessment of overall functioning). For example, nothing is noted about the signs and symptoms of major diseases (e.g., edema and shortness of breath for congestive heart failure, walking distance for claudication, or chest pain for coronary heart disease). The MDS is thus less useful to track changes in medical status per se.

The MDS has thus emerged as an omnibus instrument, designed and modified to serve several roles. At its heart, however, it is a data collection device designed to be completed by a trained nurse on the basis of information obtained by observations of the resident by a variety of parties, mainly the nurses aides who have the most contact with the residents and the professional nursing staff. (Other disciplines may be assigned to complete relevant portions. For example, social work may assess affect or physical therapy activities of daily living [ADLs].) In the interests of uniformity, the bulk of the data on all residents is derived from staff observations.*

This logistical decision has potentially profound repercussions. In effect, it treats all residents as if they were severely cognitively impaired. As a result, some areas of importance are effectively dismissed (e.g., satisfaction, meaning of activities), and others rely on presumptuous inferences based on behavioral interpretations.

The categories of data collected by the MDS are shown in Table 16.1. It is useful to contrast these with the domains usually identified as comprising the salient outcomes for nursing home residents, shown in Table 16.2, many of which represent the assessment domains addressed in the chapters elsewhere in this book. Most of these

---

*Although the MDS instructions encourage observers to encourage resident participation and input, three factors limit the likelihood of such behavior. *(1)* The source of data is primarily certified nurses aides; *(2)* No specific questions are provided to obtain systematic resident input; and *(3)* a specially designated nurse, sometimes called MDS coordinator, is responsible for gathering all the input for the MDS. He or she may fail to consult patients or key staff.

**Table 16.1.**
Minimum Data Set Domains

Cognition
Communication/hearing/vision
Physical functioning
Continence
Psychosocial well-being
Mood and behavior problems
Activity pursuit patterns
Disease diagnosis
Health conditions
Oral/nutritional status
Oral/dental status
Skin condition
Medication use
Special treatments and procedures

domains (with the possible exception of physiological status) may also be said to comprise an important portion of what has been termed *quality of life,* a central goal for nursing home care (see Chapter 7). Gathering meaningful information on many of the elements requires direct contact with each respondent. Behavioral observations offer only pale shadows at best and may grossly distort the actual situation in many instances. It would be a stretch to expect that even systematic observations alone by a trained person could generate the salient information. It is even more foolhardy to expect that casual observations on these subjects can produce adequate information on which to base a useful judgment. In effect, cognitively intact persons are disenfranchised. They are treated as if they cannot express their feelings. Although it may be possible to recognize some overt attributes of distress or discomfort, for instance, much will be missed. It is certainly not possible to distinguish meaningful activity from that which is performed in response to social pressures. The low prevalence of depression detected by the MDS in one study suggests that this approach may uncover only the more overt manifestations of affective problems (Casten et al., 1998).

Because many activities add pleasure to life only when they are done voluntarily in response to positive motivations, valuable information that addresses the components of quality of life will be missed. For example, efforts to create a measure of social quality were unsuccessful (Casten et al., 1998). When inferred depression elements from the MDS were compared with responses to standardized measures, the correlation was positive but weak (Lawton et al., 1998). Rather than inferring critical information, it would seem preferable to collect the pertinent information directly from the residents wherever possible. In effect, one would create two versions of the MDS, one for the cognitively intact residents and one for the severely cognitively impaired residents. The resident-completed version would be able to address a wider range of items. More care might be taken about which elements were inferred from the data based solely on observations.

Many of the MDS domains seem able to produce useful data. The measures of ADLs should be readily and reliably collected through observations or impressions. The behaviors associated with cognition have been assembled in a Cognitive Performance Score (CPS), which has been evaluated by comparing the results using the CPS against those obtained using standard measures (Morris et al., 1994). The material on communication, incontinence, nutritional status, oral status, skin conditions, special treatments, and medication use are all basically built on the reports of others in most clinical situations. The real Achilles heel of the MDS is its efforts to address the area usually considered to re-

**Table 16.2.** Generally Acknowledged Nursing Home Outcome Domains

Physiologic (includes skin condition and the status of specific parameters such as blood pressure and blood sugar)
Pain and discomfort*
Functional status*
Cognition*
Affect*
Meaningful social participation*
Social relationships*
Satisfaction (with care and environment)*

*Usually considered components of quality of life.

flect quality of life. Many of these domains, noted with an asterisk in Table 16.2, cannot be well probed without asking the client. In some instances, careful observational data may need to be employed when the client is too cognitively impaired to respond (see Chapter 17), but direct responses are preferable.

The developers of the MDS have created a CPS that classifies patients into one of six groups. Table 16.3 shows how MDS items have been combined to form the groups. Designated combinations of information, including whether patients are in a coma, whether they appear able to make decisions, their ability to understand, their short-term memory, and their ability to feed themselves without assistance, are matched to various levels of cognitive impairment. The actual items used in the MDS are shown in Table 16.4. They combine judgment about memory with specific items of recall that might have occurred during the previous week with judgments about decisions about daily life and reports of behaviors indicating cognitive problems. Therefore, the CPS does not actually measure cognition, but other functions associated with poor cognition.

As can be seen from Table 16.3, some items are used more than once. The CPS has been said to compare well with more established measures of cognition such as the Mini-Mental State Examination (MMSE) (Phillips et al., 1997; Morris et al., 1994; Hartmaier et al., 1995). In one study, however, the CPS was shown to agree poorly with the Global Deterioration Scale (GDS), especially in identifying more severely cognitively impaired persons (Hartmaier et al., 1994). To improve the correlation between the GDS and the CPS, the researchers developed an expanded summary measure based on the MDS, the MDS Cognition Scale (MDS-COGS). The latter uses eight items (Table 16.5) (Hartmaier et al., 1994).

Lawton and associates (1998) examined MDS data on cognition and found a single factor composed of the seven items they examined (see Table 16.5; Casten et al., 1998). When they compared the MDS-derived score with responses to standard scales, the correlations were positive and strong. The correlation with the Blesssed test was 0.66 and with the GDS, 0.59 (Lawton et al., 1998). Snowden and colleagues (1999) report a correlation of 0.45 between the CPS and MMSE in a sample of cognitively impaired residents.

Table 16.3.
Cognitive Performance Scale (CPS)

| CPS group | Coma | Decision making | Impairment count* | Severe impairment count† | Totally dependent eating |
|---|---|---|---|---|---|
| Intact (0) | No | Not severely impaired (0–2) | 0 | | |
| Borderline intact (1) | No | Not severely impaired (0–2) | 1 | | |
| Mild impairment (2) | No | Not severely impaired (0–2) | 2 or 3 | 0 | |
| Moderate impairment (3) | No | Not severely impaired (0–2) | 2 or 3 | 1 | |
| Moderate/severe impairment (4) | No | Not severely impaired (0–2) | 2 or 3 | 2 | |
| Severe impairment (5) | No | Severely impaired (3) | | | No (0–3) |
| Very severe impairment (6) { | Yes | | | | |
| | No | Severely impaired (3) | | | Yes (4) |

*Number of the following: Decision making; not independent (1–2); understood, not independent (1–3); short-term memory, not OK (1).

†Number of the following: Decision making, moderately impaired (2); understood, sometimes/never (2–3).

**Table 16.4.**
Cognitive Items from the MDS

*1. Comatose*

Persistent vegetative state/no discernible consciousness

*2. Memory*

Recall of what was learned or known
a. Short-term memory OK — seems/appears to recall after 5 minutes
b. Long-term memory OK — seems/appears to recall long past

*3. Memory Recall Ability*

*Check all that resident was normally able to recall during last 7 days*
Current season
Location of own room
Staff names/faces
That he/she is in a nursing home
NONE OF THE ABOVE

*4. Cognitive Skills for Daily Decision Making*

*Made decisions regarding tasks of daily life*
0. INDEPENDENT — decisions consistent/reasonable
1. MODIFIED INDEPENDENCE — some difficulty in new situations only
2. MODERATELY IMPAIRED — decisions poor; cues/supervision required
3. SEVERELY IMPAIRED — never/rarely made decisions

*5. Indicators of Delirium — Periodic Disordered Thinking/Awareness*

*Code for behavior in the last 7 days. Note: Accurate assessment requires conversations with staff and family who have direct knowledge of resident's behavior over this time.*
0. Behavior not present
1. Behavior present, not of recent onset
2. Behavior present, over last 7 days appears different from resident's usual functioning (e.g., new onset or worsening)
   a. EASILY DISTRACTED — (e.g., difficulty paying attention; gets sidetracked)
   b. PERIODS OF ALTERED PERCEPTION OR AWARENESS OF SURROUNDINGS — (e.g., moves lips or talks to someone not present; believes he/she is somewhere else; confuses night and day)
   c. EPISODES OF DISORGANIZED SPEECH — (e.g., speech is incoherent, nonsensical, irrelevant, or rambling from subject to subject; loses train of thought)
   d. PERIODS OF RESTLESSNESS — (e.g., fidgeting or picking at skin, clothing, napkins, etc; frequent position changes; repetitive physical movements or calling out)
   e. PERIODS OF LETHARGY — (e.g., sluggishness, staring into space; difficult to arouse; little body movement)
   f. MENTAL FUNCTION VARIES OVER THE COURSE OF THE DAY — (e.g., sometimes better, sometimes worse; behaviors sometimes present, sometimes not)

*6. Change in Cognitive Status*

Resident's cognitive status, skills, or abilities have changed as compared to status of 90 days ago (or since last assessment if less than 90 days)

*7. Behavioral Symptoms*

A. Behavioral symptom frequency in last 7 days
   0. Behavior not exhibited in last 7 days
   1. Behavior of this type occurred 1 to 3 days in last 7 days
   2. Behavior of this type occurred 4 to 6 days, but less than daily
   3. Behavior of this type occurred daily
B. Behavioral symptom alterability in last 7 days
   0. Behavior not present OR behavior was easily altered
   1. Behavior was not easily altered

*(continued)*

**Table 16.4.**

Cognitive Items from the MDS — Continued

> a. WANDERING (moved with no rational purpose, seemingly oblivious to needs of safety)
> b. VERBALLY ABUSIVE BEHAVIORAL SYMPTOMS (others threatened, screamed at, cursed at)
> c. PHYSICALLY ABUSIVE BEHAVIORAL SYMPTOMS (others were hit, shoved, scratched, sexually abused)
> d. SOCIALLY INAPPROPRIATE/DISRUPTIVE BEHAVIORAL SYMPTOMS (made disruptive sounds, noisiness, screaming, self-abusive acts, sexual behavior or disrobing in public, smeared/threw food/feces, hoarding, rummaged through others' belongings)
> e. RESISTS CARE (resisted taking medications/injections, ADL assistance, or eating)

*8. Change in Behavioral Symptoms*

Resident's behavior status has changed as compared to status of 90 days ago (or since last assessment if less than 90 days)

---

Observation should provide reasonable data for ADLs. In their analysis of the consistency of the factor score derived from the ADL measures in the MDS, however, Lawton and coworkers (1998) found that the loadings were significantly different for cognitively impaired and intact samples (see Casten et al., 1998). Looking at a sample of cognitively impaired nursing home residents, Snowden and coworkers (1999) reported a correlation of 0.59 between the MDS ADL score and the Dementia Rating Scale score for ADLs.

The reliability of the MDS has been debated. As might be expected, the developers have produced evidence to show that the tool performs reasonably well when used by trained nurses (Hawes et al., 1995). It is less clear how consistently the MDS is used in the average nursing home.

Disparaging conclusions have been reached by some researchers who reject this information as a reliable source (Teresi & Holmes, 1992), but others contend that many of the elements are adequate for research purposes (Lawton et al., 1998; Casten et al., 1998). One team of investigators questioned the usefulness of the MDS for tracking dementia-related changes (Snowden et al., 1999). Because the MDS is mandatory across the United States, it remains an attractive source of national comparative data for others.

In a reliability test of MDS among nursing homes in five states, Hawes and colleagues (1995) found that most MDS items showed good reliability when compared with the assessment of trained licensed nurses on the research staff. One item that they identified with poor re-

**Table 16.5.** Comparison of Items Used in Various Cognitive Measures Derived from the Minimum Data Set (MDS)

| Cognitive performance scale | MDS-COGS | Lawton et al. (1998) |
|---|---|---|
| Coma | Short-term memory | Short-term memory |
| Decision making | Long-term memory | Long-term memory |
| Making self understood | Location of own room | Recall room |
| *Short-term memory* | Knows he or she is in a nursing home | Recall location |
| Eating | Number of orientation items recalled | Recall season |
| | Decision making | Decision making |
| | Making self understood | Recall staff |
| | Dressing self performance | |

COGS, Cognition Scale.

liability is item B5, "indicators of delirium." They argued that overall the MDS is reliable and is a good research tool (Hawes et al., 1995). There are some problems with this assessment, however. Because the reliability was tested among nurses and not specialized personnel, such as physicians, dentists, physical therapists, psychologists, or psychiatrists, reliability estimates might be questioned. A reliability test conducted in a somewhat more typical (but still likely better than average) setting showed modest to good reliability for measures of cognition (kappa = 0.63), ADL (kappa = 0.61), time use (kappa = 0.75), social quality (kappa = 0.74), depression (kappa = 0.56), and problem behavior (kappa = 0.84) (Casten et al., 1998).

One example of questionable accuracy concerns the portion of the MDS that describes sleeping and activity patterns. In this section, staff are supposed to identify time "awake during the morning, afternoon, and evening." In a study of 27 nursing home residents, the MDS indicated that they were awake most or all of the time (i.e., nap no more than 1 hour per time period), yet these residents were observed to be sleeping almost 50% of daytime hours (Harper, 1998). In addition, charts in this study listed the medical director's diagnoses of health conditions, but not all of these diagnoses were supported by tests. For example, the diagnoses of Alzheimer's disease and clinical depression had few if any supportive tests. In institutional settings, Alzheimer's disease is often diagnosed when there is no other obvious reason for dementia. The diagnosis of depression also is difficult to confirm in research because there are few assessments from psychologists or psychiatrists in nursing home charts.

Another area where data accuracy might be a problem is with the assessment of oral/dental status (section M). Hawes and colleagues (1995) stated that this has a high reliability; however, nursing homes infrequently use dentists for this assessment. Thus, oral/dental status may often be inaccurate. Unfortunately, one never knows if chart and MDS data are accurate at a particular site. A small study of reliability of medical chart data at each research site may improve confidence in such data, although it will add to the financial and time costs.

Observations from an incontinence study also raise concerns about MDS recording. In a research project context, the MDS recordings of wetness correlated with the research staff observations but not with the wetness checks performed by nursing home staff. Moreover, the MDS recordings were insensitive to evidence of successful interventions to reduce wetness, suggesting that they are based on overall impressions more than actual observations and hence would be less useful for research purposes (Crooks et al., 1995).

The area that is likely the least contested is that addressing the performance of ADLs. The approach used is shown in Table 16.6. For each item, two separate determinations are made: (1) The resident's performance over all shifts in the last 7 days is coded on a scale from 0 (independent; no help or oversight, or help/oversight provided only one to two times over those 7 days) to 4 (total dependence), with an allowance for when activity did not occur. (This coding allows for distinctions between physical assistance and supervising an activity; see Chapter 2.) The amount of support provided is coded from 0 (no setup or physical help) to 3 (two or more persons provide physical assistance). This component recognizes the need to plan for care on the basis of the number of personnel who will be needed. Presumably the self-performance score can be used to assess progress, whereas the support score can be used for care planning.

Mood is assessed by observations. As shown in Table 16.7, these consist of verbal expressions of distress, problems with sleeping, and an appearance that is interpreted as sad, apathetic, or anxious. A separate section asks whether various pro-

**Table 16.6.**

Physical Function Measures

| | | (A) Self Performance | (B) Support |
|---|---|---|---|
| 1. | (A) **ADL SELF-PERFORMANCE**—Code for resident's PERFORMANCE OVER ALL SHIFTS during last 7 days—Not including setup)<br>0.　INDEPENDENT—No help or oversight—OR—Help/oversight if provided only 1 or 2 times during last 7 days<br>1.　SUPERVISION—Oversight, encouragement or cueing provided 3 or more times during last 7 days—OR—Supervision (3 or more times) plus physical assistance provided only 1 or 2 times during last 7 days<br>3.　EXTENSIVE ASSISTANCE—While resident performed part of activity, over last 7-day period, help of following type(s) provided 3 or more times:<br>　–Weight-bearing support<br>　–Full staff performance during part (but not all) of last 7 days<br>4.　TOTAL DEPENDENCE—Full staff performance of activity during entire 7 days<br>8.　ACTIVITY DID NOT OCCUR during entire 7 days | | |
| | (B) **ADL SUPPORT PROVIDED**—(Code for MOST SUPPORT PROVIDED OVER ALL SHIFTS during last 7 days; code regardless of resident's self-performance classification)<br>0.　No setup or physical help from staff<br>1.　Setup help only<br>2.　One person physical assist<br>3.　Two+ person physical assist<br>8.　ADL activity itself did not occur during entire 7 days | | |
| | **Bed Mobility** — How resident moves to and from lying position, turns side to side, and positions body while in bed | | |
| | **Transfer** — How resident moves between surfaces—to from: bed, chair, wheelchair, standing position (EXCLUDE to/from bath/toilet) | | |
| | **Walk In Room** — How resident walks between locations in his/her room | | |
| | **Walk In Corridor** — How resident walks in corridor on unit | | |
| | **Locomotion Off Unit** — How resident moves between locations in his/her room and adjacent corridor on same floor. If in wheelchair, self-sufficiency once in chair | | |
| | **Locomotion On Unit** — How resident moves to and returns from off unit locations (e.g., areas set aside for dining, activities, or treatments). If facility has only one floor, how resident moves to and from distant areas on the floor. If in wheelchair, self-sufficiency once in chair. | | |
| | **Dressing** — How resident puts on, fastens, and takes off all items of street clothing, including donning/removing prosthesis | | |
| | **Eating** — How resident eats and drinks (regardless of skill). Includes intake of nourishment by other means (e.g., tube feeding, total parenteral nutrition) | | |
| | **Toilet Use** — How resident uses the toilet room (or commode, bedpan, urinal); transfer on/off toilet, cleanses, changes pad, manages ostomy or catheter, adjusts clothes | | |
| | **Personal Hygiene** — How resident maintains personal hygiene, including combing hair, brushing teeth, shaving, applying makeup, washing/drying face, hands, and perineum (EXCLUDE baths and showers) | | |

grams for mood, behavior, and cognitive loss have been used in the past week. One might well wonder whether the assessor has sufficient exposure to the resident to make these judgments, as well as whether overt behaviors can be relied on to indicate mood. As already noted, this is an area where the correlations between standard measures of depression and the MDS-derived measure are weak.

Psychosocial well-being is assessed by observation as well. The assessment con-

sists of a series of judgments shown in Table 16.8. These address whether the resident displays a sense of initiative and involvement and whether there seems to be unsettled relationships and issues around past roles.

Information on preferences for activities (in terms of types and setting) is requested, but the only actual recording of activities relates to the amount of time the resident is awake and the proportion of that time he or she is involved in activities.

**Table 16.6.** — Continued

| 2. | BATHING | How resident takes full-body bath/shower, sponge bath, and transfers in/out of tub/shower (EXCLUDE washing of back and hair) Code for most dependent in self-performance and support (A) BATHING SELF-PERFORMANCE codes appear below | (A) | (B) |
|----|---------|---|---|---|
| | | 0. Independent—No help provided<br>1. Supervision—Overnight help only<br>2. Physical help limited to transfer only<br>3. Physical help in part of bathing activity<br>4. Total dependence<br>8. Activity itself did not occur during entire 7 days<br>*(Bathing support codes are as defined in Item 1, code B above)* | | |
| 3. | TEST FOR BALANCE<br><br>(see training manual) | *(Code for ability during test in the last 7 days)*<br>0. Maintained position as required in test<br>1. Unsteady, but able to rebalance self without physical support<br>2. Partial physical support during test; or stands (sits) but does not follow directions for test<br>3. Not able to attempt test without physical help | | |
| | | a. Balance while standing<br>b. Balance while sitting—position, trunk control | | |
| 4. | FUNCTIONAL LIMITATION IN RANGE OF MOTION<br><br>(see training manual) | (Code for limitations during last 7 days that interfered with daily functions or placed resident at risk of injury)<br>(A) RANGE OF MOTION　　(B) VOLUNTARY MOVEMENT<br>0. No limitation　　　　0. No loss<br>1. Limitation on one side　1. Partial loss<br>2. Limitation on both sides　2. Full loss<br>a. Neck<br>b. Arm—Including shoulder or elbow<br>c. Hand—Including wrist or fingers<br>d. Leg—Including hip or knee<br>e. Foot—Including ankle or toes<br>f. Other limitation or loss | (A) | (B) |
| 5. | MODES OF LOCOMOTION | (Check all that apply during last 7 days)<br>Cane/walker/crutch<br>Wheeled self<br>Other person wheeled<br>Wheelchair primary mode of locomotion<br>*NONE OF THE ABOVE* | | |
| 6. | MODES OF TRANSFER | (Check all that apply during last 7 days)<br>Bedfast all or most of time<br>Bed rails used for bed mobility or transfer<br>Lifted manually<br>Lifted mechanically<br>Transfer aid (e.g., slide board, trapeze, cane, walker, brace)<br>*NONE OF THE ABOVE* | | |
| 7. | TASK SEGMENTA-TION | Some or all of ADL activities were broken into subtasks during last 7 days so that resident could perform them<br>0. No　　　　　　　　1. Yes | | |

*(continued)*

### Observed Measures

Likely reflecting a strong nursing influence, skin condition and treatment are covered in great detail. As shown in Table 16.9, foot care is also addressed.

Because it relies exclusively on observations and interpretations of behavior, the MDS should perform better with cognitively impaired clients than with intact clients. At least its face validity is stronger. The studies of Lawton and others were designed specifically to address areas where observation could be useful in rating behaviors of cognitively impaired residents (Casten et al., 1998; Lawton et al., 1998). Three of these were Time Use, Social Quality, and Problem Behaviors. Table 16.10 shows the components for Time Use. Efforts to create a single factor were only modestly successful. The items did not load well for the cognitively impaired group. As a result, no efforts were made to validate it (Lawton et al., 1998).

Table 16.6.

Physical Function Measures—Continued

| 8. | ADL FUNCTIONAL REHABILITA-TION POTENTIAL | Resident believes he/she is capable of increased independence in at least some ADLs<br>Direct care staff believe resident is capable of increased independence in at least some ADLs<br>Resident able to perform task/activity but is very slow<br>Difference in ADL Self-Performance or ADL Support, comparing mornings to evenings<br>*NONE OF ABOVE* | | |
| 9. | CHANGE IN ADL FUNCTION | Resident's ADL self-performance status has changed as compared to status of 90 days ago (or since last assessment if less than 90 days)<br>0.No change　　　　　　1. Improved　　　　　　2. Deteriorated | | |

**Continence in Last 14 Days**

| 1. | CONTINENCE SELF-CONTROL CATEGORIES<br>(Code for resident's PERFORMANCE OVER ALL SHIFTS)<br>0 Continent—complete control (includes use of indwelling urinary catheter or ostomy device that does not leak urine or stool)<br>1 USUALLY CONTINENT—BLADDER, incontinent episodes once a week or less; BOWEL, less than weekly<br>2 OCCASIONALLY INCONTINENT—BLADDER, 2 or more times a week but not daily; BOWEL, once a week<br>3 FREQUENTLY INCONTINENT—BLADDER, tended to be incontinent daily, but some control present (e.g., on day shift); BOWEL, 2-3 times a week<br>4 INCONTINENT—Had inadequate control BLADDER, multiple (2+) daily episodes; BOWEL, all (or almost all) of the time | |
| | Bowel Continence | Control of bowel movement, with appliance or bowel continence programs, if employed |
| | Bladder Continence | Control of urinary bladder function (if dribbles, volume insufficient to soak through underpants), with appliances (e.g., foley) or continence programs, if employed |
| 2. | BOWEL ELIMINATION PATTERN | Bowel elimination pattern regular—at least one movement every three days<br>Constipation<br>Diarrhea<br>Fecal impaction<br>*NONE OF THE ABOVE* |
| 3. | APPLIANCES AND PROGRAMS | Any scheduled toileting plan<br>Bladder retaining program<br>External (condom) catheter<br>Indwelling catheter<br>Intermittent catheter<br>Did not use toilet room/commode/urinal<br>Pads/briefs used<br>Enemas/irrigation<br>Ostomy present<br>*NONE OF THE ABOVE* |
| 4. | CHANGE IN URINARY CONTINENCE | Resident's urinary continence has changed as compared to status of 90 days ago (or since last assessment if less than 90 days)<br>0. No Change　　　　1. Improved　　　　2. Deteriorated |

Social Quality was addressed through a series of items listed in Table 16.11. Three of the items (noted with an asterisk) proved unstable (yielded nonsignificant loadings) across exploratory and confirmatory factor analysis samples. These items also performed poorly with the cognitively impaired sample. Hence, this measure was abandoned (Lawton et al., 1998).

The MDS does not seem to generate a substantial body of scalable observations that can help to assess quality of life for cognitively impaired persons. One measure of problem behaviors is potentially useful to assess aspects of quality of life among confused residents. Problem behaviors are the most readily observable. They can be defined and are likely to be noticed, perhaps even recorded. As shown in Table 16.12, however, some of these also involve interpretation. Two factors emerged from this analysis and are shown in separate columns in Table 16.12. The first factor was eventually retained, although one item

**Table 16.7.**
Assessment of Mood

| | |
|---|---|
| 1. *Indicators of Depression, Anxiety, Sad Mood* | *Code for indicators observed in last 30 days, irrespective of the assumed cause.*<br>0. Indicator not exhibited in last 30 days<br>1. Indicator of this type exhibited up to five days a week<br>2. Indicator of this type exhibited daily or almost daily (6, 7 days a week)<br><br>Verbal Expressions of Distress<br><br>a. Resident made negative statements—e.g., "Nothing matters; Would rather be dead; What's the use; Regrets having lived so long; Let me die"<br>b. Repetitive questions—e.g., "Where do I go; What do I do?"<br>c. Repetitive verbalizations—e.g., calling out for help ("God help me")<br>d. Persistent anger with self or others—e.g., easily annoyed, anger at placement in nursing home, anger at care received<br>e. Self depreciation—e.g., "I am nothing; I am of no use to anyone"<br>f. Expressions of what appear to be unrealistic fears—e.g., fear of being abandoned, left alone, being with others<br>g. Recurrent statements that something terrible is about to happen—e.g., believes he or she is about to die; have a heart attack<br>h. Repetitive health complaints—e.g., persistently seeks medical attention, obsessive concern with body functions<br>i. Repetitive anxious complaints/concerns (non-health related) e.g., persistently seeks attention/reassurance regarding schedules, meals, laundry, clothing, relationship issues<br><br>Sleep-Cycle Issues<br><br>j. Unpleasant mood in morning<br>k. Insomnia/change in usual sleep pattern<br><br>Sad, Apathetic, Anxious Appearance<br><br>l. Sad, pained, worried facial expressions—e.g., furrowed brows<br>m. Crying, tearfulness<br>n. Repetitive physical movements—e.g., pacing, hand wringing, restlessness, fidgeting, picking<br><br>Loss of Interest<br><br>o. Withdrawal from activities of interest—e.g., no interest in long-standing activities or being with family/friends<br>p. Reduced social interaction |
| 2. *Mood Persistence* | *One or more indicators of depressed, sad, or anxious mood were not easily altered by attempts to "cheer up," console, or reassure the resident over last 7 days*<br>0. No mood indicators<br>1. Indicators present, easily altered<br>2. Indicators present, not easily altered |
| 3. *Change in Mood* | Resident's mood status has changed as compared to status of 90 days ago (or since last assessment if less than 90 days)<br>0. No change<br>1. Improved<br>2. Deteriorated |

**Table 16.8.**
Measures of Psychosocial Well-being

| | |
|---|---|
| *1. Sense of Initiative/Involvement* | At ease interacting with others |
| | At ease doing planned or structured activities |
| | At ease doing self-initiated activities |
| | Establishes own goals |
| | Pursues involvement in life of facility (e.g., makes/keeps friends; involved in group activities; responds positively to new activities; assists at religious services) |
| | Accepts invitations into most group activities |
| | *NONE OF THE ABOVE* |
| *2. Unsettled Relationships* | Covert/open conflict with or repeated criticism of staff |
| | Unhappy with roommate |
| | Unhappy with residents other than roommate |
| | Openly expresses conflict/anger with family/friends |
| | Absence of personal contact with family/friends |
| | Recent loss of close family member/friend |
| | Does not adjust easily to change in routines |
| | *NONE OF THE ABOVE* |
| *3. Past Roles* | Strong identification with past roles and life status |
| | Expresses sadness/anger/empty feeling over lost roles/status |
| | Resident perceives that daily routine (customary routine, activities) is very different from prior pattern in the community |
| | *NONE OF THE ABOVE* |

in it (socially inappropriate behavior) did not load significantly with the cognitively intact sample (Casten et al., 1998; Lawton et al., 1998). Efforts to validate this measure showed that it was significantly correlated with the Cohen-Mansfield Agitation Inventory for both day and evening shifts and with the MOSES Irritability subscale (Casten et al., 1998).

### Resident Assessment Protocols

Consistent with the goal of improving care planning, the responses to various items in the MDS trigger more in-depth assessments around specific potential problem areas. These RAPs provide more detailed information that address areas of potential concern. Table 16.13 lists the problem areas addressed by the RAPs. These, in effect, represent opportunities to pursue each of the areas evaluated in the MDS in greater detail and to add a few new dimensions. No specific additional assessment forms are used with the RAPs. Instead, a number of clinically relevant areas are sug-

gested for further exploration. The goal of a RAP is to assist caregivers in understanding a problem more deeply and developing a sound approach to addressing it, either by fixing it or by managing it. The RAPs do not provide specific steps or precise guides to what information should be collected to amplify a problematic area. Instead, they are more akin to general guidelines.

The effects of introducing the MDS in nursing home care have been hard to assess definitively. The developers used MDS data to compare care before and after the implementation and reported substantial improvement (Mor et al., 1997; Phillips et al., 1997). Even ignoring the potential bias of the investigators, however, the basic design (a simple before–after with no controls) leaves room for many questions about the extent to which demonstrated improvements in care and outcomes can be attributed to the MDS. Other changes have occurred over that period that could also influence care. For example, the regu-

**Table 16.9.**
Skin and Foot Care Elements

| | |
|---|---|
| *1. Ulcers (from any cause)* | *Record the number of ulcers at each ulcer stage—regardless of cause. If none present at a stage, record "0" (zero). Code all that apply during last 7 days. Code 9 = 9 or more) (Requires full body exam).* |
| | a. Stage 1.  A persistent area of skin redness (without a break in the skin) that does not disappear when pressure is relieved. |
| | b. Stage 2.  A partial thickness loss of skin layers that presents clinically as an abrasion, blister, or shallow crater. |
| | c. Stage 3.  A full thickness of skin is lost, exposing the subcutaneous tissues—presents as a deep crater with or without undermining adjacent tissue. |
| | d. Stage 4.  A full thickness of skin and subcutaneous tissue is lost, exposing muscle or bone. |
| *2. Type of Ulcer* | *For each type of ulcer, code for the highest stage in the last 7 days using scale in item. 1–i.e., 0 = none; stages 1, 2, 3, 4)* |
| | a.  Pressure ulcer—any lesion caused by pressure resulting in damage of underlying tissueb. |
| | b.  Stasis ulcer—open lesion caused by poor circulation in the lower extremities |
| *3. History of Resolved Ulcers* | Resident had an ulcer that was resolved or cured in last 90 days<br>0. No<br>1. Yes |
| *4. Other Skin Problems or Lesions Present* | *Check all that apply during last 7 days.*<br>Abrasions, bruises<br>Burns (second or third degree)<br>Open lesions other than ulcers, rashes, cuts (e.g., cancer lesions)<br>Rashes—e.g., intertrigo, eczema, drug rash, heat rash, herpes zoster<br>Skin desensitized to pain or pressure<br>Skin tears or cuts (other than surgery)<br>Surgical wounds<br>*NONE OF THE ABOVE* |
| *5. Skin Treatments* | *Check all that apply during last 7 days.*<br>Pressure relieving device(s) for chair<br>Pressure relieving device(s) for bed<br>Turning/repositioning program<br>Nutrition or hydration intervention to manage skin problems<br>Ulcer care<br>Surgical wound care<br>Application of dressings (with or without topical medications) other than for feet<br>Application of ointments/medications (other than to feet)<br>Other preventative or protective skin care (other than to feet)<br>*NONE OF THE ABOVE* |
| *6. Foot Problems and Care* | *Check all that apply during last 7 days.*<br>Resident has one or more foot problems—e.g., corns, calluses, bunions, hammer toes, overlapping toes, pain, structural problems<br>Infection of the foot—e.g., cellulitis, purulent drainage<br>Open lesions on the foot<br>Nails/calluses trimmed during last 90 days<br>Received preventative or protective foot care (e.g., used special shoes, inserts, pads, toe separators)<br>Application of dressings (with or without topical medications)<br>*NONE OF THE ABOVE* |

**Table 16.10.**
Time Use Components

| |
|---|
| At ease interacting with others |
| At ease with planned activities |
| At ease with self-initiated activity |
| Establishes own goals |
| Involved in life of facility |
| Accepts group activities |
| Time involved in activities |

**Table 16.12.**
Problem Behaviors Components

| |
|---|
| Wandering |
| Verbally abusive |
| Physically abusive |
| Socially inappropriate |
| Resists medication |
| Resists activities of daily living help |

latory system has become more stringent. Medical attention to nursing home patients has improved. The nature of nursing home admissions has changed.

Anecdotal reports suggest problems with carrying out the MDS evaluations. In some cases nursing homes have been said to have hired nurses specially to create MDS assessments. These nurses have no contact with the residents and hence must, at best, rely exclusively on the reports of nurses aides. Other stories describe nursing home administrators who complain that the burden of the assessments leaves no time for developing individualized care plans (a large part of the rationale for the RAI effort). Computer programs are available to convert assessments automatically into care plans, but these plans do not take into account the individual elements of a given resident. Hence, one may encounter multiple versions of the same plan in a given nursing home or among homes using the same service

The MDS 2.0 is also used as the basis for determining the amount of money nursing homes will receive from Medicare, which represents less than 10% of overall nursing home revenues. The Resource Utilization Groups (RUGs) are intended to pay more for residents who need more

care. The care needed is assessed as falling within 1 of 44 clusters. The appropriate cluster is determined by a combination of services received and the level of impairment reported on the MDS, which is now completed more frequently. Many of the RUGs payment groups are triggered by (or require) ADL scores that reflect impairment. Patients are classified into rehabilitation (based on amount of time spent and numbers of disciplines), persons requiring extensive services or special care, clinically complex problems, impaired cognition, behavior problems, or various levels of reduced physical function.

In this schema certain items seem to carry more weight. For example, depression can be a modifier to define clinically complex cases. Behavior problems raise a resident's cluster level as does functional

**Table 16.11.**
Social Quality Components

| |
|---|
| Staff conflict |
| Unhappy with roommate* |
| Unhappy with other residents |
| Conflict with family or friends |
| No contact with family* |
| Recent loss* |

*Unstable items.

**Table 16.13.** Resident Assessment Protocols Problem Areas

| |
|---|
| Delirium |
| Cognitive loss |
| Visual function |
| Communication |
| Activities of daily living functional/rehabilitation potential |
| Urinary incontinence and indwelling catheter |
| Psychosocial well-being |
| Mood state |
| Behavioral symptoms |
| Activities |
| Falls |
| Nutritional status |
| Feeding tubes |
| Dehydration/fluid maintenance |
| Dental care |
| Pressure ulcers |
| Psychotropic drug use |
| Physical restraints |

dependency and cognitive impairment. Using this approach to payment is likely to have several untoward effects on assessment and care. Whatever the concerns about the accuracy of MDS assessments previously, now that the ratings will affect payment, they are more susceptible to bias. Because they rely almost exclusively on observations and interpretations, this propensity to bias is even greater. Conceptually, case-mix payment systems create an incentive that is at least antirehabilitative. In essence, the more dependent a resident, the higher the payment. An off-setting factor in the RUGs III approach is the heavy emphasis on payments for services, especially rehabilitation, but those payments should go to only a small proportion of residents. It would be an understatement to suggest that this system is corruptible or that it will likely induce unwanted behaviors among nursing home personnel.

Skepticism not withstanding, the presence of systematic data will inevitably change the nature of the industry. Some of that change will be directed at dealing with the bureaucratic demands, but others will attempt to use the information to improve management. At a minimum, the elements addressed will become integrated into quality assessment activities and at least indirectly will shape the way questions are posed. The development of specific quality indicators based on the MDS will have an even more profound effect. Issues of data quality, based on either the way it was collected or what was collected, will likely become less pronounced as the system is more widely adopted. As attention focuses on those items targeted, more systematic data should result. Nursing home staff sensitive to these measures will likely attend to them.

The success of the MDS has led to efforts to reproduce its approach in other quarters. A version for home care (MDS-HC) has been developed, but, as discussed below, another instrument (OASIS) seems to be holding sway in that area. Another variant of the MDS is currently under de-

**Table 16.14.** Proposed Post-Acute Care Minimum Data Set Components

Diagnoses
Medical complexities
Other health conditions
Oral/nutritional status
Functional status
Bowel/bladder continence
Cognition
Vision/communication
Mood and behavior
Procedures/services
Rehabilitative prognosis
Resources for discharge (including informal care)

velopment for use in post-acute care, but again another contender is in sight (the Functional Independence Measure—FIM). Table 16.14 lists the major components of the proposed post-acute care MDS. Using the same basic instrument across sites promotes comparability and facilitates assessments of relative effectiveness and efficiency among modalities of care serving the same population. As has already been pointed out, however, simply using the same measures does not guarantee that the measures mean the same thing or are collected in the same way.

### Outcome and Assessment Information Set

A tool developed specifically for use with a home health care clientele is the Outcome and Assessment Information Set (OASIS).* It seems likely to be adopted as the mandated measure of quality for Medicare-supported home health care. The OASIS is the product of careful design, but since its implementation, design issues have gradually yielded to issues from the field with regard to simplified implementation. A tool that was initially intended to capture the nuances of subgroups by employing a branching approach has had to be sim-

*It is important to distinguish Medicare-covered home health care from other types of home care, such as that supported by Medicaid or paid for privately. Many of those services involve only homemaking types of activities and would not require the nursing-oriented approach represented by OASIS.

plified for large-scale implementation to a common format for all patients.

The initial concept behind the OASIS was to create a quality measure that would employ relevant outcomes for clinical subgroups, called Quality Indicator Groups (Kramer et al., 1990). As it has evolved as part of the Medicare home health quality assurance and improvement demonstration, the OASIS follows a consistent format for all patients. Beyond its demographic and administrative data, the form is divided into the sections listed in Table 16.15.

The handling of topics appears to be quite different from those addressed in the MDS. The emphasis of the two instruments is different. For example, the ADL section covers basically the same items as the MDS, but the specific coverage and the detail of performance data vary (Table 16.16). The OASIS is more rehabilitatively oriented; levels of performance are broken into more detail. The OASIS also includes instrumental activities of daily living (IADL) items that do not apply in the nursing home setting.

As with the MDS, the momentum created by the potential availability of a standardized data set for home health care has quickly led to consideration of using this information for purposes it was not designed for. At the top of that list is the proposal to use OASIS as a basis for prospective payment. Client characteristics defined by OASIS parameters can be statistically associated with the amounts of money paid by Medicare for their care and formulas developed to relate the two. There is no a priori reason, however, to believe that a set of parameters designed to capture elements of quality of care need be the best set to capture the factors that determine the cost of such care. Nonetheless, availability of data is likely to trump conceptual reasoning.

The MDS designed specifically for home care (MDS-HC) is more comparable than the nursing version of the MDS to the OASIS. Like the original MDS, the information is based on observations rather than patient interviews (Morris et al., 1997). Many of the sections of the MDS-HC are comparable to the original MDS, but additions have been made to recognize the home situation. Table 16.17 summarizes the types of data addressed in the MDS-HC. Some obvious differences in the home care version include coverage of IADLs, attention to informal care, preventive services, and environment. In addition, more subtle differences can be found in the degree of emphasis topics receive. For example, dental care and oral health receive less attention. Medications are addressed in more detail with more attention paid to nonpsychoactive drugs. The items included in mood and behavior are quite different, with less emphasis on those reflecting dementia. Table 16.18 shows the mood and behavior items in the MDS-HC. Skin condition is also addressed differently in the context of home care than it is in the nursing home (compare Tables 16.9 and 16.19).

These differences raise interesting questions about the comparability of the two assessments. Whereas a case can be made for using the same assessments across clients in different locations as a basis for comparing the care provided and its outcomes, this argument is weakened when the actual content of the measures differs between forms. These differences may correctly reflect the nature and prevalence of the problems expected to be encountered

**Table 16.15.**
OASIS Major Components

Living arrangements
Supportive assistance
Sensory status
Skin status
Respiratory status
Elimination status
Neuro/emotional/behavioral status
Activities and instrumental activities of daily living
Medications
Equipment management
Emergent care

**Table 16.16.**

Activities and Instrumental Activities of Daily Living Elements in OASIS

| | |
|---|---|
| *1. Grooming* | Ability to tend to personal hygiene needs (i.e., washing face and hands, hair care, shaving or makeup, teeth, fingernail care) |

0. Able to groom self unaided, with or without the use of assistive devices or adapted methods
1. Grooming utensils must be placed within reach before able to complete grooming activities
2. Someone must assist the patient to groom self
3. Patient depends entirely upon someone else for grooming needs
UK    Unknown

*2. Dressing*    Ability to Dress *Upper* Body (with or without dressing aids) including undergarments, pullovers, front-opening shirts and blouses, managing zippers, buttons, and snaps

0. Able to get clothes out of closets and drawers, put them on, and remove them from the upper body without assistance
1. Able to dress upper body without assistance if clothing is laid out or handed to the patient
2. Someone must help the patient put on upper body clothing
3. Patient depends entirely upon another person to dress the upper body
UK    Unknown

Ability to Dress *Lower* Body (with or without dressing aids) including undergarments, slacks, socks or nylons, shoes

0. Able to obtain, put on, and remove clothing and shoes without assistance
1. Able to dress lower body without assistance if clothing and shoes are laid out or handed to the patient
2. Someone must help the patient put on undergarments, slacks, socks or nylons, and shoes
3. Patient depends entirely upon another person to dress lower body
UK    Unknown

*3. Bathing*    Ability to wash entire body. *Excludes* grooming (washing face and hands only)

0. Able to bathe self in *shower or tub* independently
1. With the use of devices, is able to bathe self in shower or tub independently
2. Able to bathe in shower or tub with the assistance of another person
    (a) for intermittent supervision or encouragement or reminders *OR*
    (b) to get in and out of the shower or tub *OR*
    (c) for washing difficult to reach areas
3. Participates in bathing self in shower or tub, *but* requires presence of another person throughout the bath for assistance or supervision
4. *Unable* to use the shower or tub and is bathed in *bed or bedside chair*
5. Unable to effectively participate in bathing and is totally bathed by another person
UK    Unknown

*4. Toileting*    Ability to get to and from the toilet or bedside commode

0. Able to get to and from the toilet independently with or without a device
1. When reminded, assisted, or supervised by another person, able to get to and from the toilet
2. *Unable* to get to and from the toilet but is able to use a bedside commode (with or without assistance)
3. *Unable* to get to and from the toilet or bedside commode but is able to use a bedpan/urinal independently
4. Is totally dependent in toileting
UK    Unknown

*5. Transferring*    Ability to move from bed to chair, on and off toilet or commode, into and out of tub or shower, and ability to turn and position self in bed if patient is bedfast

*(continued)*

475

**Table 16.16.**
Activities and Instrumental Activities of Daily Living Elements in OASIS — Continued

| | |
|---|---|
| | 0. Able to independently transfer |
| | 1. Transfers with minimal human assistance or with use of an assistive device |
| | 2. *Unable* to transfer self but is able to bear weight and pivot during the transfer process |
| | 3. Unable to transfer self and is *unable* to bear weight or pivot when transferred by another person |
| | 4. Bedfast, unable to transfer but is able to turn and position self in bed |
| | 5. Bedfast, unable to transfer and is *unable* to turn and position self |
| | UK    Unknown |
| *6. Ambulation/Locomotion* | Ability to *safely* walk, once in a standing position, or use a wheelchair, once in a seated position, on a variety of surfaces |
| | 0. Able to independently walk on even and uneven surfaces and climb stairs with or without railings (i.e., needs no human assistance or assistive device) |
| | 1. Requires use of a device (e.g., cane, walker) to walk alone *or* requires human supervision or assistance to negotiate stairs or steps or uneven surfaces |
| | 2. Able to walk only with the supervision or assistance of another person at all times |
| | 3. Chairfast, *unable* to ambulate but is able to wheel self independently |
| | 4. Chairfast, unable to ambulate and is *unable* to wheel self |
| | 5. Bedfast, unable to ambulate or be up in a chair |
| | UK    Unknown |
| *7. Feeding or Eating* | Ability to feed self meals and snacks. [Note: This refers only to the process of *eating*, *chewing*, and *swallowing*, *not preparing* the food to be eaten.] |
| | 0. Able to independently feed self |
| | 1. Able to feed self independently but requires: |
| | (a) Meal set-up OR |
| | (b) Intermittent assistance or supervision from another person OR |
| | (c) A liquid, pureed, or ground meat diet |
| | 2. *Unable* to feed self and must be assisted or supervised throughout the meal/snack |
| | 3. Able to take in nutrients orally *and* receives supplemental nutrients through a nasogastric tube or gastrostomy |
| | 4. *Unable* to take in nutrients orally and is fed nutrients through a nasogastric tube or gastrostomy |
| | 5. Unable to take in nutrients orally or by tube feeding |
| | UK    Unknown |

in each setting. It is inefficient to use the same tools to collect information on clinical groups, *unless* you want to be able to make direct comparisons. It is impossible to have the best of both worlds. Claiming comparability on the basis of addressing similar constructs is insufficient and unpersuasive.

## UNIFORM NEEDS ASSESSMENT INVENTORY

Another area where the variation in practice poses problems arises around discharge from hospitals. Especially since the change in Medicare payments to hospitals under the Prospective Payment System created a climate that favors "quicker and sicker" discharges (Kahn et al., 1990), the role of the hospital discharge planner has come to resemble that of a launch coordinator. Discharge planners face enormous pressures to find new locations for patients quickly. Too often the first train leaving the station is deemed the best one, regardless of its destination.

The response to this situation has been consideration of a standard information set that would be required to be completed on each patient being discharged, the Uni-

**Table 16.17.**

Topics Covered in the Minimum Data Set Home Care Version (MDS-HC)

| | |
|---|---|
| Cognition | Diagnoses |
| Communication/hearing | Health conditions and preventive health measures |
| Vision | Nutrition/hydration |
| Mood/behavior | Dental status/oral health |
| Social functioning | Skin condition |
| Informal support services | Environment |
| Activities and instrumental activities of daily living | Service utilization |
| Continence | Medications |

**Table 16.18.** Mood and Behavior Items in the Minimum Data Set Home Care Version (MDS-HC)

| | |
|---|---|
| 1. *Indicators of Depression, Anxiety, Sad Mood* | *Code for indicators observed in last 30 days (or since last assessment if less than 30 days, irrespective of the assumed cause.* |

0. Indicator not exhibited in last 30 days
1. Indicator of this type exhibited up to five days a week
2. Indicator of this type exhibited daily or almost daily (6, 7 days a week)

a. A feeling of sadness or being depressed, that life is not worth living, that nothing matters, that he or she is of no use to anyone or would rather be dead
b. Persistent anger with self or others—e.g., easily annoyed, anger at care received
c. Expressions of what appear to be unrealistic fears—e.g., fear of being abandoned, left alone, being with others
d. Repetitive health complaints—e.g., persistently seeks medical attention, obsessive concern with body functions
e. Repetitive anxious complaints, concerns—e.g., persistently seeks attention/reassurance regarding schedules, meals, laundry, clothing, relationship issues
f. Sad, pained, worried facial expressions—e.g., furrowed brows
g. Recurrent crying, tearfulness
h. Withdrawal from activities of interest—e.g., no interest in long standing activities or being with family/friends
i. Reduced social interaction

2. *Behavioral Symptoms*

*In the last 7 days, instances when the client exhibited following behavioral symptoms. If EXHIBITED, ease of altering the symptom when it occurred.*
a. WANDERING (moved with no rational purpose, seemingly oblivious to needs of safety)
b. VERBALLY ABUSIVE BEHAVIORAL SYMPTOMS (threatened, screamed at, cursed at others)
c. SOCIALLY INAPPROPRIATE/DISRUPTIVE BEHAVIORAL SYMPTOMS (disruptive sounds, noisiness, screaming, self-abusive acts, sexual behavior or disrobing in public, smears/throws food/feces, rummaging, repetitive behavior, rises early and causes disruption)
e. AGGRESSIVE RESISTANCE OF CARE (e.g., threw medications, pushed caregiver)

3. *Changes in Behavior Symptoms*

Behavioral symptoms have become worse or are less well tolerated by family as compared to 30 days ago (or since last assessment if less than 30 days)
0. No, or no change in behavioral symptoms
1. Yes

**Table 16.19.**
Skin Condition Recording in the Minimum Data Set Home Care Version (MDS-HC)

| | |
|---|---|
| 1. *Skin Problems* | Any troubling skin conditions or changes in the last 30 days (e.g., burns, bruises, rashes, itchiness, body lice, scabies)<br>0. No<br>1. Yes |
| 2. *Ulcers*<br>*(Pressure/Stasis)* | Presence of an ulcer anywhere on the body. Ulcers include any area of persistent skin redness (Stage 1); partial loss of skin layers (Stage 2); deep craters in the skin (Stage 3); and breaks in skin exposing muscle or bone (Stage 4). [Code 0 if no ulcer, otherwise record the highest ulcer stage (Stage 1–4)]<br>a. Pressure ulcer—any lesion caused by pressure, shear forces resulting in damage of underlying tissues<br>b. Statis ulcer—open lesion caused by poor circulation in the lower extremities |
| 3. *Other Skin Problems Requiring Treatment* | *Check all that apply.*<br>Burns (second or third degree)<br>Open lesions other than ulcers, rashes, cuts (e.g., cancer)<br>Skin tears or cuts<br>Surgical Wound Sites: ☐ Throat<br>                            ☐ Abdomen<br>                            ☐ Extremities<br>                            ☐ Other<br>                            ☐ None of the above |
| 4. *History of Resolved Pressure Ulcers* | Client previously had (at any time) or has an ulcer anywhere on the body<br>0. No<br>1. Yes |
| 5. *Wound/Ulcer Care* | Number of days formal care received in last week<br>a. Antibiotics, systemic or topical<br>b. Dressings<br>c. Pressure reduction/relieving devices<br>d. Nutrition of hydration<br>e. Turning/repositioning<br>f. Debridement<br>g. Surgical wound care |
| 6. *Foot Problems* | *Check all that apply.*<br>Corns, calluses, structural problems, infections, fungi<br>Open lesions on the foot<br>Foot not inspected in last 90 days by client or other<br>None of the above |

form Needs Assessment Inventory (UNAI). Like its relatives, this form began as a two stage process. The first step involved some type of screening to determine whether the patient needed any systematic discharge planning. For those who appeared to need such effort, the second stage was a systematic approach to collecting relevant data. Here, too, it appears that the subgrouping will be lost in implementation. Instead, the same data will be collected on all patients discharged alive.

The original UNAI was developed by a committee chartered by the Health Care Financing Administration, but its product was never even field tested. A new version of the UNAI is currently being developed by many of the same group who developed the MDS. Not surprisingly, the instruments resemble each other closely. The ba-

**Table 16.20.** Uniform Needs Assessment
Inventory Components

Sociodemographics
Health status (diagnoses, conditions, cognitive/
  behavioral problems)
Functional status (activities and instrumental activ-
  ities of daily living, locomotion, communication)
Environmental factors
Nursing and other care requirements
Family and community support
Patient/family goals and preferences
Needs for continuing care

Preadmission screening
  Single form
  Common domains
  Basic problems

sic components of the UNAI are shown in
Table 16.20.

## CONCLUSIONS

Mandated measures offers an opportunity
to create a comparable database for care
across the country. The obvious critical
question is just how comparable is the information generated. Using the same format, items, and definitions is an important
first step, but substantial opportunity remains for different raters to reach different
conclusions. The further the information
synthesis and recording are from those
who make the observations, the greater is
the potential for error.

It has taken a while before all of the
mandated data have been made available
for various purposes. The requirement that
MDS data be submitted in electronic form
will make it widely accessible for different
users. Nursing homes can compare their
performance with that of their peers. Researchers can use the data to examine
aspects of care, both directly and by creatively linking MDS data to other information like medication data (Bernabei et
al., 1998).

In the nursing home area, a mandated
measure intended initially for assessing
and improving quality (the MDS) has now
been adapted to become the engine for set-

ting rates as well. The same tendency is
seen with regard to home care in the context of OASIS. In both cases, the use for
payment purposes seems likely to corrupt
the measures and hence reduce their already limited utility for assessing quality.

It is important to distinguish between
recording specific responses to questions
or discrete observations and recording systematic judgments. The latter requires
well-trained professionals and is almost always likely to produce less reliable measures because it depends on each rater's
judgment. Raters can be trained to become
more consistent. (Think about Olympic
judges.) Even so, there are differences. In
clinical practice, few raters ever receive
enough basic education or specific training
to become consistent.

When the data are collected by those
who will use them, there is an inevitable
trade-off between the quality of data and
the use made of it. The energy devoted to
data collection comes from what might
otherwise be devoted to giving care. Thus,
the burden should be as light as possible.
At the same time, it is foolish to collect
weak data, when better techniques exist.
In the case of the MDS, several domains
can be addressed with already established
measures.

The desire to create a single universal
assessment approach has forced an over-
riding reliance on observing behavior in
lieu of asking respondents directly. This
decision invariably limits the domains that
can be legitimately explored. (For example, nothing is known about residents'
preferences.) In some cases, such as cognition, the observed behaviors seem to function as reasonable proxies for direct measurement. In others, such as depression,
the effort is much less successful. Still
others, such as meaningful activities, satisfaction, and social relationships, are effectively removed from consideration. It
would be better to create two separate
streams for the MDS. Cognitively intact
residents could be addressed directly; severely cognitively impaired residents could

continue to be observed. Some areas of inquiry are eliminated for the latter group.

The initial hope for the RAI was to provide a more structured and systematic approach to data collection in nursing homes. That aim seems to have been achieved. At the same time, because the MDS was mandated, it was resisted. Nursing home staffs were likely to comply with the need to complete the form, but did so by hiring special staff or directing their energy specifically to the task. Less effort was put into actually using the data collected to improve care planning. Nonetheless, nursing home care has improved quite a bit since the MDS was implemented. Although it may not be possible to correctly credit the MDS to the extent its developers would claim, it is equally hard to dismiss its contributions. As better computer-based information systems are introduced, the data collected can be put to greater uses without requiring the staff to spend as much time manipulating them. Such a step should improve the MDS's impact on clinical care.

From the perspective of the researcher, the MDS looms as an attractive target for discussion. Some have questioned the reliability of the MDS and hence its capacity to serve as a basis for research (Teresi & Holmes, 1992). The reports of reliability based on testing under special circumstances do not necessarily generalize into acceptable performance in daily practice. It is the most universal tool available, and, with the mandate for computerized submissions, it is readily available. It seems to provide a basis for longitudinal studies, although the earlier observations about insensitivity to change (Crooks et al., 1995) and the potential for sustained halo effects, where simply directing attention to an area may produce changes, must be borne in mind. Innovative uses have already been made, such as linking the measures of pain to the use of medications from other payment sources to examine the adequacy of pain control (Bernabei et al., 1998). The same criticisms leveled against the MDS for quality apply to research purposes. Some elements seem more trustworthy than others. Those addressing quality of life components (including mood) seem the least useful, especially for cognitively intact residents.

The MDS has also been used as a basis for quality measures. Zimmerman and colleagues have proposed a series of quality indicators based on the MDS (see Zimmerman, 1984; Zimmerman et al., 1995). These are specific measures compared for purportedly homogeneous subgroups of residents at risk for the specific outcome. The term *quality indicator* reflects a reluctance to attempt real attribution. Instead, the indicators are used as screeners to identify nursing homes that deserve closer scrutiny.

## RECOMMENDATIONS

The standards for instruments must be set for specific purposes. Measures designed for establishing eligibility must be established on the basis of their capacity for predicting those who will benefit from the targeted services. Predictive validity studies are rare, and few measures have been proven to work.

The establishment of a nationally comparable data system for nursing homes offers a great opportunity, but the enthusiasm for extending this approach to all forms of long-term care must be examined carefully. It makes sense to hold all forms of care for the same population accountable for comparable outcomes, but much of the current MDS system is still weighted in attention to process dictated by professional beliefs. It will be important to examine what kind of information is most useful in various contexts. Ideally, the model called for in the original work on the OASIS, where specific clinical subgroups were first identified and measures constructed to address the relevant parameters, can be employed.

Measures that intended to establish quality, either by tracing change in status over time or by addressing specific process issues, must be shown to be both reliable and valid. The MDS, in its various versions, was designed to address both quality of care and quality of life. For the latter, it is imperative that information be obtained directly from residents whenever possible. Inferences based on behavior should be reserved for only those situations where cognitive or physical disability makes in impossible to query residents directly. In many instances, established measures already exist (many of which are reviewed in this volume) to tap relevant domains. It would make sense to use these instead of creating new approaches.

The data from the MDS can be used more creatively. Rather than simply examining actions in specific instances among defined subgroups, information like functioning and affect should be traced longitudinally. The actual patterns of change can be compared with expected changes, where the latter are derived from statistical estimations. In effect, such a procedure represents the ultimate case-mix adjustment (Smith et al., 1997).

## REFERENCES

Bernabei, R., Gambassi, G., Lapane, K., Landi, F., Gatsonis, C., Dunlop, R., Lipsitz, L., Steel, K., & Mor, V. (1998). Management of pain in elderly patients with cancer: SAGE Study Group. Systematic assessment of geriatric drug use via epidemiology. *JAMA, 279*(23), 1877–1882.

Casten, R., Lawton, M. P., Parmelee, P. A., & Kleban, M. H. (1998). Psychometric characteristics of the Minimum Data Set I: Confirmatory factor analysis. *Journal of the American Geriatrics Society, 46,* 726–735.

Crooks, V. C., Schnelle, J. F., Ouslander, J. P., & McNees, M. P. (1995). Use of the Minimum Data Set to rate incontinence severity. *Journal of the American Geriatrics Society, 43,* 1363–1369.

Harper, G. J. (1998). *Stress and adaptation among elders in life care communities.* Columbus: Ohio State University.

Hartmaier, S. L., Sloane, P. D., Guess, H. A., & Koch, G. G. (1994). The MDS cognition scale: A valid instrument for identifying and staging nursing home residents with dementia using the Minimum Data Set. *Journal of the American Geriatrics Society, 42,* 1173–1179.

Hartmaier, S. L., Sloane, P. D., Guess, H. A., Koch, G. G., Mitchell, C. M., & Phillips, C. D. (1995). Validation of the Minimum Data Set cognitive performance scale: Agreement with the Mini-Mental State Examination. *Journal of Gerontology: Medical Sciences, 50A*(2), M128–M133.

Hawes, C., Morris, J. N., Phillips, C. D., Fries, B. E., Murphy, K., & Mor, V. (1997). Development of the nursing home Resident Assessment Instrument in the USA. *Age and Ageing, 26*(Suppl 2), 19–25.

Hawes, C., Morris, J. N., Phillips, C. D., Mor, V., Fries, B. E., & Nonemaker, S. (1995). Reliability estimates for the Minimum Data Set for Nursing Home Resident Assessment and care screening (MDS). *Gerontologist, 35*(2), 172–178.

Kahn, K. L., Keeler, E. B., Sherwood, M. J., Rogers, W. H., Draper, D., Bentow, S. S., Reinisch, E. J., Rubenstein, L. V., Kosecoff, J., & Brook, R. H. (1990). Comparing outcomes of care before and after implementation of the DRG-based prospective payment system. *Journal of the American Medical Association, 264*(15), 1984–1988.

Kramer, A. M., Shaughnessy, P. W., Bauman, M. K., & Crisler, K. S. (1990). Assessing and assuring the quality of home health care: A conceptual framework. *Milbank Quarterly, 68*(3), 413–443.

Lawton, M. P., Casten, R., Parmelee, P. A., Van Haitsma, K., Corn, J., & Kleban, M. H. (1998). Psychometric characteristics of the Minimum Data Set II: Validity. *Journal of the American Geriatrics Society, 46,* 736–744.

Mor, V., Intrator, O., Fries, B. E., Phillips, C., Teno, J., Hiris, J., Hawes, C., & Morris, J. (1997). Changes in hospitalization associated with introducing the Resident Assessment Instrument. *Journal of the American Geriatrics Society, 45*(8), 1002–1010.

Morris, J. N., Fries, B. E., Mehr, D. R., Hawes, C., Phillips, C., Mor, V., & Lipsitz, L. A. (1994). MDS cognitive performance scale. *Journal of Gerontology: Medical Sciences, 49*(4), M174–M182.

Morris, J. N., Fries, B. E., Steel, K., Ikegami, N., Bernabei, R., Carpenter, G. I., Gilgen, R., Hirdes, J. P., & Topinkova, E. (1997). Comprehensive clinical assessment in community setting: Applicability of the MDS-HC. *Journal of the American Geriatrics Society, 45*(8), 1017–1024.

Phillips, C. D., Morris, J. N., Hawes, C., Fries,

B. E., Mor, V., Nennstiel, M., & Iannac-
chione, V. (1997). Association of the Resident Assessment Instrument (RAI) with
changes in function, cognition, and psychosocial status. *Journal of the American
Geriatrics Society, 45*(8), 986–993.

Smith, M. A., Atherly, A. J., Kane, R. L., &
Pacala, J. T. (1997). Peer review of the
quality of care: Reliability and sources
of systematic bias for outcome and process assessments. *JAMA, 278*(19), 1573–
1578.

Snowden, M., McCormick, W., Russo, J., Sreb-
nik, D., Comtois, K., Bowen, J., Teri, L., &

Larson, E. B. (1999). Validity and responsiveness of the Minimum Data Set. *Journal
of the American Geriatrics Society, 47*(8),
1000–1004.

Teresi, J. A., & Holmes, D. (1992). Should
MDS data be used for research? *Gerontologist, 32*(2), 148–149.

Zimmerman, D. R., Karon, S. L., Arling, G.,
Clark, B. R., Collins, T., Ross, R., & Sainfort, F. (1995). Development and testing of
nursing home quality indicators. *Health
Care Financing Review, 16*(4), 107–127.

Zimmerman, J. M. (1984). *Hospice.* Baltimore:
Urban & Schwartzenberg.

# 17

## Assessing Older Adults Who Cannot Communicate

### GILLIAN J. HARPER

Approximately 60%–80% of institution-alized and 10%–25% of community dwelling older Americans currently suffer some degree of cognitive impairment (National Center for Health Statistics, 1991, 1993; Rovner et al., 1986; Chandler & Chandler, 1988; Harper, 1985). Because the risk of Alzheimer's disease and related disorders increases with age and people on average are living longer, the total number of people with cognitive impairments is expected to increase through the first half of the twenty-first century (Schneider & Guralnik, 1990; National Institute on Aging, 1997). These predictions have lead to great concern about future assessment and care of this group (Magaziner, 1997; Teresi et al., 1994). Because elders with cognitive impairments may not be able to speak for themselves, it is a challenge to design research and clinical tools that effectively assess general health, physical function, quality of care, quality of life, and efficacy of behavioral or medical interventions. A variety of approaches to assessment of elders with dementia have been employed in clinical and research settings, but they have not been systematically compared. Each approach presents advantages and disadvantages depending on the goals of

clinical assessment and research. This chapter reviews what is known about assessing this hard to reach population using a variety of approaches.

Although cognitive impairments and dementias are often referred to as a single entity, cognitive impairment in older adults is heterogeneous in etiology and multidimensional in expression (see Chapter 4 for more detail). Older adults may become confused or unable to speak coherently due to nondementing diseases such as acute illness, metabolic disequilibrium, alcohol use or withdrawal, malnutrition, dehydration, social or environmental stressors, or depression (McPherson, 1991). Short-term reversible episodes of confusion are called *transient cognitive disorders* or *delirium*. If transient disorders are confused with dementia, a short-term episode may become a long-term health problem (McPherson, 1991). Even those with organic brain disorders show variation in impairment. Despite growing awareness of the distinction between the various forms of dementia and dementia versus delirium, cognitively impaired elders continue to be treated uniformly, but such variations should influence the choice of an assessment method.

A typical classification of adults with

cognitive impairment is "mild," "moderate," or "severe." This taxonomy is confusing because these subgroups can be relatively heterogeneous. For example, someone who is comatose can be grouped in the severely impaired category with someone who is alert but incoherent. Teresi and Evans (1996, p. 152) identified four "measurement populations": "(a) persons with impaired consciousness who are not alert; (b) persons who are arousable and alert, but unable to perform simple commands with variable ability to communicate; (c) persons who are alert, arousable, and able to communicate, but provide nonratable (e.g., rambling, incoherent) responses to questions; and (d) persons who provide ratable but incorrect responses to most test items." Additional categories can be added to this; an important one is (e) persons who are oriented on an intermittent basis. These people may give correct answers some of the time and incorrect answers at other times. Unfortunately, we do not understand the natural history (or daily patterns) of confusion. If we ask this group questions regarding function, affect, or quality of life, it is hard to know when an individual is confused and when he or she is not. This chapter briefly discusses all groups, but focuses on people who are alert (i.e., not comatose or in a persistent vegetative state).

Because individuals with dementia cannot always speak for themselves, all assessments of these people require some level of inference. Some methods require more than others. In addition, because thought processes are impaired in people with dementia, some concepts might not have meaning. For example, an individual who is unable to perform simple commands and unable to communicate might not have the capacity to conceptualize emotions such as depression, loneliness, quality of life, or stress. If they cannot conceptualize emotions, is it possible for people with cognitive impairments to feel sadness or happiness? Unfortunately, we cannot tap into the thought processes of people

who are cognitively impaired (CI). People who are cognitively impaired, however, exhibit facial expressions, body language, and communications that may be interpreted as emotion if one is willing to use such an inference for clinical or research purposes.

People with dementia may have multiple co-morbid diseases that will affect outcome measures (Warshaw, 1997). These health problems, which may be in addition to or as a result of a dementing disease, include delirium, psychiatric illness (e.g., depression), increased risk of falls, incontinence, infections, malnutrition, and chronic diseases common to older adults (e.g., osteoarthritis, cardiovascular diseases, diabetes). Physical and visual impairment complicates assessment of CI elders. Alzheimer's disease affects the visual cortex and particularly affects saccadic eye movements and flash visual-evoked potential (Mendez et al., 1990). As a result, most assessment methods of vision are inadequate for individuals with such impairments (Teresi et al., 1994). One is never sure if people with late stage dementia cannot see or just do not understand (Teresi et al., 1994). Thus, individuals with Alzheimer's disease have both age-related and disease-related impairments that may affect assessment (Uhlman et al., 1991). There also may be an overlap in symptoms of disease and affective disorders. For example, depression and dementia have several symptoms in common (Abrams & Alexopoulos, 1994). Too often, co-morbidities are ignored because it is assumed that they are part of the expression of dementing diseases, or vice versa.

## DIFFERENT APPROACHES TO MEASUREMENT

Choosing a method for assessing elders with cognitive impairments presents a conflict between quality of information and the practicality of use. Methods that allow the best information are often the most expensive. Unfortunately, accuracy, validity, and reliability of information from different sources (e.g., direct interview, observation, proxy report, and medical charts) has largely been untested (Magaziner, 1997). Thus, it is difficult to know what trade-offs one is making in choosing a particular assessment protocol. Although direct interview or observation is likely more accurate than indirect techniques (proxy reports, medical charts), the accuracy of indirect techniques is still unclear. Accuracy differs across domains of assessment. In general, there are no "gold standards" for assessing various domains among elders with CI. Such gold standards will not likely be developed because no method for assessing CI is without inference or some level of bias.

Practicality of use is an important consideration when choosing a method. Three main considerations with respect to practicality are cost, time, and ease of use. The later two considerations also affect cost. A complicated method that requires substantial training may introduce additional error and require more time and money to set up. Time-consuming techniques have to be counterbalanced with other clinical practices or research goals in terms of both time and financial constraints. Techniques that require greater amounts of time, money, and training are less amenable to clinical practice; however, they may still be of use for clinical research on interventions or program analysis. Physiological and technical assessments require the greatest amount of training and are often more expensive than other techniques. Observation techniques require a significant amount of training as well as time to establish interobserver reliability. Chart abstracting (obtaining data from written charts) can be time consuming, particularly without adequate training and will never be better than the quality of the original recording. Direct interviews and proxy reports are the cheapest techniques in terms of time, training, and money. These techniques may, however, be subject

to more bias or inconsistency due to confusion of those being interviewed or varying interpretations of proxies.

The choice of a method should reflect the level of detail and accuracy needed for a specific assessment goal. This decision should be goal or hypothesis driven, but time and money constraints may limit choices. If possible, it is best to use multiple methods of assessment to ensure quality, but this practice can be quite expensive. Multiple method approaches may help establish convergence on valid measurements through triangulation (Brewer & Hunter, 1989; Teresi et al., 1994). More information is needed on the comparability of data produced from various methods. If it is determined, for example, that proxy reports of agitation are close enough to observations, then time-consuming observations might not be necessary. Multiple approaches also allow us to measure different aspects of an issue or problem.

It is important to distinguish between impressions and systematic observations. Impressions are formed by the experience of caregivers or from unstructured observation by a clinician or researcher. Impressions gleaned by formal or informal caregivers are filtered through their experience with an older adult and their feelings toward him or her. Subjectivity and bias are inherent in assessment through impressions. Structured observations are collected in a systematic manner. Observational data are often, although not always, quantitative in nature. Typically, observations are made by researchers, but with proper training, observations can also be collected by formal and informal caregivers.

All assessment techniques require some level of inference, although there is a continuum of inference across various assessment techniques (Fig. 17.1). Even straightforward "objective" assessments require inference. We think of many aspects of assessment as objective because they are established. For example, a particular blood glucose level is associated with diabetes.

| Low | Technological assessment (polysomnography, electrocardiography) |
| | Direct assessment of the environment (sound, light sensors) |
| | Physiological measures (established relationships between blood hormone or proteins and morbidity) |
| | Physiological assessment of stress (blood pressure, cortisol, catecholamines, heart rate) |
| | Interview |
| | Direct observation (those with established social morbidities , ↓ inference) |
| | Medical chart data |
| High | Proxy interview |

**Figure 17.1.**   Continuum of inference in assessment.

This still requires inference, but it is well-established inference; a causal link between blood glucose levels and disease progression has been determined. Even these "objective" measures, however, such as diabetes diagnosis criteria, are subject to change as we learn more about morbidity and mortality related to disease states. In addition, such parameters are also subject to fluctuation due to time of day, season, activity level, and diet. Assessment becomes much more difficult when one is examining behavior and emotion. Even when doing direct assessment (interviewing individuals), one must infer meaning from responses. For example, certain symptoms may indicate depression: fatigue, insomnia, feelings of sadness, feelings of despair and worthlessness, and disinterest in daily activities. In this case, there are also established relationships between verbal responses to assessment questions and morbidity.

When assessing individuals who cannot communicate, inference becomes greater. When observing behaviors that may indicate emotions or relationships, one can never be certain of the relationships between behavior and internal "interpretation" because they cannot be confirmed. In the future, we may be able to establish "social morbidities," or social problems such as low quality of life, high levels of agitation, or poor social functioning. Certain symptoms or cues may indicate people who have poor social functioning or a low quality of life. Responses to social questions may vary according to time of day, season, and activity level and health status

of the participant. Relying on chart data or proxy responses means making inferences based on someone else's interpretation of a behavior. These realities make research of such social morbidities among CI people particularly challenging.

### Direct Interview

It is sometimes possible to interview people with cognitive impairments directly using the same interview/assessment tools that are used with oriented individuals. One may also assess older adults with CI with simplified versions of such assessment tools or by using an open-ended interview or a photograph-assisted technique. It is often possible to ask CI elders about their likes and dislikes and their own perceptions of disability and health. For a person to participate in an interview, a certain level of competence is necessary, but there is no consensus on what that level should be.

Although it may be desirable to have a standardized cut score on a cognitive assessment scale to determine competence, such a cut score may not be appropriate in all circumstances. For example, Shnelle and colleagues (1993a) demonstrated that one commonly used cut score for determining ability to comply with an incontinence intervention excludes many who are capable of participating. In addition, people who are oriented some of the time will be determined to be competent at certain times and not at others. Even when we can determine a stable cognitive score for an individual, not all domains of interest require the same level of competence. An alternative approach is to use a "run-in screen" (Schnelle et al., 1993a). With this approach, potential participants in research or intervention programs go through a test run to see if they are capable of completing the protocol. This approach was a more sensitive strategy for identifying individuals for an incontinence intervention (Schnelle et al., 1989). The use of the run-in screen, however, does make cross-study comparisons more difficult. More research is needed on competence levels to participate in interviews before any recommendations are made.

Further examination of psychometric properties of previously established scales in populations with dementia is needed. In many cases, time and money permitted, interviews should be used to augment information obtained by other techniques. This allows the inclusion of the older adults' perspectives and preferences. In addition, with transiently impaired participants, interviews should always take precedence over other methods. Because each question may require more time due to cueing, interviews are likely to take longer and result in more fatigue compared with cognitively intact older adults. Thus, it may be advisable to interview in two to four short sessions as opposed to one long interview, particularly when multiple domains are being assessed. This, of course, adds to the cost of this approach. Although basic questions about likes and dislikes are more commonly assessed by direct interview, several people have used more formal assessment instruments to measure a variety of domains, including health-related quality of life (McHorney, 1996), affect (Parmelee, Katz, & Lawton, 1989), and agitation (Levin et al., 1987), with CI participants.

## Proxy Methods

In population studies, the use of proxies allows researchers to maintain representativeness by increasing response rates of those who are unable to provide information (Magaziner, 1997). Typically, researchers or clinicians use adapted forms of questionnaires and scales intended for those without CI. There may be some domains for which the use of proxies is never appropriate (e.g., internal emotions); however, there is no agreement on which domains can or cannot be assessed via proxy reports. In most cases, proxies have been used when small numbers of individuals are not available to respond to surveys (cognitively intact participants). Little research has, however, been conducted on the use of proxies in studies where little or no information can be collected from individuals (Magaziner, 1997).

Research on noncognitively impaired participants demonstrates varying concordance between proxy and self-report. The accuracy of proxy reports depends on the informant used, the amount of exposure that a proxy has to the individual, and the presence of biases due to differences in education, care burden, and environmental/social context. Proxies tend to make inferences based on dispositional (in terms of the subject's likes and dislikes) rather than situational (based on situations that may influence behavior) information (Schwarz & Wellens, 1997). Thus, proxy data are filtered through assumptions based on past behavior of the individual rather than on the current context. When discussing CI elders, proxies may base their responses on what the individual was like before he or she became impaired rather than on consideration of the current situation. Proxy reports are closer to personal reports when they provide information on usual behaviors as opposed to extreme or rare behaviors (Schwarz & Wellens, 1997). Variables such as emotional status, pain, and subjective dimensions of health are less adequately measured by proxy reports than by more objective/observable traits (Grootendorst, Feeny, & Furlong, 1997). Some research shows under-reporting for pain and emotional problems (Grootendorst et al., 1997), while others show over-report of illness, disability, pain, and psychosocial problems (Wu et al., 1997). Both cases demonstrate the effects of biases and motivation depending on context. Although proxy interviews are often considered equivalent to direct interviews, it is essential that these two types of interviews be distinguished. Interviewing a proxy elicits the impressions of that proxy.

Who should be the informant? No one informant is necessarily best; different informants will provide different information that is filtered through their own experiences. Proxies may be family and friends (caregivers and noncaregivers) or formal caregivers. For any proxy, there must be adequate contact between the individual and the proxy to obtain quality data. When using proxies for clinical or research purposes, one needs to consider potential biases and conflicts of interest. There may be differing motivations behind proxy reports of affect, functional status, sleep, or agitation. A clinician or researcher must consider the caregivers' state of mind. It is also important to ask potential proxies about the actual frequency of contact between them and the participant.

When family caregivers spend a great deal of time with CI older adults, they are in the position to make an informed assessment. Not all caregivers, however, will provide accurate reports. For example, some spouses overestimate the amount of functional deficits of a CI elder by including those tasks that they always did for their husband or wife. For example, a wife may list inability to cook or clean as functional deficit when her husband never did these tasks as a healthy adult. On the other hand, some family members may underestimate cognitive/functional deficits because they adapt to their caregiving roles. Others may be afraid that any report of disability may place their family member at risk of being moved to a long-term care institution. Social desirability may also influence proxy reports; in other words, proxies may under-report behaviors that are embarrassing. Family or friends who are not caregivers may have less at stake but also may not be in a position to observe an individual to provide appropriate impressions.

When caregivers for CI elders feel particularly burdened, a number of sources of bias can enter into proxy-based assessment that might not be present when using proxies under different circumstances. Due to the nature of dementing diseases, many CI adults require a great deal of attention and time; both informal and formal caregivers might find caregiving particularly stressful (Kane, 1997). Thus, when using proxies for assessment purposes, we must carefully consider such potential biases and possible conflicts of interest. At least three areas should be explored for potential biases: (1) assessment of cognitive competence of proxy (many CI elders are cared for by older adults who are themselves impaired to a lesser degree); (2) assessment of health status; and (3) assessment of stress and burden (see Chapter 11).

Staff members in long-term care settings are often used as proxies in clinical practice and research. Using formal caregivers as proxies may involve a trade-off between those with the greatest amount of contact and those with more training. For example, nurse assistants have the most contact with residents of a nursing home, but they are also typically the least educated of the staff at a nursing home. They are also likely to feel the greatest amount of emotional and physical burden of caregiving. Personnel in such settings differ in levels of expertise and exposure. In addition, staff from different shifts may have variable knowledge of residents (Teresi et al., 1994). For example, if agitation primarily occurs during evening and night-time hours, day-shift staff will under-report these behaviors. Also, there may be temporal patterns of functional deficits. For example, some residents may not feed themselves during the day, but eat on their own in the evening. In these cases, proxies from different shifts will produce different reports of behavior and disability.

Staff in long-term care settings also experience caregiver burden. Perceptions of residents are influenced in a variety of ways. Sometimes residents who are demanding or confused are labeled as "difficult" or "crazy." Thus, care providers may overestimate agitation if the behavior is frustrating or if they need to justify the use of chemical and/or physical restraints. Other staff members may become "numb" and think of residents as emotionless (or not capable of emotional responses), never stressed, and living happily in their own world. These proxies will underestimate affective disorders and may overestimate expressions of positive affect. Staff may also underestimate functional limitations if they feel that a patient or resident is not trying hard enough.

The amount of burden placed on a proxy may influence assessment. If an individual is perceived as burdensome, a proxy may overestimate dysfunction or agitation. Unfortunately, burden can differ according to the role of the proxy (caregiver vs. noncaregiver) and personality of a proxy, thus preventing any consistent correction for bias. Unfortunately, with cognitively impaired individuals we have limited ability to test concordance of self-report versus proxy report. Ideally, a clinician or researcher should compare proxy reports with observations, but this effort greatly increases the cost and time of proxy methods.

The proxy approach may be acceptable for some types of information and not for others. Several studies have shown good psychometric properties for proxy-based approaches (e.g., Albert et al., 1996). When designing assessments for clinical or research purposes, one must consider the level of accuracy that is needed according to the goal of assessment. For some clinical decisions it may not be necessary to have great precision or accuracy. For example, when assessing social networks it may be enough to know that a client has a limited network and unmet needs rather than the exact number people available for assistance. When assessing agitation in home settings, if the behavior of a client has a significant impact on family caregiver, this probably indicates the need for additional services regardless of the exact frequency, duration, or stimuli.

## Observational Assessment

There are numerous methods of observation. To be useful clinically or in research, observations must be structured rather than impressionistic. Particularly when performed in a naturalistic setting, observation is very time consuming and expensive. Observational techniques may also require an extensive amount of training. If one chooses to use an observational method of assessment, the need for accuracy and precision must outweigh the expense. In addition, if such an approach is used, it is important to make sure that the method of observation chosen allows the accuracy needed for a particular purpose. Observation falls into two general approaches: laboratory and naturalistic. In laboratories, individuals are observed as they complete a specific task (e.g., dressing, following a set of instructions) or as they are exposed to specific environments or stimuli (noises or "stressful" situations). In contrast, naturalistic observation takes place in a living environment of an older adult. A laboratory approach can be performed anywhere, as long as it is controlled. The primary distinction between the two is that in a laboratory approach a behavior or experience is induced and in naturalistic observation behaviors or emotions are recorded as they happen. Laboratory observation affords more control and, thus, fewer complications than naturalistic observation. Naturalistic observation is generally more time consuming than laboratory observation but allows more realistic data collection.

### Laboratory Observation

With the laboratory approach, a clinician or researcher observes completion of specific tasks for functional assessment or observes responses to environments or stimuli (distress, behavioral/emotional responses). When assessing a functional ability, the laboratory approach addresses what individuals can do, not what they actually do. It emphasizes capability versus regular behavior. When examining responses to stimuli, one must determine a priori that a condition, environment, or stimulus is stressful or likely to induce an emotional response. A laboratory approach allows the determination of how individuals respond only under specific circumstances. This kind of observation conveys little about real-life situations or everyday behavior of an older adult with CI.

### Naturalistic Observation

With the naturalistic approach, an individual or group is observed in the "normal" environment. This technique has been used mostly for older adults living in institutions. It is more difficult to observe older adults in home environments, but qualitative methods of observation have been extensively used in retirement communities. With proper training, caregivers may be able to observe CI elders systematically (by using diaries). Overall, naturalistic observation is an underutilized method for older adults. Recently, there has been a greater interest in this approach. Observational methodology is based on child behavior research (psychology, behavioral assessment) and animal behavior or ethology (biology and anthropology: primatology/ sociocultural anthropology), that is, research with those who cannot communicate with researchers or clinicians. The basic issues are outlined in this section; for further information there are several books and articles on animal behavior, behavioral psychology, and qualitative methods (for good reviews, see Altman, 1974; Dunbar, 1976; Martin & Bateson, 1993; Bakeman & Gottman, 1997; Lerner, 1979; Gubrium & Sankar, 1994).

Although naturalistic observation is more objective than proxy reports or medical chart data, it is not without bias or inference. Meaning is always assigned to behaviors, expressions, and results. In addition, one is always concerned with changing environment or behaviors simply by being present. For example, research on nutrition has been shown to influence the kinds of things people eat (Quant, 1987).

As observers spend more time in an environment, however, most people become habituated to their presence (Bakeman & Gottman, 1997), and recorded behaviors become closer to normal behavior.

There are numerous considerations when deciding on an observation technique, including coding technique, types of measures (latency, frequency, duration, or intensity), sampling procedure (continuous vs. interval), collection technique (quantitative vs. qualitative), and method of analysis.

### Coding

When planning an observational study, one needs to develop an "ethogram" or a catalogue of behaviors/facial expressions that describe the typical behaviors of a group (Martin & Bateson, 1993). A coding scheme should be based in theory while taking the purpose of assessment into account. There are two approaches to coding: "social scheme" (functional scheme, e.g., sad, angry) or "physical scheme" (empirical description of expressions, e.g.,. forehead wrinkled; Lerner, 1979; Bakeman & Gottman, 1997). Both schemes require inference. Social schemes require inference before analysis; physical schemes require interpretation during or after analysis. For coding purposes, one should not be especially concerned with being truly objective, but that the observations are reproducible (i.e., good interobserver reliability). Codes should be distinct, or precisely defined, homogenous, and simple to identify but detailed enough to answer the question. In some cases one may want mutually exclusive categories, but this is not always necessary. Nonmutually exclusive categories are, however, more challenging to analyze.

When deciding on a coding scheme one may use a splitting or lumping approach. In some circumstances, a very detailed coding scheme may be called for, whereas more inclusive categories are useful for some analyses. One may want to use a more detailed scheme as a first step and group behaviors or expressions into larger categories later. To develop a coding scheme, it is important to do some initial unstructured observation, or one should not count first few observations in analysis to avoid "drifting" or changing of scheme after research has started (Martin & Bateson, 1993).

## Types of Measures

One can collect several kinds of measures. The measure of interest will determine sampling method:

1. *Latency*: The time from a specified event to onset of behavior
2. *Frequency*: The number of occurrences per specified amount of time
3. *Duration*: The length of behaviors
4. *Intensity*: There is no universal definition of intensity; one must make judgments of what constitutes important components of intensity (typically, people use a scale of 1 − n, e.g., *intensity* or *local rate* [psychology]: the number of acts per unit time performing discrete activity, e.g., the number of times yelling over 5-minute intervals)
5. *Sequence*: The sequence of behaviors; sequence can be recorded as real time or as the pattern of behaviors.

## Sampling

The two important components of sampling are who is being sampled and how the data are collected. General approaches include

1. *Ad libitum*: No systematic constraints are placed on when or what is recorded. One can follow a single individual or a group. Generally, one records behaviors that are most obvious. Data collected in this manner cannot be quantified (Lerner, 1979). This approach should be used only as a first step in behavioral research.
2. *Focal person*: One individual is followed at a time (continuous or specified time intervals). This is the most common approach in human behavioral research.

3. *Scan sampling*: At specified time intervals, a group of individuals are scanned, and the behavior of each individual is recorded. This approach may be particularly useful in research on social interactions or group-based interventions.
4. *Combined approach*: Simultaneous focal person and scan sampling. This technique allows examination of interactions and possible influence of others on the behavior of the individual. It may be particularly appropriate for examining agitation or quality of life (if social interaction is important to definition).
5. *Behavior sampling (all occurrence sampling)*: Each observed occurrence of a particular behavior is recorded (with or without regard to the actor).

Observations can be initiated by a timed interval or the occurrence of an event. Sampling is generally divided into continuous event recording versus timed sampling. With event recording, an observer records the time and duration (onset/offset) of a behavior or expression of interest. This method allows the determination of true frequencies and duration. With timed sampling, on the other hand, observations are based on a specified time interval; thus, duration and frequencies are estimated. The accuracy of such estimates will depend on procedure, particularly the size of time intervals.

The two basic methods of timed sampling are instantaneous and one-zero. With both, one collects data at specified time intervals. With instantaneous sampling, the behavior of interest is coded at a point in time (is it occurring or not, or what behavior is occurring). With one-zero sampling, the observer records if a behavior occurred within an interval of interest. For example, if a time interval is 5 minutes, the observer records whether an event has occurred within the 5 minutes. The frequency within the time interval is not recorded; thus, if a behavior occurred 10 times, it is recorded the same as if it had only occurred once. Instantaneous sampling produces the proportion of sample points when a behavior is occurring. This method does not allow determination of true durations or frequencies, but, if intervals are short enough for the behavior of interest, it can generate relatively good estimates (Dunbar, 1976). One-zero sampling does not give true or unbiased frequencies. With this method, observers tend to over estimate duration and underestimate frequency (Martin & Bateson, 1993). Although this technique is still used in behavioral research, it has been widely criticized. Timed sampling, in general, is not appropriate for events of short duration.

There is frequent debate over the use of timed sampling versus continuous sampling. Continuous sampling is the most accurate way of determining frequency, duration, latency, and sequencing. It is tiring for observers, however, and may result in greater error. Bakeman and Gottman (1997) state that the only advantage of timed sampling is practical ease, but others still see utility in it (Martin & Bateson, 1993). The decision to use a particular sampling procedure will depend on what one wants to examine. In many cases, timed sampling will produce excellent estimates. Because systematic observation is relatively new among elders with CI, much remains to be understood about the utility of each approach. For example, does sampling at X intervals provide a good approximation of smaller intervals or continuous sampling for different assessment purposes. Because many CI older adults in institutions spend a great deal of time inactive or sleeping, longer intervals may be adequate to capture certain variables (e.g., activity levels or patterns). On the other hand, rare events, such as agitation, may be missed if sampling intervals are too long.

## Mode of Recording

Observational data can be collected with pencil and paper, an event recorder, or a computerized recorder. For continuous sampling, computer recording is the preferred method to reduce observer burden and increase accuracy. Any recording method can be used with a timed sampling procedure. Pencil and paper are preferred in the absence of a specified ethogram (e.g., data on activities) or when there are an infinite number of states. Computerized data recording reduces the amount of time needed to analyze data because the data can be loaded directly into a spread sheet or database program. Figure 17.2 illustrates different ways observational data can be recorded.

In addition to the issues outlined above, several other factors should be considered when designing observational research. Error can occur for several reasons, including observer errors due to apprehending, observer affect, and errors in recording and computational error (Lerner, 1979). One needs to consider carefully if some times are inappropriate to observe people, such as when a participant is bathing, in the bathroom, or receiving medical care. Many view observation during these times as a violation of privacy. Unfortunately, these are also likely to be times when agitation occurs, and some information may be lost. In addition, one has to consider the best way to analyze out-of-sight observations. Finally, one has to decide how long each participant should be observed and how many times. Financial and time budgets are likely to dictate this issue; however, hypotheses and goals should also be weighed.

## Specific Observation Techniques

Behavioral observation is still a relatively undeveloped technique in research on older adults with cognitive impairments. Several different techniques have been developed.

The *Agitation Behavior Mapping Instrument* (Cohen-Mansfield, Marx, & Rosenthal, 1989) was developed specifically to examine agitation. Each participant is observed in a randomized order for 3 minutes within every hour. The observer uses a

Behavioral observation: observer check sheet

Participant ID _____ Staff ID _____ Date _____ Page # _____

| Location codes | Position Codes | Mood codes |
|---|---|---|
| r = room | s = sitting | l = laughing |
| d = dining room | u = upright | s = smile |
| h = hall | r = reclining | a = agitated |
| o = outside | | c = crying |
| hu = hub | | n = neutral |
| lr = living room | | d = distressed |
| s= solarium | | |

| Time | Location | Position | Mood | Activity | # indiv | Noise |
|---|---|---|---|---|---|---|
| 8:00 | d | s | n | Eating | 10 | Music |
| 8:05 | d | s | s | Talking | 8 | Talking |
| 8:10 | hu | u | n | walking | 0 | Call light |
| 8:15 | r | r | n | resting | 0 | TV |

Observer: _____ Date _____
Start time: _____ Stop time: _____

A=Alone  O=One-on-one  G=Group Activity
A  A  O  O  G  O  A  G  G  O
_____
_____
_____
_____

Recording the sequence of events
Source: Bakeman and Gottman (1997)

Observer: _____ Date _____
Start time: _____ Stop time: _____

| Pleasure | Anger | Anxiety |
|---|---|---|
| ✓✓✓✓ | ✓✓✓✓ | ✓✓✓ |
| ✓✓✓✓ | ✓✓✓ | |
| ✓✓ | | |

Tallying
Source: Bakeman and Gottman (1997)

Observer: _____ Date _____
Individual: _____ Tape #: _____

| Interval | Wander | Hit | Interact | TV | Sleep |
|---|---|---|---|---|---|
| 1 | ✓ | | | | |
| 2 | | ✓ | | | |
| 3 | ✓ | | | | |
| 4 | ✓ | | | | |
| 5 | ✓ | | | | |
| 6 | | | ✓ | | |
| 7 | | | ✓ | | |
| 8 | | | | ✓ | |
| 9 | | | | ✓ | |
| 10 | | | | ✓ | |
| 11 | | | | | ✓ |
| 12 | ✓ | | | | |
| 13 | ✓ | | | | |
| 14 | ✓ | | | | |

One-Zero Sampling data sheets
Source: Bakeman and Gottman (1997)

| Sample Time | A | | B | | C | | D | |
|---|---|---|---|---|---|---|---|---|
| | beh | loc | beh | loc | beh | loc | beh | loc |
| 0800 | Eat | r | Talk | d | Walk | h | Eat | d |
| 0801 | Talk | h | Walk | h | Eat | d | Walk | h |
| 0802 | | | | | | | | |
| 0803 | | | | | | | | |
| 0804 | | | | | | | | |

Scan Sample. beh = behavior; loc = location.
Source: Lerner (1979)

**Figure 17.2.** Sample data sheets.

check sheet with common agitative behavior and records if a behavior is constant (occurring five or more times) or extreme (based on averages of behavior). This technique has limited applications, requires significant training, and may not be used consistently across researchers.

*With the streams of behavior* (Lawton, Van Haitsma, & Klapper, 1996) approach, observers record facial expressions and body language at 30 second intervals in 10 minute "streams." Each participant is observed several times over several weeks, with four time periods represented (morning, early and late afternoon, early evening). Frequency or duration is estimated for each time interval and recorded in a hand-held event recorder. To code behaviors and expressions, a fair amount of time is required. Training is assisted with a video, which is available for purchase (Terra Nova Films, 1998).

*With behavior tracking* (Harper, 1998), a participant is observed over a 12–24 hour period at timed intervals (5 minutes or less). Data can be recorded with paper and pencil or with a laptop computer. At each time interval, the location, posture, activity, mood (assessed by facial expressions), noise, and number of people in the vicinity are recorded. In addition to quantitative data, qualitative data are collected in the form of field notes during observation periods and through participant observation (see below) to aid in interpretation of results. This technique provides a picture of what happens over the course of a day, but if participants are observed only once some behaviors may be missed. This technique has been used in combination with physiological techniques (e.g., ambulatory blood pressure monitoring and salivary cortisol).

*In real-time observation* (Burgio et al., 1994), a computer is used for event recording of different target behaviors. A number of variables can be recorded simultaneously (location, noise, activity, social environment, presence of restraints) with the real frequency and duration of target behaviors, such as disruptive vocalization. Elders are observed in 3 hour blocks during day-time hours, continuously within a time period. They are observed in a randomized order over several days, and no participant is observed in two contiguous blocks. This technique requires approximately 3 months of training, after which good interobserver reliability is established. This technique is flexible; the computer can be programmed to record data on any number of behaviors of interest.

There have been a number of *ethnographic studies* of elders living in communities and residential settings; however, this technique has rarely been used with demented elders (Henderson, 1994; Silverman & McAllister, 1995). In ethnographic studies, the researcher uses a technique called *participant observation*. The researcher becomes an active participant in the community to try to understand a culture or community from an "insider's point of view" (Lyman, 1994). Thus, an ethnographer may participate in planned activities, eat meals with residents, and have informal conversations with members of the community. They also spend a great deal of time observing interactions and behaviors and interviewing different members of the community (including the CI participants, if possible). Medical charts may also be read and formal assessment may be conducted for additional information. When collected from different sources, information can be triangulated to tap different perspectives. This technique is essentially a research technique; however, data collected in ethnographic research can be used in an applied manner (see Woolfson, 1997). Although this is inherently a qualitative method, it still needs to be hypothesis driven to be effective. This is a particularly good approach when examining new topics/issues to allow for the definition and measurement of new questions (Keith, 1988). Interested readers should consult books on ethnographic and anthropological techniques for a more extensive review of this topic (e.g., Bernard, 1995).

## Medical Chart Review

Medical charts are appealing sources of information because they are readily available and often easy to access. Medical charts contain a tremendous amount of information, but their quality, accuracy, and specificity vary greatly. Numerous formal assessments (e.g., mandated assessments, occupational therapy, physical therapy, speech therapy, and intake information) may be used in research contexts. With the exception of the Nursing Home Minimum Data Set (MDS), these assessments differ in format across facilities. (See Chapter 16). In addition, test results, medications, and diagnoses can be obtained. With a little more time and effort, the notes of health professionals (nurses, physicians, occupational therapists, physical therapists, speech therapists) can be abstracted to obtain additional qualitative information. Data obtained from charts, however, vary greatly in format and quality across nursing home facilities and other long-term care situations (Teresi et al., 1994). In addition, data rarely come from formal assessments.

One would expect medical charts to be accurate, but this is not always the case. Minimum Data Set data are not always based in systematic assessment or observation and have debatable reliability (Teresi et al., 1994). In addition, both formal assessments and nursing notes have a number of different authors, each with varying levels of expertise and exposure to residents. There is wide variation in completeness and accuracy. Charting tends to be based on unsystematic observation and may be done on an irregular basis. In addition, there is a tendency to chart only behavior problems and negative changes in health status, leaving the reader with a biased view of the participant. Large amounts of missing data often make analysis challenging.

## Physiological/Technological

Recently, new methods of collecting physiological markers of stress and depression have been developed that allow more widespread use in both research and clinical contexts. These include ambulatory blood pressure monitoring, salivary cortisol and immunoglobin levels, dexamethasone suppression test, and urinary or serum catecholamines tests (for good reviews, see James & Pickering, 1991; James & Brown, 1997; Pollard, 1995; Flinn & England, 1995, 1997; Harrison & Jefferies, 1977). The validity of such techniques has been well established for use with children, young adults, and middle-aged people. These techniques have been more widely used with older adults in the last few years. The validity of such approaches for CI people is still being established, but has great promise. Ambulatory blood pressure and cortisol values have been shown to vary among people with cognitive impairments and to respond to mood, behavior, and environment (Harper, 1998).

When a person is confronted with a novel or threatening situation, the body responds physiologically. Discussion of the complex neuroendocrine response to stressors is beyond the scope of this book (for a good review, see Sapolsky, 1994). To measure responses to stressors, one can examine a number of components of this integrated system, such as cortisol, catecholamine, and immunoglobin levels, heart rate, and blood pressure. Numerous advances in collection and analysis of physiological stress markers has made collection of stress markers more practical for a number of settings. This approach may not be realistic for clinical practice but is effective for clinical research.

Currently, catecholamines can be measured only from urine or blood, making this technique challenging with CI older adults. Cortisol can be measured in serum, blood spots (from finger sticks), urine, and saliva. Saliva is the method of choice because it is noninvasive and relatively easy to collect from people with CI. Several proteins of the immune system can also be collected from saliva. The easiest way to collect saliva is to have participants place a dental cotton roll in their mouth; when saturated, the cotton roll is placed in a tube called a Salivette® (Starstedt), which is centrifuged (up to 1 week later if refrigerated) and then stored at −70°C until it is assayed. There are several ways to assay cortisol from saliva, including radioimmunoassay and chemoluminescence (see Berne & Levy, 1993; Pollard, 1995; Vining, McGinley, & Symons, 1983; Hiramatsu, 1981; Worthman & Stallings, 1997).

Because blood pressure, heart rate, cortisol, and catecholamines are all subject to circadian rhythms, it important to measure them several times a day and to have consistent times for collection. In addition, blood pressure has been shown to vary with season, posture, mood, activity, and environment (James et al., 1989; James, 1991a, b; James & Pickering, 1993; Harper, 1998). Therefore, it is important to measure all these variables when blood pressure is taken. Body habitus is also associated with blood pressure; thus, at least weight, height, upper arm and midcalf skinfolds should be measured to correct for body composition in the statistical analysis. For studying stress or the effects of behavior on blood pressure, it is best to use ambulatory monitors that are worn for 24 hours. These consist of a normal blood pressure cuff connected to a small monitor ($1.1 \times 4.5 \times 3.4$ inches, 12.2 ounces) via a long tube. The monitors can be worn with a shoulder strap or connected to a belt. The most commonly used and best validated instrument is manufactured by Spacelabs Medical, Inc. These monitors have been used with CI elders and are relatively well tolerated with the exception of extremely agitated individuals (Harper, 1998). Smaller instruments are continually being developed.

### Technological Assessment

Several techniques may replace observation. These include video cameras, actigraphs (motion detectors used for sleep research and possibly agitation) and step sensors (to look at activity and restlessness). Video cameras may enable researchers to examine participants at times when it is hard to provide staff, for example, at night. If participants are particularly restless, however, stationary video cameras are likely to miss activity. In addition, video cameras may be seen as an invasion of privacy.

Actigraphs and step sensors may be good techniques for examining activity patterns. These sensors are relatively small and unobstrusive; thus they may be particularly useful for studies that require large amounts of observation time. These technologies are relatively new for use with CI older adults and require testing. Actigraphs seem to be the more reliable of the two and may enable researchers to measure general agitation (not just wandering) and sleep patterns as well. In addition, several new models of actigraphs include light sensors and/or heart rate monitors, allowing a more detailed examination of the environment in relation to behaviors and sleep patterns.

Environments can be assessed with light and noise sensors to quantify and examine potential stimuli of agitation and sleep disruption (Ouslander et al., 1998; Cruise et al., 1998). Incontinence pads that are wired to detect wetness of 10 mL can record actual episodes of night-time incontinence (Schnelle et al., 1993b). Use of such technologies is growing but is still relatively new in outcomes research with CI older adults.

### Summary of Techniques

Each technique for assessing CI elders has strengths and weaknesses. Different techniques may be excellent for assessing one domain and poor for other domains. Before choosing a technique, such drawbacks must be considered. Table 17.1 summarizes the general strengths and weaknesses of each approach. The next section discusses the use of the different techniques for several domains, including affect, function, behavioral problems, and quality of life.

### WHAT CAN WE MEASURE?

Ideally, all of the domains discussed in this book should be measurable in CI elders. Measurement of most domains is, however, a challenge among people with dementia. Many domains are assessed using a standard protocol (usually proxy interviews) or have not been measured at all. For each measurement population, we may divide domains into three groups: *(1)* domains that can definitely be assessed, *(2)*

**Table 17.1.** Strengths and Weaknesses of Methods of Assessing Older Adults with Cognitive Impairment

| Method | Strengths | Weaknesses |
|---|---|---|
| Direct interview | In many cases, individual is best informant (particularly when feelings or perceptions are assessed) | Problematic with domains requiring recall |
| | | May take more time and prompting than with noncognitively impaired |
| | In some cases, simple questions of likes or dislikes are adequate | Need to simplify questions and remind participants |
| | | Little research on psychometric properties |
| | | No consensus on level of competence necessary to complete interviews |
| Proxy | Least time-consuming and expensive approach | Requires informant with significant exposure; however, "best" sources may not always be available |
| | In many circumstances, there are well-established validities for proxy responses | Potential for conflict of interest between individual and proxy |
| | Data will be in same format for proxy and nonproxy informants, making analysis easier | Relies on good recall of events |
| | | Phone interviews with proxies are more likely to result in missing information (Corder et al., 1996) |
| | In large, population-based studies, allows inclusion of individuals who otherwise may be dropped from research | Likely to have sampling biases because some groups are more likely to have proxies than others (Corder et al., 1996) |
| | | Based on impressions, not observations |
| Laboratory observation | Good way to determine capability of older adults | Limited applications for clinical and research purposes |
| | Controlled environment for experimental research | Does not tell anything about real-life situations |
| Naturalistic observation | Can obtain accurate data on frequency, duration, latency | Expensive and time consuming |
| | More "objective" than proxy or chart reports | Challenging to analyze data |
| | Best way to examine relationships between environment and individual | May be perceived as invasion of privacy |
| | Powerful way to examine interventions | |
| | Good way to validate other approaches | |
| Medical chart review | Presumably, daily observations of staff should increase knowledge of patient/resident experience | Ideally, quality of charts should be analyzed for each site |
| | Less time consuming than observation or actual assessment | Requires good quality charts (no way to know quality without comparing with actual observations or assessments in each instance) |
| | Relatively low cost | |
| | Notes offer qualitative data (add additional information to quantitative data) | May require specialized training to read and abstract charts |
| Physiological | Powerful quantitative data | Techniques largely untested in cognitively impaired elders |
| | Potentially excellent tool for analyzing outcomes of variety of interventions | Expensive |
| | Relationship with health and illness | Most valuable when combined with observation (because sensitive to eating patterns, food intake, and sleeping patterns) |
| | Augments observational data | |

*(continued)*

**Table 17.1.** Strengths and Weaknesses of Methods of Assessing Older Adults with Cognitive Impairment — Continued

| | | Requires extensive training, particularly to analyze |
|---|---|---|
| | | People who are agitated easily may not tolerate |
| Technological | Allows accurate and precise recording of motion, environment, incontinence | May be seen as invasion of privacy |
| | Powerful quantitative data | Still relatively new |
| | | Expensive |
| | | People who are agitated easily may not tolerate |

domains that may be able to be assessed but are challenging, and *(3)* domains that definitely cannot be assessed (Table 17.2). The recommendations in Table 17.2 should be considered only as guidelines based on current research. For each subgroup, certain approaches may be appropriate while others are not. For example, we obviously cannot ask people who are comatose if they are in pain. Observation of facial expressions may, however, indicate that an individual experiences pain in specific circumstances, such as when being repositioned or transferred. For those who are confused on an intermittent basis, one should always begin by interviewing the individual and using other techniques to confirm answers. For people who fall between the comatose and relatively oriented categories, a variety of approaches may be appropriate. An individual is the best informant when it comes to feelings or perceptions, if he or she can express them. The recommended methods for several domains are discussed, and Table 17.2 presents possible approaches for a variety of domains.

This section focuses on those domains that have been extensively reviewed, including quality of life, affect, function, and agitation. Because these domains are covered in detail in other chapters, this chapter focuses on the pros and cons of various approaches rather than on the measures themselves. Other chapters review the difficulties associated with measuring the domains of quality of life, affect, and func-

tion. When examining the relative merits of approaches discussed in this chapter, it is important to remember these challenges. An additional consideration when identifying appropriate tool is the level of individual or population impairment. (The determination of cognitive skill and impairment is discussed extensively in Chapter 4.)

## DOMAINS

### Affect

Affective disorders and feelings are difficult to assess among older adults with CI because these people often cannot articulate their feelings verbally. When elders are unable to express their emotions verbally, affect must be inferred on the basis of behaviors and body language. Regardless of the source of this information (proxy, medical chart, or structured observation), inferences must be made about the meaning of individual behaviors and body languages. The nature of some diseases makes these kinds of inferences particularly challenging. For example, some diseases are associated with repetitive movements that may be incorrectly interpreted as agitation, whereas others may be associated with a certain facial expression that may be interpreted as indicating some kind of mood or affect. Regardless of ability to assess actual depression (or affective disorders), general negative affect (crying, agitation, stress, anxiety) is still important to examine. In addition, the study of affect may be an effective avenue for determining the likes

**Table 17.2.** Recommendations for Assessing Different Domains for Populations with Varying Levels of Alertness

| Domains | Comatose | Alert/unable to perform commands | Alert/ incoherent | Alert/coherent/ confused | Oriented sometimes |
|---|---|---|---|---|---|
| | | | Levels of alertness | | |
| Health (physi-ological) | + (physiological assessment, C) | + (physiological assessment, C) | + (physiological assessment, C) | + (physiological assessment, C) | + (physiological assessment, C) |
| Function | − | Challenge (O, P, C) | Challenge (O, P, C) | + (O, P, C) | + (I, O, P, C) |
| Hearing | − | − | + (O, C) | + (O, C) | + (I, O, C) |
| Vision | − | − | Challenge (O, C) | + (O, C) | + (I, O, C) |
| Nutrition | + (physiological, C, O, P) | + (physiological, C, O, P) | + (physiological, C, O, P) | + (physiological, C, O, P) | + (physiological, C, O, P) |
| Sleep | − | + (O, T/P, P, C) | + (O, T/P, P, C) | + (O, T/P, P, C) | + (I, O, T/P, P, C) |
| Pain | Challenge (O) | Challenge (O) | Challenge (O, P) | + (O, P, C) | + (I, O, P, C) |
| Cognition | − | Challenge (O, P, C) | + (O, P, C) | + (I, O, P, C) | + (I, O, P, C) |
| Quality of life | − | Challenge (O, T/P, P, C) | Challenge (O, T/P, P, C) | Challenge (O, T/P, P, C) | + (I, O, T/P, P, C) |
| Affect | − | Challenge (0, T/P, P, C) | Challenge (O, P, C, T/P) | Challenge (I, O, P, C, T/P) | + (I, O, P, C, T/P) |
| Social function-ing | − | Challenge (O, P, C) | Challenge (O, P, C) | + (O, P, C) | + (I, O, P, C) |
| Spirituality | − | − | Challenge (O, P) | Challenge (O, P) | + (I, O, P) |
| Satisfaction | − | − | − | Challenge (I, O, P) | + (I, O) |
| Values/prefer-ences | − | − | Challenge (O) | Challenge (I, O) | + (I, O)1 |

−, not recommended; +, recommended; P, proxy; I, direct interview; O, observation; T/P, technological/physiological; C, medical chart review.

and dislikes of those who cannot report internal states or preferences (Lawton et al., 1996). If we are able to meaningfully recognize positive and negative affective states, such assessment may be one way to examine the effect of interventions and study quality of life (Lawton et al., 1996).

### Approaches to Assessment

*Interview.* Moderately impaired elders may be capable of participating in standard interviews regarding depression. For example, the Geriatric Depression Scale has been found to be a valid indicator of de-

pression in mildly to moderately impaired elders (Parmelee et al., 1989). Tappen and Barry (1995) found that the Dementia Mood Picture test could be used to elicit information on emotional state even among elders with advanced dementia (Mini-Mental State Examination scores 1–11). This test combines the use of pictures of emotional expressions with questions about internal feelings. The direct assessment of affect and affective disorders has great appeal because the individual experiencing emotions should be the best informant. Although there may be several possible scales to administer with CI elders, they are still subject to interpretation because the answers to the questions may not always be straightforward (Shue, Beck, & Lawton, 1996). In addition, responses may vary with natural history patterns of confusion that are not well understood.

*Proxy.* Some affect scales are administered to both the individual with dementia and a caregiver. These include the Cornell Scale for Depression in Dementia (Alexopoloulos et al., 1988), the Dementia Signs and Symptoms Scale (Loreck, Bylsma, & Folstein, 1994), and the Dementia Mood Assessment Scale (Sunderland et al., 1988), all of which have high reliability and validity with groups of various levels of impairment. Proxies may be interviewed alone with several scales, including the Emotional Status Interview (Danner & Friesen, 1996), the Pleasant Events Schedule for Alzheimer's Disease (Teri & Logsdon, 1991), and the Family Questionnaire of the Apparent Affect Rating Scale (Lawton et al., 1996). Of course, as with any proxy report, these scales are based on unstructured observation of proxies, the accuracy of which depend on a number of factors, including frequency of contact, nature of relationship, and emotional status of the proxy. (Several good reviews regarding the validity and use of individual and proxy-based scales include Weiner et al., 1996; Teri, Logsdon, & Yesavage, 1997; and Shue et al., 1996.)

*Observation.* Several observation-based rating scales have been developed to assess depression and affect among people with dementia, including the Depressive Sign Scale of Katona and Aldridge (1985) and the Dementia Mood Assessment Scale (in combination with interviews; Sunderland et al., 1988).

Structured observation may also be used to examine more general expressions of affect among CI elders. Lawton and Colleagues at the Philadelphia Geriatric Center (Lawton et al., 1992; Lawton et al., 1996) developed an Apparent Affect Rating Scale (AARS), with 6–10 affective expressions (positive and negative) being rated during systematic observation (behavior streams). The emotions that are rated (including pleasure, anger, anxiety/fear, sadness, interest, and contentment) are defined with an ethogram of typical behaviors and rated by an observer within a defined period as never (<16 seconds), 15–59 seconds, 1–5 minutes, >5 minutes, or cannot tell for interrupted observation (Lawton et al., 1996). Behaviors associated with pleasure include, for example, smile, laugh, stroking, touching, and nodding. A similar rating scale can also be used by activity therapists and family members who can rate the frequencies of such behaviors over a longer period of time. Training research assistants to collect observational data can be done within 1 month with reliable results (kappa = 0.79–0.89) (Lawton et al., 1996). The AARS is the most systematic ethogram of emotions that has been developed to study affect among CI elders, and ratings are well correlated with standard scales of depression. Behavior streams, however, is not a good method for assessing frequency, duration, latency, or sequence of emotions and their correlates, and therefore the purpose of assessment should be carefully considered when using the AARS rating system. The ethogram can easily be used with other observational techniques such as behavior tracking or continuous recording.

*Chart data.* Some charts may contain diagnoses of affective disorders. For research purposes, these diagnoses should be used with caution given that they are often assigned by a physician rather than a trained psychologist or psychiatrist. Ideally, such diagnoses will be confirmed with a report from such personnel, but this is an inconsistent practice at best. Social services workers' or nurses' notes might document change over time with respect to mood and behavior. These are a challenge to interpret given the spotty and inconsistent nature of such reports in nurses' notes, and the absence of reports of negative affect does not necessarily indicate good mental health.

The MDS may provide more standard information on affect, particularly the section on mood and behavior and psychosocial well-being. These sections have been reported to have high reliability (Hawes et al., 1995), but they are subject to the same general problems with respect to using MDS data in research. Moreover, they are based solely on inferences (see Chapter 16). An index of depression based on MDS items (H1a Verbal Distress, H1b Nonverbal Distress, H1c Motor Agitation, H1g Suicidal Thoughts, and H2 Mood Persistence) has been developed based on factor analysis (Casten et al., 1998). It is weakly correlated, however, with standard depression scales (Lawton et al., 1998), likely as a result of difficulties in discriminating dementia and depression and biases of staff concerning the relationship between cognition and affect (Lawton et al., 1998).

*Physiological/Technological.* As discussed earlier, several physiological markers of stress can be examined as a component of affect or emotion. Stress markers appear to correlate well with facial expressions of emotion, as well as emotional and mood problems as identified in the MDS (Harper, 1998). In addition, dexamethasone suppression tests may prove useful to examine the presence of depression. They have been used with cognitively intact individuals but have rarely been used with CI elders (Rush et al., 1996). Dexamethasone suppression is not, however, universally observed among people with depression.

*Summary.* Aspects of affect that can be assessed include

- Affective disorders (depression, anxiety)
- Positive/negative affect
- Distress/stress
- Personality changes

Important aspects of choosing a method of assessment include the following:

- Consider what is an acceptable level of inference when studying affect.
- When using charted medical diagnosis, determine if a psychological assessment was performed.

- Facial expressions may be due to disease states rather than expressions of emotions.
- Absence of negative affect does not necessarily indicate presence of positive affect.
- Be aware of the potential biases that proxies may have in their impressions of emotion.

## Function

As discussed in Chapter 2, there are three major domains of functional assessment: activities of daily living (ADLs), instrumental activities of daily living (IADLs), and mobility. In the early stages of dementia, IADLs are most likely to be impaired. Physical ability to perform ADLs is unlikely to be affected until the later stages. Demented elders often forget the need for or the sequence of ADLs. Assessment of function in CI elders is important for care planning, placement, understanding the connection between cognitive deficits, identifying milestones of disease progression, and examining outcomes of behavioral or drug therapies and environmental modification (Spector, 1997). Numerous studies describe cognitive deficits associated with dementia, but there has been limited research on the relationship between cognitive and functional deficits (Mahurn, Debettignies, & Pixozzolo, 1991).

Assessment of function among cognitively impaired adults is challenging because people with CI may have both physical and cognitive disabilities. When assessing function, it is important to distinguish between physical and cognitive impairment (Beck & Frank, 1997). Elders with dementia may be physically able to complete tasks but not to think to do them and therefore need cueing and supervision. Unfortunately, it is often less time consuming and less frustrating for caregivers to complete tasks for an older adult with CI than to cue them to complete the tasks for themselves. Thus, there is often a discrepancy between capability and actual performance. Depending on the method of assessment, research or clinical assessment is likely to tap into either ability or actual performance. Such a distinction is essential, however, when using assessment to design interventions (Beck & Frank, 1997).

Typical approaches to assessment of function are self-report, proxy report, and performance measures (Beck & Frank, 1997). These approaches differ in validity, reliability, and sensitivity to change. It is also possible to assess function with observation in naturalistic settings, although there are currently no standardized methods with which to do so (Zimmerman & Magaziner, 1994). Some performance-based ADL measures have been designed specifically for people with CI. Assessments are designed to recognize early stages of dementia and clinical deficits that are related to cognitive impairments rather than motor impairments (Zimmerman & Magaziner, 1994). These tools focus on functional impairments that are common to those with dementia. Examples include the Structured Assessment of Independent Living Skills (Mahurn et al., 1991), Dressing Assessment Guide (Heacock et al., 1997), Direct Assessment of Functional Status (Lowenstein et al., 1989), and Clinical Dementia Rating Scale (Skurla, Rogers, & Sunderland, 1988).

## Approaches to Assessment

*Interview.* The same scales that are used with non-CI elders can also be used with CI persons. As with any self-report measure of function, a concern is that individuals may answer questions with respect to what they can do or what they actually do. In clinical practice, when a resident/patient responds "can't do . . . ," motivation may be also questioned. At the other extreme, individuals may have unrealistic expectations due to being cognitively impaired. For a CI person to give a valid response to questions, the individual must have both receptive and expressive communication skills (Spector, 1997). An even more challenging problem is the assessment of CI older adults' capacity to make judgments about their ability for which

there is no standard assessment method (Spector, 1997).

*Proxy.* Scales that are developed for self-report can and have been adapted to be used with proxies. Proxy-based scales include the IADL and ADL subscales of the Blessed Dementia Scale (Blessed, Tomlinson, & Roth, 1968), the Cleveland ADL scale, and the Functional Assessment Stage Scale (Reisberg et al., 1987). As with any proxy-based information, the accurate assessment of function requires that proxies have enough knowledge of the skills of the CI person. Clinical staff often report lower functional ability than patients (Zimmerman & Magaziner, 1994). Agreement is generally higher on questions about discrete observable aspects of functioning (Zimmerman & Magaziner, 1994). The source of disagreement between responses of CI elders and their proxies is often hard to determine. It may be due to the general phenomenon of proxies typically under-reporting ability, or it could be due to unrealistic evaluation of the CI individual. More research is needed to compare proxy reports with performance-based measures.

*Observation.* Specific performance-based measures are reviewed extensively in Chapter 2. These measures have the advantage of being more objective about and quantifiable of actual ability. They can also be used when a CI person cannot answer questions but can follow directions. On the other hand, there remains the discrepancy between what a person is capable of doing and what he or she actually does. In addition, CI persons may have more difficulty following directions in an unfamiliar settings where the usual context or clues are not available (Zimmerman & Magaziner, 1994). Good measures of function for people with CI should distinguish between disability due to cognitive versus physical deficits. Some scales rely on the observation of the amount of help needed to complete tasks, and again it is important to distinguish between physical assistance and cueing. Currently, most scales are not well designed to make this distinction, and cueing is difficult to measure (Spector, 1997).

*Charts.* The MDS has an ADL section that includes both ability of the resident and the amount of assistance needed with the task. These items are reported to have high reliability (Hawes et al., 1995). These data are not very detailed, however. Some nursing homes use more extensive functional assessments performed by a physical therapist or rehabilitation nurse. Such assessments are likely to vary in detail, quality, and format across institutions, making their utility minimal unless standard assessment instruments are employed.

*Physiological/Technological.* Night-time incontinence episodes may be recorded more accurately with specially wired wetness pads (Schnelle et al., 1998; Ouslander et al., 1998; Cruise et al., 1998). The use of such technology is not warranted in all situations but has shown that policies regarding night-time incontinence protocols may be overzealous (Ouslander et al., 1998). Eventually, the use of such technology may allow clinicians to tailor night-time incontinence care to minimize skin breakdown while also minimizing sleep disruption (Schnelle et al., 1998).

*Summary.* Aspects of function that can be assessed include

- Time to complete tasks
- Ability to complete tasks
- Actual functional performance
- Frequency and timing of incontinence episodes

Important aspects of choosing a method of assessment include the following:

- Be aware of the distinction between capability and actual performance.
- Be aware of motivational issues and compensating behaviors of staff.
- Consider cueing as part of the assessment.
- Use methods that distinguish physical and cognitive disabilities.

### Behavior Problems/Agitation

Behavioral problems and agitation are common problems in nursing homes and may be a considerable source of family/caregiver distress. Although estimates of prevalence vary, approximately 60% of nursing home residents are reported to have behavioral problems (Zimmer, Watson, & Trea, 1984), and approximately 90% of nursing home residents exhibit at least one behavioral problem a week (Cohen-Mansfield et al., 1989; Rovner et al., 1986; Tariot et al., 1993). Data on the prevalence of behavioral problems among community dwelling elders are not currently available.

Confusion and agitation may be further induced in facilities that commonly use chemical and/or physical restraints (Cohen-Mansfield, 1996). Mental illness is often not properly diagnosed in long-term care facilities because most do not perform formal psychiatric evaluations (Baker, 1991). Almost 60% of psychiatric disorders are not diagnosed, primarily due to failure to correctly identify neurologic or psychiatric diseases (Baker, 1991). Delirium due to acute illness may be misdiagnosed as dementia, leading to improper administration of medication and management of behavioral disturbances.

Agitation has been defined as "inappropriate verbal, vocal, or motor activity that is not explained by needs or confusion *per se*" (Cohen-Mansfield & Billig, 1986). Agitative behaviors have been divided into three major syndromes: physically aggressive behavior (hitting, kicking); physically nonaggressive behavior (pacing, disrobing, wandering); and verbally agitative behavior (constant repetitions of words) (Cohen-Mansfield et al., 1989; Teresi et al., 1994). A more complex taxonomy can be based on a multimethod assessment approach: verbal aggression/vocal agitation (screaming, moaning, complaining), physical aggression (inflicting self-harm or harm to others), affective behavioral disorder (crying, seeking reassurance, rejecting others, coldness), psychotic behavior (delusions, hallucinations, confusion), wandering, and asocial behaviors (disrupting others, disrobing, sloppy eating). Regardless of which classification system is used, agitative behaviors likely have multiple patterns of expression and etiologies (Cohen-Mansfield, 1994). Agitation is a relatively rare event, and thus assessment must include a large enough time window to capture agitative behaviors. Agitative behaviors are spotty. There is no single behavior that is observed more than 10% of the time. Research on aggression has shown that aggressive behaviors often occur less often than once a month (Marin et al., 1997; Gilley et al., 1997).

Sleep disorders may also be classified as behavioral disturbances, especially when they are associated with night-time wandering or disruptive vocalizations. Sleep disorders may be symptomatic of certain diseases, particularly Alzheimer's disease, or they may result from environmental stimuli (or lack of stimulus). Sleep apnea is particularly common among persons with dementia (Ancoli-Israel et al., 1991). In addition, the portion of the brain that regulates circadian rhythms and thus sleep patterns (superchiasmatic nucleus of the hypothalamus) may be subject to neuronal death as a part of a disease process (Hoogendijk et al., 1996). People with Alzheimer's disease who live in the community have on average 30 minutes of exposure to light (Campbell et al., 1991), whereas nursing home residents are exposed to bright light on average only 1.6 minutes per day (Ancoli-Israel & Kripke, 1989). Such low levels of light exposure can result in a disrupted circadian rhythm (Monjan, 1994). Thus, behavioral patterns and environmental circumstances may induce sleeping disturbances (Schnelle et al., 1993b). Such disturbances are likely to increase agitative behaviors during day-time and night-time hours. More research on sleep disorders among CI is needed to determine etiology.

Agitative behaviors may indicate some sort of distress for the individual, or they may not. Behaviors that are considered inappropriate by staff may seem appropriate to the actor. For example, a confused elder may constantly be taking his or her clothes off in the middle of the day because he or she thinks that it is time for bed (Cohen-Mansfield, Marx, & Rosenthal, 1992). To date, no research has been conducted that can be used to distinguish between stress-inducing versus non-stress-inducing agitation. Physiological assessment of stress in relation to agitation has great potential to make those distinctions. Preliminary research has indicated that agitation in general is associated with stress responses. In a small sample of nursing home residents, agitative behaviors were associated with increased blood pressure. In addition, those identified in the MDS as having mood or behavior problems had higher salivary cortisol and diastolic blood pressure levels, particularly in the late afternoon, evening, and night-time hours (Harper, 1998). Little is known about the causes of agitation, but research has suggested that numerous conditions may lead to agitation, including cognitive impairment, premorbid stress and fatigue, and lack of exercise, stimulation, and activity (Cohen-Mansfield et al., 1992).

Preliminary evidence suggests that particular institutional rhythms may precipitate agitation in demented individuals (Exum et al., 1993) and accidents in the general resident population (e.g., skin tears, falls; Gurwitz et al., 1994). Many institutionalized elderly suffer from "sundowner's syndrome," a period of agitation that often occurs coincident with evening meals. This may be due to a general change in sensitivity to light but is equally likely a result of in-house environmental stimuli (Exum et al., 1993; Bliwise, 1994). Early evening hours are often filled with a whirlwind of activities: meals, special activities, shift turnovers, and aid with ADLs. Such stimulation was noted by Cohen-Mansfield and colleagues (1992), who observed that residents also became more agitated on weekends and holidays (times when regular staff were more likely to be absent) regardless of time (Bliwise, 1994).

Agitative behaviors represent a particular challenge in nursing home environments because they affect not only the acting resident but also the staff and other residents. In fact, agitation in one resident often precipitates agitation in others, producing a seemingly uncontrollable and frustrating event for the nursing staff (Harper, 1998). Thus, research on agitation and its treatment is important not only at the individual level but also for institutional settings as a whole. Behavioral disturbances are associated with increased caregiver burden, patient and caregiver abuse, psychotropic medication use, and institutionalization (see Marin et al., 1997).

## Approaches to Assessment

*Interview.* The Neurobehavioral Rating Scale (Levin et al., 1987), which was originally developed for a variety of neuropsychiatric disorders, has been used with patients with dementia (Sultzer, Berisford, & Gunay, 1995). This scales appears to have potential for further use and is still under study. A few scales have been developed that are completed with a combination of individual and proxy responses. (Tariot et al., [1996] review these scales.) The use of participant response is probably not the best approach given that even mildly CI individuals may be unaware of agitative behaviors.

*Proxy.* There are numerous scales, both general behavioral measures and those developed specifically to measure agitation, to administer to caregivers. Some frequently used scales include the Cohen-Mansfield Agitation Inventory (Cohen-Mansfield, 1986), the Brief Psychiatric Rating Scale (Overall & Gorham, 1988), the Multidimensional Observation Scale for Elderly Subjects (Helmes, Csapo, & Short, 1987), the Behavior Rating Scale for Dementia (Tariot et al., 1995), the Behavioral Pathology in Alzheimer's Disease Rating Scale (Reisberg et al., 1987), the Ryden Aggression Scale (Ryden, 1988), and the Revised Memory and Behavior Problems Checklist (Teri et al., 1992). These have all been determined to have

good reliability and validity. (Good reviews of these scales are given by Weiner et al., 1996; Zaudig, 1996; and Tariot, 1996.) Given that proxy reports are less accurate with rare events (Grootendorst et al., 1997), agitation may be particularly prone to inaccurate proxy reports. These scales have been validated primarily against other scales; few have been evaluated in comparison with good structured observation and thus should still be used with caution.

*Observation.* The actual frequencies and durations of agitation can be measured only through direct observation, which is also the best way to examine the causes of behavioral problems. When this approach is used, measures of the environment should be included to determine important environmental and temporal stimuli. Agitation can be examined with respect to time, place, environmental attributes, and social context. The only way to see the direct effects of interventions is through observation. The two major groups who have examined agitation are Burgio and colleagues (Burgio et al., 1994, 1996; Burgio & Leon, 1997) and Cohen-Mansfield and colleagues (Cohen-Mansfield et al., 1989, 1992, 1995; Cohen-Mansfield, 1994, 1995, 1996). These methods are discussed in a previous section. Continuous time recording is likely to result in a more accurate picture of agitation and its correlates; however, continuous time recording and periodic observation have never been directly compared.

*Charts.* There are several areas of medical charts that discuss behavioral problems, including the MDS (mood and behavior section), nurses' notes, and a form for inappropriate vocalization/behavior, which is used to validate the use of medication. In all cases, charted agitation is based on perceptions. The use of such sources depends on the accuracy needed for a research question or clinical goal. Chart data potentially allow examination over a longer time period and may give a long-term context for behavior. Chart data have not been compared with observation to determine their accuracy.

*Physiological/technological.* Actigraphs and step-sensors, may be a good proxy for agitation (e.g., wandering, restlessness, and sleep disorders), but the validity has not been tested. We need to further examine agitation with respect to blood pressure, cortisol, and catecholamine levels. Physiological methods may show that not all behaviors considered agitation by observers are distressful or stress producing for actors. Some behaviors may be more stress producing than others. In some circumstances, behaviors that we label as agitative may be adaptive for people with CI.

*Summary.* Aspects of behavior problems and agitation that can be assessed include the following

- Frequency
- Intensity
- Etiology
- Environmental stimuli
- Temporal pattern
- Aggression
- Wandering
- Sleep disorders
- Impact on others

Important aspects of choosing a method of assessment include the following:

1. Code different behaviors separately.
2. Take into account the relative rarity of agitative behaviors in designing assessment technique and method of analysis.
3. Realize that the determination of what behaviors are appropriate depends on environmental and social context as well as caregiver's circumstances.
4. Be aware that not all behaviors may indicate distress.

### Quality of Life

Multiple domains are combined (and perhaps weighted) to provide an overall summary measure of quality of life (QOL). When people cannot reliably express themselves because of cognitive impairment, the problems of assessing any single domain are compounded. As Chapter 7 suggests, there are various schools of thought on measuring QOL. First, measures are divided into health-related QOL (either global or related to a specific health condition) and general QOL that is not conditioned on health. Whichever approach is used, typically the domains and their component items are generated through discussions with representatives of the population whose QOL is to be measured (either those with the specific disease) or older people in general.

People with dementia will be able to participate imperfectly (if at all) in such an exercise. Therefore, the biggest problem in measuring QOL is the conceptual task of deciding what conditions, circumstances, or outcomes constitute a good or poor QOL for someone with dementia at a specific stage. Value judgments are obviously needed. It is hardly an acceptable solution to ask people before they have dementia about what they would value as a good QOL if they did have the disease. It is simply impossible to enter into the unknowable experience of dementia, although inferences about what is enjoyed or not enjoyed must be drawn from observed behavior. It is even a further leap to order what is important in a good QOL.

Recently, considerable emphasis has been given to measuring well-being, including QOL, for people with dementia in nursing homes; the entire 1999 issue of the *Journal of Mental Health and Aging* was devoted to the conceptual and technical aspects of the subject (Albert and Logsdon, 1999). In considering how to define QOL, ethicist Bruce Jennings reviewed various philosophical accounts of a good life, including hedonic or pleasure theories, rational preference theories, and theories of human flourishing (Jennings, 1999). He concluded that the hedonic approach may be the only way to evaluate the QOL of a given person with dementia, but that other ways of thinking must be taken into account in a policy sense so that the life of an unhappy person with dementia is not deemed meaningless and, therefore, not worth living. Other investigators have proposed a definition that largely deals with the affective dimension; for example, Volicer, Hurley, and Camberg (1999) propose a six-factor model of QOL that includes three positive components (happy mood, engagement, and calm) and three negative components (sad mood, apathy, and agitation). In a conclusory essay, Whitehouse (1999) summarized the material in the entire volume and suggested that some attention be given to quality of dying in measuring QOL for people with dementia. Those investigators who have done pioneering work in trying to summarize QOL for people with dementia have relied on most of the methods of data collection reviewed in this chapter, as the succeeding sections show.

## Approaches to Assessment

*Interview.* One approach to measuring QOL for people with dementia is to employ the same measures used in the general population. For example, McHorney used the SF-36, a well-known QOL measure (see Chapter 7), and found, with few exceptions, that its psychometric properties were similar among CI and non-CI populations. Others have interviewed mildly cognitively impaired people using various health-related QOL measures with varying success. Not many reports can be found in the literature about the reliability of these approaches. Uman and Urman of Vital Research, Inc., have expended substantial effort in developing a multidimensional self-report measure of QOL for residents of nursing homes. They started their work with the recognition that people with dementia are heavily represented in nursing homes and sought to devise a tool that would reliably tap the "consumer's voice," including as many consumers with dementia as possible. Their instrument is called the REAL (Real Experiences and Assessment of Life). The domains they attempt to measure are help and assistance; communication with staff; autonomy and choice; companionship; safety and security; and food and environment. Using an instrument that is entirely composed of yes/no answers, they were able to obtain satisfactory results (good or high test–retest reliability) from many residents with dementia, although at the cost of reducing the responses of all residents to a simplistic level (see Uman, 1995).

Several direct interview approaches have been developed for and tested with people with Alzheimer's disease in and out of nursing homes. The easiest to use is the Quality of Life—AD Scale, a brief 13 item measure, each with a 4 point response set (Logsdon et al., 1999). The subject is asked to rate physical health, energy, mood, living situation, memory, family, marriage, friends, self, ability to do chores, ability to do things for fun, money, and life as a whole. The items are simply summed. In a sample of 77 community dwelling AD patients, only 5 were unable to complete the Quality of Life—AD Scale, and they all had Mini-Mental Status scores of less than 10. The residents' ratings were correlated with more positive scores on the Pleasant Events—AD Scale, but cognitive status itself was not predictive of QOL.

Another example is the longer D-QOL, developed by Brod and colleagues (see Brod, Stewart, & Sands, 1999a; Brod et al., 1999b). This latter tool also has five QOL domains: aesthetics, positive affect, negative affect, self-esteem, and feelings of belonging. Work with the Logsdon and Teri tool, the tool of Brod and colleagues, the direct-interview tools, and the REAL give encouragement to the idea that data can be gathered by direct report from many nursing home residents with dementia.

*Proxy.* Both health-related and general QOL measures have been studied with proxy reports from both family and staff. Often scales developed for non-CI populations are adapted for people with dementia. Most have "floor effects" for these very impaired populations because of the activity restriction common to people with dementia. The 13 item Quality of Life—AD Scale has been applied to family members of people with dementia (Logsdon et al., 1999). Although the responses were correlated with those of the CI person, they were not identical, and those family caregivers who were depressed rated their relative's QOL as worse than caregivers who were not depressed. Albert and colleagues (1999a) found poor correlation between proxy reports of QOL from a sample of caregivers in an Alzheimer's disease clinic and proxy reports from a variety of community caregivers. The poor correlation raises questions about the difficulties in training a large group of paraprofessional and family proxies to make ratings.

Some measures concentrate staff or family report on behavioral symptoms exhibited by the person with dementia. These tend to render caregiving more difficult but may not be evidence per se of a poor QOL. For instance, wandering or persevering questions may annoy caregivers but not bother the person with dementia, whereas other observable phenomena such as moaning, weeping, shouting, and handwriting have more face validity as signs of distress. Some people would consider the Multidimensional Observation Scale for Elderly Subjects (MOSES) (Helmes et al., 1987) to be a QOL measure because it taps multiple domains such as depression, anxiety, social relationships, and activity. Rabins and colleagues (1999) are now testing a multidimensional instrument for measuring the QOL of people with dementia through reports from caregivers, either family or paid. Like the MOSES, it appears to have highly specific items. It contains five domains: social interaction, awareness of self, feeling and mood, enjoyment of activities, and response to surroundings.

Some proxy measures considering positive and negative aspects of behavior have been used as reported in the literature as measures of QOL (Albert, 1997). Negative aspects have been measured by the Cohen-Mansfield Agitation Index, Discomfort Scale; positive aspects have been measured with the Pleasant Events Schedule. Both

positive and negative aspects of QOL can be captured with the Affect Rating Scale and the Progressive Deterioration Scale. When examining negative indicators, it is important to realize that the absence of negative indicators does not necessarily indicate a positive quality of life (Albert, 1997). In addition, some negative indicators may be beneficial in certain contexts. For example, wandering is commonly seen as an indicator of agitation; however, wandering may be a positive activity for many that allows an outlet for energy and helps an individual sleep better at night (Albert, 1997).

*Observation.* Lawton (1997) has examined QOL through observation, using behavior streams. He suggests that the following dimensions are relevant: expressions of affect, function, time use, social engagement, and environmental quality. He is a pioneer in the development of observational approaches to gauge affect, reporting success in achieving reliable observations with trained research assistants. Success in training nurse's aides to make these observations is more mixed (Lawton et al., 1999).

Another observational approach utilizes the Clinical Dementia Rating (Schafer et al., 1996), a global rating that evaluates multiple domains of functioning: overall QOL, happiness, physical comfort, independence, and relations with family and friends. Raters were shown videotaped interviews of a resident with mild dementia and with severe dementia. The reliability of this clinical dementia rating among trained raters seeing the same stimulus is high. The unique feature of this application was that raters were also asked to rate the utilities of the individual on the videotape using a time trade-off technique (Sano et al., 1999). (See Chapter 8 for a discussion of time trade-off methods to establish preferences.)

*Charts.* Some information that may be considered relevant to QOL, especially health-related QOL, can be found in medical charts in nursing homes. For example, the MDS items on mood and behavior, psychosocial well-being, and activity pursuit may be examined with respect to QOL. The limitations of these data noted earlier in this chapter must, however, be considered.

*Physiological/Technological.* If part of a good QOL is having low levels of stress, depression, and agitation and adequate sleep, the physiological and technological measures of these domains may be examined with the tools discussed earlier. In addition, for someone who is concerned with the relationship and response to the environment (e.g., affects of location, noise, light, and social environment on blood pressure, cortisol level, catecholamine level, and agitation), these techniques are useful.

*Summary.* Aspects of QOL that can be assessed include

- Health-related QOL
- Affect
- Social functioning
- Stress
- Sleep
- Behavioral symptoms
- Time use
- Environmental quality

Important aspects of choosing a method of assessment include the following:

- Quality of life and/or its components must be clearly defined.
- Objective measures should be separate from subjective measures.
- Absence of negative indicators of QOL does not automatically indicate positive QOL.

## CONCLUSIONS

There are multiple approaches to assessing older adults with CI, but no one perfect approach or tool. Instead, each approach has pros and cons that must be balanced according to the goals of clinical assessment and the research hypotheses. One must carefully consider the balance between quality and practicality based on as-

sessment or research goals. Formal assessment of potential biases and level of knowledge of the individual subject should be a part of proxy interviews. When using an observational approach, it is important to distinguish between structured observation and impressions. Observational methods should be designed with consideration of coding techniques, types of measures, and sampling methods in order to properly examine a domain of interest. Time and money permitting, multiple methods should be used in order to triangulate results. Although there are no gold standards in assessing CI elders, all new methods for a domain should be compared against structured (naturalistic) observation or direct assessment (nutritional, health status, and so forth).

## FUTURE DIRECTIONS

- More research is needed to compare multiple methods to determine which methods are most appropriate for each domain and for each measurement population. In addition, a balance between cost and quality should be considered.
- More research is needed on the natural history of confusion for those people in early stages of dementia to determine when direct interviews can most appropriately be conducted.
- In general, more research is needed on patient-focused measures (direct interview/assessment). This is particularly important for the development of standards to determine who is appropriate to interview for a particular domain.
- We should try to improve the quality of proxies by giving them proper training to perform structured observations on their own.
- Technological and physiological assessments have great potential; however, more research should be conducted on such assessments. In addition, with some creative thinking, more approaches are likely to be developed.

# REFERENCES

Abrams, R. C., & Alexopoulos, G. S. (1994). Assessment of depression in dementia. *Alzheimer Disease and Associated Disorders, 8*(Suppl 1), S227–S229.

Albert, S., Castillo-Castenada, C., Jacobs, D., Sano, M., Bell, K., Merchant, C., Small, S., & Stern, Y. (1999). Proxy-reported quality of life in Alzheimer's patients: Comparison of clinical and population-based samples. *Journal of Health and Aging*(5), 1.

Albert, S., Del Castillo-Castaneda, C., Sano, M., Jacobs, D., Marder, K., Bell, K., Blysma, F., Lafleche, G., Brandt, J., Albert, M., & Stern, Y. (1996). Quality of life in patients with Alzheimer's disease as reported by patient proxies. *Journal of the American Geriatrics Society, 44,* 1342–1347.

Albert, S. M. (1997). Assessing health-related quality of life in chronic care populations. *Journal of Mental Health and Aging, 3,* 101–118.

Albert, S. M. & Logsdon, R. G. (Eds.) (1999). Assessing Quality of Life in Alzheimer's Disease. *Journal of Mental Health and Aging, 5*(1), special issue.

Alexopoloulos, G. S., Abrams, R. C., Young, R. C., & Shamoian, C. A. (1988). Cornell scale for depression in dementia. *Biological Psychiatry, 23,* 271–284.

Altman, J. (1974). Observational study of behavior: Sampling methods. *Behavior, 49,* 227–265.

Ancoli-Israel, S., Klauber, M. R., Butters, N., Parker, L., & Kripke, D. F. (1991). Dementia in institutionalized elderly: Relation to sleep apnea. *Journal of the American Geriatrics Society, 39*(3), 258–263.

Ancoli-Israel, S., & Kripke, D. F. (1989). Now I lay me down to sleep: The problem of sleep fragmentation in elderly and demented nursing home residents. *Bulletin of American Neuroscience, 54,* 127–132.

Bakeman, R., & Gottman, J. (1997). *Observing interaction.* Cambridge: Cambridge University Press.

Baker, F. (1991). Behavioral disorders in skilled nursing homes. In M. Harper (Ed.), *Management and care of the elderly: Psychosocial perspectives* (pp. 24–33). Newbury Park, CA: Sage.

Beck, C. K., & Frank, L. B. (1997). Assessing functioning and self-care abilities in Alzheimer's disease research. *Alzheimer's Disease and Associated Disorders, 11*(6), 73–80.

Bernard, H. R. (1995). *Research methods in anthropology. Qualitative and quantitative approaches.* (2nd ed.). Walnut Creek, CA: Alta Mira Press.

Berne, R. M., & Levy, M. N. (1993). *Physiology* (3rd ed.). St. Louis: Mosby Yearbook.

Blessed, G., Tomlinson, B. E., & Roth, M. (1968). The association between quantitative measures of dementia and senile change in cerebral gray matter of elderly subjects. *British Journal of Psychiatry, 114,* 797–811.

Bliwise, D. L. (1994). What is sundowning? *Journal of the American Geriatrics Society, 42,* 1009–1011.

Brewer, J., & Hunter, A. (1989). *Multimethod research: A synthesis of styles.* Newbury Park, CA: Sage.

Brod, M., Stewart, A., & Sands, L. (1999a). Conceptualization of quality of life in dementia. *Journal of Mental Health and Aging, 5*(1), 7–19.

Brod, M., Stewart, A. L., Sands, L., & Walton, P. (1999b). Conceptualization and measurement of quality of life in dementia. The Dementia Quality of Life Instrument (DQoL). *Gerontologist, 39*(1), 25–35.

Burgio, L., & Leon, J. (1997). Using patient and proxy reports as outcome measures in Alzheimer's disease research. *Alzheimer's Disease and Associated Disorders, 11*(6), 179–180.

Burgio, L., Scilley, K., Hardin, J. M., Hsu, C., & Yancey, J. (1996). Environmental "white noise": An intervention for verbally agitated nursing home residents. *Journal of Gerontology, 51B,* 364–373.

Burgio, L. D., Scilley, K., Hardin, J. M., Janosky, J., Bonino, P., Slater, S. C., & Engberg, R. (1994). Studying disruptive vocalization and contextual factors in nursing home using computer-assisted real-time observation. *Journal of Gerontology, 49,* 230–239.

Campbell, S. S., Satlin, A., Volicer, L., Ross, V., & Herz, L. (1991). Management of behavioral and sleep disturbance in Alzheimer's patients using timed exposure to bright light. *Sleep Research, 20,* 446.

Casten, R., Lawton, M. P., Parmelee, P. A., & Kleban, M. H. (1998). Psychometric characteristics of the Minimum Data Set I: Confirmatory factor analysis. *Journal of the American Geriatrics Society, 46,* 726–735.

Chandler, J. D., & Chandler, J. E. (1988). The prevalence of neuropsychiatric disorders in a nursing home population. *Journal of Geriatric Psychiatry and Neurology, 1*(2), 71–76.

Cohen-Mansfield, J. (1986). Agitated behaviors

in the elderly II. Preliminary results in the cognitively deteriorated. *Journal of the American Geriatrics Society, 34,* 722–727.

Cohen-Mansfield, J. (1994). Reflections on the assessment of behavior in nursing home residents. *Alzheimer's Disease and Associated Disorders, 8*(1), 217–222.

Cohen-Mansfield, J. (1995). Assessment of disruptive behavior/agitation in the elderly: Function, methods, and difficulties. *Journal of Geriatric Psychiatry and Neurology, 8,* 52–60.

Cohen-Mansfield, J. (1996). Conceptualization of agitation: Results based on Cohen-Mansfield agitation inventory and the agitation behavior mapping instrument. *International Psychogeriatrics, 8*(3), 309–315.

Cohen-Mansfield, J., & Billig, N. (1986). Agitated behaviors in the elderly: A conceptual review. *Journal of the American Geriatrics Society, 34,* 711–721.

Cohen-Mansfield, J., Marx, M. S., & Rosenthal, A. S. (1989). A description of agitation in a nursing home. *Journal of Gerontology, 44*(3), M77–M84.

Cohen-Mansfield, J., Marx, M. S., & Rosenthal, A. S. (1992). Temporal patterns of agitated nursing home residents. *International Psychogeriatrics, 4,* 197–206.

Cohen-Mansfield, J., Werner, P., Watson, V., & Pasis, S. (1995). Agitation among elderly persons at adult day-care centers: The experiences of relatives and staff members. *International Psychogeriatrics, 7,* 447–458.

Corder, L. S., Woodbury, M. A., & Manton, K. G. (1996). Proxy response patterns among the aged: Effects on estimations of health status and medical care utilization from 1982–1984 long-term care surveys. *Journal of Clinical Epidemiology, 49,* 173–182.

Cruise, P. A., Schnelle, J. F., Alessi, C. A., & Ouslander, J. G. (1998). The nighttime environment and incontinence care practices in nursing homes. *Journal of the American Geriatrics Society, 46,* 181–186.

Danner, D. D., & Friesen, W. V. (1996). Are severely impaired Alzheimer's patients aware of their environment and illness? *Journal of Clinical Gero-Psychology, 2,* 321–336.

Dunbar, R. (1976). Some aspects of research design and their implication in the observational study of behavior. *Behavior, 58,* 78–98.

Exum, M. D., Phelps, B. J., Nabers, K. E., & Osborne, J. G. (1993). Sundown syndrome: Is it reflected in the use of PRN medications in nursing home residents. *Gerontologist, 33,* 756–761.

Flinn, M. V., & England, B. G. (1995). Family environment and childhood stress. *Current Anthropology, 36,* 854–866.

Flinn, M. V., & England, B. G. (1997). Social economics of childhood glucocorticoid stress response and health. *American Journal of Physical Anthropology, 102,* 33–54.

Gilley, D. W., Wilson, R. S., Beckett, L. A., & Evans, D. A. (1997). Psychotic symptoms and physically aggressive behavior in Alzheimer's disease. *Journal of the American Geriatrics Society, 45*(9), 1074–1079.

Grootendorst, P. V., Feeny, D. H., & Furlong, W. (1997). Does it matter whom and how you ask? Inter- and intra-rater agreement in the Ontario Health Survey. *Journal of Clinical Epidemiology, 50,* 127–135.

Gubrium, J. F., & Sankar (Eds.) (1994). *Qualitative Methods in Aging Research.* Thousand Oaks, CA: Sage.

Gurwitz, J. H., Sanchez-Cross, M. T., Eckler, M. A., & Matulis, J. (1994). The epidemiology of adverse and unexpected events in the long-term care setting. *Journal of the American Geriatrics Society, 42,* 33–38.

Harper, G. J. (1998). *Stress and Adaptation Among Elders in Life Care Communities.* Columbus: Ohio State University.

Harper, M. (1985). Survey of drugs and mental disorders in nursing homes. In R. More & T. Teal (Eds.), *Geriatric Drug Use: Clinical and Social Perspectives* (pp. 101–114). Elmsford: Pergamon.

Harrison, G., & Jefferies, D. (1977). Human biology in urban environments: A review of research strategies. In P. Baker (Ed.), *MAB Technical Notes 3.* Paris: Unesco.

Hawes, C., Morris, J. N., Phillips, C. D., Mor, V., Fries, B. E., & Nonemaker, S. (1995). Reliability estimates for the Minimum Data Set for Nursing Home Resident Assessment and care screening (MDS). *Gerontologist, 35*(2), 172–178.

Heacock, P. R., Beck, C. M., Souder, E., & Mercer, S. (1997). Assessing dressing ability in dementia. *Geriatric Nursing, 18,* 107–111.

Helmes, E., Csapo, K. G., & Short, J. A. (1987). Standardization and validation of the Multidimensional Observational Scale for Elderly Subjects (MOSES). *Journal of Gerontology, 42,* 395–405.

Henderson, J. N. (1994). The culture of special care units: An anthropological perspective on ethnographic research in nursing home settings. *Alzheimer's Disease and Associated Disorders, 8,* 140–416.

Hiramatsu, R. (1981). Direct assay of cortisol

in human saliva by solid phase radioim-munoassay. *Clinica Chimica Acta, 117,* 239–249.

Hoogendijk, W. J., vanSomeren, E. J. W., Mir-miran, M., Hofman, M. A., Lucassen, P. J., Zhou, J.-N., & Swabb, D. F. (1996). Circad-ian rhythm-related behavioral disturbances and structural hypothalamic changes in Alz-heimer's disease. *International Psycho-geriatrics, 8*(3), 245–252.

James, G. D. (1991a). Blood pressure response to the daily stressors of urban environ-ments: Methodology, basic concepts, and significance. *Yearbook of Physical Anthro-pology, 34,* 189–210.

James, G. D. (1991b). Race and perceived stress independently affect the diurnal vari-ation of blood pressure in women. *Ameri-can Journal of Hypertension, 4,* 382–384.

James, G. D., & Brown, D. E. (1997). The bio-logical stress response and lifestyle: Cate-cholamines and blood pressure. *Annual Review of Anthropology, 26,* 313–335.

James, G. D., Cates, E. M., Pickering, T. G., & Laragh, J. H. (1989). Parity and perceived job stress elevate blood pressure in young normotensive women. *American Journal of Hypertension, 2,* 637–639.

James, G. D., & Pickering, T. G. (1991). Ambu-latory blood pressure monitoring: Assess-ing the diurnal variation of blood pressure. *American Journal of Physical Anthropol-ogy, 84,* 343–349.

James, G. D., & Pickering, T. G. (1993). The influence of behavioral factors on the daily variation of blood pressure. *American Journal of Hypertension, 6,* 170–174S.

Jennings, B. (1999). A life greater than the sum of its sensations: Ethics, dementia, and the quality of life. *Journal of Mental Health and Aging, 5*(1), 95–106.

Kane, R. L. (1997). Which outcomes matter in Alzheimer's disease and who should define them? *Alzheimer's Disease and Associated Disorders, 11*(6), 12–17.

Katona, C. L. E., & Aldridge, C. R. (1985). The dexamethasone suppression test and depressive signs in dementia. *Journal of Affective Disorders, 8,* 83–89.

Keith, J. (1988). Participant observation. In K. W. Schaie & K. Warner (Eds.), *Me-thodological Issues in Aging Research* (pp. 211–230). New York: Springer.

Lawton, M. (1997). Assessing quality of life in Alzheimer's disease research. *Alzheimer's Disease and Associated Disorders, 11*(6), 91–99.

Lawton, M., Van Haitsma, K., Perkinson, M., & Ruckdeschel, K. (1999). Observed affect and quality of life: Further affirmations and problems. *Journal of Mental Health and Aging, 5*(1), 69–82.

Lawton, M. P., Casten, R., Parmelee, P. A., Van Haitsma, K., Corn, J., & Kleban, M. H. (1998). Psychometric characteristics of the Minimum Data Set II: Validity. *Journal of the American Geriatrics Society, 46,* 736–744.

Lawton, M. P., Kleban, M. H., Dean, J., Ra-jagopal, D., & Parmelee, P. A. (1992). The factorial generality of brief positive and negative affect measures. *Journal of Ger-ontology, 47*(4), 228–237.

Lawton, M. P., Van Haitsma, K., & Klapper, J. (1996). Observed affect in nursing home residents with Alzheimer's disease. *Journal of Gerontology, 51B,* 3–14.

Lerner, P. (1979). *Handbook of ethological methods.* New York: Garland STPM Press.

Levin, H. S., High, W. M., Goethe, K. E., Sis-son, R. A., Overall, J. E., Rhoade, H. M., Eisenberg, H. M., Klisky, Z., & Gary, H. E. (1987). The neurobehavioral rating scale: Assessment of behavioral sequalae of head injury by the clinician. *Journal of Neurology, Neurosurgery and Psychiatry, 50,* 183–193.

Logsdon, R., Gibbons, L., McCurry, S., & Teri, L. (1999). Quality of life in Alzheimer's disease: Patient and caregiver reports. *Journal of Mental Health and Aging, 5*(1), 21–32.

Loreck, D. J., Bylsma, F. W., & Folstein, M. F. (1994). A new scale for comprehensive psychopathology in Alzheimer's disease. *American Journal of Geriatric Psychiatry, 2L,* 60–74.

Lowenstein, D., Amigo, E., Duara, R., Guter-man, A., Hurwitz, D., Berkowitz, N., Wilkie, F., Weinberg, G., Black, B., Gittel-man, B., & Eisdorfer, C. (1989). A new scale for the assessment of functional sta-tus in Alzheimer's disease and related dis-orders. *Journal of Gerontology: Psycho-logical Sciences, 44*(4), 114–121.

Lyman, K. (1994). Fieldwork in groups and in-stitutions. In J. Gubrium & A. Sankar (Eds.), *Qualitative Methods in Aging Re-search* (pp. 155–170). Thousand Oaks, CA: Sage.

Magaziner, J. (1997). Use of proxies to measure health and functional outcomes in effec-tiveness research in persons with Alzhei-mer's disease and related disorders. *Alzhei-mer's Disease and Associated Disorders, 11*(6), 168–174.

Mahurn, R. K., Debettignies, B. H., & Pix-ozzolo, F. J. (1991). Structured assessment of independent living skills: Preliminary re-port of performance measure of functional

ASSESSING THOSE WHO CANNOT COMMUNICATE

abilities in dementia. *Journal of Gerontology, 46,* 58–66.

Marin, D. B., Green, C. R., Schmeidler, J., Harvey, P. D., Lawlor, B. A., Ryan, T. M., Aryan, M., Davis, K. L., & Mohs, R. C. (1997). Noncognitive disturbances in Alzheimer's disease: Frequency, longitudinal course, and relationship to cognitive symptoms. *Journal of the American Geriatrics Society, 45*(11), 1331–1338.

Martin, P., & Bateson, P. (1993). *Measuring behavior. An introductory guide.* Cambridge: Cambridge University Press.

McHorney, C. A. (1996). Measuring and monitoring general health status in elderly persons: Practical and methodological issues in using the SF-36 health survey. *Gerontologist, 36,* 571–583.

McPherson, S. A. (1991). Transient cognitive disorders in the elderly. In M. Harper (Ed.), *Management and care of the elderly. Psychosocial perspectives* (pp. 180–188). Newbury Park, CA: Sage.

Mendez, M. F., Mendez, M. A., Martin, R., Smyth, K. Z., & Whitehouse, P. J. (1990). Complex visual disturbances in Alzheimer's disease. *Neurology, 40,* 439–443.

Monjan, A. A. (1994). Sleep and dementia: Measurement issues. *Alzheimer's Disease and Associated Disorders, 8*(1), 223–226.

National Center for Health Statistics (1991). *Mental illness in nursing homes: United States, 1985.* Washington, DC: U.S. Government Printing Office.

National Center for Health Statistics (1993). *Health data on older Americans: United States, 1992* (Vital and Health Statistics Series 3: No. 27). Washington, DC: U.S. Government Printing Office.

National Institute on Aging (1997). *Progress report on Alzheimer's disease, 1997.* Silver Spring, MD: Alzheimer's Disease Indication and Referral Center.

Ouslander, J. G., Buxton, W. G., Al-Samarrai, N. R., Cruise, P. A., Alessi, C., & Schnelle, J. F. (1998). Nighttime urinary incontinence and sleep disruption among nursing home residents. *Journal of the American Geriatrics Society, 46*(4), 463–466.

Overall, J. E., & Gorham, D. R. (1988). The Brief Psychiatric Rating Scale (BPRS): Recent developments in ascertainment and scaling. *Psychopharmacology Bulletin, 24,* 97–98.

Parmelee, P. A., Katz, I. R., & Lawton, M. P. (1989). Depression among institutionalized aged: Assessment and prevalence estimation. *Journal of Gerontology: Medical Sciences, 44*(1), M22–29.

Pollard, T. M. (1995). Use of cortisol as a stress marker: Practical and theoretical problems. *American Journal of Human Biology, 7,* 265–273.

Quant, S. A. (1987). Methods for determining dietary intake. In F. E. Johnston (Ed.), *Nutritional Anthropology* (pp. 67–84). New York: Alan R. Liss.

Rabins, P., Kasper, J., Kleinman, L., Black, B., & Patrick, D. (1999). Concepts and methods in the development of the ADRLQ: An instrument for assessing health-related quality of life in persons with Alzheimer's disease. *Journal of Mental Health and Aging, 5*(1), 33–49.

Reisberg, B., Borenstein, J., Franssen, E., Salob, S., & Sateinberg, G. (1987). BEHAVE-AD: A clinical rating scale for the assessment of pharmacologically remediable behavioral symptomology in Alzheimer's disease. In Altman (Ed.), *Alzheimer's disease problems, prospects, and perspectives* (pp. 1–16). New York: Plenum Press.

Rovner, B., Kafonek, S., Filip, L., Lucas, M., & Folstein, M. (1986). Prevalence of mental illness in a community nursing home. *American Journal of Psychiatry, 143,* 1446–1449.

Rush, A. J., Giles, D. E., Schlesser, M. A., Orsulak, P. J., Parker, C. R. J., Weissenburger, J. E., Crowley, G. T., Khatami, M., & Vasavada, N. (1996). The dexamethasone suppression test in patients with mood disorders. *Journal of Clinical Psychiatry, 57,* 470–484.

Ryden, M. (1988). Aggressive behaviors in persons with dementia who live in the community. *Alzheimer's Disease and Related Disorders, 2,* 342–355.

Sano, M., Albert, S. M., Tractenberg, R., & Schittini, M. (1999). Developing utilities: Quantifying quality of life for stages of Alzheimer's disease as measured by the Clinical Dementia Rating. *Journal of Mental Health and Aging, 5*(1), 59–68.

Sapolsky, R. M. (1994). *Why zebras don't get ulcers.* New York: W.H. Freeman and Company.

Schafer, K., Sano, M., Mackell, J., Ernesto, C., & Morris, J. (1996). Clinical monitoring of rating scales in multicenter trials. *Controlled Clinical Trials, 17,* 57S.

Schneider, E. L., & Guralnik, J. M. (1990). The aging of America: Impact on health care costs. *Journal of the American Medical Association, 263*(17), 2335–2340.

Schnelle, J., Powell, M., Newman, D., & Ory, M. (1993a). A subject screening strategy for nursing home residents: Run-in versus mental status testing. *Behavior, Health and Aging, 3,* 13–21.

Schnelle, J., Traubhber, B., Sowell, V., Newman, D., Petrilli, C., & Ory, M. (1989). Prompted voiding treatment of urinary incontinence in nursing home patients: A behavior management approach for nursing home staff. *Journal of the American Geriatrics Society, 37*, 165–171.

Schnelle, J. F., Cruise, P. A., Alessi, C. A., Al-Samarrai, N., & Ouslander, J. G. (1998). Individualizing nighttime incontinence care in nursing home residents. *Nursing Research, 47*, 197–204.

Schnelle, J. F., Ouslander, J. G., Simmons, S. F., Alessi, C. A., & Gravel, M. D. (1993b). The nighttime environment, incontinence care, and sleep disruption in nursing homes. *Journal of the American Geriatrics Society, 41*, 910–914.

Schwarz, N., & Wellens, T. (1997). Cognitive dynamics of proxy responding: The diverging perspectives of actors and observers. *Journal of Official Statistics, 13*, 159–180.

Shue, V., Beck, C., & Lawton, M. P. (1996). Measuring affect in frail and cognitively impaired elders. *Journal of Mental Health and Aging, 2*, 259–271.

Silverman, M., & McAllister, C. (1995). Continuities and discontinuities in the life course: Experiences of demented persons in a residential Alzheimer's facility. In J. N. Henderson & M. D. Vesperi (Eds.), *The culture of long term care: Nursing home ethnography* (pp. 197–221). Westport: Bergin & Garvey.

Skurla, E., Rogers, J. C., & Sunderland, T. (1988). Direct assessment of activities of daily living in Alzheimer's disease: A controlled study. *Journal of the American Geriatrics Society, 36*, 97–103.

Spector, W. D. (1997). Measuring function in daily activities for persons with dementia. *Alzheimer's Disease and Associated Disorders, 1*(6), 81–90.

Sultzer, D. L., Berisford, M. S., & Gunay, I. (1995). The neurobehavioral rating scale: Reliability in patients with dementia. *Journal of Psychiatric Research, 29*(3), 185–191.

Sunderland, T., Alterman, I. S., Yount, D., Hill, J. L., Tariot, P. N., Newhouse, P. A., Meuller, E. A., Mellow, A. M., & Cohen, R. M. (1988). A new scale for the assessment of depressed mood in dementia patients. *American Journal of Psychiatry, 145*, 955–959.

Tappen, R. M., & Berry, C. (1995). Assessment of affect in advanced Alzheimer's disease: Dementia Mood Picture Test. *Journal of Gerontological Nursing, 21*, 44–46.

Tariot, P. (1996). Behavioral manifestations of dementia: A research agenda. *International Psychogeriatrics, 8*(1), 31–38.

Tariot, P. N., Mack, J. L., Patterson, M. B., Edland, S. D., Weiner, M. F., Fillenbaum, G., Blazina, L., Teri, L., Rubin, E., Mortimer, J. A., et al. (1995). The Behavior Rating Scale for Dementia of the Consortium to Establish a Registry for Alzheimer's Disease. The Behavioral pathology Committee of the Consortium to Establish a Registry for Alzheimer's Disease. *American Journal of Psychiatry, 152*(9), 1349–1357.

Tariot, P. N., Podgorski, C. A., Blazina, L., & Leibovici, A. (1993). Mental disorders in the nursing home: Another perspective. *American Journal of Psychiatry, 150*(7), 1063–1069.

Tariot, P. N., Porsteinsson, A., Teri, L., & Weiner, M. F. (1996). Measurement of behavioral disturbance in chronic care populations. *Journal of Mental Health and Aging, 2*, 213–227.

Teresi, J., & Evans, D. (1996). Cognitive assessment measures for chronic care populations. *Journal of Mental Health and Aging, 2*, 151–174.

Teresi, J., Lawton, M. P., Ory, M., & Holmes, D. (1994). Measurement issues in chronic care populations: Dementia special care. *Journal of Alzheimer Disease and Associated Disorder, 8*(Suppl 1), S144–S183.

Teri, L., & Logsdon, R. G. (1991). Identifying pleasant activities for Alzheimer's disease patients: The pleasant events schedule-AD. *Gerontologist, 31*, 124–127.

Teri, L., Logsdon, R., & Yesavage, J. (1997). Measuring behavior, mood, and psychiatric symptoms in Alzheimer's disease. *Alzheimer's Disease and Associated Disorders, 11*(6), 50–59.

Teri, L., Truax, P., Logsdon, R., Uomoto, J., Zarit, S., & Vitaliano, P. P. (1992). Assessment of behavioral problems in dementia: The revised memory and behavior problems checklist. *Psychology and Aging, 7*(4), 622–631.

Terra Nova Films (1998). *Recognizing and responding to emotion in persons with dementia.* A training film videotape produced by the Philadelphia Geriatric Center (1-800-779-8491).

Uhlman, R. F., Larson, E. B., Koepsell, T. D., Rees, T. S., & Duckert, L. G. (1991). Visual impairment and cognitive dysfunction in Alzheimer's disease. *Journal of General Internal Medicine, 6*, 126–132.

Uman, G. (1995). *Measuring consumer satisfaction in nursing homes: A Phase 1, Small Business Innovation Research (SBIR) Grant Study.* Paper presented at the Annual Meeting of the Gerontological Society of America, November 8, 1995 (available from Gwen Uman, Partner, Vital Research, 8380 Melrose Ave, # 309, Los Angeles, CA 90069).

Vining, R. F., McGinley, R. A., & Symons, R. G. (1983). Hormones in saliva: mode of entry and consequent implications for clinical interpretation. *Clinical Chemistry, 29,* 1752–1756.

Volicer, L., Hurley, A., & Camberg, L. (1999). A model of psychological well-being in advanced dementia. *Journal of Mental Health and Aging, 5*(1), 83–94.

Warshaw, G. (1997). Assessing physical status in Alzheimer's disease research. *Alzheimer's Disease and Associated Disorders, 11*(6), 66–72.

Weiner, M. F., Koss, E., Wild, V., Folks, D. G., Tariot, P., Luszcynska, H., & Whitehouse, P. (1996). Measures of psychiatric symptoms in Alzheimer's patients: A review. *Alzheimer's Disease and Associated Disorders, 10,* 20–30.

Whitehouse, P. (1999). Quality of life in Alzheimer's disease: Future directions. *Journal of Mental Health and Aging, 5*(1), 107–111.

Woolfson, P. (1997). *Old Age in Transition.* Westport: Bergin & Garvey.

Worthman, C. M., & Stallings, J. F. (1997). Hormone measures in finger-prick blood spot samples: New field methods for reproductive endocrinology. *American Journal of Physical Anthropology, 104,* 1–21.

Wu, A., Jacobson, D., Berzon, R., Revicki, D., van der Horst, C., Fichtenbaum, C., Saag, M., L, L., Hardy, D., & Feinberg, J. (1997). The effect of mode of administration on Medical Outcomes Study health ratings and EuroQol scores in AIDS. *Quality of Life Research, 6,* 3–10.

Zaudig, M. (1996). Assessing behavioral symptoms of dementia of the Alzheimer's type: Categorical and quantitative approaches. *International Psychogeriatrics, 8*(2), 183–200.

Zimmer, J. A., Watson, & Trea, H. (1984). Behavioral problems among patients in skilled nursing facilities. *American Journal of Public Health, 14,* 1118–1121.

Zimmerman, S. I., & Magaziner, J. (1994). Methodological issues in measuring the functional status of cognitively impaired nursing home residents: The use of proxies and performance-based measures. *Alzheimer's Disease and Associated Disorders, 8*(1), 281–290.

# III
## Conclusion

# 18

# Accomplishments, Problems, Trends, and Future Challenges

ROSALIE A. KANE

This book presents a wide assortment of assessment tools. The last chapter examines the state of assessment for the elderly as the new millennium begins. What have been the collective areas of accomplishment by gerontological researchers and practitioners? What problems need to be solved, and what content areas need attention? How can we characterize current trends in the assessment of older people, and what challenges is the future likely to bring?

## SINCE 1981

In the preface we described our 1981 effort in three ways: making a strong case for systematic assessment; summarizing existing measures; and providing user warnings to guide in selecting measures and interpreting their results. This chapter begins by revisiting those themes in light of what has transpired in the almost two intervening decades.

### The Case for Systematic Assessment

More than ever, a strong case can be made for systematic assessment. Without efforts to measure a content area, clinicians are unlikely to take it seriously, and researchers are unlikely to advance knowledge about it. We hold this truth too self-evident to belabor. It must be added, however, that assessment technology cannot be content to do only the easiest things. As M. Powell Lawton notes (personal communication), our best concepts are the hardest to measure. Areas like spirituality and preferences, treated in this book, and other areas not directly treated (e.g., autonomy, sense of individuality, dignity, the good death, freedom from fear) are extremely difficult to conceptualize, let alone measure, but the effort needs to be made. Only then can we determine whether the services that we provide, the way we provide them, and the places where we provide them make a difference in matters of elemental importance.

Mandating systematic assessment will be insufficient, even if a particular tool is chosen. Those making the assessments need to be committed to the importance of the endeavor and educated and competent in the use of the tools. It is easier for a program to settle on an assessment tool than to find a way to use it consistently over time and across assessors. We will return to issues of application later in this chapter, because they pose a formidable hurdle.

## The Measures Themselves

Measures have proliferated with no sign of abatement. Every year, literally hundreds of posters are presented at the annual meetings of the Gerontological Society of America and the American Geriatrics Society displaying new wrinkles on how to assess familiar topics and making assessment forays into previously unmeasured areas. The chapters in Part I show that the developmental stages for measuring the various topics differ enormously. Table 18.1 summarizes the state of assessment in each of the topical areas included in Part I, emphasizing developments since the manuscript for the 1981 book was completed about two decades ago. Issues and caveats are discussed in the text in the next section, which elaborates on the content of Table 18.1.

## Issues and Caveats

### Functional Measures

Measures of functional status—activities of daily living (ADL), instrumental activities of daily living (IADL), and, to a lesser extent, mobility—are so numerous that in Chapter 2 Pearson proposed a moratorium on new tools in favor of clarifying the properties and relative merits of the existing ones. The ADLs and IADLs have been called the *lingua franca* of geriatrics. It is rare to find a clinical geriatric program that makes no attempt to assess functional status; and functional measures, at least ADL measures, are included in most research studies. As a dependent variable or outcome sought, some would argue that functional status assumes paramount importance because maintaining, improving, or slowing decline in functioning is what services for older people are all about. As an independent variable—that is, something that might influence the outcomes being measured, functional status is almost as ubiquitous as the inevitable age, gender, marital status, and ethnicity. It is an al-

most universally applied "case-mix adjustor." Baseline functional status is (and should be) taken into account when investigators examine other outcomes in the social and psychological spheres or when they examine changes in functional status itself.

With so many tools, does it matter which one is selected? The answer, within limits, is "not really." The same basic result can likely be achieved with any number of functional assessment tools. Clearly, a tool that yields more detail should be used for rehabilitation purposes. More important is achieving clarity within the clinical team, among the case managers who do assessments, and among the research teams about the use that is to be made of the information and selecting a strategy accordingly. It may be more important to know what individuals are *able* to do, or it may be more important to know what they *actually* do. Perhaps it is necessary to know both, in which case both questions need to be asked. It may be important to know what the individuals *believe* they can do, which has led to questions such as "if nobody was able to help you with _____, could you do it yourself?" Difficulty in performance and untoward consequences related to this performance area have been built into some of the tools and may be important for a program or a study.

Regardless of the decisions made on the issues just laid out, which will influence the choice of tool, at least three areas should be dealt with:

1. A time frame must be incorporated and stuck to consistently. Typically this is a choice made by the rater rather than inherent in the measure, but it must be decided in advance whether the time frame is yesterday, in the last week, or in the last month and whether the performance being measured is the best, the worst, or the usual that occurred in that time frame. When demonstrated performance is used, obviously this question is moot and the performance

**Table 18.1.**

Progress and Challenges in 12 Content Areas for Assessing Older People

| Summary of state of assessment | Challenges and next steps |
|---|---|
| **Function** | |
| A large number of tools exist to assess ADL and IADL, with a major proliferation and refinement of older tools in last 20 years. This work has evolved steadily since the late 1950s and is widely accepted as the basis for physical rehabilitation. Self- report, proxy report, observer ratings, and demonstration approaches are available. Distinctions between measuring capability and performance have been made. Almost any study of older people includes some measure of physical functioning. | ADL/IADL tools have been used to determine eligibility for services and case-mix adjustments for provider's payment levels. These uses can compromise validity. <br><br> Some concern that ADL/IADL measures undercount people with cognitive impairment who are capable of tasks but need to be reminded or supervised. |
| **Health and Physiological Measures** | |
| Steady development of brief scales to measure specific topics like fall risk, malnutrition, pressure sores, and so on. Measures of pain and discomfort have greatly evolved since 1980. The brown bag assay to examine medications has become common. This general area of development makes it possible for lay people, including older people themselves, to provide systematic information to health care professionals. | Pain measurement is challenging because of its subjective nature. <br><br> Debate about appropriateness of using proxies to measure pain in end-of-life studies. <br><br> Scoring approaches not always clear — e.g., how to reduce a list of medications and their dosages or a list of signs and symptoms or a history of health care utilization to a meaningful summary. |
| **Cognition** | |
| One of the best developed content areas. Many performance measures are available and often used for laboratory research of cognitive and experimental psychologists. Psychometric properties tend to be known. A great variety of somewhat interchangeable direct-interview cognitive screening tools exist. Also the last 20 years have seen refinement of systematic batteries of measures to stage Alzheimer's disease — in the end, these require observer ratings by interviewers or judges. Measures of cognitive performance are highly sensitive to the circumstances of the test and the attitudes and physical state of the person being tested. | Possible that some measures pick up distinctions without clinical significance. The trend toward linking assessments to practical life tasks is an important corrective. <br><br> Orientation and memory as measured by short screening tests may not fully predict life problem solving or ability to reliably report satisfaction. Some re-thinking needed about going exclusively to proxies based on these tests. <br><br> Positive areas of cognitive functioning such as wisdom, humor, and creativity are not as well developed. |
| **Affect** | |
| Measures of depressive and anxious affect have increased in number. There is a positive trend away from rating scales to direct interview tools. Psychometric properties tend to be known. Reliable observational tools available to assess affect for people who cannot communicate. Positive affects being measured as well as absence of negative affect. Efforts to measure hope and optimism have expanded. | Distinctions between affective state and personality trait still difficult. <br><br> Some emotions (e.g., loneliness or anger and resentment) have had much less measurement work, and they tend not to be used in general clinical practice with old people or gerontological research and program evaluation despite their relevance to the topics being studied (e.g., effects of various long-term care arrangements). |
| **Social Functioning** | |
| Measures of social networks, social support, social activities, and coping have increased. They are increasingly designed with social roles of older people in mind. No gold standards have as yet emerged, however. Subjective well-being and life satisfaction are still being measured by the same durable measures used 20 years ago. | There is still no widely accepted classification of general assessment areas within social functioning (which could include expanded IADL measures in the activity area and psychological measures in the coping area). Many tools are long and descriptive without psychometric properties established. |

*(continued)*

**Table 18.1.**

Progress and Challenges in 12 Content Areas for Assessing Older People—Continued

| Summary of state of assessment | Challenges and next steps |
|---|---|
| Quality Of Life (QOL) | |
| Distinctions are made between health-related QOL (either general or tied to specific diseases) and broad QOL. Measures have tended to be developed for other populations and applied to older people. There is excessive reliance on variants of SF-36. Some work has been done recently to conceptualize QOL for people with dementia. | The term QOL has sometimes been applied to any measure that seems to tap and summarize multiple, differing dimensions. Vast differences exist among QOL measures, varying from narrow to broad. More work needed on measuring QOL in people with dementia. Sometimes unexamined value judgments are buried in QOL measures. |
| Values and Preferences | |
| General approaches to measure the strength and relative importance of various values have been available for decades and are not particularly centered on older people. Some efforts have been made in the last 20 years to develop approaches and items to measure end-of-life values and preferences, preferences for features of long-term care, and preferences related to choice and control. Psychometric properties are not well established. | Basic work still needed on conceptualizing what should be assessed in this topic area and developing and testing instruments. In long-term care practice, professionals are reluctant to approach assessing preferences systematically. Hard to find a practical measure that is theoretically sound. Methodological problems are great because of tendency to adjust preferences based on current experience. |
| Satisfaction | |
| Consumer/customer satisfaction measures for health care providers and plans have been developed; many are not specific or sensitive to needs of those older people who have chronic health problems and high need for care. Some satisfaction tools have been developed for long-term care programs. Researchers have been considering ways to overcome positivity biases by the way questions are phrased. Some efforts have been made to incorporate importance into preferences. Norms hard to develop when response rates are low. | The validity of satisfaction measures is compromised if individuals are intimidated, if they lack an information base for distinguishing between good or poor care, and if they have accommodated to objectively substandard conditions. This area better developed for health programs than housing programs or life conditions. Some satisfaction measures are applied as marketing tools without much attention to sample frame or response rates. To develop properties of the measures, this must change. |
| Family Caregivers | |
| Great expansion of assessment capability, from almost no tools in 1980 to a wide variety of tools now, some of which have been used repeatedly and whose psychometric properties are known. Caregiver measures are often developed on populations of people caring for people with dementia, however. Measures of caregiver "burden" are particularly well developed; recent trends have been to assess positive features and effects of family caregiving. | Need for more attention to assessing caregiver inputs—frequency, type, and quality—to be used as independent variables. Need better measures of caregiver burden that avoid social desirability. The care-receiver perspective on family caregiving is somewhat missing; the person receiving care is seldom been used as a respondent on family care. Primary family "caregivers" are used as proxy informants to assess their relative, and their own caregiving experience is also assessed. Sometimes the report of "behaviors" of the relative is used as a measure of family burden rather than as data about the functioning of the older person. |

*(continued)*

**Table 18.1.** — Continued

| Religion, Religiousness, and Spirituality | |
|---|---|
| Great expansion of assessment efforts from low baseline 20 years ago. Since the mid-1990s the efforts were accelerated by the National Institute on Aging and the Fetzer Institute Working Group. Psychometric properties rarely go beyond alpha reliability for scale development, and norms are rarely available. | Distinguishing between religion and spirituality is still a problem in many measures. |
| | Measures of religious practices (for independent variable use) may not generalize well across religious groups. |
| | Large number of brief tools have been suggested by the Fetzer Working Group but need testing in large-scale studies. |

| Environments | |
|---|---|
| In geriatrics and gerontology (as opposed to architecture and environmental studies), environmental assessments have concentrated on long-term care environments (e.g., nursing homes, assisted living, Alzheimer's care units) or on safety checks for home environments as places for people with disabilities. Rating tools have been developed with acceptable reliability. | Need for measures that are based on objective, observable indicators rather than judgments. |

ADL, activities of daily living; IADL, instrumental activities of daily living.

is for the time period observed. Although much attention has been given to the generalizability of test performance in measures of cognition, the same attention has not been devoted to measures of physical performance, although they too will be influenced by fatigue, boredom, anxiety, and transient conditions of health status and context.

2. The instructions and definitions should distinguish being unable to perform a function because of memory problems that make the person forget to do it or forget how to do it without supervision for safety. In some instances, it will be sufficient to add this need for reminding and/or supervision into the general definition, but in some instances it may be important to have a separate column to measure the functional abilities and one to measure the extent to which reminding and supervision are needed

3. A very common problem is to confound the need for assistance with the amount of assistance given or, worse, to use the amount of assistance received to measure the need. This happens sometimes for convenience; for example, case management programs need to

know the amount of help received and, thus, the "functional assistance shortfall" in order to make a plan. In the interests of a shorter assessment form, they often combine assistance with capacity or performance.

In short, matters are somewhat the same as they were 20 years ago for selecting a measure of ADL/IADL, although there are many more measures from which to choose. There still is considerable interchangeability among choices, and it is still crucial to work on the fine-print decisions about the measure.

One newer practical problem has surfaced, which does not have a good answer but needs to be recognized. When studies compare outcomes of nursing home residents with those at home or in a new residential setting, a key question concerns whether functioning is enhanced in one program or the other. So as not to disfavor nursing homes, such studies often leave out most IADL functions and bathing because rules and customs require that bathing and medications be assisted, and the environments offer little opportunity for cooking, cleaning, and other IADL functions. By leaving these functions out, however, researchers have compromised their ability to show the possible superiority of alternative settings. A related problem occurs with case-mix adjustment. It is essential to take into account baseline functioning in order to compare change over time for groups of older people. But, if older people in one setting are permitted and even encouraged to be independent and do things for themselves, they look more functional at baseline and they are assumed to reflect a population with less disability than, for example, the nursing home population. This problem is not solved by following an admission cohort. Functional dependency is so sensitive to environment that soon after admission the people with equal capabilities are bound to look different in vastly different environments.

## Physiological Functioning

As Chapter 3 has shown, assessment of physiological functioning has become more developed in the past decades and is now replete with tools to create some objective way of classifying common clinical problems like fall risk, nutritional status, pressure sores, and so on. The self-reported health measure—a single question whereby the individual characterizes his or her own health from excellent to poor—remains remarkably predictive of mortality and other outcomes. Many more tools are now available to measure pain and discomfort, although interpretation is still difficult because of the subjectivity of the topic. The field is divided between those who would never accept a proxy rating of someone else's pain and those who believe it is necessary and important to get some approximation of the pain experienced by those who are dying or those who cannot speak and accept the ratings of staff or relatives as the best we can do.

## Cognitive Functioning

The great length of the chapter on cognitive functioning bears testimony to the at-

tention given to this domain. Tools to measure cognitive functioning have often been developed by and for the use of experimental psychologists. As such, the tools often entail demonstration of abilities, and their norms and psychometric properties are usually known. As Table 18.1 suggests, instruments are less well developed to tap upper-level functioning such as logic, creativity, and wisdom; but even here, tools are available.

As with ADL measures, within limits, it probably does not matter which cognitive screening test is used; many are interchangeable, although some seem less likely to alienate the older person being tested. More important is how to interpret the results of a cognitive screening test. We may be too prone to use them to exclude direct input from older persons, deeming them unreliable. For example, it is typical to seek a proxy in a research study for anyone who falls below some preset Mini-Mental State Examination score. More work is needed to see whether people below those scores can answer questions about their daily activities and preferences reliably and (in the case of the former) accurately. (In our own studies, we have encountered anomalies in cognitive screens; for example, an individual who missed all the easier questions about where he was perfectly recollected the day, month, and year of his birth and subtracted series 3's correctly.) When such a screen is performed at the end of an interview to provide a case-mix adjustment, should the entire seemingly cogent interview be discounted? If such a screen had been performed at the beginning of an interview to sort the sample, perhaps the result would have been better (because of the fatigue factor), although alienating the respondent is always a concern.

Cognitive screens must also be applied consistently and relentlessly to yield the score. A survey center director with much experience administering such tools reports that she has heard respondents suddenly recall the president and cry out "It's

Clinton!" 10 minutes later in the middle of another question. It would seem to reflect considerable memory skill to keep searching for that elusive name, yet the individual would not be credited with the right answer under the rules of administration for most mental status tests. It does seem self-evident that the importance of today's date slips away when all days are the same and no appointments loom ahead. Also, we have instructed interviewers to give a correct score to the person with the presence of mind to consult a date on a wristwatch or look at a calendar, but this strategy obviously penalizes those who do not have such aids. The debate will continue to rage between those who favor an "objective" measure of cognitive performance and those who prefer to test cognitive function in the context of practical applications.

## Emotion and Mental Health

Once again, there has been growth in depression screening tests. Perhaps in the last 20 years, there also has been more acceptance of question-and-answer tests to gauge emotional well-being rather than strict reliance on a clinical interview by a qualified mental health professional. The major growth area has been in observational scales to examine emotions such as anger, sadness, and anxiety. To use these clinically, a commitment to making multiple observations at standard times is necessary, although work is needed to determine how many observations in, for example, the Apparent Affect Rating Scale are needed for reliable results. As was the case 20 years ago, the lines between an emotion and a personality trait are blurred.

## Social Functioning

Considerable agreement has now been reached about acceptable measures of social networks and of social support (variables that are often found as independent variables in research studies). Social well-being, which implies a value judgment, is much more difficult to measure because there is no unified body of theory that suggests the right blend of activity, stimulation, and relationships that constitutes social well-being. Moreover, this area is particularly sensitive to cultural and individual variations. The perception of meaningful relationships, of being loved by and loving others, of being trusted by and trusting others, seems pivotal to social well-being, which is probably why the questions about the reciprocal presence of a confidante (someone you trust and turn to, someone who trusts and turns to you) remain as a marker of the work that still remains to be done in this area.

The social functioning construct remains highly susceptible to societal values. Being among people is generally viewed as better than being alone, but many people prefer solo tasks like reading or doing puzzles over a group activity. Is watching a movie in a crowd more socially integrating than watching TV at home? Whereas there is growing evidence to suggest that having someone with whom to relate (even a pet) has some protective effect, there is scarce reason to argue that level of protection increases with the number of friends.

## Quality of Life

The term *quality of life* is used in a great variety of ways. Historically, the term was introduced as a counterpart of health status ("but what about quality of life?"). As such, it can be as narrowly as incorporating disease-free intervals, symptom control, and improved functioning to supplement measures of survival. At the other extreme, a good or poor quality of life can be a broad concept, encompassing all the domains discussed in Chapters 2 to 6 — functional, health, cognitive, psychological, and social domains. These domains can be further subdivided to include finances, housing, and general quality of the environment. A debate is being waged about how best to incorporate objective and subjective (i.e., perceived quality of life) elements into a measure and whether structural elements of the physical or built environment should be included. Whether and how to assess the quality of life of people with moderate or severe dementia is also an issue.

Quality of life measures are basically multidimensional measures with varying degrees of comprehensiveness in inclusion of domains. As such, the individual elements or domains must meet the standards required for any measure. The additional and perplexing problems concern how to aggregate and weight the information — that is, what to take most seriously and how to decide. Quality of life has become the politically correct adjuvant to almost any study of outcomes of care. Economists have seized on quality of life measures to create quality-adjusted life years, which place a different value on survival at varying levels of QOL. Rarely, however, do we examine what goes into these quality-adjusted life years and how valid are the implications. The well are prone to discounting the value of a disabled life, but many people with disabilities seem to cling to their lives all the same.

### Values and Preferences

Even more than religiousness and spirituality, the values and preferences area is underdeveloped when it comes to applications designed to be relevant to the care of frail older people. In the half-empty/half-full tradition of the glass, however, it is encouraging that development of some of these tools are underway. The current practice climate that promotes consumer control and autonomy has influenced the direction of that development.

The elegance of design too often comes at the cost of using very artificial solutions. The field needs a simple mechanism to tap preferences systematically if we are ever to incorporate this information into practice or even to develop individually weighted summary scores for research.

### Satisfaction

Satisfaction sometimes is related to the realization of preferences. As Chapter 9 suggests, however, satisfaction bears a re-

lationship to expectations as well. Satisfaction tools are likely to be self-completed, especially when the respondents are family members of frail elderly people. The satisfaction of a client will be sensitive to how the tool is administered and who administers it — those who are dependent on a service are particularly likely to be hesitant to criticize it. At the end of the 20th century, customer satisfaction has become a buzzword in long-term care. Two cautions are needed for this enterprise. First, customer satisfaction should not be equated with quality of life because the former is a narrower concept linked to expectations. Second, as Smith emphasized in Chapter 9, satisfaction data for a program are meaningless unless based on an appropriate sample frame and a high response rate.

### Religiousness and Spirituality

Although it is fashionable to include spiritual well-being as a fourth dimension of well-being (along with the physical, psychological, and social spheres identified by the World Health Organization), we have made only baby steps toward determining how to measure it. The work of the Fetzer Institute Working Group is promising in that regard, especially for suggesting ways to measure, usually as independent variables, religion and religious practices. As Chapter 10 illustrates, psychometric work and published norms are rare in this arena of measurement. Moreover, some of the scales to measure spirituality and sense of meaning seem extremely hard to score and interpret apart from the religious denomination in which they originated. We concur, however, with many of the investigators in this area that the time has come to apply measures of religiousness and spirituality in a more widespread way and, by doing so, learning more about their properties.

### Family Caregiving

Until now all content areas discussed in this chapter have applied to older people being assessed. The family caregiver material in Chapter 11 is meant to assess the performance and well-being of family members (or friends) who give care to older people. The tools in this area are plentiful, and one positive trend is that some tools now measure the positive effects associated with caregiving rather than the burdens alone. Much of the instrument development has been done with dementia in mind, and it is often a subtle matter to disentangle measuring the behavior of people receiving care (e.g., their wandering or aggressive behavior) from measuring the difficulties that behavior creates for a family caregiver (which is a matter of perception or appraisal). The dominant paradigm for family care has been the primary family caregiver, who may or may not be supported by other family members, and our measurement tools and research designs have somewhat been forced into that model. Finally, as the chapter identifies, tools are not yet developed to assess family caregiving from the perspective of and in the voice of the person receiving the care. That is a necessary developmental area.

## Environments

Chapter 12 is the furthest removed from assessment of the older person (more so than the preceding one since many family caregivers are actually old). It treats the assessment of physical and social environments in which older people function. Elaborate approaches are available, the best known being Moos' Multiphasic Environmental Assessment Protocol (MEAP), which in its entirety is too difficult to apply even in many research contexts. In general, these tools have been developed, in part, by occupational therapists and others who are assessing the safety and functionality of the living environment with an aim to improving it and by researchers who may need a tool for a particular purpose. The latter genesis has led to considerable work on assessing the environment of Alzheimer's disease special care units in nursing homes, a matter of

well-funded research interest in the 1990s. We see a general need to improve environmental assessment tools, refining them to the point where they are reliable in the hands of unspecialized trained assessors. This calls for minimizing subjective ratings and emphasizing specific observations. Obviously, how an environment is *used,* including the rules and conventions that govern its use, is also an important area of assessment.

## TRENDS AND CHALLENGES

### Computerization

The advent of the computer and the rapid trend toward miniaturization will make computer technology ever more accessible to facilitate assessments. While the largest experience with using computers probably lies with computer-assisted surveys, it is easy to envisage how computers will change the nature of assessment. At the simplest level, computers can be used to collect data. Programming them to use branching logic can reduce the time of interviews. They can make calculations and flag missing or inconsistent findings. Computerized data can form the basis for flow charts and graphs to show change in status more dramatically.

It is now feasible to use computers to help older people monitor their own status on a regular basis and to transmit these findings to a central location for analysis. Such an approach will allow for closer monitoring. It is feasible to include automatic instructions on how to respond in case of an observed deviation from the person's expected course. This step will make older people more empowered and allow them to play a bigger role in managing their own care. They can directly enter and download input into central data banks for analysis.

Some see this geometric expansion in access to data as a threat to privacy. The idea that Big Brother is watching and can now monitor a variety of personal habits and behaviors is uncomfortable. Some means must be found to protect people's privacy while gaining information Just as an inter-disciplinary team needs to work in at atmosphere of trust, so too must a system of care provide adequate safeguards to ensure that personal information is not abused.

## Training in Assessment

We cannot take for granted that people, even well-educated professionals, will use assessment tools consistently over time or consistently compared with other users. It is by no means certain that the assessments will be used as they were intended to be used. This issue was discussed in Chapter 1, but we return to it here because of its importance. So much attention is given to the development of tools, but so little to consistent training in the use of these tools. When case managers are trained in the use of assessment tools for home-based care programs, they are likely to receive fairly detailed instructions on how to fill out forms and calculate scores, but little on how literally to ask questions, what constitutes a necessary probe for clarification or completeness, and what constitutes a bias. They are rarely trained on how to get beyond the practical difficulties that may arise: an angry respondent, a suspicious respondent, a sad respondent, or a garrulous respondent. They receive little training in how to deal with the older person's emotional reactions or their own — to deal with the latter, they often skip over sensitive areas. They also have little instruction on how to manage time and how to explain the importance of the assessment, its uses, and its time parameters. Role playing is an essential ingredient of training, as is doing assessments that are observed and critiqued.

When comprehensive assessments are used in clinical contexts, the common complaint is that there is not enough time to conduct them. It is not unusual for nurses and social workers to say that the assessment interferes with their work; it is rare for them to say that the assessment guides and informs their work. In nursing homes, where the Resident Assessment Instrument including the Minimum Data Set (MDS) is mandatory, it is rare to find that facilities incorporate that task into their daily work in a way that promotes more structured encounters with residents and more opportunity for all staff to read and use the latest assessment. Rather, there is a trend toward hiring separate MDS coordinators and allocating time away from the clinical context to "do the MDSs." Charting is viewed as a task separate from collecting the information needed for care, and the MDS is too often seen as charting rather than assessment.

In her autobiographical work, *The Shadow Man*, Mary Gordon presents a vivid example of effective probing in the sense of clarification. A physician to whom she had taken her mother, a nursing home resident with Alzheimer's disease who now "speaks from the desert," did not have time to administer a standard depression tool so Mary was asked to administer the questions and circle her mother's answers on the form.

When I first ask her the questions, she answers everything positively. She is satisfied with her life, she isn't bored, she is hopeful, she's in good spirits, she doesn't worry. I think I understand something. I ask her if she thinks that saying there is anything wrong with her life means that she's complaining, that she's ungrateful for what she had, that she's a weakling, a crybaby. Of course, that's what I think, she says, looking at me from the desert. I tell her that's not the way it is; they need to know how she really feels for their work. It's their business to get an accurate picture, I tell her. "You have to do it for them." I never tell her who "them" is and she never asks. "Okay, if it's their business," she says.

She answers the questions slowly. She isn't satisfied with her life, she isn't happy, she often feels helpless, she often feels downhearted and blue, she feels her situation is hopeless. She frequently feels like crying. On the other hand, she doesn't feel her life is empty, she is hopeful about the future, she is not afraid that something bad is going to happen, she thinks it is wonderful to be alive. Her most heartfelt response is to the question "Do you feel pretty worthless the way you are now?" "Oh, yes," she says, "completely worthless." (Gordon, 1996, pp. 213–214).

In this example, the daughter had the patience to cast the assessment correctly and ended up receiving thoughtful responses. It is especially interesting that her mother's responses did not change from automatic positive to automatic negative.

Assessment tools are also undermined when those using them do not understand why they are using them or perceive them as a program requirement with little real significance. Therefore, the training needs to incorporate sensitization to the purposes of the tool.

### Cultural Relevance

Fueled by both demographic shifts (specifically, the rapid growth of older persons among various minorities) and a growing awareness of the importance of cultural differences, substantial attention has been directed toward the need for culturally sensitive measures. Early efforts were crude. For example, the Short Portable Mental Status Questionnaire (SPMSQ) mental examination uses corrections for education and race.

Efforts to translate standard measures into other languages quickly reveal that the translation implies much more than simple words. For measures like ADLs and IADLs, functioning may rely on the availability of various environmental supports. Preparing a meal is quite different, for example, if one first has to hunt for the food or chop the firewood. Using the toilet may involve a substantial journey. Certain phrases have drastically different meanings in other languages. Some concepts, like caregiver burden, may be socially unacceptable in some cultures.

While a beginning has been made in this cross-cultural realm, much work remains to be done. These efforts go hand in hand with other needs to ensure that educational materials are culturally relevant and that clinicians are trained at least to respect other cultures, to understand the cultural boundedness of many comfortable practices, and to avoid offending those of other cultures.

## PERSPECTIVE OF BEING ASSESSED

It is important to turn around the microscope and consider how the assessment affects those being assessed. This corrective is needed to set up the circumstances of the assessment, including ensuring that the assessment task does not close off communications the older person wants to make, that it is done in ways and at times that are acceptable to the older person, and that it is explained to the older person why the questions are being asked and who will see the results. An exercise in imaginative empathy is important, too, for approaching the assessment tasks in the spirit of humility. One cannot capture the essence of a human being through a standardized assessment tool, and it is the height of hubris to imagine one can. It is possible, however, that assessment tools will pave the way for better understandings and better practices that permit each unique human being to flourish. A spirit of humility also keeps in the forefront the understanding that the domains and items in assessment tools reflect only the part of experience that professionals and researchers have thus far thought worthwhile to measure to provide better care and to measure the results. We need to constantly re-examine whether we are making the right choices.

## REFERENCES

Gordon, M. (1996). *Shadow man: A daughter's search for her father.* New York: Random House.

# Index